# RESEARCH AND EVALUATION IN COUNSELING

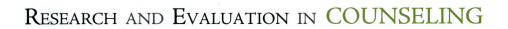

# RESEARCH AND EVALUATION IN COUNSELING

## Bradley T. Erford

*Loyola University Maryland*

## SECOND EDITION

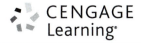

CENGAGE
Learning·

Australia • Brazil • Mexico • Singapore • United Kingdom • United States

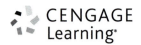

*Research and Evaluation in Counseling,*
**Second Edition**
Bradley T. Erford

Product Director: Jon-David Hague

Product Manager: Julie Martinez

Product Assistant: Kyra Kane

Media Developer: Audrey Espey

Associate Marketing Manager: Shanna Shelton

Art and Cover Direction, Production Management, and Composition: PreMediaGlobal

Manufacturing Planner: Judy Inouye

Cover Image: LdF/Getty Images

For product information and technology assistance, contact us at
**Cengage Learning Customer & Sales Support, 1-800-354-9706.**

For permission to use material from this text or product, submit all requests online at **www.cengage.com/permissions.**
Further permissions questions can be e-mailed to
**permissionrequest@cengage.com.**

Library of Congress Control Number: 2013949990

ISBN-13: 978-1-285-45489-4

ISBN-10: 1-285-45489-8

**Cengage Learning**
200 First Stamford Place, 4th Floor
Stamford, CT 06902
USA

Cengage Learning is a leading provider of customized learning solutions with office locations around the globe, including Singapore, the United Kingdom, Australia, Mexico, Brazil, and Japan. Locate your local office at **www.cengage.com/global.**

Cengage Learning products are represented in Canada by Nelson Education, Ltd.

To learn more about Cengage Learning Solutions,
visit **www.cengage.com.**

Purchase any of our products at your local college store or at our preferred online store **www.cengagebrain.com.**

Printed in the United States of America
2  3  4  5  6  7  18  17  16  15

*This effort is dedicated to The One: the giver of energy, passion, and understanding, who makes life worth living and endeavors worth pursuing and accomplishing, the Teacher of love and forgiveness.*

# CONTENTS

CHAPTER **6**   Qualitative Research Designs   105

CHAPTER **7**   Quantitative Research Design in Counseling   126

CHAPTER **8**   Practical Counseling Research Approaches: Using Action Research and Single-Subject Research Designs   153

## Section III    Collecting and Analyzing Data in Counseling Research and Evaluation   217

### CHAPTER 11    Collecting Data   218

CHAPTER **12**    Describing Data    236

CHAPTER **13**    Deriving Standardized Scores    261

CHAPTER **14**    Statistical Hypothesis Testing    274

*by Richard S. Balkin and Bradley T. Erford*

# PREFACE

The evolving profession of counseling has entered the age of accountability, regardless of one's specialization or practice venue. Managed care and school reform have become important forces that drive decision making in contemporary society. Given this context, the more a professional counselor knows about counseling research, and research and evaluation procedures, the more informed, effective, and efficient one's treatment of clients and students will be.

A second driving force comes from within the counseling profession itself. After many years of identity exploration and discussion, the counseling profession has agreed on a basic core of education and training standards to which all professional counselors should adhere. This book addresses the core curricular assessment requirements of the Council for Accreditation of Counseling and Related Educational Programs (CACREP), thereby providing state-of-the-art information on research, statistics, and evaluation that all professional counselors must know. *Research and Evaluation in Counseling* is different from other counseling books, however, in that it is written *by* a counselor educator and professional counselor *for* professional counselors.

The text is partitioned into three sections. Section I provides important foundational issues and information about research, including the philosophies behind approaches to inquiry, basic concepts, ethical and legal implications, counseling outcome research, characteristics of research studies, and an introduction to the process of locating, reviewing, and writing research.

Section II provides in-depth explorations of the major methodological issues of which all professional counselors should be aware to consume or conduct effective research. Readers are introduced to essential approaches, designs, and data analysis procedures in qualitative research methodology. Readers are also presented with quantitative approaches and designs and procedures, including single-subject research designs (SSRD) that are useful in documenting individual client progress for clinical accountability and action research useful in evaluating and changing ongoing program initiatives. Section II also reviews how to develop, implement, and analyze needs assessments and program evaluation procedures leading to documentation of accountability in programs and client outcomes.

Section III covers basic data analysis procedures in detail, including how to collect data and transform raw scores into standardized scores. Chapter 15 provides a hands-on introduction to SPSS, a commonly used statistical package that allows professional counselors to easily construct databases and conduct basic and advanced statistical analyses. Descriptive statistics are discussed in detail, including graphing methods and measures of central tendency and variability. To prepare the reader for inferential statistics, an introduction to statistical inference and hypothesis testing is offered, followed by the major statistical procedures used for determining statistical inference: univariate statistics (e.g., *t*-test and ANOVA), correlation, regression, and chi-square. Chapters 18 and 19 are designed for the advanced student or professional counselor who may have more complex empirical designs requiring more sophisticated methods of analysis, including strategies for transforming skewed or nonlinear data sets into more normalized distributions so that parametric inferential statistics based on linear model assumptions (e.g., univariate, correlation, and regression) may be applied. When normalized data samples are not possible, or when data are categorical (e.g., nominal and ordinal), nonparametric statistics may be applied. Advanced multivariate procedures are reviewed, including multiple regression, multivariate analysis of variance (MANOVA), factor analysis, and other less commonly used multivariate methods.

In short, *Research and Evaluation in Counseling* (2nd ed.) is the most comprehensive introductory research, evaluation, and statistics text ever written specifically for professional counselors.

# Acknowledgments

Special thanks go to the outside accuracy reviewers who carefully scrutinized the entire manuscript and whose comments led to substantive improvement in the final product:

Susan Boes, *University Of West Georgia*
Timothy Coppock, *Gannon University*
Perry Francis, *Eastern Michigan University*
Chris Hennington, *Lubbock Christian University*
Evelyn Lyles, *University Of Maryland*

I also thank the reviewers of the first edition of this text: Richard Wantz, Wright State University; Peter Manzi, Buffalo State College; and Brenda J. Freeman, Northwest Nazarene University. I am immensely appreciative to individual chapter authors from the first edition of this text:

CHAPTER 1 The Nature of Research and Inquiry
*Gary R. Galluzzo, Jacquelyn Hilldrup, Danica G. Hays, and Bradley T. Erford*

CHAPTER 2 Characteristics of a Research Study
*Carl J. Sheperis and Bradley T. Erford*

CHAPTER 3 Locating, Reviewing, and Writing Research
*Susan H. Eaves, Sara Craft, Carl J. Sheperis, Debbie K. Wells, and Bradley T. Erford*

CHAPTER 5 Qualitative Approaches to Research
*Deborah R. Newsome, Danica G. Hays, and Teresa Christensen*

CHAPTER 6 Qualitative Research Designs
*Danica G. Hays and Deborah R. Newsome*

CHAPTER 7 Quantitative Research Design in Counseling
*Carl J. Sheperis, Yun Hui Gardner, Bradley T. Erford, and Marie F. Shoffner*

CHAPTER 8 Using Single-Subject Research Designs to Document Client Outcomes
*Carl J. Sheperis and Jonathan D. Miller*

CHAPTER 10 Program Evaluation and Needs Assessment for Best Practices and Accountability
*Randall L. Astramovich, Wendy J. Hoskins, and Bradley T. Erford*

CHAPTER 11 Using *SPSS* for Introductory Statistical Analyses
*Gordon Brooks*

# ABOUT THE AUTHOR

**Bradley T. Erford**, PhD, LCPC, NCC, LPC, LP, LSP, is a professor in the school counseling program of the Education Specialties Department in the School of Education at Loyola University Maryland. He was president of the American Counseling Association (ACA) for 2012–2013. He is the recipient of the ACA Research Award, ACA Extended Research Award, ACA Arthur A. Hitchcock Distinguished Professional Service Award, ACA Professional Development Award, and ACA Carl D. Perkins Government Relations Award. He was also inducted as an ACA Fellow. In addition, he has received the Association for Assessment in Counseling and Education (AACE) AACE/MECD Research Award, AACE Exemplary Practices Award, AACE President's Merit Award, the Association for Counselor Education and Supervision's (ACES) Robert O. Stripling Award for Excellence in Standards, Maryland Association for Counseling and Development (MACD) Maryland Counselor of the Year, MACD Counselor Advocacy Award, MACD Professional Development Award, and MACD Counselor Visibility Award. He is the editor of numerous texts, including: *Orientation to the Counseling Profession* (Pearson Merrill, 2010, 2014), *Crisis Intervention and Prevention* (Pearson Merrill, 2010, 2014), *Group Work in the Schools* (Pearson Merrill, 2010), *Group Work: Process and Applications* (Pearson Merrill, 2011), *Transforming the School Counseling Profession* (Pearson Merrill, 2003, 2007, 2011, 2015), *Professional School Counseling: A Handbook of Principles, Programs and Practices* (pro-ed, 2004, 2010), *Assessment for Counselors* (Cengage, 2007, 2013), *Research and Evaluation in Counseling* (Cengage, 2008, 2014), and *The Counselor's Guide to Clinical, Personality and Behavioral Assessment* (Cengage, 2006); and coauthor of several more books: *Mastering the NCE and CPCE* (Pearson Merrill, 2011, 2015), *35 Techniques Every Counselor Should Know* (Pearson Merrill, 2010, 2015), *Educational Applications of the WISC-IV* (Western Psychological Services, 2006), and *Group Activities: Firing Up for Performance* (Pearson Merrill, 2007). He is also the general editor of *The American Counseling Association Encyclopedia of Counseling* (ACA, 2009). His research specialization falls primarily in development and technical analysis of psycho-educational tests and has resulted in the publication of more than 60 refereed journal articles, 100 book chapters, and a dozen published tests. He was a representative to the ACA Governing Council and the ACA 20/20 Visioning Committee. He is a past president and past treasurer of AACE; past chair and parliamentarian of the ACA—Southern (US) Region; past chair of ACA's Task Force on High Stakes Testing; past chair of ACA's Standards for Test Users Task Force; past chair of ACA's Interprofessional Committee; past chair of the ACA Public Awareness and Support Committee; cochair of the National Awards Committee; past chair of the Convention and Screening Assessment Instruments Committees for AACE; past president of the Maryland Association for Counseling and Development (MACD); past president of Maryland Association for Measurement and Evaluation (MAME); past president of Maryland Association for Counselor Education and Supervision (MACES); and past president of the Maryland

Association for Mental Health Counselors (MAMHC). He was also an associate editor of the *Journal of Counseling and Development*. Dr. Erford has been a faculty member at Loyola since 1993 and is a Licensed Clinical Professional Counselor, Licensed Professional Counselor, Nationally Certified Counselor, Licensed Psychologist, and Licensed School Psychologist. Prior to arriving at Loyola, Dr. Erford was a school psychologist/counselor in the Chesterfield County (VA) Public Schools. He maintains a private practice specializing in assessment and treatment of children and adolescents. A graduate of The University of Virginia (PhD), Bucknell University (MA), and Grove City College (BS), he teaches courses in Testing and Measurement, Lifespan Development, Research and Evaluation in Counseling, School Counseling, and Stress Management.

## Contributing Author

**Rick Balkin**, PhD, is an associate dean and associate professor on faculty at the Texas A&M University-Corpus-Christi. He has practiced in psychiatric hospitals, outpatient clinics, and community mental health centers since 1993. Dr. Balkin holds professional licenses in Texas and Arkansas and has a specialization in supervision. He is also a Nationally Certified Counselor. Dr. Balkin is active in the American Counseling Association and the Association of Assessment in Counseling and Education. His primary research interests include counseling outcomes, program evaluation, counseling adolescents, and gender and ethnic differences in counseling. Dr. Balkin most often teaches clinical coursework and research components. He is currently the editor of *the Journal for Counseling & Development* and is a past editor of *Measurement and Evaluation in Counseling and Development*.

# SECTION I
# Foundational Issues in Counseling Research and Evaluation

Section I addresses important foundational issues of research and evaluation in the counseling profession. Chapter 1 introduces the reader to the scientific inquiry and investigation process, including important ethical and legal considerations. Chapter 2 reviews the fundamental characteristics of research studies, familiarizing the reader with the research process while summarizing the expanded content delivered in subsequent chapters of this book. Graduate students in counseling programs must frequently learn to locate research studies, prepare literature reviews, and even write a thesis, research report, research proposal, or capstone project. Chapter 3 is meant to provide the basic information professional counselors need to begin this process. Finally, Chapter 4 presents a concise summary of counseling outcome research to inform the reader about some of what we already know works in counseling and to pique one's curiosity to pursue what is yet unknown or is still emerging knowledge within the counseling profession.

# The Nature of Research and Inquiry

## CHAPTER 1

Our current understanding of inquiry and research has developed over many centuries. This initial chapter defines much of the terminology the reader will encounter throughout the rest of this book and provides insights into positivist, postpositivist, and postmodern paradigms, including an emphasis on social justice, which shape the nature of research and inquiry in counseling and related disciplines today.

# The Nature of Knowing

How do you *know* that you know? There are many ways to answer this question, each based on a particular philosophical tradition. Our senses, or **sensory experiences**, have long been recognized as one way we come to know something or to treat it as a portion of knowledge upon which we rely or act. Our senses are powerful research tools that guide us through life with bits and pieces of knowledge that we learn to trust. After we pick up a few rocks, we realize that rocks are hard and actually hurt when we apply them with force to the side of our heads. Sensation received, lesson learned! In the practice of counseling, what clients "sense" about themselves is often the content of the interaction with a professional counselor. Clients include in their sessions what they've observed about others as well as themselves and use that information as the basis for understanding thoughts and feelings, actions taken, and decisions made.

**Traditions** and **faith** are another source of knowledge. They help us construct knowledge that gives us a sense of confidence and trust in ways very similar to sensory experiences. Societal, cultural, and religious traditions powerfully shape some of what we count as knowledge. How one is raised, in what culture, and with what religious practices provide foundations for knowledge so powerful that one often cannot discern their influences on how one behaves and acts in daily life. Children raised in rural areas assume some "knowledge" about life that children raised in inner cities cannot assume, and, just as important, the reverse is true: Urban children assume a knowledge that rural children often cannot grasp. Their separate cultures don't lend themselves well to teaching out-of-culture experiences; that is, it is difficult to teach urban children about rural life and rural children about urban life. One often must experience the life events relevant to a specific context to understand it. Likewise, growing up in an urban Chinese city leads to a significantly different acculturative experience than growing up in an urban American city, or rural Tanzania versus rural Appalachia. This concept is particularly relevant to the training of professional counselors, as multicultural/systemic counseling is now known as the "Fourth Force of Counseling." Professional counselors must understand and act upon the diverse perspectives clients bring to a counseling setting to help them adjust to their environmental milieus.

A third way of knowing comes from trusting in those whom we consider authorities—someone, or something, that we believe to be more knowledgeable than we are. That **authority** might be this book, a professor, a parent, or some of those traditions and beliefs we rarely question. In times of personal uncertainty, we often appeal to those authorities to provide us with knowledge, wisdom, and the decision-making process that we cannot seem to access ourselves; we trust what those we respect tell us.

At the same time, it is not uncommon for us to integrate the knowledge we gain from those authorities with the other ways of knowing, such as our senses, our beliefs, and the ways we were raised. We take what an authority tells us and use that new knowledge to explore some other phenomenon in our lives. All of these ways of knowing can be characterized as "personal." They allow, and sometimes even encourage, us to include ourselves in our observations and believe the knowledge created to be valid until a new experience proves it otherwise. As we move away from these more personal ways of knowing, however, we get closer to the "science" side of knowing, the less personal and more detached side.

Among the scientific ways of knowing are the more objective ways, including *formal logic* and *systematic inquiry*. Both the field of logic and the field of systematic inquiry rely on a set of acquired skills and rules for inquiring into some phenomena or events. These rules encourage one to assess senses, beliefs, and feelings against these more objective or external standards to create the science of any discipline. As such, science is the use of systematic inquiry processes to yield trustworthy information that we call knowledge. In a sense, logic and scientific inquiry historically discourage us from allowing our personal ways of knowing to influence what we study and how we study it. The human science fields, of which counseling is one, are advanced through the scientific investigations conducted by researchers in very systematic ways. These systematic ways include learning a series of steps designed to make our studies as objective and as free from personal bias as possible. When the researcher demonstrates an arm's-length distance from the study, its findings, and its conclusions, we tend to treat the study as generating new knowledge we can trust and can use for further research and practice. For example, if a counseling researcher wants to know whether a new technique or approach to the treatment of client trauma is effective, the researcher can use more objective scientific procedures, rather than personal observations or beliefs. Importantly, while the use of personal observations and beliefs may suffice for personally convincing the researcher, it may not carry much weight with other counselors, who may want more objective "proof." The use of standardized and objective scientific procedures may be viewed by other counselors as more convincing evidence that the new trauma counseling technique or approach is indeed effective.

So the ways of knowing range from the personal, or subjective, to the impersonal, or objective. The history of scientific inquiry suggests that the latter more objective and systematic scientific inquiry has been the more accepted way of knowing when building professional fields, such as counseling and psychology. Most people believe that there is more truth in objectivity than there is in subjectivity. The field of research methodology, however, is not even close to putting this distinction to rest.

## Philosophies of Science

Ponterotto (2002, 2005) described inquiry as a scientific pursuit guided by five core philosophies: ontology, epistemology, axiology, rhetoric, and methodology. These areas, or philosophies of science, have been influenced somewhat by the evolution of quantitative and qualitative approaches to research throughout history. Moreover, these philosophies of science guide the researcher in selecting a paradigm(s) (outlined in the next section) in which to couch their inquiry.

**Ontology** refers to the nature of reality; specifically, it involves an understanding of the things that constitute the world. What can we know about the reality of a phenomenon? Is reality objective or subjective? Is reality universal or context specific? What factors influence reality, if any at all?

**Epistemology** refers to the study of how knowledge is acquired in the context of the researcher–informant relationship (Ponterotto, 2005). What is the path to knowledge? How does the method by which knowledge is acquired affect data collection? Is knowledge limited? Is knowledge contextual?

**Axiology** refers to the role of values in research, including the idea of researcher bias and reflexivity (Ponterotto, 2005). What is the role of values in each aspect of the research process? How are research questions laden with values of the researcher, informants, and/or setting, if at all? To what degree should values be minimized within research?

**Rhetoric** refers to the way by which data analyses are presented (Creswell, 2012). Should results be presented in numerical form? Should data be presented in narrative form? Should data be described by categories or themes? What type of voice (i.e., first, second, or third person) should the researcher use? What terminology should be used to describe the rigor of the study?

**Methodology** refers to the processes and procedures of inquiry (Ponterotto, 2005). This philosophy emerges from reflection on the other philosophical assumptions and relates to how one conceptualizes the research design (Creswell, 2012). Which research design (e.g., grounded theory, true experimental, phenomenology, quasi-experimental, case study method, single subject, and ethnography) is most appropriate for a study? Should multiple designs be used? How will data be collected (e.g., interviews, observation, tests, and audiovisual material)? Are mixed methodologies (i.e., qualitative and quantitative approaches) appropriate?

A second way of conceptualizing a philosophy of science involves the terms "inductive" and "deductive reasoning." In **inductive reasoning**, a researcher begins by observing real and practical data that are evident in the environment to better understand the data or even develop a theory to better explain the observations of the data. For example, a researcher may notice how different teachers interact with and discipline their school-aged students and even conduct interviews with the teachers and the children to better understand and describe what is happening, why, and the intended and unintended results or the interactions. Inductive approaches tend to be more descriptive and correlational to "construct a theory" and often are linked to qualitative approaches for knowledge generation. Thus, the researcher studying teacher–student interactions may eventually be able to "induce" a theory of teacher–student disciplinary interactions. In **deductive reasoning**, a researcher begins with an established, or at least a tentative, theory and through an in-depth study of how that theory purportedly operates, develops and tests hypotheses of how certain facts of the theory will operate or relate to observable variables. The manipulation of these variables creates data that are then examined and determined to either support or not support the hypothesis. Then the cycle is repeated. These results are then used to confirm, disconfirm, or modify the theory. In the teacher–student interaction example, the researcher could test the hypothesis that teachers who demonstrate predominantly democratic/authoritative disciplinary styles yield significantly better student academic outcomes than teachers with authoritarian/autocratic disciplinary styles. Notice how this deductive process starts with a preexisting theory and tests that theory by collecting data to answer a question stemming from that theory. Figure 1.1 illustrates this cyclical, complementary process of inductive and deductive reasoning.

In addition to addressing various assumptions in inquiry, each philosophy of science relates to and builds upon the others (Creswell, 2012). Professional counselors who are engaged in research should reflect on these questions throughout their studies to help

**Figure 1.1**

The cyclical inductive and deductive reasoning process.

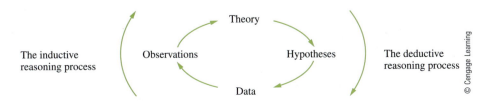

The inductive reasoning process

Theory

Observations

Hypotheses

Data

The deductive reasoning process

© Cengage Learning

solidify which paradigm(s) is(are) most suitable. Now that the philosophical dimensions of scientific inquiry have been examined, we turn our attention to research paradigms.

## How Real Is Real? Research Paradigms

Research paradigms are principles and assumptions related to philosophies of science that guide how counseling researchers design their inquiries (Creswell, 2012; Guba & Lincoln, 2005). Although paradigms may overlap in research practice, each may also be valid independently (Ponterotto, 2005). Three major categories of paradigms (i.e., frameworks for research designs) are evident in research approaches: empiricism, positivism and postpositivism, and postmodern paradigms.

### Theories of Empiricism

Many people advance objectivity over subjectivity because of the research traditions that used scientific inquiry to seek the greatest good for the greatest number of people. Dating back to the Renaissance and the Age of Reason in the 17th century, inquiry shifted away from examining personal experiences—the senses, faith, and feelings—as the primary sources of knowledge creation and replaced it with empiricism, a philosophical movement that claimed all knowledge came from experiences that can be tested against the experiences of others and not from the more personal senses. Empiricism dominated scientific thinking during the 1600s to 1800s in the natural and social sciences. Virtually all research in the human science fields is empirical because at some point the researcher must show some form of external validation of the findings—that the findings apply to others outside the current research setting. We are so accustomed to external validation that it is often hard for us to appreciate how much we rely on it for knowledge. A substantial criticism of empiricism is that human senses often belie a true understanding of reality. For example, it is a common occurrence that two human beings will experience the same event, but each will have different ideas about what happened or what it means. Likewise, our U.S. justice system, which uses eye witness accounts, is replete with instances in which human senses were shown to be selective and deceived the observer.

### Positivism and Postpositivism

For all of its success in challenging earlier definitions of knowledge creation, empiricism gave rise to a more refined philosophical tradition of inquiry that has dominated since the late 1800s. Traditionally, positivism and postpositivism are primary paradigms of quantitative research that seek cause–effect understanding among variables that can be identified and isolated within an objective manner (Ponterotto, 2005). Positivism, a paradigm closely aligned with the hypothetico-deductive method, focuses on hypothesis testing of existing theory. Positivism involves a search for nature's laws through observation and comparison via experiments that seek to explain phenomena through cause-and-effect relationships. Positivists challenged empiricism as still allowing too much subjectivity into inquiry, arguing that knowledge is acquired through experience and the observation of facts, to the exclusion of feelings, emotions, and senses. By drawing a clear line between the researcher and the study, positivists introduced even greater objectivity than empiricism, assuming that more objectivity would increase the amount of trust one could place in the study and results. This tradition has proven very successful in the physical and natural sciences, which have been advanced by maintaining objectivity as a hallmark of good scientific inquiry.

The positivist tradition includes the well-known practice of creating experimental and control groups to determine the comparative effects of a treatment on the participants under study. Positivists assert that phenomena can be predicted and controlled, and, thus, theory may be verified via statistical control (Ponterotto, 2005). For example, consider a pharmaceutical company that has invented a new drug to reduce the symptoms and effects of depression in adults. To test the drug, researchers administer the drug to randomly assigned groups of adult participants who are prescreened for a diagnosis of depression. The objective of the study is to determine how well the new antidepressant medication reduces the symptoms of depression. One group receives the antidepressant, and the other receives a placebo (an inert or inactive treatment, such as a sugar pill that looks like the new antidepressant medication) or maybe a rival product that is already available by prescription for the treatment of depression (a comparison treatment). In both cases, the participants under study do not know whether they are receiving the antidepressant, the placebo, or the comparison product. Through the random assignment of participants to the treatment and control groups, the researchers try to control as much as possible for any preexisting biases based on participant characteristics, and by masking the experimental drug and the placebo or comparison drug, they try to control for any participant biases that might occur during the study (e.g., if participants know they are getting the placebo instead of the antidepressant medication, they will probably report no change in mood states or may even stomp off and leave the study). These steps in the research design process are intended to decrease the subjectivity and therefore increase the objectivity of the study. The positivist tradition seeks, through experimentation, to minimize the subjectivity that naturally occurs in the study's participants so that the researchers can be more confident in their results on the effects of the antidepressant. This confidence is drawn from the controls placed on the study and is paramount in positivist scientific inquiry. Without it, we might never be sure that the antidepressant is safe and can be prescribed without worry.

In more recent years, the positivist tradition has been challenged because of its limitations, and this has given rise to a postpositivist movement. Developed as a rebuttal to positivists' claim that a fully comprehensible reality exists, **postpositivism** asserts that researchers can only *approximate* a universal truth (Guba & Lincoln, 2005). Postpositivists acknowledge that theories are meant to be tested for exceptions and disproven and that research should rigorously attempt to disprove a phenomenon to strengthen our understanding of it (Ponterotto, 2002, 2005).

Counseling researchers who adhere to the positivist and postpositivist paradigms believe that an objective and standardized researcher–informant relationship is possible. Further, they assert that research relationships have little or no influence on the results and methodology, thus minimizing enmeshment and avoiding bias. Further, both positivists and postpositivists maintain that values do not belong in the research process. They may employ methods that involve structure and manipulation to help explain a phenomenon in a generalizable manner. For instance, experimental and/or quasi-experimental designs that use random assignment or predesigned interviews or surveys in search of a collective experience are indicative of positivist and postpositivist ideology. When presenting results, both positivists and postpositivists attempt to remain emotionally neutral from the data, and rhetoric is objective (Ponterotto, 2005).

All research methods reveal some findings and conceal others; that is the nature of systematic inquiry. As much as we wish, no study can answer every question that arises. All researchers make trade-offs when they design a research study, and the good researcher knows how to recognize those trade-offs, consider the implications for the results, and think about how to improve upon the study for the future. Positivist practices reveal very well what can bring the greatest good to the greatest number of people—for example, in the antidepressant study mentioned above, the antidepressant reduces the symptoms and effects of depression more quickly than the placebo or the rival product. Positivist practices, however, do not reveal what the participants experienced during the study or why they reacted to the treatment the way they did. At best, the positivist tradition can tell us what happened, but it cannot tell us why. There is an "understory" to the experimental results that can reveal even more, and most of that understory includes the introduction of subjectivity as a rediscovered way of knowing. And this is the primary criticism that gave rise to the more recent postmodern paradigms.

### Postmodern Paradigms

In reaction to the positivist way of knowing, and even to the postpositivist tradition, a postmodern paradigm developed. **Postmodern paradigms**, a group of theories that include constructivism, critical theory, and feminism, are often used in qualitative approaches to research (Creswell, 2012; Guba & Lincoln, 2005). Postmodern approaches are also concerned with social justice and the understanding and application of context to the creation of knowledge. Proponents of **constructivism** argue against positivist perspectives that originated from the Enlightenment period, specifically that humans progress linearly via rational thought independent of context and that a universal truth may be discovered by using the scientific method. Additionally, constructivists critique earlier paradigms because they believe reality should never be labeled as objective, as the voices of the researcher and informants are biased and seated in different cultural experiences and identities. As such, pure objectivity is unattainable; a singular "truth" does not exist. Because an interactive dialogue between the researcher and informants is instrumental in co-constructing findings, constructivists view interpretation as a primary component of research (Bogdan & Biklen, 2006; Creswell, 2012; Ponterotto, 2005). Multiple realities, all equally valid, exist because different individuals develop unique constructions within unique social interactions. As a very simple example, the next time you are in a group of friends or classmates, ask, "What is your favorite color?" The diversity will amaze you. If you next ask, "Why is it your favorite color?" you will begin to understand the complexity of human beings and the diversity of opinions and realities that arise from their lived experiences. Thus, one goal of research from the constructivist paradigm is to understand the lived experiences of informants through dialogue and reflection. Further, the process of conducting qualitative research, a primary research methodology embraced by constructivists, acknowledges the power differential among researchers and informants (Bogdan & Biklen, 2006).

The constructivist way of knowing, which involves constructing rather than discovering meaning from experiences, is a reaction to what positivist research practices cannot explain well. Because constructivism is grounded in the idea that knowledge depends on the participant's frame of reference, it reintroduces subjectivity into the equation of conducting research in ways even more personal and powerful than the postpositivist tradition. Returning to the antidepressant study example, in the constructivist tradition, the researchers may want to interview the participants to discover what other things they've noticed about themselves as a result of being a participant in the study—what are commonly called side effects, but what could also be subjectively noticed positive or negative consequences. Note that these positive or negative consequences are simply noticed by the participants as co-occurring with treatment and cannot be linked causally to being a study participant. In this way, researchers are not only measuring whether the symptoms and effects of depression have subsided, but in the constructivist perspective, they are looking for any problems their treatment may have caused, such as headaches, sleeplessness, dry mouth, change in appetite, and the like, and any positives the treatment may have contributed, such as more stable mood, relationships, appetite, sexual desire, sleep, etc. These data allow the participants to reveal quite different information than a positivist, or objective, study might by allowing the participant to offer more personal data. Usually, these take the form of interviews or completion of questionnaires about these side effects. It is very important to future clients, doctors, counselors, and the drug company that the drug be effective for most people with as few side effects as possible. The challenge of such research is to determine both the benefits of the drug as well as its shortcomings.

As a second example, imagine that a team of counseling researchers is interested in understanding the grief process in children. Counseling researchers who subscribe primarily to a constructivist paradigm would ask children who have experienced a recent loss what helped them through the various stages of grief, as well as how the child grieved. In these dialogues, the team would co-construct the grief process and co-interpret ways in which children manage and overcome grief. Further, the research team would assume that children's worldviews as related to this phenomenon originate from cumulative social experiences. Constructivism assumes multiple realities, which adds a richness of perspective, but this richness makes it difficult to generalize to larger populations or diverse groups. For instance, in the grief example, the perspectives of the children in the sample may reflect only those perspectives of that group of children, rather than generalize to other children or children from diverse cultures or nationalities. While postpositivist researchers focus on and are concerned with promoting generalization, researchers using constructivism and other postmodern approaches are less concerned with generalizability.

Like constructivism, **critical theory** accepts the tenet that reality is socially constructed. Critical theorists, however, acknowledge that an individual's reality is embedded in power relations within social interactions (Ponterotto, 2005). Critical theory as a paradigm is multifaceted and action oriented, with the common goal of using research as a criticism of cultural ideology as a way to eliminate oppression (Creswell, 2012; Hays & Singh, 2012). As such, research is viewed as a political endeavor that should facilitate social action to benefit the powerless in society. Further, it accuses the research process from other paradigms of silencing the powerless groups in society. Critical theory seeks to examine how social power is reproduced in various settings and events (Bogdan & Biklen, 2006). Thus, the role of the researchers' values is significant in designing the methods and promoting change through the inquiry. One can easily see how critical theory is a force for social justice in the societal context.

In our example of children and grief, counseling researchers who behave as critical theory advocates would also be interested in promoting change and shifting power dynamics. Additionally, they would be careful to select children whose voices normally might not be heard or be accessible in counseling research, such as those from minority or lower socioeconomic statuses whose families cannot afford or might be less likely to seek counseling. Thus, counseling researchers using this paradigm would be creative in gathering information from inaccessible individuals to guide theory related to this phenomenon. They could use these data to create programs that would more fully address a broad range of children who are experiencing grief. Social justice and social action are prime drivers behind critical theory. One can also easily see that diverse theoretical variations are likely to emerge from postpositivist, constructivist, and critical theory approaches, leading to rich discussions and attempts to converge and differentiate emerging theoretical propositions.

The paradigm known as **feminism** emphasizes the role of affect within phenomena, the researcher–participant relationship, and the political implications of research (Bogdan & Biklen, 2006; Creswell, 2012). Using gender as its framework, counseling researchers analyze and reconceptualize the role that gender plays in phenomena and/or settings.

Further, feminism in qualitative inquiry seeks to dismantle the patriarchal structure that is currently dominating the counseling profession by critiquing current applications of research with the goal of empowerment, social action, and social justice. Professional counselors who work under the critical theory or feminist paradigm may use methods similar to constructivists but may assume that oppression plays a critical role in a research inquiry.

In addition to implementing social change by challenging the current status quo in society in general and in research more specifically, counseling researchers who adhere to a feminist paradigm would also explore the role of gender in counseling and research relationships. In the grief process and children research example, counseling researchers who use a feminist paradigm might be interested in exploring how grief is experienced and managed differently according to gender, as well as how gender role socialization influences the way children experience grief. Furthermore, counseling researchers might forthrightly discuss the research relationship with participants to demystify the process and treat the inquiry more like a collaborative dialogue, with everyone involved having equal status in the process. Thus, the feminism research approach promotes social justice and social action, helping to shift the focus from a historical male-centric or patriarchal lens to one that celebrates the roles female culture and affect play in our understanding of the human experience. Importantly, feminism does not seek to denigrate the role that males play in society, just to equalize and celebrate the contributions of male and female gender roles.

Professional counselors who adhere to postmodern paradigms view the researcher as an instrument in qualitative inquiry, a tool that is changed by the research process. They conceptualize the researcher–informant relationship as a necessary component of data analysis in that researchers' interactions serve to develop and confirm findings with informants. Moreover, postmodern counseling researchers question earlier studies' findings in light of new theories (Hays & Singh, 2012). Because the relationship is inseparable from other aspects of the research process, researchers' values are recognized as unavoidable and significant in qualitative inquiry. Additionally, critical theorists and feminists believe that research values or bias should influence research process and outcome, thus inviting social activism and contributing to social justice. Postmodernists use interviews and fieldwork to emphasize detailed descriptions of findings rather than try to condense the results into a general summary. When presenting results, postmodernists are more likely to use first-person rhetoric, present data in a narrative format, and provide detailed descriptions regarding research bias and reflexivity (Creswell, 2012; Ponterotto, 2005).

These two traditions should not be thought of so much as opposite ends of a continuum as a more rounded conception of the multiple ways new knowledge can be created. To use a trite expression, they are two sides of the same coin. Both the postpositivist and the postmodern traditions rely on systematic inquiry to advance our knowledge of the field and on validating the findings before reporting them to other researchers and practitioners. And they use quite different methods to do so—but more on that in Chapters 5–7.

## Paradigmatic Postscript: The Search for Truth, Knowledge, and Understanding

Of all the animal species we humans are unique in our ability to contemplate our origin. We are the only living beings capable of asking why we are here, how things work, and how we function. The quest for this knowledge began as early as recorded history when the great philosophers began their search for truth through their senses, feelings, and faiths. The most dominant among them believed that truth was the knowledge of the divine and that the divine was the source of all truth. Unfortunately, the positivist methods that rose as a reaction to the sensory ways of knowing have not been able to prove the existence of the divine, a quest that continues for some today, and the quest for truth was replaced with the quest for knowledge, something that the positivist methods did comparatively well. The first disciplines to most efficiently use this newer exploration were the hard or pure sciences, especially mathematics, physics, and chemistry. Borrowing heavily from what many consider the "purest" science—mathematics—physicists conducted experiments of all kinds in attempts to understand how things worked and, in a sense, to answer the preceding questions.

Physics dominated the advancement of research design for the next century, and in the late 1800s the first social science, psychology, began to emerge. Psychology, the first field to study humans as systematically as physics studied nature, adopted the positivist traditions so well developed over the 19th century in the sciences. Throughout the 20th century, other social sciences were developing, and the early researchers in these fields—economics, political science, sociology, and education—also adopted the mathematics-based positivist practices that worked so well for the Western world's discoveries of the 19th century. But the findings from the positivist traditions that applied to humans were not as satisfying as they were in those fields that did not study human beings. Over the course of the 20th century, what began as a search for truth and then a search for knowledge became a search for understanding *how* humans worked. If one could understand human beings, then perhaps one could begin to identify ways to improve the conditions in which humans find themselves, whether those conditions are physical, emotional, social, or economic. The positivist traditions were not revealing enough, and by the end of the 20th century, the postmodern paradigms began to emerge. This most recent tradition has the capacity to replace the quest for understanding truth with the quest for understanding how people make meaning of the conditions in which they find themselves. In this view, *truth* may be the meaning that people ascribe to things and to themselves, which in some ways swings back full circle to the great philosophers.

How we see the world informs what we see. As both a research field and a practice, counseling has struggled with the divide between these two research perspectives. We know the "general effects" of findings from the positivist tradition, but we also see clients who don't fit the theory as well as we'd like. For professional counselors, understanding and embracing these research traditions are experiences that arise with each client we see. We seek to apply the general principles from the positivist research to individuals and their inherent subjectivity. In the end, understanding the systematic process of research informs us as researchers and practitioners in a fluid human science field as we try to help others bring meaning and health to their own lives.

# The Hallmarks of Scientific Inquiry

Early in the evolution of scientific inquiry, the French philosopher and mathematician Rene Descartes introduced the notion that following a systematic process was essential to understanding the world around us. Over the next few centuries, that orderly and systematic process came to be known as the *scientific method*, and it is marked by three essential features: objectivity, generalizability, and replication. **Objectivity**, as discussed earlier, connotes that the hand and mind of the researcher are removed as far as possible from the research itself. That is, the thoughts, opinions, and expectations of the researcher do not influence the findings that result from the data-gathering process; otherwise, the result would be a very biased definition of knowledge. **Generalizability** is another way to define the quest for the greatest good for the greatest number of people. As shown in the preceding example of the antidepressant medication, researchers strive to determine how widely their findings apply by identifying a **population** they would like to study (e.g., adults with depression). Because they cannot include in the study every person in the nation or world who has depression, researchers draw a representative sample of people who have depression. This **sample** is a subset of the target population to be studied. The researchers then use systematic procedures by (randomly) choosing from the drawn sample to create groups of participants who represent that larger class of people or population. If the researchers accurately choose their sample of participants from the larger population, the researchers can be confident that the sample closely represents the population, giving the researchers a more manageable study and the ability to generalize their findings to all other depressed adults.

As another example, if a researcher wants to study obesity in adolescents, the researcher cannot study the entire population of adolescents who are obese. So, working with local agencies and practitioners, the researcher can locate a group of these adolescents who live in the area and ask them to participate in the study. Then, through a systematic procedure, the researcher can draw a subset or sample of individuals that will make the research manageable. How accurately this procedure produces a representative sample will determine the extent to which the researcher can generalize to all other adolescents with obesity. In short, the researcher cannot study the population, so selects a sample, operates on it, and then generalizes the sample results to the larger population. Theoretically speaking, if the sample was selected properly and appropriate safeguards used, the sample results should generalize to the population and provide external validity.

The third hallmark of scientific inquiry is replication. **Replication** is the consistency of findings from one study to the next. Imagine conducting a study, obtaining the results, and then conducting the study again and again. All things being equal, the findings from the first, second, and subsequent studies should be very similar. If they are, then replication has been achieved, and one can trust the findings. But if the findings from the studies do not match, one cannot assume that new knowledge has been created, and "it's back to the drawing board!" It is only after several studies produce the same results that the findings can be considered sound and trustworthy. Objectivity, generalizability, and replication are three of the traditional hallmarks of scientific inquiry. They are drawn primarily from the positivist tradition, but they have come to define what we think of as "good science" or quality research. Note, however, that these concepts are always undergoing revisions and reconsiderations. Therefore, one cannot consider them as fixed forevermore. Astute researchers and practitioners remain attuned to them and use them as barometers for assessing the quality of any research study. Researchers always review a study to determine how much subjectivity was allowed in, whether in the data-gathering methods or the interpretation of the results. The importance of maintaining objectivity through the concept of validity or validating the findings against other research or even the perspectives of the participants is discussed further on.

When it comes to generalizability, it is not uncommon to ask, for example, whether a particular treatment that was tested only on adults will work equally well on adolescents. In trying to find the greatest good for the greatest number of people, we constantly want to know what works and whether it will work with a different population. In this example, it is another way of asking, "Does this treatment generalize to adolescents?" Again, in the positivist tradition that has shaped the nature of scientific inquiry, the more generalizable the findings, the more productive the scientific investigation.

Replication is the assurance of constancy. Two studies that use similar samples and similar procedures should produce similar results. If they do not, it is difficult to have faith in the treatment or the research method. We want to see the same findings from multiple studies because only then we can confidently apply them to other studies or even to the larger world of practice.

Good researchers will apply these concepts every time they read a study. A lack of objectivity, generalizability, or replication should be a warning that more research is needed before we can wholeheartedly accept the results.

# Reliability and Validity

If we are to trust a study's findings, there must also be reliability and validity. **Reliability** is the estimate of how consistently the scores from instruments used to gather the data performed or how closely they approximated the "true" score. For example, when you step on your bathroom scale, you believe it is reliable because every time you weigh yourself, you get a very similar weight, or score. Now imagine that you have been doing some serious dieting. On Monday you weigh yourself, and the scale registers 150 pounds, but then on Tuesday it reads 130 pounds! While your first reaction may be stunned ecstasy, soon thereafter you probably will have doubts about your trusty scale's reliability. It is no different with psychological, personality, or observation instruments, or with interviewing techniques. Researchers try to derive scores from the data-gathering instrument that are as reliable as possible by not changing the instrument from one data-gathering event to another. Most standardized assessments (e.g., SATs, GREs) are considered highly reliable instruments because they produce similar scores from one administration to another. Those who design data-collection instruments are required to assess the reliability of derived scores by using particular statistical calculations for estimating reliability, and they must report these results in a research study. In contrast, instruments that yield unreliable scores, or even instruments that yield reliable scores but were used in ways that compromised their reliability, produce research findings that are unequally reliable. Imagine that you have always gotten an accurate reading from your bathroom scale, but if you weigh yourself at different times on different days, *you* are compromising its reliability. If you weigh yourself in the morning before you eat breakfast one day and weigh yourself in the evening after a large meal another day, the weights you get cannot be considered an accurate "score." The scale has no way of knowing about the inconsistency of your routine; it only knows its own consistency. When we are confident that the instruments we use in our research yield reliable scores, we can have faith in the results.

**Validity** is the degree to which a study's conclusions are consistent with the data used. In other words, the findings are judged valid if the researchers do not draw conclusions beyond what resulted from the data. The validity of a study's findings can also be doubted if the researchers interpret inaccurately. Say a counselor researcher wants to study how newly married couples handle the first years of marriage. She interviews 10 couples over a five-year period and uses the same set of questions at each session so she knows she has an instrument that will generate reliable scores—in this case, the interview. She gathers the data from the five years and discovers that all the couples reported the same four stages of growth. As long as she connects those four stages directly to the data, we can consider her findings to be valid. But say she went on to draw conclusions about the *future* of the marriages; this would mean that she went "beyond the data," and therefore her conclusions would be less valid. This does not mean that her predictions about the future may not turn out to be correct, just that the current data do not support those predictions. In a sense, then, validity is another measure of consistency. In this case, however, it is how consistent the researcher is in interpreting the findings and giving them meaning within the context of the literature rather than the kind of consistency associated with reliability. Scores derived from the instruments (the questions) may be reliable, but how the researcher interprets the findings affects validity.

# The Role of Theory

Using theory helps researchers understand and place into context the findings they generate from their studies. A **theory** can be seen as a lens through which researchers view the phenomenon they want to study. At the design stage of the study, the theory helps the researchers make a prediction about how the participants will respond to the treatment, which then allows the researchers to state their research hypotheses or write their research questions. Thus, theory provides the conceptual framework for the hypothesis that the researchers want to investigate. In this way, researchers test the power of a theory by drawing hypotheses and stating research questions. The clearer and more robust the theory, the better it explains the results of the study.

You are probably already familiar with a behavioral theory called "classical conditioning," which is commonly associated with Ivan Pavlov (of "Pavlov and his slobbering dogs" fame). Pavlov demonstrated that animals have a natural response to a predictable stimulus, such as a dog salivating when it smells or sees food. Similarly, noted psychologist, B. F. Skinner applied behavioral principles to humans to study how well behavior theory explained how humans learned to perform a wide variety of tasks. Behavior theory, however, is only one of many theories. As a lens, a theory helps to predict how people will behave, and it provides a foundation for the explanations for people's behaviors. Researchers build or add to the predictive ability of a theory with each study they conduct based on that theory. The stronger the theory, the more likely it can explain behaviors, feelings, or thoughts. A robust theory can tell us a great deal about human behavior, and it can help us understand the world a little better. It is theory that allows us to make educated guesses, or hypotheses, when we conduct a research study and work with clients or students.

Once the data are collected, though, theory plays another role. The theory being tested through the hypothesis now provides the framework for interpreting the data, and it shapes the researchers' explanation of the data. A theory is like those lesser or more absorbent paper towels in the TV commercials. The findings from the study are placed on the paper towel to test the strength of the theory. The stronger the theory, the more findings it can hold, or the more behaviors it can explain. Theories with low powers of explanation leave us feeling unfilled, confused, and sometimes with a mess that needs explaining and clean up! Robust theories explain a lot and can hold up to a great deal of scrutiny. More important, however, researchers build theories by testing them in different settings. A theory gains its robustness by the variety of findings it can validly explain. New theories are created or modified when the existing theories cannot adequately explain how people behave and why. But no theory can ever explain 100 percent of the observations.

Theories are lenses for making predictions and interpreting results. They provide a research study with a conceptual framework that advances the literature and our ability to explain phenomena. Theories are generalizations about people that are always being tested and always being challenged for their strength in helping to understand the world. The development and validation of theory is the primary goal of scientific inquiry.

# Types of Research

On some levels, research is difficult to categorize. The typology presented in this section may seem oversimplified to the experienced researcher, given its utilitarian nature, but it is important for the novice to understand that research is practiced for multiple purposes. As noted in the preceding section, one of those purposes of research is to develop theories that help to explain behaviors, thoughts, attitudes, and so on. Research that seeks to build theory is called **basic research**. Consider the researcher who wants to determine if social learning theory (Bandura, 1977a) explains how many close friends college students report having. The researcher designs an instrument based on social learning theory to give to the students to determine how they make friends in college. He then analyzes the data to see how well the theory predicts and explains close friendships. In this way, the research is testing the power of social learning theory to explain friendships among college students.

By comparison, **applied research** takes basic research one step further into the world of practice. Using the preceding example, the applied researcher puts the college students into a newly designed peer counseling program that, based on previous research using social learning theory, the researcher believes will increase the number of friends they make by providing them with skills to develop closer friendships. The researcher identifies the population of college students and then draws two samples. One sample is assigned randomly to the experimental peer counseling setting, and the other is assigned to a control setting of counseling that is not drawn from social learning theory. Both samples of participants fill out a questionnaire in which they report how many close friends they have in college. The students in the experimental group complete the peer counseling exercises over a period of several weeks. At the end, both groups complete another questionnaire in which they are asked again to report how many close friends they have. If the training based in the principles of social learning theory is valid, the researcher expects to see an increase in the number of friends for the students in the experimental group compared with those in the control group. This study is the application of a sound theory that is now being used to change people's behavior, rather than only to test the power of the theory to explain behavior.

More recently, a trend called **action research** has been emerging. Action research does not build theory the same way basic research does nor does it apply theory in any particular way. Here, the researcher is often a practitioner who has an immediate problem he or she would like to understand better. In this case, the practitioner, an elementary school counselor, wants to understand how students choose their friends at the beginning of the school year, because the school community feels it is important to establish a socially engaging and productive learning environment. At the beginning of the school year, the researcher has the students complete a questionnaire about what they look for in a friend. He also gathers data by observing how students interact during recess. After six weeks of data gathering, he is able to plot a chart showing which students have made friends and which have not. He then has each student complete a sociogram indicating which classmates are considered good friends. He then gives the students another questionnaire: "What I like about my best friends in this school." By the tenth week of school, he is ready to draw some observations on how well the desired characteristics of friends match those whom the students named as close friends. In this way, he is conducting an action research project that does not build theory or apply a specific theory but does give the professional school counselor some insights into the dynamics in the classroom through a theoretical lens. The ultimate goal, however, is to create programmatic interventions in the school that increase opportunities for students to widen their circle of friends and to build more trust in the school community, thereby improving school climate.

Although quite simplified, these three types of research are all important to the advancement of our understanding of the world. Each brings its own pieces to the puzzle of understanding ourselves, and each type provides understanding from a different angle. Basic research builds theory, applied research tests to see how far the theory can be extended for the purposes of generalizability, and action research is the application of theory to a local setting that does not allow for generalizability but does create local insight toward the improvement of practice.

# Variables

An important concept in this book is that of the variable. A **variable** is any behavior or trait that varies under different conditions (i.e., can exist in more than one level or state). For example, similar to behaviors, eating, strength, and satisfaction are all variables because they can vary from one setting to another. Most personality traits are variables, including happiness with a relationship, various types of intelligence, and levels of stress, among many, many others. Height and weight are both variables because human beings vary in height (measured in inches or centimeters) and weight (measured in pounds or kilograms). Researchers want to measure variables or the effects of one variable on another because it helps them to build theory about how we behave or to understand who we are.

In research, there are many different kinds of variables, but the two most important are independent and dependent variables. **Independent variables** are those believed to affect the behavior or status of another variable. For instance, any counseling session is an independent variable in the life of the client because it is intended to affect client behavior. All treatments, including counseling, medications, interventions, training programs, and even books you are reading (such as this one), often act as independent variables in our lives. They intend to change us in some way, to cause us to be different. How we become different depends on how well the independent variable works. Most independent variables can be manipulated by the researcher, although some independent variables are **organismic variables**—that is, characteristics of an individual that cannot be directly manipulated. Fox example, sex is an organismic variable because (with a few exceptions) participants can be categorized as either male or female. In such cases, researchers cannot "randomly assign" a sex to a participant, but they can categorize or group all participants as males or females and then randomly assign females and then males to various other treatment conditions. In behavior studies, the independent variable is sometimes referred to as the **stimulus variable**. In correlational studies, the independent variable is often referred to as the **predictor variable**.

**Dependent variables**, in contrast, are those that "depend on" the independent variable for their response. Imagine you are taking a medication to reduce your cholesterol. Whether you are taking the active drug or not is the independent variable, and your blood cholesterol levels are the dependent variables because they *depend on* the drug to affect them. Using the preceding example, the counseling session is the independent variable, and the ability to self-regulate is the dependent variable because the nature of the client's needs requires the counselor to increase the client's self-regulatory practices through the sessions. Sometimes the dependent variable is also referred to as an **outcome variable**, **criterion variable** (in correlational research), or **response variable** (in behavioral research). Dependent variables are measured or observed, not manipulated. It is very important to become proficient at identifying independent variables (IVs) and dependent variables (DVs) in research studies. As practice, identify the IVs and DVs in the following situations: (1) Does frequency of counseling affect counseling outcome? (2) Is depression reduced by different levels of medication? (3) Can achievement be predicted by intelligence and maternal education level? One handy way to do this is by inserting the variable names into the question "What is the effect of [IV] on [DV]?" Although this question is oversimplified (and certainly not all studies are causal), it tells you which variable is producing the effect (the IV) and which is being affected (the DV).

Another way to conceptualize variables is by using the terms "categorical" and "quantitative variables." **Categorical variables** are variables whose response choices can be categorized—for example, sex (male, female), candidates for political office (Mendez, Jackson, Aziz), or geographical regions of the United States (Northeast, Midwest, South, West). In other words, categorical variables are similar to nominal scale variables— variables that name but do not order or quantify the choices. **Quantitative variables** are variables that can be represented on a numerical scale and are not exclusively categorical—for example, distractibility, height, or place finished in a race. Generally, ordinal, interval, and ratio scale measures are quantitative variables (see Chapter 11).

# Types of Research Methods

Just as there are different types of research (e.g., basic, applied, and action research), there are also different types of research methods. **Research methods** involve the processes researchers employ to collect data and the procedures used to analyze the data to reach conclusions. Researchers choose among the following methods and select the one that will provide the best data to address the research question. Researchers do not begin with a method and then fit the problem to it; it is precisely the opposite. The most reliable and valid data-gathering and data-analysis methods are fit to the research hypothesis or research question. This section only briefly examines the major methodologies used in counseling research, but each is discussed in more detail later in the book.

In broad terms, there are two types of research methods: **quantitative methods**, which rely on mathematical calculations to characterize the data collected to address the research question, and **qualitative methods**, which rely on words, or narrative description, rather than numbers and calculations, to characterize the data collected to address the research question. The distinction between these two methods is very important.

Quantitative research methods generate numerical data and are generally used in studies that seek objectivity rather than subjectivity. Ordinarily, the results are meant to be generalized from the sample being studied to the population it represents (e.g., college students with a personality disorder, mothers and/or fathers experiencing a significant loss, cancer survivors, students' ratings of a professor). Quantitative methods generally maintain objectivity by using instruments that are theory based and that require the participant to reply in a standardized format (e.g., personality inventory, survey instrument, intelligence test).

In contrast, qualitative research methods do not seek to generalize the findings but rather try to focus on the contexts and meanings from which people draw—for example, when experiencing a significant loss, or surviving cancer, or managing a personality disorder. Qualitative methods do not usually derive numerical data, instead relying on participant verbalizations to try to include the subjectivity that is represented by feelings, emotions, and attitudes. This is accomplished by asking the participants to state their responses to the data-gathering instruments in their own words rather than on an instrument where the responses were designed by the researcher. Thus, rather than a standardized measurement to assess a personality type, a qualitative researcher might interview the participants or give them a set of tasks to complete that allows them to put their emotions into their solutions. In this way, the participants are representing themselves rather than letting an objective instrument do it for them. For example, one may feel constrained by a university's course evaluation instrument because it doesn't ask the questions you would like to write the answers to. The front of the form usually seeks quantitative data, whereas the back of the form often gives students the opportunity to write a few sentences in a more open-ended, expressive format. This is the kind of narrative on which qualitative research methods are based and serves as an important distinction between quantitative and qualitative methods.

Another distinction between quantitative and qualitative methods is that because quantitative methods seek to generalize from the sample to the population, they are trying to confirm an effect or relationship. That is, researchers often turn to quantitative methods as the theory becomes more robust because, as just noted, the more robust the theory, the greater its explanatory power. In contrast, qualitative methods seek to understand how people make meaning of such effects or relationships among events. If quantitative methods are more confirmatory, then qualitative methods are more exploratory. Our conceptions of science have not allowed us to see the results of qualitative studies as anything but a representation of the setting in which the study was conducted. We cannot generalize from a study of the family structures of the urban poor in Brooklyn, New York, to the family structures of all urban poor in the nation. Qualitative research methods are very powerful in exploring settings for possible new theories, but eventually we need research studies that use quantitative methods to generalize the results from that original locale. Contemporary social science fields have come to understand the necessity of both quantitative and qualitative methods to understand human dynamics. Each will be explored in more detail in Chapters 5–7.

For now, it is essential to understand that quantitative and qualitative methods are two sides of the same coin. Each method both reveals and conceals some aspects of the participants being studied. In more recent times, the human science research community has come to accept how revealing and concealing research methods are. As such, there has been a rise in "mixed methods" research—that is, a quantitative study with objective measures combined with case study data that tries to uncover what the instrument might not reveal. The field of research is stronger for this emerging sense of wholeness when studying the fluid nature of humans as participants, and the methods on both sides of this coin continue to evolve to further our understandings of humans.

# Ethical Issues in Research in Counseling

Simply stated, ethics in most human science research are concerned with protecting the rights and welfare of the participants being studied. In the field of counseling, however, it goes a bit further to include respecting the dignity of the study participants. In all human research undertaken in the United States, the participants are protected by codified laws and regulations, and the astute professional counselor looks closely at the *Code of Ethics* published by the American Counseling Association (2014). Research in counseling is a bit more distinct because poor research practices may impugn the dignity of the human participants, researchers, and even the entire profession. It is essential to understand from the outset that concern for human dignity must transcend all other considerations when conducting research in counseling. Many of these protections are guaranteed and assured by a code of ethics that is maintained by a human subjects review board. These protections include the avoidance of harm, which may include undue stress, and negative reactions to medicinal or interpersonal interventions. The counseling researcher must be scrupulously aware of any effects that the treatments are having on research participants. Most institutions of higher education and private research institutions have written human subjects review procedures and panels that approve applications and review compliance with these procedures. The provisions of the ACA *Code of Ethics* (2014) can be found at http://www.counseling.org/knowledge-center/ethics. These are relatively simple rules of ethics to follow and should remain at the fore in the minds of counseling researchers.

Researchers must take care when conducting any type of research, because the participants involved are humans, and often children. It is necessary to obtain approval from Institutional Review Boards (IRBs), before beginning research. Various organizations, including the American Counseling Association (2014) have set forth ethical standards for conducting research with humans. The ethical principles of autonomy, nonmaleficence, and beneficence are of the utmost importance. **Nonmaleficence** means to do no harm while **beneficence** means to promote the welfare of those involved. Research participants have the right to **autonomy**, meaning that they have the ability to make their own well-informed decisions. Participants should not be coerced or forced into participation in research. This principle ties in with the importance of informed consent.

**Informed consent** means that a participant must have full knowledge of the potential risks, benefits, procedures, and purpose of the study. Participants must also be made aware that they are free to withdraw their participation at any time during the study without penalty. Children and those with cognitive limitations are not deemed able to provide informed consent, so researchers should obtain written consent from their parents or guardians. Researchers should still strive to provide information about the study to the child in vocabulary that the child can understand and to seek assent from the child participant. Table 1.1 provides a sample informed consent form.

However, what if you were conducting a study where giving away the purpose of the study at the beginning would influence or bias the results? **Deception** in research is justified when the potential benefits outweigh the risks and there is no alternative way to achieve the desired results. When using deception, it is essential for the researcher to explain the nature and purpose of the deception immediately after the study concludes. This explanation of the study's purpose, called **debriefing**, is necessary in all studies but is especially important in studies where deception is used. The researcher should also use this time to ensure that the participant has not sustained any physical or psychological harm as a result of participation in the study.

Sometimes some level of risk or harm is not avoidable in the study. For instance, it is likely that participants will feel embarrassed when asked about their sexual experiences, but if the benefits of the study outweigh this risk, the researcher can handle this situation by electing to conduct the study in a private setting, ensure confidentiality, and take steps to help the participant feel more comfortable at the conclusion of the study. Weighing the benefits of the study for the participants and humanity in general against the risks for the participants is the best way to determine whether the study is ethical or not. If the benefits greatly outweigh the risks and there is no less invasive procedure, the study can be deemed ethical. In the United States, participants can only participate in research that poses greater than minimal risks if there is a direct benefit to the participant or if the research produces knowledge about a condition that is generalizable to future participants (Blake, Joffe, & Kodish, 2011).

| **TABLE 1.1**    Sample informed consent form. |
| --- |

I, _____[participant's name]_____, agree to participate in a study to develop a new rating scale assessing a wide variety of emotional perceptions that is being conducted by _____[name of principal researcher(s)]_____ of _____[institutional affiliation]._____    The general purpose of this study is to determine what average performance is for participants of different sexes or ages on the various constructs measured to more accurately identify emotional difficulties people may be having. To study this, the investigator will need to collect responses from more than 1,500 adults. The investigator is interested only in statistical analysis of all 1,500 forms and your singular test results. As a participant, I understand that

1. I will be expected to complete the rating scale, which will take approximately 10–15 minutes.
2. Completion of the test is purely voluntary. I am under no obligation to complete it. I am free to stop participating at any time without penalty.
3. Some temporary stress or discomfort may be experienced as a result of providing answers to questions about emotional issues. Most adults answer questions similar to the ones you will be responding to without difficulty, but if any of the items should cause you concern or distress, you have

the right to refrain from answering any questions or to discontinue this test.

4. My signature on this form does not waive my legal rights of protection.
5. All information is guaranteed to be **confidential**. Only the principal investigator and his assistants will have access to my responses. My data will be used only for the purposes of this study and will remain in a locked office. Please be assured that your identity will not be identifiable from the protocol. All responses from all participants will be pooled for the analysis of the study and reported as group values. Therefore, your responses will remain totally **anonymous** after coding.
6. I agree that any information obtained from this research may be used for publication or education, provided that I am in no way identified.
7. If I have any questions or problems that arise in connection with my participation in this study, I should contact the project director at ____[provide contact information here]____ .
8. This study has been explained to me, and I understand that I am voluntarily consenting to participate.

_____          _____
Date                                 Signature of Participant

_____          _____
Date                                 Signature of Investigator

_____          _____
Date                                 Witness*

THIS PROJECT HAS BEEN REVIEWED BY THE ___[institution's name]___ HUMAN SUBJECTS REVIEW OFFICER ___[phone number]___ .

*If investigator does not witness participant's signature, the person administering informed consent should indicate name and sign.

© Cengage Learning

Confidentiality is not just guaranteed in some studies; it is a necessary component of all ethically sound research. Researchers must take steps to safeguard the confidentiality of the information gained by blinding or disguising the identity of participants in coding and reporting. If a researcher wishes to identify a research participant in a subsequent publication, the researcher must first gain explicit written permission from the participant to do so. Sometimes situations will arise in which a researcher learns confidential information that the researcher feels should be shared. For instance, upon finding out that an adolescent participant has HIV, the researcher would likely want to ensure that the adolescent receives appropriate help and treatment. The best way to go about this would be to encourage the adolescent to disclose this information herself and provide the adolescent with resources and support. There has been much debate about whether researchers should report suspected maltreatment of children participating in their studies. Allen (2009) has examined both sides of the ethical debate and concluded that researchers should be mandated reporters of child maltreatment, just as many other teaching and counseling professionals are. Allen feels that the importance of protecting vulnerable populations overrides the importance of protecting the integrity of scientific studies.

It is important to keep in mind that all of these guidelines of informed consent, protection from harm, and confidentiality are just guidelines. It is the responsibility of the researcher to determine how these guidelines best apply to their studies. The researcher must take necessary steps to appropriately uphold these guidelines. It is incumbent on the researcher to continually evaluate the ethics of the study throughout the experiment to make adjustments if necessary. For example, if participants with posttraumatic stress disorder (PTSD) are showing incredible gains through the experimental treatment, it may be unethical to continue to withhold treatment from the control group.

Finally, researchers must bear in mind the importance of cultural sensitivity. This means that researchers must obtain informed consent in culturally appropriate ways to ensure that multicultural participants understand what is being asked of them. Researchers must also choose culturally appropriate designs and tests and refrain from using tests that have been shown not to yield valid scores for the multicultural population in question. Furthermore, it is the responsibility of the researcher to gain culturally sensitive knowledge and attitudes. The researcher needs to understand which aspects of human development are universal and which are culture specific to appropriately design and interpret the results of studies. Being aware of and avoiding ethnocentric biases and overgeneralizations of within-group homogeneity are important requirements for conducting culturally sensitive research. Finally, researchers should strive to include members of various minority groups in their samples to broaden the applicability of their findings to various groups. Much counseling research has been performed exclusively on White, middle-class Americans, so we must remember that the findings do not necessarily apply to all multicultural groups. We should strive to conduct studies to determine if the findings are in fact corroborated or differentiated.

Remember that while maintaining the integrity of research designs and the pursuit of knowledge is important, we must always balance these benefits with the personal rights and privacy of the individual participants. Research with human participants can be challenging to conduct in ways that do not harm the participants, but we must strive to meet this challenge to both gain new knowledge and protect the participants who help us gain it.

A final ethical issue pertains to the importance of keeping abreast of new information in the counseling field. Practitioners must be aware of new knowledge and techniques to be competent service providers. It is the ethical responsibility of counselors to stay up to date on new information to provide the best possible services to their clients. By providing evidence-based, effective practices for clients, counselors are both minimizing risks for clients and promoting the good of clients (Barsky, 2009). Counselors should use these best practices as guidance, using professional discretion rather than strict adherence to guidelines. This way, the counselor uses empirically based practices while also taking into account the client's culture and preferences. The ethical counselor-researcher should become intimately acquainted with the ACA *Code of Ethics*; so please take a few minutes at this point of reading this book to peruse and understand Section G: Research and Publication (ACA, 2014; see http://www.counseling.org/knowledge-center/ethics).

## Advancing Knowledge in Counseling

If any group of professionals in the human sciences needs to practice "research-type" thinking, it is professional counselors. Professional counselors need a "scientist–practitioner" disposition to capture both the need for a scientific foundation for practice, as well as to denote the connections among theories and research intended for professional practice. This is not to say that as a practicing counselor you are obligated to publish research, but it does mean that professional counselors have an array of theories about humans, and they should apply them in a research sense to their clients to understand them better and to bring them to a healthier place.

In this regard, the scientist-practitioner must embrace a wider repertoire of theory-based and research-based practices that rely less on a devotion to one research method or another. The field of counseling has been advanced both through the confirmatory nature of the quantitative or postpositivist research traditions and the exploratory nature of the qualitative or constructivist tradition. As a practicing professional, you are expected to keep abreast of the latest findings in the field by reading counseling research journals, evaluating the research you read with the content of this text in mind, and discerning what research-based knowledge you can apply to your practice with your clients. As a scientist-practitioner, this is the least you can do to remain current in an ever-changing world, but you can go even further to contribute to the literature by using the concepts and methods in this book and participating in or facilitating research studies. Much more on the topic of advancing knowledge in counseling will be presented in Chapter 4: Outcome Research in Counseling.

# Conclusion

This chapter introduced the concepts and terms that guide counseling research. It provided key terms that will be explained in greater detail throughout the text and presented research in the context of knowledge production, including knowledge as the meaning people make, or construct, of their surroundings. This chapter also placed scientific inquiry as a human activity that is shaped by the changing conceptions of humans, including what they know and how they act so the beginning student in counseling can distinguish points of entry into the field as a scientist-practitioner. It is hoped that as you read the chapters throughout the remainder of this book on each method, the kinds of data they generate, and how they are used you will reflect on what knowledge is and how it is accumulated in the best interests of understanding the human experience. As you do, here are some key points to keep in mind:

1. Research is concerned with the search for truth. Truth, however, can be as subjective as it is objective. There is always more to learn.

2. Research is a systematic process of collecting and analyzing data to test a research hypothesis or address a research question.

3. Empiricism is the foundation for systematic scientific inquiry that seeks to build theory through objectivity, generalizability, and replication.

4. To assist the research enterprise, a variety of research methods have been created. Quantitative methods seek knowledge through the pursuit of objectivity. Qualitative methods allow the perspective of the research participants to shape the data.

5. Many factors can threaten the validity of a research study, from the consistency of the data-gathering instruments, the nature of the participants in the study, to the conclusions the researcher draws from the data.

6. The role of theory is to ground the study and provide a lens through which the data and findings can be analyzed.

7. A study's ethical dimensions must be preserved and maintained to protect the participants in the study from mistreatment, and the responsible scientist-practitioner in

the field of counseling refers routinely to the *Code of Ethics* of the American Counseling Association (2014).

8. Research is a human endeavor. The work of researchers reflects all the strengths and weaknesses of human beings, and all research studies can be improved.

*Now go to the Student Workbook found on cengagebrain.com that accompanies this text for additional application and review activities.*

# Characteristics of a Research Study

## CHAPTER 2

In recent decades, counseling has greatly advanced as a profession. Most of the progress is a result of the research counseling has generated. To prove its usefulness and effectiveness in the helping professions, professional counselors must continue to conduct research that advances knowledge of human behavior. Although not all professional counselors become researchers, each must possess the skills to critically analyze research results to provide the best services possible to clients and students.

While the number of qualitative research articles is on the rise (Erford, Miller, Schein, McDonald, Ludwig, & Leishear, 2011), much of the research in counseling is conducted on larger groups of people and involves measurements that can be counted—what we call quantitative methods. Quantitative research deals mainly with data represented as numbers. It assumes that facts and feelings can be separated and that a single reality can be measured. The quantitative researcher's role is viewed as more of a detached observer. Basically, through observation and manipulation of variables, quantitative researchers look for relationships among variables to explain relationships and possible causes.

Quantitative approaches to research are synonymous with the scientific method and so they are called empirical or scientific research. Whether researchers use quantitative or qualitative methodology, they follow specific guidelines when designing a study, collecting data, and performing subsequent analyses. This gives us a systematic process to obtain information or investigate a phenomenon. The scientific method is basically the testing of ideas to find the answers to a particular research problem or question—and the systematic, standardized approach allows subsequent researchers to replicate or expand upon the study at hand. Using the scientific method in a study makes the results more credible and is the most effective way to establish accurate and reliable facts or principles.

Planning research should not be viewed as a linear process but rather as a parallel or simultaneous one. Systematic research inquiry is not without error, and it often requires researchers to retrace their steps, and sometimes go all the way back to the drawing board, to create a more appropriate study. I usually explain the presence of error in a research study by reminding people that when you begin the study you start out controlling 100 percent of the variance or results. But every decision you make along the way chips away, or cleaves, portions of the variance you control. For example, imagine that you are going to measure depression as your dependent variable. You have a choice between two depression instruments: one is a very accurate measure of validity and the other is only moderately accurate. You are probably better off choosing the more accurate measure because even though it is not perfect, it will give you better control over the outcome (i.e., helps you control for experimental variance). This makes it more likely that at the end of the study you will be able to better detect an important result if it exists. In other words, error is like static. If you have a clear signal, it is easy to hear your favorite song. But the more static (error) there is, the harder it is to hear the tune.

As you can easily tell, following a systematic, rather than haphazard, process helps advance a field of inquiry. The general characteristics of the research process presented in this chapter are the statement of the research problem or question, literature review, formulation of a hypothesis, definition of variables, and determination of sample, methodology, procedures, data collection, data analysis, interpretation, results, discussion, and implications/applications. However, an important caveat is that these characteristics, while common to both quantitative and qualitative research methodologies, are ordinarily found more frequently in quantitative research methodology. These two research traditions do vary substantially, as will become clear in subsequent chapters of this book. It is also important to understand that the information in this chapter is the introductory, 30,000-foot view of these characteristics. Much deeper treatments of most of these characteristics will reappear as the chapters unfold.

# Statement of the Research Problem or Question

Researchers begin with a problem they want to solve or a question they want to answer. Identification of a clear problem or question is the foundation of any quality research project. Although this may seem very simple, it is impossible to advance the counseling profession without knowing what research has already been conducted, what gaps exist in the research literature, and what has not yet been investigated. By examining others' research endeavors, an investigator can develop a rationale for one's own work. In other words, the research question should be substantial enough to justify the time and energy required to investigate it. In addition, any legal and ethical implications for conducting the research should be considered at this stage, *before* too much time or too many resources have been invested.

The wording of a research question is important; it usually implies that certain methods or analyses will logically follow. Research questions are ordinarily phrased in very general terms and may or may not make specific reference to the variables of interest. For example, an empirical study I published in 1999 (Erford, 1999) explored the research question of whether time-out was effective in reducing noncompliant episodes in elementary aged children with oppositional defiant disorder (ODD). Years earlier I used time-out when disciplining my own children and often recommended it to the parents and teachers of youth who were defiant. I noticed (noticing usually makes me wonder why, which helps me ask the question) that while the traditional procedure (e.g., sitting in the corner for 5–10 minutes) was effective, sometimes children continued to make noise or move around, or ask questions when they were supposed to be sitting quietly in the corner. I started to experiment with modifications to time-out, which resulted in the construction of a contingency delay model—basically I constructed "Dr. Erford's 7 rules of the time-out chair" and issued penalty minutes for violations of any of the rules. This seemed to work *much* better, but all I had was anecdotal evidence from parents and teachers, and my own observations. So I asked myself, "Is the contingency delay model more effective than regular time-out or even just doing nothing when kids refuse to comply with directions, or have a conniption?"

In the end, research questions help to focus the researcher's literature review and lead to the development of specific research hypotheses. Some examples of research questions are "Which counselor characteristics affect client outcomes in counseling?" "How does interest and competency relate to career satisfaction?" "Which family dynamics help facilitate resiliency in children and adolescents?" These are very broad questions, and a great deal of refinement and detail are needed before we are ready to answer the question. But first, we need to dive deep into our repository of accumulated knowledge—the extant literature! I mean, for goodness sake, someone may have already studied and answered my question!

# Literature Review

Although design, data collection, and analyses are critical components of any research study, any research effort would be futile without a comprehensive review of the literature, which can refine a research question and help formulate a viable hypothesis to be tested. A literature review involves analyzing all relevant articles, journals, books, and other available sources of quality information that pertains to the researcher's current research topic. Through literature review, we can examine the efforts of others who have studied similar research problems to observe what they have learned and develop a rationale for how the proposed study could add to the existing base of knowledge. The literature review should present the most current and relevant existing information on the topic under investigation. Usually this means reviewing literature within about the past 10 years, although classic sources and quality studies may have been conducted decades ago. By reviewing the literature, many researchers can identify a theory or framework through which they will analyze a problem and interpret results.

A thorough review of the literature can stand alone as a publication in professional journals and can serve as a useful resource for researchers who are investigating that particular topic. For example, Hinton, Sheperis, and Sims (2003) reviewed the literature on factors that contributed to delinquency (e.g., developmental issues, gender-related issues, and environmental factors) and effective approaches for treating it (i.e., those that employ direct and indirect client and community services and tend to be action oriented, multifaceted, preventive and remedial, culturally sensitive, and systemic in nature). The purpose of their review was to evaluate the differences between traditional methods of treatment for juvenile offenders and systemic models of intervention to help readers deal with the challenges of therapeutic intervention within the juvenile offender system. This literature review would give researchers who were interested in the components of effective treatment of juvenile offenders a starting point for developing research questions and refining their approach based on previous efforts.

In the time-out example (Erford, 1999), I reviewed the literature and found that while a lot had been written about behavioral techniques like time-out, few actually systematically evaluated the effectiveness of time-out, and none evaluated the effectiveness of the contingency delay model. I had asked a good question and now had the evidence to suggest the question was supported by the extant literature as viable. Of course, if multiple studies had already been conducted on my topic, I could have moved to a different topic, replicated a previous study, or extended upon the previous study to further our understanding about the use of time-out with school-aged children. Chapter 3 provides an in-depth discussion of procedures for locating, reviewing, and constructing literature reviews.

## Formulation of Hypotheses

Once a problem has been examined through a comprehensive literature review, the researcher refines the research question so that the new study being conducted will contribute to the literature by offering new and more current information about that problem. This is generally done by developing a research hypothesis. A **hypothesis** is a tentative explanation for a phenomenon and is used as the basis for further investigation. It can also be considered a prediction, an educated guess, or a statement of what specific outcome the researcher expects. In this step, we must consider and establish the variables (i.e., factors, characteristics, and conditions) that are under investigation. Like the research question, developing the hypothesis(es) is critical to designing the appropriate procedures to collect data and extract meaning from the results.

Quality hypotheses are concrete formulations of behavioral phenomena. In formulating a hypothesis, researchers establish concrete criteria that can be observed and subsequently tested. For example, Eaves, Emens, and Sheperis (2008) wanted to examine the effects of a systematic counseling intervention on clients' self-report of symptoms. The researchers hypothesized that clients who received a counseling intervention using

**Figure 2.1**

Flowchart of research purposes, types of hypotheses, and statistics indicated.

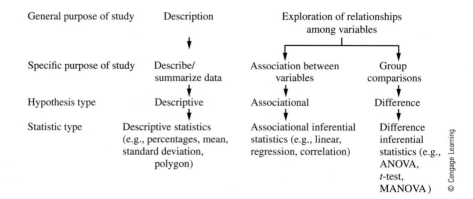

the data-based problem solver model (see Chapter 8) would report significantly less distress over the course of five counseling sessions as measured by the *Brief Symptom Index (BSI)* (Derogatis, 1993). In this case, client distress was quantified through the standard scores of the *BSI*, and the researchers were able to use statistical analyses to determine the significance of differences across participants.

Often, research questions and hypotheses are categorized according to purpose, such as descriptive, associational, or difference (see Figure 2.1). Basic descriptive hypotheses or questions summarize participant scores on a single variable, usually by presenting measures of central tendency (i.e., mean, median, and mode) and variability (e.g., standard deviation and range), or percentages of each category (e.g., 12 percent of the sample had high anxiety). Some descriptive questions might be "What is the sample's average GPA?" or "What percent of the sample is depressed?" Associational hypotheses or questions explore how scores on an independent variable (called the predictor variable) relate to scores on some dependent variable (called the criterion variable), with both variables ordinarily composed of continuous scales. An example of an associational hypothesis might be "Is there a relationship (correlation) between degree of rapport and counseling outcome?" An example of a hypothesis that lends itself to regression analysis is "Is graduate school GPA an indicator of career success for professional counselors?"

Group comparison questions and hypotheses generally lead to research approaches that use randomized experimental, quasi-experimental, and causal-comparative designs. In such designs, categories of the independent variables (e.g., levels of rapport) are used to divide participants into groups (e.g., high rapport and low rapport), which are then compared to determine if they differ on the dependent variable (counseling outcome). An example of a group difference hypothesis is "Do participants in the high-rapport group obtain better treatment outcomes than participants in the low-rapport group?" (addressed using a *t*-test). When more than two levels of the independent variable (e.g., low, medium, and high rapport) are presented, the hypothesis might be "Is there a difference in counseling outcome among clients in the low-, medium-, and high-rapport conditions?" (addressed using the ANOVA). So *how* you ask the question or phrase the hypothesis has particular implications for the types of study design, procedures, and data analyses required.

Hypotheses can also be classified as nondirectional and directional. A **nondirectional hypothesis** predicts that a difference will occur without indicating which group will perform higher. Likewise, a nondirectional associational hypothesis will not predict whether the relationship between variables in an associational hypothesis will be positive or negative. Some examples of nondirectional hypotheses are "A relationship exists between participant GPA and SAT-Reading scores" and "The counseling outcomes among participants with different levels of therapist–client rapport will vary." A **directional hypothesis** predicts not only the difference (or relationship) but the direction as well. Some examples are "A positive correlation exists between participant GPA and SAT-Reading scores" and "Participants with high counselor–client rapport will experience higher counseling outcomes than participants with low counselor–client rapport."

Although measuring differences or associations is important when trying to support a hypothesis, the researcher must also develop hypotheses that are falsifiable. According to Furlong, Lovelace, and Lovelace (2000, p. 17), "Falsifiable hypotheses are ones that data could clearly disprove because the hypothesis itself identifies events that *cannot* occur if the hypothesis is true." For example, professional counselors might speculate that children with attention-deficit/hyperactivity disorder (ADHD) who receive psychopharmacological intervention would perform better academically than such children who do not receive intervention. This hypothesis clearly implies that psychopharmacological intervention is beneficial for those with ADHD. If research was conducted on this hypothesis and the researchers discovered that no difference in academic performance between the two groups was observed, then the hypothesis has been disproved. In research, professional counselors often use the terms **null hypothesis** ($H_0$) (e.g., predicting no differences [or relationships] will be observed between or among groups) and **alternative hypothesis** ($H_1$) (e.g., predicting that differences [or relationships] will be observed between or among groups). These terms are common in statistical hypothesis testing that is associated with inferential studies, and they will be discussed in much more detail in Chapter 14.

In the time-out study example (Erford, 1999), I needed to establish a statistical hypothesis because I was going to test it empirically using a test of difference. My null hypothesis was, "There is no difference in noncompliant episodes among wait list, regular time-out, and the contingency delay model group members over time." My alternative hypothesis was, "There is a difference in noncompliant episodes among wait list, regular time-out, and contingency delay model group members over time." Note that the statistical hypothesis is precisely worded and even identifies the dependent variable, conditions, design, and likely statistical test used to answer the question. (Can you identify them yet?) But before we run the experiment, we need to tighten up the definitions behind those pesky variables. Remember, if the definitions are loose and nebulous, it will be difficult to know what they are, how to measure them, and how to replicate the study. In other words, precisely worded hypotheses and nice tight definitions reduce static (error) and help get a clear signal (result).

## Definitions

When conducting research, it is important to establish and define the meanings of all the key terms used in the study. Definitions can be either conceptual or operational. **Conceptual definitions** are those found in the dictionary. If you want to know what depression or noncompliance means, the dictionary is the place to go. More critical to research studies, however, are **operational definitions**, which outline the precise steps required to measure a variable accurately.

Operational definitions not only help the researcher to be more concrete about the variables and constructs (this will be important for determining validity later), but will also be useful to researchers who attempt to replicate the results. For example, a researcher might be interested in what effects graduate study in counseling has on the stress levels of students. Conceptually speaking, *stress* is an ambiguous term and can mean different things to different people. So in this case it would be important to define *stress* in terms of scores on the *Inventory of Coping Reactions* (Carver, Scheier, & Weintraub, 1989), changes in blood pressure, or even the number of self-reported negative life events that might have occurred over the past year. Thus, this definition of *stress* is measurable, includes common criteria for the concept of stress, and describes the measurement tools needed to obtain data. Operationally defining a variable helps others replicate and expand upon your study. If everyone measures depression differently, everyone is studying a different concept (i.e., different kinds of apples). When everyone is using the same operational definition, everyone is studying the same thing (i.e., the same type of apples). In the time-out study (Erford, 1999), regular time-out and the contingency delay models were described in extensive procedural detail, as was "noncompliant episode." Here are some guidelines for evaluating operational definitions:

1. Is each definition adequate?
2. Does each definition provide a complete description of the important dimensions of each variable?
3. Are the definitions accurate?
4. Are the definitions of the variables universally agreed upon?
5. Are the definitions clear?
6. Are the terms of measurement and devices described adequately?

# Sampling

A **sample** refers to the individuals who will participate in the study. The **population** is the larger group of individuals to whom the results of the study (based on the sample) are to be generalized. Samples are drawn or selected from populations, and the selection process is critical to the generalizability of a study's eventual findings. Researchers must carefully describe the methods and procedures that will be used to collect the sample because that will affect the degree to which inferences can be made about the population (Patten, 2009). Researchers have developed a variety of sampling methods, including convenience sampling, simple random sampling, stratified random sampling, cluster sampling, purposeful sampling, snowball sampling, and multistage sampling. These will be reviewed in detail in Chapter 7.

# Instrumentation

Selecting the appropriate apparatus is critical to conducting effective research. The term **apparatus** refers to any scales, tests, or assessment instruments that are used in the collection of data. A detailed description and a rationale for use of the instrument(s) should be provided in any published research study. Researchers often turn to published reviews of instruments to aid in their selection. Examples of test reviews can be found at http://buros.unl.edu/buros/jsp/search.jsp or http://www.theaaceonline.com/resources.htm

Most published research studies will contain a section on instrumentation. Authors attempt to provide a rationale for their choice of instruments in this section by reporting information related to normative samples, reliability and validity data, and overviews of scales and subscales. For example, Constantine (2002) studied the relationship between racism attitudes, White racial identity attitudes, and multicultural competence in 99 school counselor trainees. As part of this research, Constantine used a demographic form and three standardized instruments (i.e., New Racism Scale, White Racial Identity Attitude Scale, and Multicultural Counseling Knowledge and Awareness Scale). For each of the scales, Constantine reported the purpose of the instrument, the number of items, the range of scores, means scores, and coefficients alphas. Through review of her instrumentation section, it is evident that the scales chosen would be beneficial in examining the relationships among her identified variables.

# Procedures

Replication of research results strengthens the reliability of data. For any replication to occur, researchers must document procedures meticulously. The term **procedures** refers to the detailed description of the process of the study (e.g., what, when, where, how, and with whom) and a description of the materials used in the study. The general design or methodological process the researcher will use should be discussed here.

For example, Sheperis (2001) recruited professional counselors from schools and agencies to participate in his research project where his instrument (BARIS) would be administered in group situations. These assistants were instructed to read the instrument aloud to the group to compensate for any physical disability or inability to read. They also were trained to avoid bias in presentation by reading each item in a controlled, neutral tone and with a consistent pace. The assistants were directed to report any problems regarding the administration or completion of the instrumentation. They also were instructed to avoid discussion of individual items. Upon completion of the respective administrations, the assistants visually scanned instruments to check for responding errors. Participants were asked to complete any items omitted, if they so desired at that time. Such attention to detail clarifies how the study was conducted and facilitates future replication by other researchers.

Sometimes the procedures are very specific, even to the point the researcher gives verbatim directions. This helps to standardize the procedures so that any other researcher can replicate the study. This happens in clinical trials when researchers use published standardized treatment manuals. It also helps practitioners to know exactly what to say and do when using the procedures with a client, thus enhancing generalizability when implementing the procedure in real-life practice. In Erford (1999), the researcher provided flow charts indicating how to implement the modified time-out procedure, even placing in quotations what the clinician or parent should say during implementation. Helping the research consumer know what to do and how to do it standardizes the research procedure and helps practitioners more easily transfer the study into real-life practice.

# Data Analysis

**Data analysis** is the process of analyzing collected data and describing any statistical procedures conducted. Chapters 11–19 provide the specifics of a wide variety of data analysis procedures. When data from an entire population are analyzed, the descriptive tools (e.g., mean and standard deviation of the population) are referred to as parameters. When data from a sample are analyzed, the descriptive tools (e.g., mean and standard deviation of the sample) are referred to as statistics. (Remember: *P*opulations yield *p*arameters; *s*amples yield *s*tatistics.)

Statistical methods are categorized into descriptive and inferential types. **Descriptive statistics** describe and summarize data. **Inferential statistics** help predict the probability of occurrence of some causal event or association with some degree of confidence and allow this prediction to be generalized back to the population from which the sample was drawn. For example, a researcher may use an inferential statistic to determine if one counseling approach is more effective than another on a given sample. The result may allow the counseling profession to improve the overall quality of client care when this sample result is generalized and applied to the population of all clients receiving clinical care.

Inferential statistics are further subdivided into parametric and nonparametric tests. **Parametric tests** (e.g., *t*-tests and ANOVA) are used to evaluate hypotheses when the dependent variable is measured with an interval or ratio scale and when certain other assumptions are met (e.g., normally distributed scores, homoscedasticity). **Nonparametric tests** (e.g., chi-square, Mann-Whitney *U*) are used to evaluate hypotheses about the shapes of distributions and are only applied to nominal or ordinal data. Under normal circumstances, parametric tests are more powerful than nonparametric tests.

Accurate and precise data analysis is critical to the research process. Obviously, the more sophisticated the type of statistical technique used, the more expert the researcher must be. Frequently, counselor researchers will participate in a research team, with at least one team member having considerable expertise in advanced statistical methods. Such collaborations allow complex counseling questions to be studied using very sophisticated procedures.

# Results

The results section provides a detailed summary of the collected data after statistical analysis. Novice researchers often confuse this section of a research report with the interpretation or discussion section. In the results section of a report, the researcher should present the resulting data analysis in a meaningful manner (i.e., tables, correlation matrices, and graphs). All tables and figures should be constructed according to the guidelines of the American Psychological Association (APA). No interpretation is done at this point in a manuscript.

# Discussion/Interpretation

Although it is tempting to discuss the interpretation of data in the results section, it should be reserved for the discussion or interpretation section of the report. Here a detailed summary of the probable explanation(s) of the observed phenomena, trends, and anomalies are presented. In this section, researchers try to make sense of the data, discuss the significance of the results, suggest how the results may relate to previous studies, and report any possible limitations. Researchers should always refer back to their initial hypothesis in a discussion of the results. In drawing conclusions, it is extremely important that the researchers draw only conclusions that are supported by the data. Objectivity, generalizability, and replication are all affected when the researcher "goes beyond" the data and makes unsubstantiated conclusions.

Pan and Lin (2004) provided an example of a discussion summary in their study of members' perceptions of leader behaviors, group experiences, and therapeutic factors in group counseling. To relate their findings to previous studies, the researchers likened their discovery that participants cited cohesiveness and instillation of hope as the most important therapeutic factors to results found by Shechtman and Perl-Dekel (2000). In discussing limitations to their work, Pan and Lin (2004, p. 189) said the following about the results of their study:

> [They] may reflect Yalom's (1985) argument that differences in the therapeutic factors were mostly associated with the type of group and the stage of group development. Nevertheless, because minimal differences of means were found between the mid-ranked factors, conservative interpretations should be made to explain these differences.

In relating their work back to their original hypotheses, Pan and Lin (2004, p. 189) said the following:

> As expected, this study found significant positive correlations between group members' views of leaders' behaviors and members' group experiences. The results were congruent with the research findings of Pan and Lin (2000), who suggested that the perceptions members have about their leaders might alleviate members' symptoms, enhance their psychological functioning, and influence members to change.

These passages are good examples of how the current study (i.e., Pan & Lin, 2004) built upon previous work and could easily be linked back to the theoretical underpinnings that spurred the generation of the hypothesis.

# Implications for Practice and Future Research

One final element that a researcher should address in a report or manuscript is the implications for practice and future research. Although research is important in its own right, most consumers of research want to know how the results apply to *them* (i.e., how can they use it in their counseling sessions). Also, because most studies are based on previous efforts to some degree, researchers often address the degree to which the findings of their study add or fail to add to the current problem or issue under investigation. This final section can range up to several pages of text and is the part of the article that practitioners often find most helpful. To improve professional counseling, researchers should be meticulous and exact in this final section. Likewise, researchers often suggest the next research steps needed to extend upon the findings of the current and previous studies.

# Conclusion

In this chapter, we examined an 11-facet process for conducting research. Other books and articles may report different steps in this process, but what is most important is that the process must be systematic, objective, stable over time, and produce conclusions that are drawn directly from the findings while remaining free of unsubstantiated opinions.

*Now go to the Student Workbook found on cengagebrain.com that accompanies this text for additional application and review activities.*

# Locating, Reviewing, and Writing Research

## CHAPTER 3

Writing scientific literature is a skill that must be learned. Writing for scholarly consumption is fundamentally different than other styles of writing, such as constructing extended response essays or writing to influence. This chapter presents the steps necessary to write a review of counseling literature, including identifying a topic of inquiry; locating literature pertinent to the topic; critically evaluating selected literature; and organizing quality, relevant literature. Some tips for successfully writing the review are provided with a focus on the American Psychological Association (APA, 2010) style guidelines.

Professional counselors both evaluate existing research and produce new research to expand on and improve the professional practice and knowledge of the counseling discipline. The way counseling research results are disseminated has a great impact on how the knowledge is applied. Yet no matter how sound a research query might be, a study is no better than the document in which it is presented. It is only a waste of time and effort when the enlightening results of a well-designed and conducted study are shrouded by a poorly written report. Although an informative and concise report is critical to quality research, the art of writing can be the most difficult step in the research process to teach (Heppner, Kivlighan, & Wampold, 2008).

Fortunately, writing is a skill that can be learned and perfected with knowledge, practice, and feedback. This chapter outlines the writing process and its role in counseling research. Before we begin, however, it is important to address the issue of psychological readiness. Professional counselors must possess both the attitude and the intellectual knowledge to be successful writers.

Often the greatest barrier to producing an effective written research report is one's own feelings or attitudes about writing. Many researchers possess the skill, knowledge, and expertise to compose various types of written documents, but a lack of self-confidence or self-discipline—like chronic procrastination—can greatly hamper success. When this happens, a counseling student or researcher must be willing to take responsibility for such shortcomings and find a way to overcome them. Some deterrents to productivity include the lack of prioritizing, time, space, or support from others; disorganization; negative or illogical self-talk; and difficulties with coauthors. If, however, *you* are the greatest obstacle, you must acknowledge and own this and develop a plan that will motivate you (Heppner & Heppner, 2004). Successful authors are disciplined, knowledgeable, skillful, focused, and attentive to detail. No one is born with these talents and characteristics; learning to write effectively requires hard work, practice, and a lot of critical feedback from writers who have mastered the craft. Indeed, Malcolm Gladwell, in his book *Outliers: The Story of Success* (2008), popularized the "Rule of 10,000 hours," an interesting hypothesis (but certainly not a static rule or law) that proposed that one needs to engage in meaningful, focused practice for about 10,000 hours to achieve an expert level of performance. As this pertains to professional writing, five years of full-time, focused writing should do the trick! There is a corollary maxim we have all heard, "Practice makes perfect," which of course is not true. It should read thus: "Perfect practice makes perfect." While many are striving for neither perfection nor expertness in professional writing, there are a number of important hints and rules that can help you make a smoother transition to writing for scholarly consumption in the field of professional counseling.

# The Scope and Purpose of Reviewing the Literature

The first section of a research report is referred to as the literature review, a summary of the existing literature on the research topic. Composing a literature review is often a daunting task for students and neophyte researchers. One of the primary obstacles is the belief that literature reviews must be enormous. Yet, in fact, the length of the review depends on its purpose. A literature review for a dissertation, for example, is normally very lengthy, but the average literature review of a dissertation in a quantitative project is only about 25 draft text pages. Generally, literature reviews for quantitative journal articles are very brief (often only four to eight draft pages), but qualitative literature reviews can be much longer. So the study purpose and target audience determine the length of the document.

A quality literature review's main purpose is to integrate information from a variety of sources to demonstrate the benefits and drawbacks of prior research efforts and present a clear rationale for the intended project. Because each literature review has a page limit, it is important to be concise and to leave out unnecessary material. Unless the topic is unusually complex, more is not necessarily better; brevity and concision are key elements in skillful scholarly writing. You should carefully evaluate each resource's relevance to your report before you include it. For example, is the article directly related to the topic (i.e., primary resource), or is it just general information that supports the argument (i.e., secondary source)? Literature can be found in journal articles, authoritative books, and other similarly reputable documents that contain older and more current information on a particular issue. Web sites should be avoided unless the source is authoritative (e.g., Centers for Disease Control [CDC], U.S. Census Bureau, and National Institute of Mental Health [NIMH]). The literature review should not only summarize this information but do it in an organized fashion, corroborating a need for the proposed study. Readers should be able to determine what previous work was conducted on this topic, what major findings were gathered, what important conclusions can be drawn, what contradictions may be evident, any problems with the prior research, and the future directions that will be taken (Creswell, 2012; Heppner & Heppner, 2004).

A well-developed review of the literature gives the reader a clear explanation of the rationale for the current study and why more research in the proposed area is warranted (e.g., the study does not duplicate research already available). In other words, the literature review justifies the study if it establishes the importance of the research and proves that it emerges from notable prior research. Finally, a quality literature review reflects the author's knowledge of the topic and the author's ability to locate relevant research, evaluate it effectively, and use it to organize a study (Fraenkel, Wallen, & Hyun, 2011; Heppner et al., 2008; Patten, 2009).

No matter what the topic, writing a literature review includes the following five steps. These steps can serve as a guide for where to begin and how to know when you are finished.

1. Identify the topic of inquiry.
2. Locate literature pertinent to the topic.
3. Critically evaluate the selected literature.
4. Organize quality and relevant literature.
5. Write the literature review.

# Identifying a Topic of Inquiry

Before you evaluate research for how it might be relevant to your study, explore previous published research studies for some other useful elements. If you begin with a broad and general topic idea but have not yet settled on a specific theme, reviewing the literature can help you narrow your scope. In fact, this process, known as the inductive method, can be the best way to identify a possible research topic because it will help you come up with your own ideas. Pay particular attention to the sections on limitations of the current study and suggestions for future research (Heppner & Heppner, 2004; Patten, 2009). Often, authors of previously conducted research suggest topics for future exploration that are natural extensions of their studies, so a topic has basically already been created for you. Much of the preliminary literature search might already be done, and all you have to do is expand on the previous study. In addition, perusing counseling journal tables of contents will often lead to interesting articles and topics to pursue. Finally, reading a research compendium like Chapter 4 can give the student or novice researcher some background information on what we know works in counseling, thus providing the needed grist for the scholarly mill.

As your curiosity becomes the impetus for your ideas, you may consider exactly duplicating (replicating) a study to confirm the results. Or you might consider changing certain features of the previous study, such as those suggested in the limitations and future research sections, and conducting a modified replication or extensional study. Actually, the purpose of most research is to expand on or improve upon existing research. For example, one study may demonstrate that a counseling technique may be helpful in the treatment of anxiety and suggest that modifications to that technique may be even more effective; until someone studies those suggested modifications, the question remains unanswered. You may also notice discrepancies in findings and decide to pursue a resolution to the conflicting reports. Some studies may report a particular pattern of data, whereas others may address a different factor or even a contradictory one. Research that explains these inconsistencies can be extremely beneficial for the field of study, as a means of both advancing our practical understanding of the phenomenon as well as determining how different research methodologies (however subtle) and samples (however similar) can explain disparate results. Finally, you may arrive at a creative idea that is not an expansion of an already conducted study but is actually an entirely new direction for inquiry. Although you may feel that this is the best way to contribute to the research, the opposite may be true. For instance, Strangor (2011) strongly advocated basing topic ideas on existing research because that way the field would advance "more rapidly because it contributes to the accumulation of a unified and integrated body of knowledge" (p. 27). When you can find literature that is relevant to your idea, it tells you that others considered your topic important. So whichever approach you take, evaluating research should help you to select a topic (Patten, 2009; Strangor, 2011).

Evaluating published research has other advantages. If you are interested in measuring certain variables, the literature will be able to tell you which research designs and instruments were used successfully in the past. By exploring which investigations have hit a dead end, you can avoid unproductive lines of inquiry. By analyzing a reputable researcher's style and organization, you can learn a lot about the art of writing research reports (Heppner & Heppner, 2004; Patten, 2009). Many studies are unsuccessful due to poor methodology or instrumentation. The wise researcher learns from the mistakes and successes of others and builds on their accomplishments.

# Locating Literature Pertinent to the Topic

Once you have narrowed your topic, you can begin a more specific literature search. You can minimize frustrations, wasted time, and monotony by concentrating on the practical aspects of the literature search. Students frequently complain that they are able to locate only a few articles that are relevant to the topic. If you have this problem, either your topic is too specific or you haven't done a thorough-enough search. On the other hand, some students feel overwhelmed when they find over 200 articles on their topic. If that is your experience, your topic is probably too broad or you have located some articles that are not particularly relevant to your study. In any case, you must be prepared to refine your topic and your search.

Many students become distressed at the prospect of discarding what originally looked like promising literature. Actually, this is a good thing because it shows that you are reading the literature critically and making progress as a researcher. In fact, one recommended method is to first conduct a search of the literature, locate the articles that seem the most relevant, examine those articles carefully, and discard those that do not apply. Then start at the beginning again with a narrower focus to winnow the prospects even further.

Another potentially fruitful way to search for pertinent literature is by author instead of topic. As you read articles, you will probably discover that certain authors have contributed greatly to your topic of interest. You can then go back and search their publications for additional information specific to your study (Heppner & Heppner, 2004).

Before searching the literature, it may be helpful to consult a basic reference book, such as an encyclopedia. The *Encyclopedia of Counseling* (American Counseling Association, 2009) is a good place to start when you don't know a lot about a counseling topic. These and other specialized reference books are available in most university libraries and are good starting points for overviews or summaries of a topic, names of important people in the field, or definitions of terms used in that topic. Sometimes, authoritative web sites are also helpful in providing general information about a topic.

This first step is more for learning something about the topic than for isolating pertinent research. Once you have done this and know a little more about the topic, you can decide exactly what aspect is of interest to you. At this point, it may be a good idea to write the topic as a question to get a clearer idea of the concepts involved. For example, you might ask, "Does the personality of the supervisor affect the supervisee's acceptance of direction during the counselor supervision process?" This question demonstrates two main concepts: (1) the personality of the supervisor and (2) the supervisee's acceptance of direction. Then you can start refining your search by identifying key words that fall into these two concepts: (1) personality, counseling, supervisor, supervision, or (2) supervisee, compliance, working alliance. You can broaden the scope to include the domains of mental health counseling, school counseling, and supervisory working alliance assessments. As you think about the topic more critically, consider how a writer would organize it:

1. *Advocate*—supports a certain position
2. *Educator*—instructs others on a subject
3. *Interpreter*—compares the pros and cons of studies
4. *Investigator*—looks into causes and links

Use the journalists' starting points of *who, what, when, where,* and *why* to generate possible research questions: "*Who* are the influential authors in personality or supervision?" "*What* is the connection between supervisor personality and the working alliance?" "*When* is instruction by a supervisor most effective or *when* does supervision likely occur during counselor training?" "*Where* does one find the pertinent interaction between supervisor and supervisee data to review?" "*Why* is the positive working alliance in the supervisory process beneficial to the supervisee or more broadly to the counseling profession?" When you search the literature, you are looking for the answers to these questions.

Now that you have compiled some key terms and questions, you can start searching for relevant literature. Often, the key to a thorough and effective search involves knowing what resources are available. The most helpful sources are your librarian, online library catalogs, online journal databases, Internet search engines, and sources from reference lists of promising articles (Creswell, 2012). We will examine each of these, but it may be even more helpful if you are using your computer to investigate these sources as you read the following section. Hands-on application is the best way to learn this material.

The best and most authoritative source of information is your reference librarian, who can guide you in your quest of finding the information you need. Not only do reference librarians provide instruction and advice in the uses and locations of the physical library's resources, but they also usually maintain a home page that:

1. tells you how to access services, such as interlibrary loans and policies for reserving books;
2. supplies information about library instruction, including seminars, workshops, and survival skills for graduate students;
3. provides links by subject area to resources such as corporate and statistical research centers;
4. provides information about institutional review board (IRB) training;
5. contains a list of helpful databases;
6. contains a list of electronic journals;
7. provides links to additional library sources (e.g., Galaxy, Worldcat, and SFX).

Galaxy, Worldcat, and SFX are several of the available subject directories that let you browse through any library's collection—in other words, they are online library catalogs. Worldcat can access libraries all over the world. Because of its size, publications are categorized by type (i.e., book, journal, newspaper). An icon next to each entry tells you which library has it so that you can request an interlibrary loan.

You can also locate literature with a database specific to the topic, such as EBSCO, ProQuest, ERIC, or other searchable databases available through university libraries. You can do either a basic search or an advanced search. For a basic search, be as specific as possible with key words, qualifying words, and phrases to avoid ambiguity (e.g., instead of just "counseling," key in "counseling supervision" or "counselor supervision"). To obtain search results that contain only the exact words in the exact order specified, put quotation marks around the key words. If you don't want to end up with hundreds or thousands of results, connect two specific words or phrases with a capital *AND*.

For an advanced search, you can narrow the search and be more specific by typing in key terms a certain way. On the drop-down menu, choices such as author, title, article type, publication date, source, range of dates, publication type, and language are listed, and the specific terms you are interested in can be connected with *AND*. Because different search engines and databases use different search methods, click on Help in each database to learn how to search most effectively. Again, your reference librarians can be a huge help.

If you want to narrow your search further by omitting certain key words, you can insert a plus sign (+) before the word you want to keep and a minus sign (−) before the word you want to leave out—for example, "supervision + counseling − nursing." Use the minus sign with caution. Sometimes it will exclude documents that contain both the desired and the rejected words.

The "Boolean operator set" can also be used to search for literature. The Boolean operator *AND* will limit results to only documents that contain both words—for example, "counseling AND supervision." You can also use it more than once: "counseling AND supervision AND personality AND working alliance." The Boolean operator *NOT* limits your search by excluding certain words—for example, "counseling AND supervision NOT nursing."

In the initial stages of your search, you may want to expand it somewhat. You can do this with the Boolean operator *OR*. For example, if you key in "counsel OR counselor," you will get many more results. Like AND, you can use it more than once:

"counseling OR counselor OR supervision OR working alliance." This would supply any document that contained any one or more of these terms.

Another way to broaden your search is by using only lowercase letters. This will show you all the documents that contain the term in any case: all lowercase, all uppercase, or capitals and lowercase. Truncating a word to its basic stem and inserting a symbol, usually an asterisk (*), after it will show you documents that contain any variation of that stem word. For example, if you're unsure whether to search under "supervisors," "supervision," or "supervisory," you can key in "supervi*." Of course, if you key in "super*," you may get results that contain words like "superintendent," "Superman," or "superconductor," which aren't any help to you at all.

All of these limiters, expanders, search syntaxes, and connecting words can be used with any search engine on the World Wide Web, such as the popular Google.com. You can see which characters are useful to truncate words, control vocabulary, identify descriptors, enclose phrases, and list connector words. Most search engines are case sensitive and will only pick up exact matches if uppercase is used.

At this point in your search you must decide if you want to save, print, or e-mail the information you have gathered. Often, a vendor feature is available whereby you can store saved searches. You can choose an ID and a password to access it at a later date and decide if you want to use it. You can save articles to a folder on your hard drive or on a computer disk. There is also an area where you can store photos or videos. If you decide to print out documents, often you can print it as a PDF or HTML file. PDF is preferred because it includes text as well as visuals like graphs or pictures in the original typeset format. HTML is more printer-friendly because it contains only text.

The final ready source of literature is the list of references an author has cited in manuscripts. Pay close attention to the references listed in your readings and jot down any studies that sound relevant to your topic. When it appears that you have already investigated the authors' references from several of your most recent primary source articles, you probably have exhausted your literature search.

## Different Types of Literature

Now that we have covered *how* to locate literature, we can examine the types of literature that our searches have yielded. Although online library catalogs and online journal databases are the research tools most often used today because of their breadth of material and ease of use, there are many other resources that can prove invaluable, including handbooks, reviews, indexes, books, journals, field interviews, and Internet resources.

### Handbooks, Reviews, and Indexes

**Handbooks** summarize important contributions to research in a specific area and are published in most fields every two to five years. These summaries, usually written by leading experts in the field, often provide extensive references and give a thorough glimpse of the topic. Useful summaries can also be found in encyclopedias, statistical indexes, and annual reviews. For example, *Professional School Counseling: A Handbook of Theories, Programs, and Practices* (2010), a second edition compendium of 96 chapters edited by Erford, focused on topics of interest to school counselors. **Statistical indexes** report trends that are useful in writing problem statements or literature reviews. **Annual reviews** comprehensively summarize the most recent literature in a particular area and are, as the name implies, published annually. *Career Development Quarterly* famously publishes an annual review of the most important and influential articles related to career development and counseling that appeared in print the previous year (see Erford & Crockett, 2012; Hartung, 2010). In addition to reading the summaries, you should look at the reference lists here, too (Creswell, 2012; Heppner & Heppner, 2004). Notice that much of this information is available online, but Internet resources should be avoided unless they are from authoritative sources (e.g., CDC, NIMH, and Substance Abuse and Mental Health Services Administration [SAMHSA]) and have been vetted by peer review. Anyone, regardless of expertise, can establish a web site and post virtually anything for public display. The discerning scholar avoids such sources to preserve the integrity of the scholarly endeavor.

## Books and Journal Articles

Books and journal articles are typically the most frequently cited references in a literature review. Books can be helpful to the extent that they synthesize the literature, but those that offer summaries of specific studies or present new research are the most useful. Of course, while summaries of previous studies are helpful, one should always strive to find the original study for use as a primary source. Thus, books are often secondary sources of information, with the book author telling you what the author of the primary study said. This is sometimes an exercise in "degrees of separation," like when someone whispers a message into someone else's ear, who whispers into another person's ear, and so on. The message usually changes more substantially the further you get from the primary (first person) source. This is an important caution when constructing a literature review: go to the primary source whenever possible!

**Refereed journal articles** typically contain highly specialized information about a study that has been reviewed by experts in the field (i.e., peer reviewed), which makes its content more credible. Refereed journal articles are usually the best sources of scholarly information available in the counseling field. Well-known journals in the counseling field include the *Journal of Counseling & Development*, *Career Development Quarterly*, *Measurement and Evaluation in Counseling and Development*, *Counselor Education & Supervision*, *Professional School Counseling*, and the *Journal of Mental Health Counseling*. In addition to books and articles, unpublished works (e.g., dissertations and conference presentations) can be used for pertinent information. However, such works should be used sparingly because they often represent literature summaries and, thus, are secondary sources (one degree of separation) and not subject to extensive, blind peer review—a process that serves as quality control. However, searching the reference list of a recent dissertation or thesis for relevant studies can be a very fruitful tactic.

When choosing literature, always consider scope and content. Not all information is reliable, authoritative, timely, objective, or supported by evidence. Consider the source of the information and decide if it is relevant. First, identify the audience (e.g., broad-based and commercial, scholarly), the scope (e.g., survey-style overview, in-depth analysis), and the role or purpose (e.g., informant, educator, investigator, and advocate). When you explore a document, identify the author and the author's credentials, determine the accuracy of the information, check the date of the study, determine if it is written in an organized manner, and see if the conclusion supports the hypothesis. Remember that just because it is published, it is not necessarily reliable. Regarding timeliness, ordinarily a source published within the past 10 years is considered recent.

In general, the reliability of published information often depends on the author's credentials, experience, and accomplishments. Although timeliness is relevant, the article's publication date may not be that significant, depending on what information you are looking for. Magazine articles may be current, but they tend to become dated quickly. Scholarly journals and books frequently have the most staying power as long as current resources are not important to your study. For example, if a professional counselor wanted to research current trends in multicultural supervision, it would be less appropriate to survey research that is more than 10 years old. However, if an author was discussing appropriate statistical techniques for data analysis, it may be important to include some of the seminal efforts in that area that may date back half a century or more. Consider the following proposition:

> In recent years, there has been an influx of research on sexual abuse trauma, PTSD symptomatology, and the efficacy of cognitive behavioral interventions (Edmond, Rubin, & Wambach, 1999; Farrell & Hains, 1998; Hall & Henderson, 1996; King, et al., 2000a; King, et al., 2000b; Nishith, Hearst, Mueser, & Foa, 1995; Palm & Follete, 2001; Parnell, 1999; Shapiro & Maxfield, 2001).

In this case, the author is informing the reader about current trends related to cognitive-behavior therapy with sexual abuse survivors. Although the statement that cognitive-behavior therapy is effective with sexual abuse survivors may be true, notice that all of the citations are more than 15 years old. This lack of current (i.e., "In recent years …") resources makes the reader question the validity (or at least the current relevance) of the argument.

### Field Interviews

**Field interviews** may be included in literature reviews, but they should be subjected to the same criteria as written reports. To evaluate the usefulness of a field interview, you must first determine who the appropriate subjects are for the report and then get their permission, in writing, to use their information. Researchers should evaluate interviews for hard facts or some solid quotes, checking for any hearsay evidence or whether time has perhaps distorted the interviewee's memory. After establishing the timeliness and comprehensiveness of the interviewees' responses, researchers should obtain permission to use the names of everyone involved and to ensure the reliability of their responses.

### Internet Resources

We are living in a digital age and time of globalization. This presents us with both advantages and challenges. Anyone can "google" just about any query and derive dozens if not thousands of "hits" via the Internet. However, the Internet is a "buyer-beware" venture (even though most of the information is free, and worth every penny!), and researchers must be cautious about the use of nonrefereed sources of information. Using authoritative sources is fine; the CDC, SAMHSA, NIMH, and the U.S. Census Bureau are just a few of the government-sponsored web sites that many counselors find helpful. These web sites promote the dissemination of refereed works, thus exercising a quality control mechanism similar to peer-reviewed journals.

A newer development in the digital age that deserves substantial measured caution is the use of wikis. A wiki is a web site that allows users to add content and edit and clarify information that is available for widespread (and usually free) dissemination. The benefits of such a service are potentially quite valuable for general consumption, but the challenges are equally troubling—especially when information is not reviewed or vetted by experts. At this point, wikis and other online information sources should be avoided by researchers producing scholarly reviews and studies. For general information purposes, wikis can provide informative entrees into topics that are difficult to understand and navigate.

## Critically Evaluating the Selected Literature

Publication in scholarly journals is often a long and difficult process that involves extensive blind review by editorial board members. Although the review process helps to create a quality literature base, some articles still have flaws. In other words, the blind review publication process tends to improve the ultimate scholarly product but does not guarantee that the research is sound. Thanks to freedom of speech and freedom of the press, nearly anything can be printed or posted on the Internet. Thus, even articles in reputable journals require careful evaluation. Before assessing the article, you should read the author's definitions of the terms used because some statements may be true only if a term is defined a certain way; that is, different authors may conceptually or operationally define the same term in different ways. These definitions may also supply some insight into any biases in the research process. You should be aware of the researcher's assumptions and weigh the premises of his or her arguments *before* you use the work's findings in your study. Be cautious and skeptical when drawing conclusions, and consider all the evidence. Part of your training as a professional counselor is to think critically and abstractly, and evaluate all of the information you encounter. Finally, consider alternative interpretations of research findings; often, results can have multiple explanations (Rathus, Nevid, & Fichner-Rathus, 2005). Studies should be examined for quality, and any that have serious methodological flaws should be used sparingly (Heppner & Heppner, 2004). When you compile resources for a literature review, rely most heavily on refereed journal articles, and then sparingly proceed to other journal articles, books, conference papers, dissertations, and theses as appropriate and necessary (Creswell, 2012).

While thoroughly evaluating the quality of a work, you also must decide whether it is relevant to your study. Studies that contain all the current variables you are interested in should receive preferential treatment in the literature review. These sources should be described in greater detail and be more thoroughly critiqued. Studies that have at least one of the variables you are interested in may still be important if they contribute to an understanding and justification of the current study. Do not include irrelevant studies or irrelevant details about studies. During the process, stop and ask yourself *why* you are including that study. If you don't know the answer, it is unlikely that your readers will. A great literature review streamlines the sources and information to paint a picture for the reader of the most relevant information available. As you read the literature for relevance and quality, try to form a mental image of how each piece of information will fit into the overall review. Afterward, you can create on paper a literature map or an outline that will provide a framework for the finished product (Creswell, 2012).

# Organizing Relevant, Quality Literature

Once you have evaluated the literature for relevance to the current study and for quality, you can begin to organize the review. It is usually a good idea to begin with the most recent article and work backward; many of the more recent articles will cite the earlier articles, and this should give you a general understanding of previous work. When reading the research, systematically analyze the articles to make better use of your time. At this point, you are doing two things: (a) categorizing into a system through note taking and (b) refining a framework that you will use when you write your review (Creswell, 2012; Heppner & Heppner, 2004).

Categorizing involves making summary notations of the common sections in most research sources for the purpose of a written review. Each notation should be a condensed version of the most important features of the research report. Summary notes may be taken on paper, note cards, or a computer—whichever you consider most efficient and helpful. Different authors (Creswell, 2012; Fraenkel et al., 2011) have their own preferences for categorization systems. Heppner and Heppner (2004) suggest the

**Figure 3.1**

Literature map: Steps to conducting a literature review.

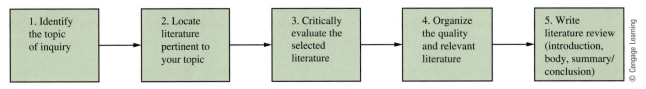

following: (a) full citation, (b) research problem, (c) dependent and independent variables, (d) hypotheses or research questions, (e) summary of literature review, (f) sample, (g) methodological concerns and limitations, (h) instrumentation, (i) research design, (j) findings, (k) direct quotes, (l) references to find, (m) suggestions for future research, and (n) questions about the research.

Depending on your topic, you may have to revise this format to fit your particular needs and circumstances. The most important thing is to make careful notes about the issues and topics that will be most helpful in consolidating and synthesizing the literature when you are ready to write. Taking a little time to do this now will save you a lot of time later and will greatly contribute to the quality, depth, and overall organization of the literature review (Heppner & Heppner, 2004). To avoid plagiarism, make sure that the notes you make are paraphrases of the literature and appropriately cited. Most unintentional plagiarism probably occurs because writers copy the text word for word from a source and then do not change it later in the editing process. Sometimes this is incidental, but the ultimate responsibility for avoiding plagiarism rests with you, the writer!

Refining a framework involves turning your visual image of an outline into a concrete literature map. A **literature map** is a figure or drawing that displays the research literature visually. This will help you to organize key topics and common material so that you can formulate the most convincing argument for your study. During the organization process, you should try to visualize how the final product will look. Now you must determine where each piece of information in the review will go (Creswell, 2012; Heppner & Heppner, 2004). Figure 3.1 shows what a brief literature map for this chapter might look like.

# Writing the Literature Review

Now that you have identified a topic and located, evaluated, and organized the pertinent literature, you are finally ready to start writing. This is where you will convince readers that you are a knowledgeable and skilled author competently pursuing an important area of inquiry. A literature review typically has three sections: an introduction, a body, and a summary or conclusion, although these facets are not usually labeled as such. Note that in APA Style (2010) all three of these components are usually contained within the section of an empirical article simply referred to as the "Introduction."

## The Introduction

The **introduction** should convince the reader that the topic is important and interesting. Compelling statistics, a brief practice-based scenario, or dramatic, albeit factual, statements related to the topic will get the reader's attention. This is where you want to present the rationale for the study as well. This introductory section is not the place to do a complete review of the literature, but it should include an overview of the most important findings that have led to the present study. A brief discussion about the potential implications of the proposed study is warranted as well, although that should be examined in much more detail at the end of the research report in what is typically referred to as the "Discussion" section. The introduction should contain a clear, concise statement about the purpose of the study and what the reader can expect to see (Fraenkel et al., 2011; Heppner & Heppner, 2004).

## The Body

The **body** should briefly explain the primary and related findings of the literature review. Although preceded by a separate introductory section, the body is made up of several segments. After an introductory paragraph that tells the reader what to expect, it is further divided into sections, and sometimes subsections, depending on its length.

The sections or headings in the literature review depend on how the resources were organized. Each paragraph should begin with a topic sentence that prepares the reader for the content of the entire paragraph. The paragraph should end with an appropriate transition that links the previous and upcoming information in the following paragraph or section. The reader should be able to tell just by reading the topic and transition sentences what the review is about. Although these structural elements may sound elementary, they give the body a concise and logical structure that makes it easier for readers to understand the topic. Remember that you are guiding your readers through your research process (Fraenkel et al., 2011).

In addition to the structural elements in the body, the entire review should have a funnel effect—in other words, it should begin with a broad focus and end with a narrow focus, leading naturally to your research question(s) or hypothesis(es). For instance, if the study is about testing the treatment effects of person-centered therapy with survivors of child abuse, you might begin with the broader issue of child abuse, then go to the topic of person-centered therapy, and then conclude with prior research on therapy modalities used with child abuse and issues shown to improve with the use of person-centered therapy. You should also include any literature related to the effects of person-centered therapy with child abuse survivors. This will highlight common and discrepant characteristics in the literature, which will be discussed in the final section—the summary or conclusion (Heppner & Heppner, 2004).

## The Summary or Conclusion

The last section of the literature review is the **summary** or **conclusion**, where the funnel becomes the narrowest. The main purpose of the summary is to confirm the rationale for the study. Any connections between the proposed research and existing research and the contributions the proposed study will make to the field should be emphasized here (Heppner & Heppner, 2004; Patten, 2009).

Essentially, the summary ties together the main points of the review and gives the reader a succinct depiction of what is known to date. Any conclusions reached in the body should be repeated here to instill in readers the importance of the study (Fraenkel et al., 2011; Heppner & Heppner, 2004).

When you think about these three sections, it might help if you conceptualize them as Heppner and Heppner (2004, p. 90) did: "Common practice is to tell the reader what you are going to do, do it, and tell them what you did." This sounds a lot like the old axiom on public speaking, "Tell them what you are going to say, say it, and then tell them what you said." Boxes 3.1–3.3 provide brief examples of literature reviews leading to both quantitative and qualitative methodological studies.

**BOX 3.1    Sample literature review leading to a quantitative study.**

# Yoga as a Treatment for Childhood Anxiety

## Anxiety in the Lives of School-Aged Students

Anxiety has been defined as a negative mood state that occurs in anticipation of a perceived threat (Wood, 2006). Anxiety is most often used to describe an unpleasant emotional state or condition that is characterized by subjective feelings of tension, apprehension, and worry (Murata et al., 2004). The DSM-IV-TR (APA, 2000) noted that the following symptoms can denote anxiety in children: restlessness, easily fatigued, difficulty concentrating, irritability, muscle tension, sleep disturbance.

Anxious behavior appears to be common in both male and female children of all ages (Strauss, Frame, & Forehand, 1987). Research indicated gender differences in anxiety, with girls reporting higher prevalence and intensity of fears and anxiety than boys (Austin & Chorpita, 2004). Furthermore, anxiety was among the most common psychiatric disorders in adolescents, with as many as 20 percent of adolescents in the general population diagnosed as having an anxiety disorder (Essau, 2005).

Anxiety affects children in many ways. Children who had high teacher ratings of anxiety were viewed by teachers as being less happy, showing a higher prevalence and severity of somatic complaints, and demonstrating more problematic peer relations (Strauss et al., 1987). These researchers also reported that anxious children were significantly less popular than nonanxious children and more frequently socially rejected by their peers. Wood (2006) reported that children who were highly anxious often were overly reticent, avoided peer interaction, or acted in a less-competent manner around peers because of preoccupation with threat and an inability to focus on the social cues at hand. Essau (2005) also noted that anxiety tended to co-occur with other disorders, such as substance abuse, and that adolescents with significant levels of anxiety were highly impaired in various life domains, such as in school, at home, and in social activities.

Of key interest in the present study, research has consistently shown that school performance was affected by anxiety. Wood (2006) reported that past studies demonstrated an association between child anxiety disorders and poor academic performance, indicating that over the course of a school year, children with anxiety disorders often performed below their ability level. Cross-sectional studies supported this claim by showing associations between child anxiety disorder status and school performance (Wood, 2006). Research has also shown that teachers perceived anxious children as demonstrating significant deficits in academic performance relative to nonanxious children (Strauss et al., 1987).

Researchers have further documented the need for interventions to help children manage their symptoms of anxiety in order to improve school performance. While some authors have questioned the necessity of treatment for anxiety in children primarily because of its transience and pervasiveness, others concluded that the significant problems in adjustment experienced by children with anxiety warrants therapeutic intervention (Strauss et al., 1987). Wood (2006) further noted, "Given the hypothesized role that high anxiety plays in poor school performance and social maladjustment, an intervention that substantially reduces anxiety might indirectly improve these outcomes" (p. 345). Indeed, researchers have long suspected a link between lowered levels of anxiety and higher academic performance among highly anxious children. For example, Zipkin (2001) found that students in a more relaxed (nonanxious) state were able to concentrate more easily, allowing for improved academic performance.

## The Effectiveness of Yoga

Against this backdrop, there is a growing body of evidence that yoga is an intervention that substantially reduces anxiety. Zipkin (2001, p. 286) defined yoga as "an ancient and complete system of physical, mental, and spiritual development which incorporates physical postures (asanas), breath control, mental concentration, and deep relaxation." Yoga incorporated physical postures, breath control, mental concentration, and deep relaxation to positively affect mental states (Peck, Kehle, Bray, & Theodore, 2005). Yoga treatment is part of a growing awareness that patients are more than just minds, as indicated by Maslow describing the individual as an integrated, organized whole,

*(Continued)*

*(Continued)*

whose body and mind could not be separated (Clance, Mitchell, & Engelman, 1980).

A wealth of research documented the positive health effects of practicing yoga, particularly in terms of countering symptoms of anxiety. Yoga techniques have historically been found to enhance well-being, mood, attention, mental focus, and stress tolerance (Brown & Gerberg, 2005). Some studies reported reductions in stress and other psychological symptoms (Waelde, Thompson, & Gallagher-Thompson, 2004). Lavey et al. (2005) reported that participation in a yoga program was associated with significant improvements in five of the negative emotions subscales on the *Profile of Mood States* (i.e., Tension-anxiety, Depression-dejection, Anger-hostility, Fatigue-inertia, Confusion-bewilderment). During yoga, the coordination of body movements and stretching, in combination with deep breathing, improved the body's overall circulation, resulting in lowered tension as well as increased levels of blood and oxygen throughout the entire body that in turn affected the central and autonomic nervous systems (Peck et al., 2005). The practice of yoga appeared to stimulate the parasympathetic system which resulted in a sense of calm. Yoga practice has also been shown to reduce middle school children's state anxiety, heart rate, headaches, and general tension and stress symptoms. Yoga participants often discovered greater physical flexibility but also a corresponding increase of mental and emotional flexibility in daily life (Roth, 1997). Yoga was found to relieve stress and tension, dissipate excess energy, relieve tiredness and lethargy, lengthen attention span, improve and maintain general physical health, develop sharper concentration and greater mental clarity, and cultivate better interpersonal relationships (Zipkin, 2001).

Even with the growing body of evidence showing the health benefits of yoga, more causal research still needs to be conducted to document yoga's effectiveness as an intervention or treatment for anxious children. Peck et al. (2005) reported that future studies need to examine the causal effects of yoga on indices such as stress management and general well-being.

## References

American Psychiatric Association. (2000). *Diagnostic and statistical manual of mental disorders* (4th ed., text revision) (DSM-IV-TR). Washington, DC: Author.

Austin, A. A., & Chorpita, B. F. (2004). Temperament, anxiety, and depression: Comparisons across five ethnic groups of children. *Journal of Clinical Child and Adolescent Psychology, 33*, 216–226.

Brown, R. P., & Gerberg, P. L. (2005). Sudarshan Kriya yogic breathing in the treatment of stress, anxiety, and depression: Part II—Clinical applications and guidelines. *The Journal of Alternative and Complementary Medicine, 11*, 711–717. doi: 10.1089/acm.2005.11.711

Clance, P. R., Mitchell, M., & Engelman, S. R. (1980). Body cathexis in children as a function of awareness in training and yoga. *Journal of Clinical Psychology, 36*, 82–85.

Essau, C. A. (2005). Frequency and patterns of mental health services utilization among adolescents with anxiety and depressive disorders. *Depression and Anxiety, 22*, 130–137. doi: 10.1002/da.20115

Lavey, R., Sherman, T., Mueser, K. T., Osborne, D. D., Currier, M., & Wolfe, R. (2005). The effects of yoga on mood in psychiatric inpatients. *Psychiatric Rehabilitation Journal, 28*, 399–402.

Murata, T., Takahashi, T., Hamada, T., Omori, M., Kosaka, H., Yoshida, H., & Wada, Y. (2004). Individual trait anxiety levels characterizing the properties of Zen meditation. *Neuropsychobiology, 50*, 189–194.

Peck, H. L., Kehle, T. J., Bray, M. A., & Theodore, L. A. (2005). Yoga as an intervention for children with attention problems. *School Psychology Review, 34*, 415–424.

Roth, B. (1997). Mindfulness-based stress reduction in the inner city. *Advances, 13*, 50–58.

Strauss, C. C., Frame, C. L., & Forehand, R. (1987). Psychosocial impairment associated with anxiety in children. *Journal of Clinical Child Psychology, 16*, 235–239.

Waelde, L. C., Thompson, L., & Gallagher-Thompson, D. (2004). A pilot study of a yoga and meditation intervention for dementia caregiver stress. *Journal of Clinical Psychology, 60*, 677–687.

Wood, J. (2006). Effect of anxiety reduction on children's school performance and social adjustment. *Developmental Psychology, 42*, 345–349.

Zipkin, D. (2001). Relaxation techniques for handicapped children: A review of literature. *The Journal of Special Education, 19*, 283–287.

*Source:* This literature review was originally written by Kimberly Flyr in July 2006. Reprinted with permission.

**BOX 3.2    Sample literature review leading to a qualitative study.**

## Meeting the Unique Needs of the High School Student-Athlete: A Case Study

Student-athletes may be one of the least recognized subcultures that exist in high schools today. Often characterized as "dumb jocks" while concurrently resented for their perceived popularity, this group is often misunderstood. As a group, student-athletes are applauded for their successes and simultaneously resented for their privileges. These stereotyped attitudes can serve to dehumanize student-athletes and do not properly reflect their full complexity as individuals (Valentine & Taub, 1999). Student-athletes tend to be subjected to prejudice and discrimination in a similar manner to other groups thought of as "minority cultures" (Sedlacek & Adams-Gaston, 1992). Student-athletes tend to have a unique culture that sets them apart from traditional students, with different life experiences that may present problems when relating to their peers. Even the term *student-athlete* indicates the distinctiveness of these students. No other group within the school is referred to with this hyphenated role identity. Musicians are not labeled student-musicians; thespians are not described as student-thespians (Goldberg & Chandler, 1995).

As a subculture, student-athletes possess many positive characteristics. In a study of leadership skills, Dobosz and Beaty (1999) concluded that student-athletes demonstrated significantly greater leadership ability than did students who did not participate in athletics. Student-athletes also were more self-confident and self-reliant. According to Goldberg and Chandler (1995, p. 39), participation in athletics, "can have a positive impact on educational aspirations and academic achievement; and may encourage athletes to stay in school, thereby benefiting from the formal learning environment."

Although there are many positive attributes associated with student-athletes, they also encounter numerous challenges. As athletic participation becomes a life focus, the individual growth and development of other areas of the student-athlete may be neglected or inhibited (Miller & Wooten, 1995). Professional school counselors must understand the life-experiences student-athletes face as they attempt to satisfy the stage-relevant developmental tasks of (a) identity formation, (b) personal competency, (c) growth of interpersonal relationships, and (d) future goal and career planning (Goldberg & Chandler, 1995). To properly address the developmental needs of the student-athlete, professional school counselors must also understand the complex demands of athletic participation. Because student-athletes must maintain dual roles as students and as athletes, there may be psychological and social implications that can result in failure to attend to daily responsibilities and difficulties as they work through these developmental tasks (Cole, 2006).

Additionally, as they chase their athletic dreams, many student-athletes are unable to properly balance academics and sports (Parmer, 1994). Time becomes a precious commodity. They must juggle their academic course load, practices, games, travel for away-games, family commitments, and participation in social events (Watt & Moore, 2001). Because of the intense time commitments, student-athletes have limited flexibility in their schedules (Jordan & Denson, 1990). The combination of academic and athletic requirements can be overwhelming for even the most academically gifted students (Carodine, Almond, & Gratto, 2001). Professional school counselors need to be watchful for signs of undue stress and prepared to intervene as appropriate. For student-athletes to reach their full athletic and academic potential, they must be physically and mentally healthy (Broughton & Neyer, 2001).

## Insights Into the Collegiate Athletic Process

For many student-athletes, their ultimate goal and focus is obtaining an athletic scholarship and competing at the collegiate level. For some student-athletes this dream will become a reality; for many others it will not. Early on in the process, professional school counselors should educate students and parents by helping them understand that scholarships are not as abundant as they believe and the competition is extraordinary. Additionally, they must understand that college recruiters

*(Continued)*

(Continued)

are doing a job: bring the best athletes to their college. Their concern is not necessarily what is best for the student-athlete. It becomes the responsibility of the student-athlete, family, and professional school counselor to help the student-athlete determine if a particular college is an appropriate choice (Koehler, 1995).

It is also important that the student-athlete have a realistic picture of what life will be like as a collegiate student-athlete. When an athlete commits to playing a sport in college, it is often a year-round obligation. At the most competitive level, playing sports is like holding down a full-time job while attending school (Liedtka, 2006). Athletes spend a tremendous amount of time with their teammates, often to the exclusion of other friends and family. They often live in special housing, eat together, and may attend classes together (Goldberg, 1991). It is important that a student-athlete select a college where they feel comfortable and accepted by not only the coaching staff, but also the entire team. When a student-athlete visits prospective colleges, the professional school counselor should urge the athlete to ask questions of both the coaches and the players. It is imperative to get a real sense of what the team and the college will be like.

For professional school counselors to adeptly handle the needs of the student-athlete, it is essential that professional school counselors are familiar with all of the necessary language, terms, and regulations. Terms such as unofficial visit, letter of intent, and verbal commitment may be confusing, at first, but it is important that professional school counselors educate themselves and become familiar with all aspects of the recruiting process (Liedtka, 2006).

In addition, professional school counselors must become familiar with the regulations of the National Collegiate Athletic Association (NCAA). The NCAA has a Clearinghouse that reviews a students' coursework and determines whether they meet the eligibility requirements. Student-athletes must attain a minimum score that is a combination of their high school grade point average and standardized test scores (Liedtka, 2006). If student-athletes do not meet these requirements, they are not eligible to play collegiate athletics. Therefore it is essential that a professional school counselor be knowledgeable of these regulations and counsel students accordingly. The importance of this has come

to the forefront lately as several students have sued their school district when they lost scholarships due to NCAA ineligibility. Although a professional school counselor has yet to be held liable, the courts have stressed the need for counselors to practice with care and caution (Stone, 2006).

In addition to making sure that a student meets all NCAA requirements, the school counselor must also ensure that the student has completed all necessary testing required by the colleges. Because student-athletes are being recruited, their timeline for college admission is often different than that of the traditional student. A recruited athlete may be asked to make a verbal commitment during their junior year of high school and sign an official letter of commitment by the fall of their senior year. In order for a scholarship offer to be made, all necessary testing must be completed ahead of time. This almost always includes the SAT and/or the ACT college entrance exams. In addition, many colleges are now requiring SAT subject tests. If all required testing has not been completed, an official scholarship offer cannot be made.

## Role of the Professional School Counselor

The professional school counselor should serve as the coordinator or collaborator in the college selection process for a student-athlete. They can be the advisor for what Goldberg (1991) referred to as the "athletic triangle" of athlete, coach, and parent. This can be extremely useful because often the coach is not part of the teaching staff. The professional school counselor can bring all interested parties together and make sure that everyone is moving in a direction that will best serve the needs of the student-athlete.

When there are several interested parties involved in the recruiting process, it is easy to forget that the student-athlete is going to college primarily to get a college education. The professional school counselor may need to continually remind all stakeholders of this. It is important that the college selected be a good fit both athletically and academically. Because a college coach can sometimes have academic standards lowered for a potential student-athlete, it is often possible that what may be a good fit athletically may be a mismatch academically. The professional school counselor may be

(Continued)

*(Continued)*

the lone voice of reason. It is unlikely that a student who only performed at an average level in high school will be successful at a highly competitive college. It may be hard for a student-athlete or his or her parents to comprehend this when a college is offering a scholarship, but a professional school counselor who is concerned with the best interest of the student must be willing to voice such concerns. One question that the counselor should ask of the student repeatedly is "Would I attend this school if I weren't playing a sport?" (Liedtka, 2006).

Although the rules of the NCAA mean that all interested parties must be concerned with high school academic performance and constantly monitor a student's progress, the high school counselor must not lose sight of the future career development needs of the student-athlete (Goldberg & Chandler, 1995). With so much of the college selection process focused on finding a good match athletically, it is important to be mindful of the student's future career goals. It is common for the student-athletes to be so focused on playing at the collegiate level, that they lose sight of the fact that college is the vehicle for them to help plan for the future, one that most likely will not contain athletics. Professional school counselors should encourage student-athletes to complete career assessments and explore vocations that match their personalities and strengths (Cole, 2006). Students should research the offered academic programs at colleges that are recruiting them and ensure that there are suitable programs.

Graduating from high school and starting to make future career plans can be a scary and exciting time for students. For student-athletes, the stakes are even higher because college scholarships are often involved. The needs of student-athletes are often very different than those of the traditional student. The world of athletic recruiting is one that many counselors are not familiar with. Because athletics are involved, it is necessary to involve the coach in the decision-making process. Unfortunately, high school student-athletes are often unprepared to make the necessary decisions. They must operate on a different time line than the traditional student in terms of college testing and college selection. They must be concerned not only with their academic future, but also their athletic future.

# References

Broughton, E., & Neyer, M. (2001). Advising and counseling student athletes. *New Directions for Student Services, 93*, 47–53.

Carodine, K., Almond, K. F., & Gratto, K. K. (2001). College student athlete success both in and out of the classroom. *New Directions for Student Services, 93*, 19–33.

Cole, K. W. (2006). Supporting student athletes. *School Counselor, 43*, 28–33.

Dobosz, R. P., & Beaty, L. A. (1999). The relationship between athletic participation and high school students' leadership ability. *Adolescence, 34* (133), 215–220.

Goldberg, A. D. (1991). Counseling the high school student-athlete. *School Counselor, 38*, 332–340.

Goldberg, A. D., & Chandler, T. (1995). Sports counseling: Enhancing the development of the high school athlete. *Journal of Counseling & Development, 74*, 39–44.

Jordan, J. M., & Denson, E. L. (1990). Student services for athletes: A model for enhancing the student-athlete experience. *Journal of Counseling & Development, 69*, 95–97.

Koehler, M. (1995). Student athletes and high schools: Let's shift the focus. *Clearing House, 68*, 158–159.

Liedtka, K. (2006). College sports: A team effort. *School Counselor, 43*, 14–21.

Miller, G. M., & Wooten, H. R. (1995). Sports counseling: A new counseling specialty area. *Journal of Counseling & Development, 74*, 172–173.

Parmer, T. (1994). The athletic dream and the black male student: Primary prevention implications for counselors. *School Counselor, 41*, 79–83.

Sedlacek, W. E., & Adams-Gaston, J. (1992). Predicting the academic success of student-athletes using SAT and noncognitive variables. *Journal of Counseling & Development, 70*, 724–727.

Stone, C. (2006). College advising and the courts. *School Counselor, 43*, 6–7.

Valentine, J. J., & Taub, D. J. (1999). Responding to the developmental needs of student athletes. *Journal of College Counseling, 2*, 164–179.

Watt, S. K., & Moore, J. L., III. (2001). Who are student athletes? *New Directions for Student Services, 93*, 7–18.

*Source:* This literature review was originally written by Cynthia Michael in July 2006. Reprinted with permission.

**BOX 3.3    Sample literature review leading to a mixed-methods study.**

## The Need for Gay Straight Alliances in Rural High Schools

Adolescence is characterized by many developmental benchmarks, one of which is evolving sexual identity. Youth who identify as lesbian, gay, bisexual, or transgender (LGBT) must navigate through a world where heterosexuality is presumed to be the norm. For sexual minority students attending rural schools, it can be an extremely problematic time. Rural communities tend to hold more conservative values than urban counterparts. These traditional attitudes, often based on religious beliefs, may lead to decreased tolerance for anything viewed as outside of the accepted community standard (McCollum, 2010). Consequently, there may be few, if any, support services for sexual minority youth. Studies have shown that LGBT youth are at increased risk for isolation, depression, suicidal ideation, and substance abuse (Espelage, Aragon, Birkett, & Koenig, 2008). However, they have also demonstrated that positive school climates and parental support can mitigate these negative outcomes.

The purpose of this manuscript is to compare through qualitative instruments the adolescent experiences of LGBT students from urban and rural areas, and to examine the effects of the presence or lack of Gay Straight Alliances (GSA's) on those experiences. Quantitative analysis will then examine respective levels of depression and anxiety as a measure of overall mental health of gay and lesbian youth.

## Context of LGBT Issues in Schools

Few studies have compared the experiences of adolescent LGBT students in rural areas with those of LGBT students in urban settings (Poon & Saewyc, 2009). However, the ill-effects of bullying and discrimination of sexual minority students are well documented. Whether in urban or rural areas, these youth are often subjected to abuse and harassment from multiple individuals in their lives including families, schools, and the surrounding communities at a rate higher than their heterosexual peers (Varjas et al., 2006). Students who are or are *perceived* to be LGBT (Satterly & Dyson, 2005)

often endure pervasive abuse in the form of verbal harassment, having rumors spread about them, being grabbed or touched in sexual ways, and even physical assault (Goodenow, Szalacha, & Westheimer, 2006).

McCullum (2010) posited that in rural settings schools can be an especially demoralizing and discouraging place for students whose sexual identity falls outside the community norms. Youth in rural districts are more likely to be verbally and physically victimized even more than those in "urban districts with a history of bullying problems" (p. 33). LGBT students in rural communities may also experience greater social isolation than their urban peers (Poon & Saewyc, 2009). They lack the opportunity to identify with peer groups (which may be nonexistent) and access to information and resources for support. School administrators who try to implement programs that affirm LGBT presence, may get resistance from parents and school boards who find such topics inappropriate to address (Frank & Cannon, 2009). A direct consequence of such policies is that rural sexual minority adolescents are twice as likely to use alcohol, tobacco, and other drugs and to have early sexual experiences as their urban counterparts. In addition, rural sexual minority girls reported more symptoms of depression than urban LGBT girls (Poon & Saewyc, 2009).

As bad as the situation is for LGB students in these rural districts, the situation is even more disheartening for adolescents who identify as transgender (McGuire, Anderson, Toomey, & Russell, 2010). Many protections designed for LGB individuals do not include gender expression. Youth who display gender non-conformity experience greater victimization (verbally and physically), more isolation, and more mental health problems than their fellow LGB students. Transgendered youth are at greater risk of poor academic performance, missing school, or even dropping out. Protective factors for these students include gender neutral rest rooms and locker rooms, accommodations for gender identity in extra-curricular activities (sports, dances, etc.), and acknowledgment of name and pronoun changes in school records and by faculty. Studies have also shown the positive effects of supportive teachers and mentors on the academic and social development of transgender.

*(Continued)*

*(Continued)*

## School Climate

School climate, "the general atmosphere of a school campus" (Walls, Kane, & Wisneski, 2010, p. 310), reflects the attitudes and beliefs of the community as a whole (McCollum, 2010). Many members of rural communities take pride in their conservative religious and social values. They may be distrustful of anyone whose lifestyles or identities are not normative. These attitudes can lead to negative school climate. Negative school climate is all too common in rural districts, and often leads to academic disengagement, career and vocational disparities, and emotional distress (Walls et al., 2010).

## Gay, Lesbian, & Straight Education Network (GLSEN) 2009 School Climate Survey

The GLSEN 2009 School Climate Survey (GLSEN, 2010) seems especially relevant in light of the recent rash of suicides of students enduring chronic bullying due to their perceived sexual orientation/expression. The survey of 7,261 middle and high school students found that in the past year, nearly 9 out of 10 sexual minority students experienced harassment at school. Almost two-thirds felt unsafe at school and nearly one-third missed at least a day of school because of safety concerns. The study also found that students who were more frequently harassed had a half a grade lower than those who were less harassed. In addition, increased levels of victimization lead to increased depression and anxiety and decreased self-esteem. This is consistent with the research on bullying and victimization of LGBT students.

In spite of the alarming statistics uncovered by this study, the School Climate Survey also reported some positive results and hope for improving the environment for LGBT students. The survey reported that:

> Having a Gay-Straight Alliance in school was related to more positive experiences for LGBT students, including: hearing fewer homophobic remarks, less victimization because of sexual orientation and gender expression, less absenteeism because of safety concerns and a greater sense of belonging to the school community … The presence of supportive staff contributed to a range of positive indicators including fewer reports of missing school, fewer reports of feeling

unsafe, greater academic achievement, higher educational aspirations and a greater sense of school belonging … Students attending schools with an anti-bullying policy that included protections based on sexual orientation and/or gender identity/expression heard fewer homophobic remarks, experienced lower levels of victimization related to their sexual orientation, were more likely to report that staff intervened when hearing homophobic remarks and were more likely to report incidents of harassment and assault to school staff than students at schools with a general policy or no policy. (GLSEN, 2010, p. 1).

However, despite the reported benefits, less than half of sexual minority students had a GSA at their school and slightly more than half could identify supportive educators or other allies. Even more alarming, less than a fifth of LGBT students attended a school that had a comprehensive anti-bullying policy. This is evidence of the great need for more systemic supports for this student population in order to increase academic performance and decrease psychological stress.

## Effects of Homophobic Bullying

Homophobic bullying had a damaging effect on the psyche of sexual minority children. Nonheterosexuals seem to experience psychiatric disorders at a higher rate than their heterosexual counterparts (Craig, Tucker, & Wagner, 2008). There is evidence of increased risk of internalizing symptoms among sexual minority youth. They are twice as likely as heterosexuals to have a lifetime mood disorder and/or anxiety disorder (Hatzenbuehler, McLaughlin, & Nolen-Hoeksema, 2008). Studies have shown that these individuals have "higher incidences of substance abuse/use, promiscuity, truancy, suicide, sexual and physical abuse, isolation from family and friends, homelessness, and pressure to abide by gender conforming norms" (Whitman, Horn, & Boyd, 2007, p. 145).

Feelings of isolation and lack of safety also have academic consequences. According to Whitman et al. (2007), LGBT students often miss class or entire days of school, which leads to poor academic performance and lower grades not indicative of their true abilities. They held that it is no surprise then that lower GPA's lead to lower academic aspirations, making these students less likely to pursue a college education.

*(Continued)*

(Continued)

## Systemic Barriers

Although school systems have recently been concerned with including cultural diversity issues in their curriculum, often sexual minorities are not included in that paradigm. Further, LGBT individuals are the only cultural minority to grow up outside of their own cultural group (Frank & Cannon, 2009). The invisibility of sexual minority role models in family and school settings robs the youth of the opportunity to learn effective coping skills in a hostile environment (Frank & Cannon, 2009; Varjas et al., 2008) and the ability to enlist support in their plight.

One study shows that many school administrators, especially in rural areas, are uninformed regarding LGBT issues, with some reporting that they know of no sexual minority students in their school (Pace, 2004). These same administrators felt that their school was a safe place for LGBT students. In addition, eight out of ten teachers reported having negative feelings toward lesbians and gays, and only one-third of school counselors felt that LGBT issues were appropriate topics to address with students. Not surprisingly, a very small number of LGBT students come out to their school counselors.

Research also showed that teachers and administrators may actually promote or maintain bullying behaviors toward LGBT youth. Many students reported that when witnessing harassment of sexual minority students, most teachers did not intervene (Kennedy & Covell, 2009; Valenti & Campbell, 2009). In fact, many school officials either did not intervene on behalf of the LGBT youth, or were themselves abusive or hostile toward LGBT youth (Craig et al., 2008).

The reasons for the unwillingness to intervene are unclear. One explanation is that rural communities in general hold more conservative values, which may explain negative attitudes or misconceptions about non-heterosexual orientation (Poon & Saewyc, 2009). McCollum (2010) gave several explanations for these educators "not rising to the challenge" (p. 34). Lack of awareness on the part of administrators can be a big part of the problem. While anti-bullying policies are in place in every school district, the language may not be specific to sexual orientation/gender expression. In addition, bigoted attitudes among the staff may prevent some teachers from even acknowledging that anti-gay harassment qualifies as bullying.

Job security is also a very real fear among rural educators (McCollum, 2010). It could be that some educators fear being shunned by colleagues or harassed by parents for addressing such issues. In some rural districts, merely bringing up the subject of homosexuality can threaten careers. Some school counselors or teachers may fear a backlash from angry parents when trying to incorporate the topic in sex education or instituting a GSA. There is also the very important issue of gay educators themselves. Ten percent of teachers are gay but they are not always willing to self-identify (Valenti & Campbell, 2009). Especially in rural areas, educators who are sexual minorities fear losing their job if they are outed. Many of these teachers totally separate their private and professional lives, limiting interactions with students, colleagues, and parents. These self-imposed restrictions add to the isolation of both LGBT teachers and students, furthering the invisibility of positive gay role models.

## Protective Factors and the Impact of GSA's

Despite the bleak picture that most of the current literature paints of the LGBT youth experience, there is evidence that circumstances can improve for this population. A few studies have suggested that "GSA's have the potential to make a positive impact on the educational experiences of sexual minority youth" (Walls et al., 2010, p. 311). Protective factors such as individual support and/or an inclusive campus climate can mitigate some of the negative effects of minority membership. GSA's offer support by providing information on coming out and relationships in general, helping to foster mentor relationships with supportive faculty, developing coping strategies for a hostile environment, and offering a safe space to connect with peers.

Walls et al. (2010) documented the many benefits of GSA membership. Improved educational outcomes in the form of class attendance, better study habits, and greater educational aspirations were reported. An improved campus climate led to feelings of greater safety and fewer reports of harassment. Mental health benefits were noted as well. GSA members have reported greater levels of comfort with their identity. "Achieving comfort with one's minority status is correlated with improved well-being and life satisfaction" (Craig et al., 2008, p. 250). This leads to a sense of

(Continued)

*(Continued)*

belonging in the school and a decrease in risky health behaviors. In addition, for many LGBT youth the presence of a GSA was therapeutic, whether or not they were members (Walls et al., 2010). Some study participants noted that although they were not ready to identify themselves through membership, just knowing the group was there was an extremely encouraging factor in their identity development.

Valenti and Campbell (2009) reported that "GSA involvement by LGBT youth greatly increase their positive interaction with the school" (p. 231). It increased their sense of belonging and helped them "explore aspects of themselves in a safe environment" (p. 231). Many other important protective factors have the potential to greatly improve the quality of life for an LGBT student. Kennedy and Covell (2009) strongly advocated that teachers be trained and required to include homosexuality as a part of the health curriculum. The need for such education is particularly great in light of the long-term effects of homosexual bullying. McGuire et al. (2010) outlined the following protective factors: intervention by school personnel when harassment occurs; policies prohibiting discrimination on the basis of sexual orientation/expression; establishment of GSA's; and information about and inclusion of LGBT issues. McCollum (2010) suggested the following: supportive teachers posting a safe zone sign; including the history of LGBT people who have made contributions to history, science, athletics, and the arts as a part of the curriculum; organizing in-service training for administrators to help create safer schools; and if a GSA is present, offering to act as advisor or making other contributions. Finally, having the support of one or both parents cannot be underestimated in terms of its positive effects. Studies have shown that LGBT adolescents with parental support suffered fewer mental health problems than those with less support (Espelage et al., 2008).

## Conclusion

There is a dearth of research regarding the particular plight of LGBT adolescents in rural school districts. However, it is abundantly clear that this population endures an enormous amount of psychological distress due to the pervasive, often systemic, harassment and discrimination launched at them by a hostile environment. The consequences of such injustices are severe and long

lasting. LGBT adolescents display poor academic performance, social isolation, and mental illness at a rate higher than their heterosexual counterparts.

The research also has demonstrated that with the implementation of protective factors, these students can improve academically, socially, and psychologically. Such factors include the presence of GSAs, supportive teachers and parents, role models, and inclusive policies. This will require collaboration among parents, teachers, administrators, staff, and community members. Also, further study will be needed to gauge the effects of such interventions. However, if current research is any indication, it will be well worth it in terms of the improved academic, career/vocational, personal/social, and psychological gains for sexual minorities. The purpose of this study was to compare the adolescent experiences of LGBT students from urban and rural areas and to examine the effects of the presence or lack of GSAs on their lives. Respective levels of depression and anxiety will also be measured as indicators of mental health.

## References

Craig, S. L., Tucker, E. W., & Wagner, E. F. (2008). Empowering lesbian, gay, bisexual, and transgender youth: Lessons learned from a safe schools summit. *Journal of Gay & Lesbian Social Services, 20,* 237–252.

Espelage, D. L., Aragon, S. R., Birkett, M., & Koenig, B. W. (2008). Homophobic teasing, psychological outcomes, and sexual orientation among high school students: What influence do parents and schools have? *School Psychology Review, 37,* 202–216.

Frank II, D. A., & Cannon, E. P. (2009). Creative approaches to serving LGBTQ youth in schools. *Journal of School Counseling, 7, 35,* 1–25.

Gay, Lesbian, & Straight Education Network. (2010). *2009 National school climate survey.* Retrieved from http://www.glsen.org/cgi-bin/iowa/all/library/record/2624.html?state=research&type=research

Goodenow, C., Szalacha, L., & Westheimer, K. (2006). School support groups, other school factors, and the safety of sexual minority adolescents. *Psychology in the Schools, 43,* 573–589.

Hatzenbuehler, M. L., McLaughlin, K. A., & Nolen-Hoeksema, S. (2008). *Journal of Child Psychology and Psychiatry, 49,* 1270–1278.

*(Continued)*

*(Continued)*

Kennedy, C., & Covell, K. (2009). Violating the rights of the child through inadequate sexual health education. *International Journal of Children's Rights*, *17*, 143–154. doi: 10.1163/092755608X278939

McCollum, S. (2010). Country outposts. *Teaching Tolerance*, *38*, 33–35.

McGuire, J. K., Anderson, C. R., Toomey, R. B., & Russell, S. T. (2010). School climate for transgender youth: A mixed method investigation of student experiences and school responses. *Journal of Youth and Adolescence*, *39*, 1175–1188. doi:10.1007/s10964-010-9540-7

Pace, N. J. (2004). Gay, rural, and coming out: A case study of one school's experience. *The Rural Educator*, *25*(3), 14–18.

Poon, C. S., & Saewyc, E. M. (2009). Out yonder: Sexual-minority adolescents in rural communities in British Columbia. *Research and Practice*, *99*(1), 118–124.

Satterly, F. A., & Dyson, D. A. (2005). Educating all children equitably: A strengths-based approach to advocacy for sexual minority youth in schools. *Contemporary Sexuality*, *39*(3), 1–7.

Valenti, M., & Campbell, R. (2009). Working with youth on LGBT issues: Why gay-straight alliance advisors become involved. *Journal of Community Psychology*, *37*, 22–248. doi: 10.1002/jcop.20290

Varjas, K., Dew, B., Marshall, M., Graybill, E., Singh, A., Meyers, J., & Birckbichler, L. (2008). Bullying in schools towards sexual minority youth. *Journal of School Violence*, *7*(2), 59–86. doi: 10.1300/J202 v07n02_05

Varjas, K., Mahan, W. C., Meyers, J., Birckbichler, L., Lopp, G., & Dew, B. J. (2006). Assessing school climate among sexual minority high school students. *Journal of LGBT Issues in Counseling*, *1*(3), 49–75. doi: 10.1300/J462v01n03_05

Walls, N. E., Kane, S. B., & Wisneski, H. (2010). Gay-straight alliances and school experiences of sexual minority youth. *Youth and Society*, *41*, 307–332. doi: 10.1177/0044118X09334957

Whitman, J. S., Horn, S. S., & Boyd, C. J. (2007). Activism in the schools: Providing LGBTQ affirmative training to school counselors. *Journal of Gay and Lesbian Psychotherapy*, *11*(3/4), 143–154. doi: 10.1300/J236 v11n03_08

*Source:* This literature review was originally written by Sylvana Alsamadi in July 2012. Reprinted with permission.

## Tips for Writing the Literature Review

Now that you know *what* to write about, we'll discuss *how* to write it. Quality writing is essential to a credible research report. Although it is not possible to cover all the fundamentals of good writing, we will examine the most important rules

As a researcher, being informative is an absolute necessity, especially when writing a research report that is designed to inform the reader. You should provide enough information so that the reader is enlightened but not smothered with unnecessary details. Always strive for both brevity and clarity (i.e., write concisely). Try to make your point without embellishment, overstatement, or using an emotional plea. Ask yourself these questions: (1) Is this information necessary for the reader to understand the study? (2) Is the information in each paragraph consistent with the topic? (3) Are the central points supported without digressions? (Furlong, Lovelace, & Lovelace, 2000; Heppner et al., 2008)

Authors should be forthright and discuss the fundamental nature and true essence of a study. In other words, do not misconstrue the findings of others or report the findings in a way not originally intended in an attempt to justify your study. Likewise, when pointing out contradictory evidence, do so carefully. Do not be overcritical of others' work, even if it refutes the current line of thinking. Support for the topic should naturally spring from the existing literature. If not, one should consider the importance of, or reasons for, conducting the current study at all (Heppner et al., 2008).

Although we have already talked about organization and logic, they are important in how you write, too. The literature review is a presentation of one's position, not just a regurgitation of previous findings. Research questions should be justified based on the literature reviewed. The reader should be able to see how the conducted research logically stems from the studies that are discussed in the review. Always remember that readers may have very little knowledge of the subject matter, so what may be a logical progression to you may not be as obvious to your readers (Heppner et al., 2008).

Finally, it is fair to say that if you never begin, you will never finish. Procrastination haunts every writer at one time or another. Write! And then write some more. Most authors have to rewrite several times before they produce a quality review. Some people write the first version quickly and then revise it several times. Others write carefully the first time so they don't have to spend a lot of time on revisions. Whatever the method, all writers can benefit from the feedback of others, so ask your colleagues, instructors, or advisors to read and critique your material (Heppner et al., 2008).

In addition to these four general rules, some further guidelines may prove helpful. Anticipate audience questions while you are writing. Ask yourself what reactions or questions they might have. Typical advisor questions might be, "What evidence do you have to support this statement?" "What is the point of this section?" and "What does all this mean collectively?"

Although there is a huge difference between professional jargon and colloquial language, it can be very difficult to write between the two. **Professional jargon** refers to the technical and specialized vocabulary that is specific to one's field or discipline. This type of terminology can be especially useful when you are trying to communicate specialized understanding of a construct, but it can also confuse and discourage the reader if it is used aimlessly. If you are going to use professional jargon, use it sparingly and define it for the reader. **Colloquial language** is common, everyday language used in informal speech, and although easier to understand (and quite entertaining in text messages and e-mails: e.g., "U gonna go 2 d party?"; "You coming to the game?"), it is inappropriate in scholarly writing. You want your writing to be scientific and formal, not creative or informal, so use professional language, but don't go to extremes (Heppner & Heppner, 2004). Table 3.1 summarizes some helpful tips for improving writing style. Here are some final tips when writing your literature review:

1. Provide conceptual definitions of major terms.
2. Use direct quotations sparingly.
3. When several authors have made the same point, group them together.
4. Discuss major studies in more detail than less-relevant studies.
5. Follow a particular style manual, such as APA (Patten, 2009).

**TABLE 3.1**   Strategies to improve writing style.

| | |
|---|---|
| Tip #1: Write from an outline. | Tip #2: Reread your own copy after setting it aside for a few days. |
| 1. Helps identify main ideas and subordinate ideas. | 1. Highlights faults and errors in logic. |
| 2. Adds discipline to writing. | 2. Lets you "hear" problems in the text. |
| 3. Maintains continuity and pacing. | Tip #3: Ask a colleague to review and critique the draft. |
| 4. Discourages tangential excursions. | 1. Gets the perspective of another person. |
| 5. Points out omissions. | 2. Helps identify errors in logic or assumptions. |

© Cengage Learning

# Writing in APA Style

Too often, student literature reviews simply report the findings from each study in a sequential manner, from paragraph to paragraph. This is a disastrous writing style! Every paragraph begins with a reference to a particular study, summarizes the study, and then moves on to the next paragraph, where the same pattern is repeated. Although the basic information may be covered, this type of writing does not encompass the quality of analyzing, synthesizing, and critiquing expected of knowledgeable and skilled writers and researchers. Rather, a high-quality review not only describes the existing literature but it also critiques it in such a way that the reader has a much better understanding after he or she has read it (Heppner & Heppner, 2004).

Using the preceding style in each paragraph may be tempting because trying to think of ways to synthesize the wealth of available literature can be a lot more work. Yet one useful method is constructing a framework for the literature review. For example, examine the literature for consistencies between studies, comparable or parallel findings, or common themes. (If you have used the categorization system, this should be easy for you.) You will often find that many studies used a similar methodology. Or you may discover that a classic study was the impetus for a particular line of query or the inspiration for a new line of research. Sometimes previous research can be integrated into chronological order to show the historical progression of the topic. Exploring the impact of a single variable across a group of studies can be an effective way to make a resolute statement about a body of research. The most important thing is to think in a critical and analytical manner, looking for themes to assist in writing an organized and coherent literature review (Heppner & Heppner, 2004).

APA style (historically known as the Harvard method) is widely used among professional counselors, counselor educators, and counseling students, and it represents correct writing for any member of the field. Adherence to APA Style (APA, 2010) requires more than just knowing how to compose references. Professional counselors should pay careful attention to this style throughout the manuscript and refer to the manual for rules about the writing process. In fact, reading the *Publication Manual of the APA* is an excellent way to improve your writing skills and familiarize yourself with APA procedures. Remember that literature reviews are critical evaluations of material that has already been published. The purpose of a literature review is to examine the progress made toward clarifying the problem. Following are some general comments about how to construct a manuscript in APA Style (2010). These comments are far from comprehensive and students should purchase and read the *Publication Manual of the APA* (2010).

- When describing previously conducted research, APA uses third person, past tense. Present tense may be used during narrative transitions.
- The document should be typed, double spaced, and printed on good quality paper with a letter quality printer.
- All margins (left, right, top, and bottom) must be 1.0 inches.
- It is preferable to use Times New Roman 12-point font.
- Only justify the left margin.
- Do not divide words at the end of a line with a hyphen. (Turn off the automatic hyphenation system in your word-processing program.)
- Indent the first line of every paragraph.

- If necessary, use Level 1, 2, or 3 headings for subdividing the sections of your article. For example:

  Level 1 should be:
  **Centered, Uppercase and Lowercase Bolded Heading**
  Level 2 should be:
  **Flush Left, Bolded, Uppercase and Lowercase—Side Heading**
  Level 3 should be:
  **Indented, bolded, lowercase paragraph heading ending with a period.**

- Quotations should be avoided as the purpose of the literature review is for you to summarize the relevant extant literature. Students should restate and paraphrase information and use appropriate citations to avoid plagiarism.

- "Plagiarize" means to pass off the words and ideas of another person as one's own or without crediting (or quoting) the source of the idea or information. Students must appropriately cite and reference all information. Words used verbatim from another source must be enclosed within quotation marks (i.e., " ").

- Quotations of more than 40 words must be displayed in a double-spaced block with no quotation marks. Indent five spaces from the left margin and type the entire quotation within the indented margin.

- There are numerous appropriate ways to cite sources within the text of your literature review. The important thing is to keep the cited information together, rather than breaking it up [e.g., Smith (2015) indicated…, *not* Smith determined that … maternal smoking (2015)]. Appropriate citation styles include:

  Smith (2015) indicated that …

  … maternal smoking (Smith, 2015).

  In a recent study of maternal smoking (Smith, 2015), it was determined that …

  In 2015, Smith …

- Multiple sources can be used to document a specific fact or point. When doing so, the sources must be presented in alphanumeric order, as in the following example:

  > Numerous authors discussed the detrimental effects of maternal smoking on the developing fetus (Jones, Jenkins, & Smith, 2015; Matthews & Bennett, 2014; Smith, 2015).

- Do not use secondary citations. Use the original source in all possible instances.

- When citing the same source within the same paragraph multiple times, APA Style allows the author to drop the year of publication after citing it with the year the first time [Smith (2010), then just Smith].

- Note that if a source is used within a paragraph and no subsequent sources are used, you do not need to repeatedly recite the source throughout the paragraph. It is assumed that all subsequent discussion within the paragraph is related to or an extension of the original citation. However, if an intervening different citation is used, you must recite the original author later in the paragraph to credit that author with the subsequently revealed information.

- Use the "et al." convention appropriately. When citing six or more authors, always use the et al. convention (e.g., Johnson et al., 2015). When citing three to five authors, always write out all authors the first time (e.g., Smith, Blarney, Merrill, & Lynch, 2015), then use the et al. convention for all subsequent citations in the remainder of the manuscript (e.g., Smith et al., 2015).

### The Title Page

- The title summarizes the main idea of the paper and should be concise; a recommended length for the title is 12–15 words.
- The author's name should be listed as first name, middle initial, and last name (e.g., Bradley T. Erford).
- Institutional affiliation should be listed under the author's name (e.g., Loyola University Maryland).
- The running head, an abbreviated title of less than 50 characters, including punctuation and spaces, is inserted within the page header in capital letters in the flush-left position.
- The page header also includes the page number in a flush-right position. Number title page 1.

### The Abstract

- A brief (<120 words, 960 characters) summary of the review article.
- State the topic in one sentence, if possible.
- Briefly summarize salient points, conclusions, and the implications or applications of your conclusions.
- Number the abstract page 2.

### The Text of the Review Article

- Define and clarify the problem.
- Briefly summarize previous investigations to inform readers of the current state of research on the topic. Use an integrative summary writing style. Do *not* provide a summary of the samples, statistics, methods, etc., of each article. Focus on summarizing the findings across studies to support your salient points, conclusions, and implications.
- Identify relations, contradictions, and gaps in the current literature.
- Suggest future steps necessary to further clarify or solve the problem.
- The review article is ordered according to relationship of content, rather than the step-by-step chronology characterizing a research article.
- Number the first text page 3 and subsequent pages chronologically.

### References

- All text citations must be listed in the References section.
- All listed references must be cited in the text.
- References are useful because they allow other investigators to easily locate your resources.
- Number the Reference pages as chronological continuations of the text.
- *Note:* Many journals now obtain a digital object identifier (doi) number, which should be added to the end of the reference.
- Reference journal articles as follows:

Two or more authors of a journal article format:

Sandberg, K., & Erford, B. T. (2013). Choosing assessment instruments for bulimia practice and outcome research. *Journal of Counseling & Development*, *91*, 366–378. doi: 10.1002/j.1556-6676.2013.00107.x

Book reference format:

Erford, B. T. (2013). *Assessment for counselors* (2nd ed.). Belmont, CA: Cengage Wadsworth.

Edited book reference format:

Erford, B. T. (Ed.). (2014). *Orientation to the counseling profession: Advocacy, ethics, and essential professional foundations* (2nd ed.). Columbus, OH: Pearson Merrill.

Chapter in an edited book format:

Heller Levitt, D., Darnell, A., Erford, B. T., & Vernon, A. (2014). Theories of counseling. In R. Byrd, & B. T. Erford (Eds.), *Applying techniques to common encounters in school counseling: A case-based approach* (pp. 7–42). Columbus, OH: Pearson.

Smith, L. F. (2003). Review of the Test of Early Reading Ability, Third Edition. In B. S. Plake, J. C. Impara, & R. A. Spies (Eds.), *The fifteenth mental measurements yearbook.* Retrieved from http://www.unl.edu/buros/bimm/

Here is a list of common errors identified by the APA, specific to the literature review, and the correct use of the applicable APA rule. This list is not intended to be a substitute for familiarity with the *APA Publication Manual* in its entirety.

*Neglecting to include the page number in a citation for a direct quotation.* The in-text citation should be as follows: (Jones, 2000, p. 60).

*Incorrect citation of electronic references.* The citation for a specific Web document should include the author, date, title of document, and complete Web address:

Kaczynski, A. T., Wilhelm Stanis, S. A., Besenyi, G. M., & Stephanie Child, S. (2013). *Differences in youth and adult physical activity in park settings by sex and race/ethnicity.* Retrieved from http://www.cdc.gov/pcd/issues/2013/12_0276.htm

*Use of passive self-references.* Ordinarily, APA Style uses third-person past tense. Currently, self-referents may be used, but they must be active, not passive. "The present author" or "the researchers" can now be replaced with "I" or "we." Passive sentence construction should also be avoided. For example, "The experiment was designed by Gould (2015)" is written in the passive voice. A better sentence structure is "Gould (2015) designed the experiment."

*Incorrect spacing.* Only one space should follow a period, initial, and other end punctuation.

*Confusing abbreviations.* Abbreviations should be used only when the term appears frequently throughout the manuscript. The entire term should be written the first time it is used. For example, although you know that ACA stands for the American Counseling Association, it is still important to provide the complete name the first time it is mentioned for readers who may be unfamiliar with it—for example, "The American Counseling Association (ACA) conducted a study …"

*Giving life to inanimate objects.* Human characteristics should not be attributed to things that are not human. This common error is a result of the form of the scientific model. For example, authors may write, "A review of the literature showed a need for further research on cognitive behavioral therapy with survivors of sexual abuse." "Literature" is an inanimate object and does not have the ability to "show" anything. It would be much better to say, "Evident in the literature was a need for research on cognitive behavioral therapy with survivors of sexual abuse."

*Inappropriate vocabulary usage.* Three pairs of terms that are frequently used incorrectly are *affect/effect, that is/for example,* and *infer/imply.*

*Incorrectly writing numbers.* Numbers below 10 should be spelled out in words. Numbers with two digits should be represented with numerals. Some exceptions are always using Arabic numerals for places in a series (page 2), times (8 a.m.), dates (3/30/2020), or ages (4 years old). If a sentence begins with a number, it is always written out ("Thirty participants were sampled"). Better yet, lead the sentence with the noun and place the numeral in a secondary position (e.g., "Of participants, 30 were sampled using ...")

*Incorrect adverb use.* Avoid common pitfalls of using incorrect adverbs such as *secondly* and *lastly.*

*Confusion regarding* **seriation**. Lowercase letters within parentheses [e.g., (a)] should be used when presenting a list of brief items within a paragraph or sentence, especially when the items on the list are not sequential. Numbers (e.g., 1) should be used when the items begin a new paragraph within a series.

*Bias in language.* Put the person before the disability—for example, "a person with a hearing impairment," not "a deaf person," or "a person with a disability," not "a disabled person." Avoid words such as *patients*, *invalids*, *subjects*, *cripple*, *deformed*, *senile*, *elderly*, *crazy*, and so forth. Capitalize racial/ethnic groups and use the more specific rather than the general term (Cherokee versus Native American). *Sexual orientation* should be used in lieu of *sexual preference*. Men and women with a same sex sexual orientation are referred to as gay males and lesbians, respectively. When referring to specific sexual encounters, use the terms *female-female behavior*, *male-male behavior*, or *same-gender behavior*. The words *man* and *he* should be used only when discussing males. Be clear about the way you refer to gender identities.

## Length, Headings, Tone, and Presentation

Although effective writing skills are critical to developing a quality manuscript, it is equally important to present written material in an organized and logical fashion. **Headings** help the reader to understand the organization of the paper. For example, most research articles contain an introduction, a review of the literature, a methods section, a results section, and a discussion of findings. Because these are standard headings, readers of research articles can break down the various elements of a study more readily and can follow along more easily. Aside from the obvious benefits of headings to the readers, headings can help the writer, too. Think of your major headings as a beginning outline for the writing process. (This is why it is important to decide on the main headings *before* you start writing.) Headings will help you to organize the document and maintain a logical process.

The tone of your writing should be based on the **target audience**. Knowing your audience will help you to decide on a formal or less formal voice. Regardless of audience, you should avoid overly colorful or stylistic writing. In general, the tone of your writing should be scientific rather than literary. The writing style, however, must adhere to the rules of the *APA Publication Manual* (APA, 2010). The APA Style Guide permits the use of first person and the editorial *we*. Although it is important to avoid extensive first-person narratives, it is acceptable to say, "We reviewed the literature related to counselor supervision" instead of "The researchers reviewed the literature related to counseling supervision." Thus, although the tone should be scientific, the style of the entire manuscript does not have to be third person, as is the case with traditional scientific models. The traditional voice in scientific writing dictates that the writer minimize oneself and focus only on the content. Writers use facts and arguments as the dialogue or rhythm of the article. Of course, when referring to studies conducted by others, third-person past tense should be used because the studies were conducted by others (third person) at some point in the past (past tense).

Present findings and ideas directly and in a professional manner. Establish your voice and evaluate notes to determine how the pieces described will be reassembled. The manner of writing should remain open and direct without excessive restructuring of the topic. As we have seen, sentences, paragraphs, and headings must follow a logical and orderly pattern. It is important to remember that your manuscript should logically flow along the lines of the argument presented.

**Transition words** (e.g., *then, next*) provide additional readability to the document by increasing the coherence of writing. It is important to see how various elements of the review connect to the others. Transitional expressions and other types of connectors become important navigational elements, such as cause–effect links (e.g., *therefore, consequently*), and contrast links (e.g., *however, nevertheless, although*).

## Strategies for Improving Writing Style and Some Final Tips for Writing Successfully

Readers are encouraged to create an outline when they write. An effective literature review is a synthesis of research from more than one field or study. Because the material accumulated can become overwhelming, it is important to have a map to guide the process. The resulting synthesis of information will provide a unique interpretation of the argument. As you review resources and write the literature review, continue to ask yourself, "What is the purpose?" and "Am I demonstrating that purpose?".

Remember that a quality literature review contains identifiable main ideas and subordinate ideas. As with any other form of writing, establish a line of communication that includes a proposition, and then validate and support the argument, making it acceptable to the reader. In other words, display discipline in writing by discussing the various aspects of the research in an organized manner. A step-by-step approach fine-tunes your abilities as a writer to search for the information and synthesize it into an organized presentation. Finally, consider the following sundry advice when writing a manuscript:

- Spell out words; do not use contractions.
- Use *and* in the body of the text and an ampersand (&) when citing authors in parentheses.
- Do not divide words using a hyphen.
- Left justify text only. Do not right or fully justify text.
- Use abbreviations and acronyms sparingly. Always spell out the entire term the first time it appears.
- Use Arabic numerals to express numbers 10 and above and words to express numbers below 10.
- Convert run-on sentences (two complete sentences not joined with an *and, or,* or *but*) into two complete sentences.
- A sentence fragment cannot stand alone, so connect it to another clause or sentence to make it complete.
- Use commas between complete sentences, such as before the *and, or, but,* or *for which*.
- Insert commas on both sides of a parenthetical facet (e.g., It was, in fact, hard to imagine).

- Use a comma after an introductory clause (i.e., containing a subject and verb) when the clause begins with the following words: *when, although, unless, until, after, because,* or *since* (e.g., Although nearly six feet tall, Lee weighed only …).
- Surround an appositive with commas (e.g., My father, an extremely generous man, was …).
- When commas surround a nonessential clause (e.g., My partner, whom I've known since college, is …), the clause is considered "extra information" and the commas can be omitted (e.g., My partner whom I've known since college is …).
- Avoid unclear pronouns (e.g., *it, this, which,* or *that*).
- Make sure to use parallel sentence structure.
- Be sure the noun and verb agree (e.g., We were [not "We was"] going to go shopping).
- Do not shift between first and third person.
- Stay in the active tense (e.g., Jones had numerous opportunities to complete the study, *not* Jones has had numerous opportunities to consider completing the study).
- Use of a colon in a sentence is only appropriate if it completes the thought that precedes it (e.g., The obvious impediments were as follows: …).
- Make sure that quotation marks follow the comma or end mark (e.g., "Jones was dead?" ).
- Avoid beginning a sentence with *also, but,* or *and.*
- Place *only* immediately before what "only" is meant to qualify (e.g., It was only noon. *Not,* It only was noon).
- Avoid using *so* when you mean *so that* (e.g., She ran long distances so that she could …).
- Hyphens are needed to make an adjective for the noun that follows (e.g., a 14-year-old teenager).
- Use *farther* when the distance is measurable and *further* when the distance is not measurable.
- Do not use "etc." in formal writing; use "for example" or "e.g." and give two to three examples.
- Capitalize proper nouns. Do not capitalize generic nouns.
- Appropriately use *affect/effect.* Ordinarily, *affect* is a verb, and *effect* is a noun. (e.g., How does studying affect your test scores? What effect does studying have on your test scores?)
- Use the Oxford comma before the final element in a series of adjectives or nouns (e.g., I love to eat apples, pears, and oranges) to prevent misreading.
- If a paragraph does not make the point you wish to make, restructure the paragraph. It sometimes adds precision of language and meaning by moving phrases or sentences to different locations.
- Use *as if* instead of *like* (e.g., She felt as if she was going around and around).
- Do not split the infinitive. *To* should not be separated from the verb. Instead of "to not stay," use "not to stay."
- Appropriately use *in* and *into*; *into* is used when there is movement from outside to inside something.

- If *not only* is used, follow it with *but also* (e.g., Not only are they getting smaller, but they also are using less energy).
- Avoid clichéd language (e.g., Jones completed the study in the knick of time).

Finally, remember that your work can contribute to the field. If you are interested in pursuing publication, work with an experienced professor or colleague to submit the paper, thesis, or dissertation for professional review.

## Conclusion

A literature review is intended to be a compilation of pertinent existing documents that informs readers about the past and current state of knowledge on a given topic. A review logically details the need for the study that ensues, shows the reading audience that you are knowledgeable about your topic, and demonstrates that other studies have not addressed the same topic in exactly the same way. It is not expected that the beginning student or researcher will easily encompass all goals of writing immediately. Professional writing is a complex skill that takes much practice and feedback. Work closely with established authors, writing drafts, receiving feedback, and rewriting.

*Now go to the Student Workbook found on cengagebrain.com that accompanies this text for additional application and review activities.*

# Outcome Research in Counseling

Now that we have examined the nature and characteristics of research studies and the correct construction of a literature review, we are ready to take the whirlwind tour of counseling outcome research. Outcome research involves the literature on counseling effectiveness: what works and what doesn't. This chapter reviews the counseling outcomes literature both generally and in four specific areas: theoretical approaches, client–counselor characteristics, career interventions, and interventions with school-aged youth.

## CHAPTER 4

# Outcome Research: The Relationship Among Training, Research, and Practice

The mental health needs of our population are substantial, with no signs of abating. One in 100 children had a substantiated report of child maltreatment, and the same percentage of children perpetuate a serious violent crime (Federal Interagency Forum on Child and Family Statistics, 2012). Nearly one in four adolescents reported a binge drinking episode during the previous two weeks or use of illegal drugs during the previous month. More than 8 percent of adolescents and adults experienced a major depressive episode during the previous year and an additional 6 percent reported serious emotional or behavioral difficulties. In total, it was estimated that about one in five U.S. adults, children, and adolescents have a diagnosable mental disorder, but as few as one in five of these potential clients receive mental health services. The majority of these potential clients never seek help, for a variety of reasons, but it is clear that professional counselors must be well prepared to address the myriad concerns of these individuals if and when they do present for counseling. Although many view the mental health needs of our society as individualized and addressable on a case-by-case basis, a more systemic, social justice/action approach is needed to get at the root causes of mental illness and provide a more systemic, preventive, wellness-based approach to addressing the current mental health issues on a societal level.

Professional counselors must acknowledge that the identification and use of research to improve counseling effectiveness is not only a core curriculum requirement of counselor education programs (CACREP, 2009) but an ethical responsibility (ACA, 2014) as well. ACA has gone so far as to insist that ethical counseling is not possible without a working knowledge of the **outcome research** and research- and evidence-based practices. Furthermore, in this era of accountability it is critical to the continued existence of the counseling profession that professional counselors understand and be knowledgeable of what does and does not work with clients, what techniques and approaches result in positive changes for a diverse clientele.

Still, outcome research receives much less attention than it deserves, and the results of outcome research are often ignored by practitioners for various reasons. Sexton, Whiston, Bleuer, and Walz (1997, pp. 10–15) identified seven myths about outcome research. Each of these criticisms has been used by practitioners, and even some educators, to disregard relevant findings in the extant literature while allowing practitioners substantial leeway to engage in practices that are more "comfortable," both theoretically and personally, rather than more effective. Although some of these criticisms may have had some merit in the past, the study of outcome research in counseling has evolved to the point that such myths have been either abandoned or discounted:

1. Outcome research doesn't provide anything relevant to the practitioner.
2. Research results cannot be trusted.

3. Research studies examine minute detail, not clinical problems.
4. Outcome research only looks at group differences; practitioners need help with individual clients.
5. Research only seeks statistical significance; practitioners need to know what makes a practical difference.
6. Research focuses on evaluating theory; practitioners need clinical discoveries of new methods.
7. Research doesn't provide anything that can be used in practice.

From these myths and criticisms, it is painfully obvious that a schism has existed within the counseling profession: the research/practice split. The **research-practice disconnect** has existed for decades, but it has closed substantially over the years as practitioner demands for more relevant outcome research have been heard by counseling researchers. But more to the point, accountability movements within managed mental health care and education have forced the issue. In contemporary counseling settings, professional counselors must convince the public and third-party payers that they are providing therapeutically *and* cost-effective services.

Sexton et al. (1997) proposed an integrated process of training, research, and practice that would cultivate a substantial knowledge base to address the concerns of all involved. Note that in this proposed model, practitioners and educators feed relevant, practical questions into the knowledge base that can be conceptualized and researched, leading to more relevant and practical training and practitioner-based information. Then clinicians can integrate these new, more relevant findings into clinical practice, and trainers can integrate the findings into state-of-the-art counselor education programs and in-service training modules. This model is collaborative and collegial rather than contentious or adversarial. Practitioners, educators, and researchers learn from each other and collaborate to ask and answer important research questions that elevate professional practice.

Sexton et al. (1997) provided an excellent examination of the integration of training, research, and practice, and two facets of that discussion warrant special mention here. First, educators and trainers must be compelled to provide counselors-in-training with treatment approaches that have been empirically validated and tailored to fit the needs of individual client characteristics. Second, researchers must understand the difference between clinical efficacy (tightly controlled experimental conditions that may not generalize) and effectiveness studies (what works in pragmatic, naturalistic circumstances), the latter being of primary concern to practitioners because practitioners focus on effectiveness within diverse clinical settings.

Key to this discussion is the ideal of the scientist-practitioner model, which will be reviewed in substantial detail in Chapter 8, properly embedded in the discussion of action research and single subject research, which are both practical research applications for counselors in the field. As you read the rest of this chapter, try to formulate your own questions about the counseling field. These questions may form the basis for important, practice-informing inquiry. The discussions in later chapters can then be applied to design qualitative or quantitative studies and subsequent statistical analyses that can answer your questions.

# Studying Outcome Research

The topic of outcome research in counseling is huge, and entire books have been written on just this area of the literature. The size of the literature base varies by counseling specialty area and topic, as some topics (e.g., client characteristics) have been studied in detail across disciplines and specialties for decades (Sexton et al., 1997), whereas others (e.g., school counseling) have received little attention until very recently (Whiston, Feldwisch, & James, 2015). Unfortunately, much of the outcome research literature is spread across countless journals and in single studies, limiting the generalizability of findings. The purpose of this chapter is to provide an integrative, albeit cursory, view of what is known to be effective so that professional counselors can enhance counseling skills and practice ethically and efficiently. An important caveat: Some of the presented literature may appear somewhat dated, but nonetheless is important because it represents the classic studies that shaped our understanding of the field of study.

Outcome research typically involves three types of methodology: clinical trials, qualitative reviews, and meta-analytic reviews. **Clinical trial studies** appear frequently in the research literature and are very helpful because of their reliance on comparison groups (e.g., control, placebo, treatment as usual, alternative treatment), standardized treatment protocol, and the use of outcomes measure. Clinical trials, however, offer only a single result based on quantitative methodology, and different studies on the same topic may yield variable, or even contradictory, results. Thus, this chapter reviews only a few of the thousands of single-study, clinical trial reports available in the literature.

Instead, vast accumulated quantities of studies can be identified and collapsed into summary reviews, using both qualitative and quantitative methodologies. Each of these approaches presents with various strengths and weaknesses. **Qualitative analysis** is perhaps the most common and involves researchers examining and summarizing robust trends and findings across studies, clients, and contexts. Like all experimental methods, qualitative reviews can sometimes present biased conclusions, so criteria and procedures should be put into place to ensure that the information is processed systematically and conclusions are robust and replicable (Erford, Miller, Duncan, & Erford, 2010).

The third approach, **meta-analysis**, is a specific quantitative technique that allows empirical studies to be collapsed into a meaningful quantitative index, known as an effect size (ES). An **effect size** for experimental studies is calculated by subtracting the mean of the control group from the mean of the experimental group and then dividing by the standard deviation of the control group (or the pooled variance of the control and experimental groups, $SD_p$): $[M_e - M_c]/SD_c$. The effect sizes from various comparable studies can then be averaged (usually weighted according to the sample size) and compared to a criterion-referenced effect size range to indicate the strength of the finding. Cohen (1988) stated that an *ES* of 0 indicates no effect of treatment, *ES* = .20 indicates a small effect of treatment, *ES* = .50 indicates a medium effect of treatment, and *ES* = .80+ indicates a large effect of treatment. Note that effect sizes are simply the number of standard deviations above or below the (control group) mean in which a given treatment score lies (e.g., *ES* = 1.00 means the treatment mean was one standard deviation [SD] above the control group mean). Thus, if the variances of the treatment and control group distributions are similar, one can conclude that the average client in the treatment group performed better than a given percentage of the control group participants. For example, an *ES* = 1.00 means that the average client in the treatment group attained an outcome better than 84 percent of the control group participants.

Another way of expressing effect sizes in correlational research involves the computation of the Pearson *r*. In these instances, effect size interpretations are *r* = .10 (small), *r* = .30 (medium), and *r* = .50 (large). Of course, there are additional formulas for effect size estimates, but these are the two primary statistics found in the literature. Table 4.1 provides a summary of some available meta-analytic outcome research studies on counseling effectiveness that are mentioned in this chapter.

**TABLE 4.1**  Selected meta-analytic studies from the extant literature.

| Source | Outcome Explored | Population | *ES* |
|---|---|---|---|
| *Effectiveness of Counseling with Adults (or Heterogeneous Samples)* | | | |
| Bachar (1998) | Counseling effectiveness | Heterogeneous | .80 |
| Cuijpers (1998) | Outreach programs for depression | Elderly | .77 |
| Lambert et al. (1993) | Individual counseling effectiveness | Heterogeneous | .82 |
| McRoberts et al. (1998) | Individual versus group counseling | Heterogeneous | NS |
| | Depression (individual > group) | Heterogeneous | .29 |
| Mitte (2005) | Cognitive behavior therapy (vs. control) | Adults with anxiety | .82 |
| | Cognitive behavior therapy (vs. control) | Adults with depression | .76 |
| Robinson et al. (1990) | Individual counseling effectiveness | Clients with depression | .83 |
| | Group counseling effectiveness | Clients with depression | .84 |
| Tilliski (1990) | Individual counseling effectiveness | Heterogeneous | 1.35 |
| | Group counseling effectiveness | Heterogeneous | 1.35 |
| *Client/Counselor Characteristics* | | | |
| Horvath & Symonds (1991) | Working alliance and outcome | Heterogeneous | .26* |
| Martin, Garske, & Davis (2000) | Therapeutic alliance and outcome | Heterogeneous | .22* |
| Orlinsky, Grawe, & Parks (1994) | Counselor skill and outcome | Heterogeneous | .20 |
| Shirk & Karver (2003) | Therapeutic alliance and outcome | Children and adolescents | .24* |
| *Career and Educational Planning* | | | |
| Oliver & Spokane (1988) | Career interventions | Overall | .82 |
| Whiston, Tai, Rahardja, & Eder (2011) | Educational planning | K–12 students | .27 |
| Whiston, Sexton, & Lasoff (1998) | Career interventions | Overall | .45 |
| *Youth and School-based Interventions* | | | |
| Bennett & Gibbons (2000) | Cognitive behavior interventions on antisocial behaviors | Minors | .48 |
| Bratton, Ray, Rhine, & Jones (2005) | Play therapy | Minors | .80 |
| Kazdin, Bass, Ayers, & Rodgers (1990) | Counseling effectiveness | 4–18 years | .88 |
| LeBlanc & Ritchie (2001) | Play therapy | Minors | .66 |
| Prout & Prout (1998) | School counseling program effectiveness | Minors | .97 |
| Stage & Quiroz (1997) | Decreasing disruptive behaviors | Minors | .85 |
| Weisz et al. (1995) | Counseling effectiveness | 2–18 years | .71 |
| Whiston et al. (2011) | School counseling program effectiveness | Minors | .46 |
| Wilson, Gottfredson, & Najaka (2001) | Prevention programs for problem behaviors | Minors | ~.10 |
| Rongione et al. (2010) | Alcohol use (waitlist) (single group studies) Drug use (waitlist) (single group studies) | Teenagers | .02 .26 .29 .21 |
| Vaughn & Howard (2004) | Substance use | Teenagers | >.20 |
| Erford, Erford et al. (2011) | Depression (waitlist) (single group studies) | Minors | .55 .36 |
| Weisz, McCarty, & Valeri (2006) | Depression | Teenagers | .34 |
| Erford, Paul, Oncken, Kress, & Erford (in press) | Oppositional behavior (waitlist) (single group studies) | Minors | .68 .63 |

*(Continued)*

**TABLE 4.1** *continued*

| Source | Outcome Explored | Population | *ES* |
|---|---|---|---|
| Erford, Kress et al. (in press) | Anxiety (waitlist) (single group studies) | Minors | .48 .42 |
| Trask, Walsh, & DiLillo (2011) | Psychological effects of child abuse | Minors | .54 |
| Kowalik, Weller, Venter, & Drachman (2011) | CBT on pediatric PTSD | Minors | .20 to .33 |
| In-Albon & Schneider (2007) | CBT and anxiety | Minors | .86 |
| Silverman, Pina, & Viswesvaran (2008) | Individual CBT for anxiety Group CBT for anxiety | Minors | .44 .41 |

*Note:* * means *ES* calculated using Pearson *r*.

CBT, cognitive behavioral therapy; PTSD, post-traumatic stress disorder.

© Cengage Learning

Notice how the process mitigates certain flaws in some studies by summarizing the results across numerous studies into a meaningful, generalizable result. Meta-analysis has been widely used in counseling and educational research, but is not without its critics and methodological shortcomings. Still, it is a helpful technique that enjoys widespread use. With these procedural details as context, you are ready to dive right into the research outcomes literature. Enjoy!

# How Effective Is Counseling?

Thousands of studies over the past half century have explored the question of counseling effectiveness, and the short answer is: very effective. This conclusion is consistently reached for both individual and group counseling, and for children and adults, whether the reviews of extant literature are narrative or empirical meta-analyses. Ordinarily, meta-analytic reviews report effect sizes of .70+ for individual and group counseling interventions over control groups, and about .40+ over placebo treatments (Bachar, 1998; see Table 4.1). An effect size of .70 means that the average client who is receiving counseling displayed a better outcome than 76 percent of control group participants (i.e., +.70 standard deviations above the mean is the 76th percentile rank). Furthermore, most studies indicate little or no difference between individual and group counseling effectiveness.

Of course, some evidence does exist that factors outside of the counseling relationship and treatment may account for improvement in client symptoms. In fact, Lambert, Masters, and Ogles (1991) reported that factors outside of counseling may account for as much as 40 percent of client improvement. This is bolstered by studies indicating that up to 90 percent of some populations may experience spontaneous remission rates (range of 0–90 percent), although higher rates of remission are associated with mild issues and shorter durations (Lambert, 1976; Mann, Jenkins, & Belsey, 1981). Still, even these studies indicate that counseling adds substantially to outcomes in most clients.

A fair and related question is whether counseling can harm clients. According to Sexton et al. (1997), a small percentage of clients do get worse during the course of treatment. It appears that about 6–12 percent of clients experience negative effects during counseling (Beutler, Frank, Schieber, Calvert, & Gaines, 1984; Henry, Schacht, & Strupp, 1986), although the effects cannot be attributed to counseling alone. Factors that may contribute to negative client outcomes include lack of counselor skill, quality of the therapeutic alliance, or inappropriately applied treatments (Lambert & Bergin, 1994).

Now that our question "How effective is counseling?" has been answered, we can turn our attention to the facets of counseling that produce successful treatment outcomes. Interestingly, most of the available research indicates that, in general, counseling is effective regardless of the theoretical approach espoused by the counselor (Sexton et al., 1997), although some approaches appear to have treatment advantages for some conditions and some client types. For example, cognitive behavior therapy appears to result in better treatment outcomes than other theoretical approaches for anxiety and phobic problems and equal to the effects of antidepressant medications (Mitte, 2005). Interestingly, when the allegiance of the experimenter is accounted for, most theoretical approach differences usually disappeared!

To complicate matters, over 400 different permutations of therapies currently exist (Kazdin, 2011), many of which have not been subjected to empirical study. Sexton et al. (1997) provide an excellent review of the outcome research related to several commonly used theoretical approaches, including experiential, client-centered, cognitive-behavioral, behavioral, and psychodynamic. The overwhelming evidence that these varied approaches are more or less equivalently effective leads to the tentative conclusion that "common factors" may exist across therapeutic approaches that account for a large proportion of counseling effectiveness.

Aside from theoretical orientation, a number of other factors related to counseling effectiveness have been studied. Treatment length is often thought of as a contributing factor to therapeutic outcome, with some practitioners concluding that more is better. Howard, Kopta, Krause, and Orlinsky (1986) concluded that about 50 percent of improvement occurred by the eighth session, 75 percent by the half-year mark, and 85 percent by the end of the first year of counseling. This is somewhat in keeping with the philosophy of brief, solution-focused counselors who indicate that if substantial change will occur, it will do so by the eighth session. It is probably safe to conclude that the more severely disturbed a client is at the beginning of counseling, the more benefit he or she will derive from a longer course of treatment. Likewise, mildly impaired clients appear to make good progress in fewer sessions (Lambert & Bergin, 1994). So more is not always better, but clients who terminate or drop out of counseling during the first several sessions often stop before substantial and enduring gains have been achieved.

Clients who drop out of counseling, thus prematurely terminating treatment, are problematic regardless of setting, presenting problems, or therapeutic approaches. Of clients referred for counseling, nearly 49 percent never turn up for the first session (Phillips & Fagan, 1982). Of those who do show up for the first session, most terminate counseling by the eighth session (Garfield, 1994). Keep in mind that most of the studies related to premature termination are based on clients who volunteer for counseling. A classic study of the National Institute of Mental Health (NIMH; Elkin et al., 1989) indicated that 69 percent of children and youth had fewer than 6 visits, and only 12 percent had more than 10 visits.

Initial impressions and counseling activities may facilitate relationship building and reduce dropout rates. The outcomes literature indicates that clients are less likely to drop out prematurely if professional counselors (a) administer complete psychological evaluations; (b) are perceived as trustworthy and competent; (c) are perceived as skillful; (d) convey respect, directiveness, and a strong alliance (Mohl, Martinez, Ticknor, Huang, & Cordell, 1991); and (e) establish mutually agreed-upon goals and roles. Of course, the match between the client and professional counselor is of critical importance to rapport, therapeutic commitment, and eventual outcome. Table 4.2 provides some specific facets of counseling and reported effect sizes.

**TABLE 4.2**    Selected effect sizes for specific facets of counseling effectiveness.

| Study | Characteristic | Population | *ES* |
|---|---|---|---|
| Hoag & Burlingame (1997) | Group outcome: disruptive behavior | Minors | .69 |
| | Group outcome: anxiety/fear | Minors | .62 |
| | Group outcome: adjustment to divorce | Minors | .51 |
| | Group outcome: social skills | Minors | .49 |
| | Group outcome: depression | Minors | .46 |
| | Presenting problem: depression | Minors | .72 |
| | Presenting problem: behavior disorder | Minors | .56 |
| | Presenting problem: social | Minors | .32 |
| Mitte (2005) | CBT and anxiety | Heterogeneous | .82 |
| | CBT and depression | Heterogeneous | .76 |
| | CBT and quality of Life | Heterogeneous | .89 |
| Erford et al. (2013) | Bulimia (counseling) | Adolescents and adults | .81 |
| | (self-help) | | .58 |

# Which Client and Professional Counselor Factors Contribute to Successful Outcomes?

Over the years, research has consistently demonstrated that counseling of all types is effective. Now, researchers are concentrating on isolating common client and professional counselor characteristics that influence or create successful therapeutic outcomes. If all, or at least most, approaches to counseling are generally effective, and different approaches may hold advantages in addressing some types of client problems better than others, it makes sense that personal characteristics of clients and professional counselors may play some role in treatment efficacy. Unfortunately, these results have been far less satisfying than studies of direct treatment effects. In general, the effect sizes of client and counselor characteristics on treatment outcome from meta-analytic studies appear small, and many studies indicate little if any discernible effects (see Table 4.1).

This has led some researchers to suggest that exploring the "fit" or interaction among different client concerns, treatment approaches, client characteristics, and professional counselor characteristics may be a fruitful area for future research (Sexton et al., 1997). For example, if it is clear that cognitive behavior therapy is effective for clients with depression, is it possible that matching differing client characteristics and counselor characteristics can boost treatment efficacy? This is an important question that deserves much attention from practitioners, researchers, and counselor educators. For now, the remainder of this section will explore what is currently known about the contribution of client and professional counselor factors to successful treatment outcomes.

Much of the research in this area of the literature is correlational and has focused on client demographic information and motivation for counseling. Studies indicate that treatment outcome is unrelated to client gender, socioeconomic class, race, or age.

In contrast, and not surprisingly, level of disturbance when seeking counseling (e.g., mild, moderate, severe) has been consistently linked with outcome, with more severe clients making less progress than mildly afflicted clients (Orlinsky, Grawe, & Parks, 1994). The role of client expectancy in counseling has also received mixed results with early studies by Frank (1959), Friedman (1963), and Goldstein (1960) that show that higher initial expectation was related to higher clinical outcome, and later studies (Garfield, 1994) that show little relationship. Some have hypothesized that initial expectancy may be important to outcome indirectly by allowing clients to become invested in counseling, thus serving as a mediating variable; Lambert et al. (1991) indicated that about 15 percent of therapeutic outcome was related to client expectations.

Characteristics of professional counselors also have been well studied, again by using primarily correlational procedures. Interestingly, the research is very supportive of the observation that some professional counselors are more effective than others, regardless of the treatment approaches used (Crits-Christoph & Mintz, 1991; Lambert, 1989). At least indirectly, this seems to indicate that some professional counselor characteristic(s) must be operative. The consideration of professional counselor demographic variables (e.g., sex, age, race) has yielded mixed results, generally due to unsound methodology and the correlational nature of the research (Sexton et al., 1997). For example, African American clients preferred African American counselors, and Hispanic clients preferred Hispanic counselors, but such preference did not result in improved outcomes (Whiston & Sexton, 1993). Such preferences may, however, result in fewer clients leaving counseling prematurely, so the longer exposure to counseling may yield more positive long-term gains.

Likewise, professional characteristics of counselors appear to make little difference in treatment outcome. Meta-analyses that investigated treatment outcomes among disciplines (e.g., professional counselors, psychologists, social workers, marriage and family therapists) indicate no differences between and among professional mental health provider groups (Erford et al., 2011, 2013). Perhaps, most interesting, a number of studies indicate that there is no relationship between training or experience and treatment outcome (Christenson & Jacobson, 1993; Erford, Erford et al., 2011; Erford et al., 2013; Weisz, Weiss, Alicke, & Klotz, 1987). This result was not always consistent, however, as Lyons and Woods (1991) determined that experienced therapists displayed better outcomes than less experienced therapists, and Stein and Lambert (1995) determined that professionally trained counselors have better outcomes than the untrained. Interestingly, Stein and Lambert (1995) concluded that the experience levels of trained therapists had no differential treatment effect with mildly impaired clients, but they became a more important determining factor when treating more severely disturbed clients. Of course, the opposite has also been demonstrated, as in Svartberg & Stiles's (1991) meta-analytic study that concluded that counselor effectiveness decreased with experience. This is not as anomalous as it may seem, as will be demonstrated in the following section on the outcomes literature related to career interventions. This observation has led many to consider the importance of "counseling skill" as the operational construct, not training or experience. Thus, a highly skilled counselor with minimal experience will often generate better clinical outcomes than a less skilled counselor with decades of experience.

Beutler, Machado, and Neufeldt (1994) argued that training, practice, experience, and supervision do not always result in counseling skill. Indeed, the literature is replete with studies that failed to account and control for this important source of variance (Moncher & Prinz, 1991), although some (Orlinsky et al., 1994) reported a small effect size of .20 for counseling skill and treatment outcome when skill level was controlled.

The focus on counselor skill has led to a current impetus in counseling on the introduction and validation of **treatment manuals** into professional practice. These manuals standardize treatment of certain conditions by providing a research-based (and hopefully empirically validated) approach, providing the accountable professional counselor with a "recommended treatment regimen." The use of treatment manuals is encouraged by managed care providers, and several professional associations and researchers have championed the concept. Preliminary evidence on the use of treatment manuals in counseling has concluded that either no difference in effectiveness of the manual over no manual treatments exists (Robinson et al., 1990) or adherence to manual procedures results in a better treatment outcome (Luborsky, McClellan, Woody, O'Brien, & Auerbach, 1985). Henry, Strupp, Butler, Schacht, and Binder (1993), however, indicated that adherence to treatment manuals may actually result in a decline in relationship and supportiveness. That is, manuals may enhance professional counselor technical proficiency while simultaneously negatively affecting important therapeutic alliance factors. This makes sense if one considers that Lambert et al. (1991) concluded that about 30 percent of therapeutic outcome was due to the strength of the therapeutic alliance and only 15 percent due to the approach or technical skill of the clinician. If one sacrifices the alliance by focusing on a mechanistic treatment regimen, it stands to reason that client outcomes may be diminished.

The relationship between professional counselors' personal traits and treatment outcome has also been studied. The counselor's self-confidence and personal adjustment have been found to be significantly related, albeit inconsistently, to outcome (Sexton & Whiston, 1991). Also, Sexton et al. (1997) concluded that, at best, only a slight relationship exists between a professional counselor who is receiving personal therapy and treatment outcome for their clients; no doubt this research is confounded by the various reasons a counselor may choose to seek therapy (e.g., self-actualization, deeper personal insight into countertransference, supportive family counseling for a disruptive child, marriage therapy, and substance use). It is probably safe to conclude that counselor maladjustment only hinders treatment outcomes for their clients when it results in serious impairment (Sexton et al., 1997) and negatively affects the therapeutic alliance.

Finally, several meta-analyses (e.g., Martin, Garske, & Davis, 2000; Shirk & Karver, 2003) have explored the therapeutic alliance as a factor in treatment outcome, and all have determined small effect sizes (see Table 4.1). **Therapeutic alliance** has ordinarily been defined as a collaborative relationship between client and professional counselor in which an affective bond and agreement on treatment goals have been established (Martin et al., 2000). Interestingly, the American Psychological Association Division 29 Psychotherapy Task Force (Steering Committee, 2002) enumerated seven relational variables termed "promising and probably effective": (1) positive regard, (2) congruence/genuineness, (3) repairing alliance ruptures, (4) self-disclosure, (5) quality of relational interpretations, (6) management of countertransference, and (7) feedback. These facets of therapeutic relationships and skill have been studied in the literature for decades and provide a new validation challenge for researchers interested in studying the therapeutic alliance, its interaction with treatment approaches, and treatment outcomes.

In sum, then, some client and professional counselor factors may be somewhat important in predicting treatment outcomes, but in all but a few cases, these effects are negligible to small. Sexton et al. (1997, p. 81) concluded, "There is no single counselor or client characteristic, no single theory, or no technique that can account for the success of good counseling." They and many other researchers look to interactions among these facets (i.e., client–counselor similarity, client–process matching, and client problem–treatment matching) as ripe areas for future outcome research.

# Outcome Research on Career and Educational Planning Interventions

Career interventions are implemented with school-aged students through adulthood and involve systematic interventions aimed at helping individuals understand career values, beliefs, interests, competencies, and life-role salience, culminating in a plan of action to achieve vocational direction and success. In K–12 schools and universities, individual planning involves a systematic coordination of activities designed to assist students in determining personal goals and plans for the future (American School Counselor Association, 2012). To date, the most comprehensive (and fascinating) review of career counseling outcome research was written by Sexton et al. (1997). Several qualitative reviews (Swanson, 1995; Whiston & Oliver, 2005) provide narrative evidence of the effectiveness of career interventions. In the counseling outcome literature, two meta-analyses have been conducted that generally support career interventions with effect sizes ranging from small to large, although the two studies vary to some degree on the specific effectiveness of some characteristics. Oliver and Spokane (1988) reviewed 58 studies (7,311 total participants) conducted between 1950 and 1982 that focused on career counseling interventions. In an extension of the Oliver and Spokane study that precisely replicated the previous study's meta-analytic methodology, Whiston, Sexton, and Lasoff (1998) analyzed the results of an additional 47 studies conducted between 1983 and 1995 (4,660 total participants). Because the Whiston et al. study replicated the Oliver and Spokane methodology precisely, professional counselors now have an outstanding summary of the effectiveness of career interventions over a 45-year period! Table 4.3 provides a summary of effect sizes for the outcomes measured in these two studies. These two meta-analytic studies are fascinating and must-reads for any professional counselor who is providing career intervention services. Overall, 83 percent of studies of career intervention reported at least some positive effects (Sexton, Whiston, Bleuer, & Walz, 1995).

Specifically, note that treatment appears moderately effective regardless of length of treatment. Career interventions appear moderately to highly effective in individuals from middle school through adulthood but not with elementary-aged students, who, developmentally speaking, are just becoming aware of vocational interests and choices and ordinarily only have a passing interest in the world of work. Surprisingly, counselors-in-training produced slightly better outcomes than experienced professional counselors, but trained professional counselors and counselors-in-training far outperformed "counselor-free" (e.g., self-help) interventions. Individual counseling interventions and career classes appear to yield the best results, but small group counseling, workshops, and group test interpretations were also moderately effective. Computerized interventions yielded small to moderate effect sizes, whereas counselor-free interventions resulted in little discernible difference from control group conditions. The ineffectiveness of counselor-free interventions has been validated in a study by Whiston, Brecheisen, and Stephens (2003) and previous studies by Garis and Niles (1990) and Niles and Garis (1990), all of which concluded that clients gained from the use of computerized career interventions when coupled with counselor-led interventions but not without the guidance of a professional counselor. Not surprisingly, Lenz, Reardon, and Sampson (1993) reported that participants with high scores on Social and Enterprising scales of the *Self-Directed Search* displayed a lower preference for computerized career interventions, perhaps preferring more people-oriented interventions. Importantly, Galassi, Crace, Martin, James, and Wallace (1992) indicated that task-focused career counseling was significantly more preferred than person-centered approaches.

**TABLE 4.3**   Effect sizes (ES) for selected Oliver and Spokane (1988) and Whiston et al. (1998) meta-analysis outcome variables.

| Oliver & Spokane *ES* | Whiston et al. *ES* | Characteristic |
|---|---|---|
| .82 | .45 | All studies combined (unweighted) |
| *Length of treatment* | | |
| .31 | .61 | Single session intervention |
| 1.01 | .53 | 2–7 sessions intervention |
| .65 | .74 | More than 8 sessions intervention |
| *Age of client* | | |
| −.01 | .04 | Elementary school students |
| 1.28 | .42 | Middle school students |
| 1.02 | .31 | High school students |
| .85 | .59 | College students |
| .82 | .54 | Adults |
| *Experience of counselor* | | |
| .72 | .51 | Experienced counselor |
| .83 | .81 | Counselor-in-training |
| .31 | .29 | Counselor-free |
| .38 | .60 | Other (usually facilitator or group leader) |
| *Treatment Types* | | |
| .74 | 1.08 | Individual counseling |
| .62 | .73 | Group counseling |
| .76 | .36 | Group test interpretation |
| .75 | .36 | Workshop |
| 2.05 | .54 | Class |
| .59 | .45 | Computer intervention |
| .10 | .12 | Counselor-free |
| *Cost for Services [Computed as: (Effect size) × (n participants) ÷ (hours)]* | | |
| .52 | .92 | Individual counseling |
| 2.00 | .87 | Group counseling |
| 4.35 | 2.1 | Workshop |
| 2.74 | 4.9 | Class |
| | 5.5 | Computer |
| | −4.4 | Counselor-free |
| 2.45 | 1.40 | Accuracy of self-knowledge |
| *Specific Treatment Outcomes* | | |
| .97 | .73 | Securing job or probability of hire |
| .40 | .38 | Certainty/decidedness |
| .88 | .88 | Career-related knowledge |
| 1.03 | 1.30 | Skills (interview, writing, and problem-solving) |
| 1.05 | .55 | Career maturity |

© Cengage Learning

When it comes to cost-effectiveness, workshops and classes appeared to yield the biggest gains owing to the number of participants that can be simultaneously accommodated. Likewise, group counseling (large effect) appears to have an advantage over individual counseling (medium to large effect), although all far exceeded the cost-effectiveness of counselor-free interventions. Consistently high outcomes were observed in a client's accuracy of self-knowledge, career-related knowledge, and job-related skills. Thus, professional counselors and counselors-in-training have a relatively robust research base to back up claims of effective career interventions (Oliver & Spokane, 1988; Whiston et al., 1998). Sexton et al. (1997) pointed out that further treatment effectiveness in the career counseling domain could be enhanced if practitioners and counselor educators would develop treatment manuals with standardized procedures that are empirically validated, similar to what has been done for numerous mental health conditions.

A third meta-analysis (Whiston, Tai, Rahardja, & Eder, 2011) that involved 10 studies that specifically targeted educational planning interventions with school-aged youth arrived at an overall effect size of .27 (small). But the effect size for the three studies involving middle school students was 1.01, perhaps indicating that educational planning activities can be most efficient with young adolescents. Baker and Taylor (1998) reported a moderate effect size for the use of career activities facilitating school-to-work transitions. Finally, Whiston and Sexton (1998) reported that educational planning and career interventions were helpful to and valued by students from diverse backgrounds, including cultural minorities, the gifted, and students with learning disabilities.

# The Effectiveness of Counseling Children and Adolescents and School-Based Interventions

Many professional counselors provide services to school-aged youth. Some professional counselors provide services through private practice or agency services that generally involve traditional individual or group counseling services. Professional school counselors are employed by schools and provide direct and indirect counseling services at the school sites. Importantly, the services offered by professional school counselors are diverse and complex, going well beyond traditional individual and group counseling services to include consultation/collaboration with teachers, parents, and administration; career development and educational planning services; developmental classroom guidance lessons; implementing conflict resolution and peer mediation programs; and development and assessment of comprehensive school counseling programs.

Several diverse meta-analytic studies have been conducted in schools, clinics, and research laboratories that explore the general effects of individual counseling with children and adolescents. Casey and Berman's (1985) meta-analysis resulted in an effect size of .71, meaning that the average treatment group participant performed better after treatment than 76 percent of control group participants (i.e., .71 standard deviations above the control group mean is the 76th percentile). Weisz et al. (1987) reported an $ES = .79$; Kazdin, Bass, Ayers, and Rogers (1990) reported an $ES = .88$; LeBlanc and Ritchie (2001) reported an $ES = .66$ (specific focus on play therapy); and Weisz et al. (1995) reported an $ES = .71$. Taken together, these meta-analytic studies, which included more than 300 individual studies of school-aged youth, indicate the effects of general individual counseling are medium to large. Again, these studies did not differentiate among youth who were counseled in schools, agencies, private practice, or research laboratories, or by level of counselor experience, but the general conclusion supports the use of counseling with school-aged youth (Kazdin, 1991, 1993, 1994).

The effectiveness of individual counseling with school-aged youth is heartening, but caution is warranted in applying adult interventions blindly to cases involving children. Developmental considerations must be constantly appraised. For example, a counseling intervention appropriate for an adult or adolescent with depression may be ineffective or even harmful to a young child with depression.

A number of studies have explored the effectiveness of the broader range of school-based interventions, and Table 4.4 shows the results from several meta-analytic studies of primarily school-based interventions. Several qualitative reviews of the literature have been conducted over the past few decades. Whiston and Sexton (1998) indicated that, in general, positive changes in students result from the broad ranges of services performed by professional school counselors. The conclusion of an earlier qualitative review by Borders and Drury (1992) was even more favorable as observed through significant student improvements in academic performance, attitudes, and behaviors. A qualitative review focused on elementary-aged students (Gerler, 1985) concluded that student affective, interpersonal, and behavioral characteristics are positively affected by school counseling programs. St. Clair (1989) suggested that middle school students benefited from school counseling services that included behavior management, self-relaxation, and daily progress reports. In a qualitative study of low-performing K–12 students, Wilson (1986) concluded that school counselor strategies and interventions resulted in higher grade point averages across all levels of education.

Unfortunately, few meta-analytic studies have been conducted on school counseling services. One notable recent exception was Whiston et al. (2011), who reviewed 117 studies published since 1980 and yielded an overall unweighted $ES = .46$ (weighted $ES = .29$). Other meta-analytic studies focused on more specific aspects of a comprehensive developmental school counseling program. Sink and Stroh (2003) indicated that elementary students who attended schools with a comprehensive school counseling program had slightly higher achievement scores. Both Sprinthall (1981) and Baker, Swisher, Nadenichek, and Popowicz (1984) concluded that primary prevention programs were at least moderately effective. Prout and DeMartino (1986) and Prout and Prout (1998) conducted the only meta-analyses of individual counseling specifically within the school context and concluded that effect sizes for counseling services in schools were medium and large, respectively.

Attention to outcome research on school counseling effectiveness continues to lag behind other specialty areas of counseling, particularly that of career and individual counseling (Whiston et al., 2015) and is replete with methodological limitations. These methodological limitations are due, at least in part, to the complexity of assessing highly variable, complex, comprehensive programs. Thus, these conclusions about the effectiveness of school counseling interventions should be viewed with caution.

Some outcome research has focused on specific types of school-based interventions rather than a comprehensive program. Whiston et al. (2011) conducted a meta-analysis to evaluate developmental classroom guidance activities and concluded that this intervention had primarily small effect sizes across the K–12 curriculum. More focused studies found classroom guidance to be effective in addressing personal/affective issues (Rowley, Stroh, & Sink, 2005), wellness (Omizo, Omizo, & D'Andrea, 1992), academic achievement (Lee, 1993), social competence (Weissburg, Caplan, & Harwood, 1991), school attitude and behavior (Schlossberg, Morris, & Lieberman, 2001), and combinations of academic, social, and self-management skills (Brigman & Campbell, 2003; Campbell & Brigman, 2005). It is important to point out that many professional school counselors are using curricular materials and programs that are not well studied (Rowley et al., 2005). Thus, even greater effectiveness may be obtained by using empirically validated instructional materials and supplements. Indeed, the evaluation of instructional materials and procedures used in developmental guidance programs is an area of the research and evaluation literature that deserves tremendous attention from empirically oriented practitioners and researchers.

| TABLE 4.4 | Selected effect sizes for specific facets of counseling effectiveness for youth and school-based interventions. |
|---|---|

| Study | Characteristic | Population | ES |
|---|---|---|---|
| Wilson, Gottfredson, & Najaka (2001) | Prevention programs for problem behaviors | Grades K–12 | ~.10 |
| | Delinquency | K–12 | .04 |
| | Alcohol/drug use | K–12 | .05 |
| | Dropout/attendance | K–12 | .16 |
| | Other problem behaviors | K–12 | .17 |
| | Overall | Grades K–5 | .05 |
| | Overall | Grades 6–8 | .09 |
| | Overall | Grades 9–12 | .14 |
| Stage & Quiroz (1997) | Decreasing disruptive behavior (overall) | K–12 | .85 |
| | Using punishment | Minors | .58 |
| | Using token economy | Minors | .90 |
| | Using response cost | Minors | .53 |
| | Using differential reinforcement | Minors | .95 |
| | Using group behavior modification | Minors | 1.02 |
| | Using individual counseling | Minors | .31 |
| | Using parent training | Minors | .60 |
| | Decreasing disruptive behavior—students with ADHD | | .78 |
| | Students in regular education | | .72 |
| | Students with mental retardation | | .78 |
| | Students with serious emotional disturbances | | .98 |
| | Students with learning disabilities | | .97 |
| Bratton, Ray, Rhine, & Jones (2005) | Nondirective play therapy | Minors | .92 |
| | Directive play therapy | Minors | .71 |
| | Group play therapy: professional led | Minors | .73 |
| | Individual play therapy: professional led | Minors | .70 |
| | Filial trained play therapy: parent led | Minors | 1.05 |
| | Play therapy for behavior problems | Minors | .81 |
| | Play therapy for social adjustment | Minors | .83 |
| | Play therapy for family relationships | Minors | 1.12 |
| Whiston et al. (2011) | School counseling program effectiveness | K–5 students | .25 |
| | | 6–8 students | .39 |
| | | 9–12 students | .34 |
| | Group guidance curricular activities | K–5 students | .29 |
| | | 6–8 students | .41 |
| | | 9–12 students | .39 |
| | Responsive services (group and individual) | K–5 students | .40 |
| | | 6–8 students | .22 |
| | | 9–12 students | .34 |
| | Peer mediation (knowledge) | Minors | .39 |
| Rongione et al. (2010) | Alcohol use (waitlist) | Teenagers | .02 |
| | (single group studies) | | .26 |
| | Drug use (waitlist) | | .29 |
| | (single group studies) | | .21 |
| Vaughn & Howard (2004) | Substance use | Teenagers | >.20 |

*(Continued)*

**TABLE 4.4** *continued*

| Study | Characteristic | Population | *ES* |
|---|---|---|---|
| Erford et al. (2011) | Depression (waitlist)<br>(single group studies) | Minors | .55<br>.36 |
| Weisz, McCarty, & Valeri (2006) | Depression | Teenagers | .34 |
| Erford, Paul, Oncken, Kress, & Erford (in press) | Oppositional behavior (waitlist)<br>(single group studies) | Minors | .68<br>.63 |
| Erford, Kress et al. (in press) | Anxiety (waitlist)<br>(single group studies) | Minors | .48<br>.42 |
| Trask, Walsh, & DiLillo (2011) | Psychological effects of child abuse | Minors | .54 |
| Kowalik, Weller, Venter, & Drachman (2011) | CBT on pediatric PTSD | Minors | .20<br>−.33 |
| In-Albon & Schneider (2007) | CBT and anxiety | Minors | .86 |
| Silverman, Pina, & Viswesvaran (2008) | Individual CBT for anxiety<br>Group CBT for anxiety | Minors | .44<br>.41 |

ADHD, attention-deficit/hyperactivity disorder.

Responsive services (e.g., individual counseling, group counseling) have also received some attention in the school-based outcomes literature. Some researchers have concluded that individual counseling is more effective than group counseling (Nearpass, 1990), whereas others reached the opposite conclusion (Wiggins & Wiggins, 1992; Wilson, 1986). What is clear is that both are at least somewhat effective in remediation of problems displayed by children and adolescents. For example, Whiston et al. (2011) conducted a meta-analysis of 58 studies of school populations, assessing the effectiveness of primarily group counseling interventions and derived an overall effect size of .35. In more focused studies, Littrell, Malia, and Vanderwood (1995) concluded that brief, solution-focused approaches to individual counseling were effective with adolescents, and Thompson and Littrell (1998) reached a similar conclusion when counseling students with learning disabilities. Likewise, Erford, Miller et al. (2011) demonstrated the effectiveness of counseling for depression, Erford et al. (2013) for bulimia, and Erford, Kress et al. (in press) for anxiety with school-aged children. Group counseling was also determined to be effective for a wide range of school-based behaviors, including discipline problems, social skills training (Whiston & Sexton, 1998), adjustment to divorce (Omizo & Omizo, 1998; Pedro-Carroll & Alpert-Gillis, 1997; Pedro-Carroll, Sutton, & Wyman, 1999), and relaxation (Bauer, Sapp, & Johnson, 2000; Kiselica, Baker, Thomas, & Reddy, 1994).

Some outcome research focused on specific problem areas identified by educators, especially disruptive behavior. Efforts to reduce disruptive classroom behavior using behavior modification techniques have generally been effective. Stage and Quiroz (1997; see Table 4.4) reported an effect size of .78, indicating that 78 percent of treatment group participants outperformed the average control group participant. Medium to high effects were noted regardless of the type of behavior modification technique studied. For example, token economies and response cost procedures (Stage & Quiroz, 1997) were very effective, as were time-out procedures using contingency delay procedures (Erford, 1999). When intervening with aggressive students, Wilson, Lipsey, and Derzon (2003) concluded that behavioral counseling was more effective (i.e., large effect size) than peer mediation programs (i.e., small effect size). Erford, Paul et al. (in press) conducted a meta-analysis of oppositional outcome studies confirming this result.

Research on conflict resolution and peer mediation programs in schools indicated that "although their number is growing, few reliable studies of the effects of violence prevention and conflict resolution education programs have yet appeared" (Burstyn & Stevens, 2001, p. 146). Whiston et al. (2011) indicated a small effect ($ES = .39$) of peer mediation programs on improving student knowledge of how to address conflict-laden problem situations, but little is known about the effects of these programs on actual student behaviors. Indeed, Wilson et al. (2003) found little improvement in aggressive behaviors because of peer mediation programs, and Lewis and Lewis (1996) noted this could be because many, if not most programs are supervised by noncounselors with little or no training. Gerber and Terry-Day (1999) and Lewis and Lewis (1996) concluded that insufficient empirical support exists to warrant the widespread use of peer mediation and conflict resolution programs in schools and that a great deal more study is needed in this area. Whiston et al. (2015) indicated that two problems recur in the peer mediation research. First, many of the studies of peer mediation do not systematically sample student participants. Second, many evaluation studies of peer mediation programs do not anchor the finding to theoretical frameworks upon which the programs were designed. As a result, little helpful research has been conducted that allow professional school counselors to state with confidence that the programs are theoretically sound and have desirable effects. Much more attention is needed to these methodological and theoretical considerations if our understanding and use of peer mediation and conflict resolution programs in schools is to move forward.

Research on school-based prevention programs for problem behaviors have yielded mixed results. Wilson, Gottfredson, and Najaka (2001) concluded that effect sizes were either not significant or very small when primary prevention programs were studied. They found that these programs were more effective at the high school level ($ES = .14$) than at elementary ($ES = .05$) or middle schools ($ES = .09$; see Table 4.4), especially for dropout and attendance issues ($ES = .16$). In general, effect sizes for prevention programs for delinquency ($ES = 0.04$) or alcohol/drug use ($ES = 0.05$) were not significant. Wilson et al.'s meta-analytic conclusions stand in contrast to a substantial number of qualitative, quasi-empirical, and true experimental studies that, as stand-alone studies, claim substantial effectiveness for prevention programs, especially drug prevention programs (Botvin, Schinke, & Orlandi, 1995; Durlack, 1995; Gottfredson, 1997, 2001; Gottfredson, Wilson, & Najaka, 2001; Rongione, Erford, & Broglie, 2011; Tobler & Stratton, 1997) and programs aimed at reducing delinquent or conduct problems in school-aged youth (Catalano, Arthur, Hawkins, Berglund, & Olsen, 1998; Erford, Paul, Oncken, Kress, & Erford (in press); Gottfredson et al., 2001; Hawkins, Farrington, & Catalano, 1998; Lipsey & Derzon, 1998; Samplers & Aber, 1998; Stage & Quiroz, 1997). Also related to prevention programs, Baker et al. (1984) concluded that programs that implemented communication and psychoeducational skills were effective. Less effective were programs emphasizing substance abuse prevention, moral education, and coping skills training. Perhaps key to the differential effects is Tobler and Stratton's (1997) observation that interactive programs were more effective than noninteractive programs; that is, how the program is delivered and how engaged the students are in the program lessons may contribute substantially to a program's effectiveness.

Although some research exists to suggest that school-based counseling services are effective, "the research is neither vast nor methodologically strong" (Erford & Wallace, 2010, p. 38). Much greater consistency in targeted outcomes, instruments, and methodology is required to move this area of the outcome research literature forward.

# Implications for Professional Counselors

So where does this leave us as professional counselors? Obviously, a good deal of helpful research has been accumulated over the years. Much research, however, is still needed to skillfully implement and scientifically understand the practice of counseling. And that is where you as a member of the next generation of professional counselors can take the profession to new heights.

Perhaps most critically, students and practitioners must collaborate in research studies whenever possible. As a student, assist professors and field researchers by volunteering time and services. The research enterprise is often a long, time-intensive process, and "many hands make light work." In the process, you will pick up research and evaluation skills that may lead to valuable future action research activities. As a practitioner, engage in focused action research and program evaluation with your clients and collaborate with researchers to help with active outcome research agendas. Many practitioners think, "What could I possibly do to help?" or "How could my two or three clients with this particular issue be of any help in a research study?" Much helpful research is accomplished through aggregation of research samples and results. Simply making your worksite or willing clients available as a pool of potential participants can lead to a wealth of information when pooled together with others. Professional school counselors and community agency counselors can be of particular help given the large populations of potential participants they work with. The important point is to get active in research studies while you are still a student to understand the process and stay active when you take your rightful place as a professional counselor in the field. Most researchers will acknowledge that the two facets of the research process that practitioners can be most helpful with are access to participants and data collection.

As advocates for the profession, all professional counselors must take a role in seeking increased funding for research in at least three primary areas: (a) finding out what works in counseling, (b) how best to communicate this information to practitioners and counselors-in-training, and (c) basic research in counseling and related areas. Funding generally comes from three sources: government agencies, private foundations, and universities and professional associations. Advocating for generous funding from these sources will pay huge future dividends in terms of effective counseling practices with children and adults.

Professional counselors should read and use outcome research to inform and improve the effectiveness of their practice. Some excellent counseling journals publish outcome research in an easily accessible style, whereas others require a bit of sophistication to discern relevant practice information. When you encounter a helpful result or resource, summarize it and pass this research on to other colleagues. Serving as a conduit of information to your colleagues can be incredibly beneficial to their clients and the profession.

Finally, professional counselors are well advised to focus specifically on the core conditions of effective helping. Lambert (1991) concluded that 30 percent of therapeutic outcome is because of these core conditions, 15 percent due to the specific technique, 15 percent due to client expectations, and 40 percent due to factors outside of the counseling setting. Although a professional counselor can certainly become very skilled at a given technique, twice as much variance is attributed to core therapeutic conditions, such as the counselor–client alliance. Likewise, professional counselors should take advantage of the remaining 40 percent (due to outside factors) by considering multiple systems, culture, and context when planning interventions. Such planning can help focus clients on sources of intrinsic resiliency and environmental resources to bolster therapeutic outcomes.

# Conclusion

Thousands of research studies have explored the effectiveness of various facets of counseling. Still, much remains unknown. This chapter briefly reviewed the extant literature on counseling outcome research with an emphasis on summarizing what works and what does not. No theoretical approach to counseling has demonstrated superiority over any other, although some approaches show more promise with certain issues and under specific conditions. This observation has led some researchers to conclude that much of the effectiveness of counseling interventions may be due to core therapeutic conditions common to most if not all counseling approaches, including factors related to establishing an effective therapeutic alliance.

Career counseling interventions have received a good deal of attention in the extant literature and appear to be quite effective across a wide range of treatment types, age, and outcomes. Interestingly, nearly all types of career intervention that involve a professional counselor are effective, whereas those who use individuals who are not trained as counselors appear ineffective or may even produce negative outcomes. Career interventions generally were not effective with elementary students but were effective with middle school students through adults. Interventions requiring two or more sessions appeared much more effective than "one-shot" interventions.

The outcome research on counseling interventions with school-aged youth is among the more poorly studied areas. As for adults, individual and school counseling interventions appear to be at least moderately effective. Comprehensive school counseling programs appear somewhat effective in improving student academic performance, social skills, and behavior, but less so when the focus is on prevention programs, especially related to substance abuse and delinquency. Research on peer mediation and conflict resolution programs is still inconclusive. These programs do appear to raise student levels of information, but little evidence exists that these programs lower levels of conflict and aggression in schools.

Several implications and suggestions for how professional counselors can help bridge the research-practice gap and tap into a wealth of continuing outcome research were offered. Professional counselors should collaborate with researchers and conduct their own action research and evaluation studies, as well as advocate for increased funding for counseling research. Professional counselors should also read, summarize, and disseminate research on effective counseling practice to other practitioners. Finally, professional counselors should focus on the core conditions when establishing a therapeutic alliance, as these relational facets account for nearly one-third of therapeutic outcome variance.

*Now go to the Student Workbook found on cengagebrain.com that accompanies this text for additional application and review activities.*

In Section II, the reader is introduced to numerous methodological issues that shape the nature of counseling research and evaluation. As seen in Chapters 5–7, these methodological approaches are ordinarily categorized as qualitative and quantitative research procedures. In Chapter 8, special attention is provided to action research and single-subject research designs, which are being used with increasing frequency by professional counselors in clinical practice, often at the insistence of managed health care organizations. In the final two chapters in this section, we address topics more commonly associated with program evaluation. Chapter 9 provides an introduction to the conduct of a needs assessment, a critical element of program development and goal setting. Chapter 10 addresses accountability and program evaluation of counseling programs, which have become more highly emphasized and valued in recent years because of educational and health care reform movements.

# Qualitative Approaches to Research

The practice of counseling is always changing. Sometimes, counselors encounter client populations and situations about which little is known. In such instances, an important first step in helping these clients is to describe in rich detail and understand what they are going through, and then try to conceptualize the issue or develop a tentative explanatory theory. As explained in Chapter 1, qualitative methods are tailor-made for theory induction! This chapter explains the general process of developing a qualitative approach to research. First, characteristics of qualitative research are presented. Second, steps in developing a research design are discussed, including selecting a research problem and developing research questions, selecting a sample and sampling method and entering a research setting, determining the researcher's role, employing various data collection methods and management tools, and establishing trustworthiness for a qualitative study.

The use of **qualitative research** designs is increasing in counseling practice and research as professional counselors continue to explore complex constructs and engage in outcome research. Recent changes in academic standards (i.e., Council for Accreditation of Counseling and Related Programs [CACREP], 2009) set forth for counseling programs promote knowledge about various research methodologies including qualitative approaches. CACREP (2009) standards state that professional counselors "understand qualitative and quantitative research methodologies, including the criteria of the worthiness of each, in order to measure learning processes and outcomes, assess environments and organizations, and measure program effectiveness" (p. 22). In essence, professional counselors who are engaged in clinical work and research should be familiar with qualitative research design, the relationship between practice and research with respect to qualitative inquiry, and related issues of research rigor.

An increase in qualitative approaches to research is imperative as the counseling profession addresses the need to understand constructs and groups that historically have not been thoroughly studied. Heightened interest in the value of qualitative approaches may be a result of an increased focus on culture and power in counseling process and outcome, as well as the idea that an operational definition of various constructs may be impossible given their complexities.

Survey data revealed that professional counselor trainees view qualitative approaches to research as a holistic process that serves to create a research identity (Reisetter et al., 2004). Qualitative approaches are perceived as congruent with personal and professional worldviews, theoretical frameworks, and counseling skills. Further, certain qualitative methods, such as interviewing and participant observation, parallel the skills used by professional counselors in clinical interviewing and within counseling sessions. Thus, qualitative approaches to counseling research may serve to connect counseling practice with research.

# Characteristics of Qualitative Research

Qualitative research design is an interpretive and naturalistic approach that stresses how social experience is created and given meaning (Denzin & Lincoln, 2011). Qualitative research design involves an investigation of people and processes within a particular context for a sustained amount of time to obtain culturally embedded meaning, resulting in a rich description of people, events, and settings (Bogdan & Biklen, 2006). In counseling, qualitative research may involve interacting with clients to explore their perspectives on issues such as mental health, cultural norms in counseling, and satisfaction with the counseling relationship. Qualitative designs typically stress the socially constructed nature of reality, focus on situations and intimate relationships, acknowledge that research inquiry is value laden (Denzin & Lincoln, 2011), and reexamine meanings, processes, symbols and thick descriptions of phenomena (Berg & Lune, 2011). Thus, as professional counselors and counseling researchers gather data, they place equal value on various client meanings of situations and processes, and question and challenge themselves on how their assumptions may influence their findings.

Qualitative inquiry tends to be an **inductive process** by which data are used to construct theory and/or lead to a deeper understanding of an issue or phenomenon (Bogdan & Biklen, 2006). For example, a team of counseling researchers may be interested in identity development within intimate relationships among adolescent females. The team may reach a tentative conclusion through conducting and analyzing a series of interviews and observations that peers are a salient influence on adolescent identity development. This conclusion may be compared to existing theory or data to further understand how social networks affect intimacy among adolescents. Thus, qualitative inquiry and resulting data may create, advance, or dispute existing theory within various aspects of counseling practice.

Qualitative approaches to research are often used because of the nature of the research question (i.e., *how* or *what* questions), the need to explore a phenomenon that cannot be easily identified or explained, and to provide detailed information regarding a construct, event, or population within its natural setting (Creswell, 2013). For instance, counseling researchers may want to identify ways in which males and females conceptualize child abuse. They may collect data through naturalistic methods (e.g., observations and informal interviewing during social interactions) to better understand how gender may impact how child abuse is defined and described. The researchers may also be interested in how gender and personal experiences with childhood trauma may influence the nature of responses. This research question would be suitable for qualitative inquiry because researchers would be interested in describing the phenomenon by gaining insight into males' and females' beliefs, definitions, and experiences related to child abuse.

Qualitative and quantitative inquiries are similar in that both focus on understanding relationships between constructs in a systematic, scientific manner. (See Table 5.1 for a comparison of qualitative and quantitative methods.) Both methods can be rigorous, minimizing the impact of external influences such as extraneous independent variables and **researcher bias**. Qualitative approaches, however, differ from quantitative research in several important ways. For instance, quantitative research tends to refer to isolation and measurement of variables via statistical control within large-scale sampling and emphasizes researcher objectivity and a drive toward precision via deductive reasoning. Qualitative research tends to be more open ended, integrates the researcher's voice, and uses smaller samples to gather rich data (Berg & Lune, 2011; Ponterotto, 2005).

For example, imagine that a researcher is interested in factors that affect achievement motivation among middle school students. From a quantitative perspective, the researcher could select a couple of variables that achievement motivation theories espouse as related to a success orientation, such as internal locus of control and parental involvement. Then the researcher may construct a pretest and posttest design, identify measures that will assess these two variables, and administer the measures to a large stratified sample to generalize the findings to middle school students. In contrast, if a qualitative framework was used to examine factors related to achievement motivation, the researcher may employ purposive sampling and conduct focus group interviews for a select few cases without preidentifying potential moderating factors. Importantly, qualitative and quantitative inquiry may be congruent in that research designs may combine

| **TABLE 5.1** Characteristics of qualitative and quantitative research methods. | | |
|---|---|---|
| | **Qualitative Methods** | **Quantitative Methods** |
| Purpose | To describe and understand the ways that people give meaning to their own and others' behavior; to understand social phenomena as they occur naturally. | To study relationships, cause-and-effect; may manipulate variables, situations, or conditions to study complex phenomena. |
| Ontological Assumptions | Primarily postmodern (e.g., constructivism, critical theory, feminism). | Positivist and postpositivist. |
| Epistemological Assumptions | Knowledge is actively constructed; consequently, people's internal constructions are examined. | Knowledge arises from observations of the physical world. |
| Research Design | Designs may be selected in advance and may evolve during the study. | Developed prior to the study. |
| Approach | Inductive; used to develop concepts and theory. | Deductive; tests theory. |
| Hypotheses | Research questions, not hypotheses, guide the study. | Hypotheses (null and alternative) are established in advance. |
| Data Collection | Individual or group interviews and/or observation, archival data. | Standardized instruments, surveys, rating scales, checklists. |
| Sampling | Purposive (expert informant), small samples. | Random techniques, large samples. |
| Nature of Data and Analysis | Data primarily are words. Narrative description and interpretation are used for analysis. | Data primarily are numbers. Statistical tests are used for analysis. |
| Use of Results | To holistically describe phenomena, generate theory, and increase understanding of a particular individual or group. | To generalize to a population. |

© Cengage Learning

or use both areas of inquiry at various points of a study. This is called **mixed methodology inquiry**. Action research (see Chapter 8) frequently uses qualitative or mixed methods data collection and analysis methodology. Thus, with the achievement motivation inquiry, the researcher could conduct a large-scale survey, collect qualitative interview data to test against the larger sample findings, adapt the study to reflect the findings from both perspectives, and continue exploring the phenomenon with either or both qualitative and quantitative methods.

# Designing Qualitative Research

Given the strength of qualitative research in exploring and describing phenomena, it is important to consider the following key components when designing rigorous qualitative inquiry:

- Identifying the problem and developing research question(s).
- Selecting a population of interest and entering a research setting.
- Determining the researcher's role and researcher bias.
- Selecting a sampling method.
- Using various data collection methods and management tools.
- Establishing trustworthiness throughout the study.

When designing a qualitative study, researchers should consider the benefits and costs of the investigation for both the participants and themselves. That is, what are the time and financial costs and benefits for all parties? These considerations will help focus the study and determine the intrusiveness of methods and procedures.

## The Research Problem

One of the more difficult tasks of using qualitative research in counseling is identifying a focus for a study and research questions that will seek to answer a specific research problem. Researchers should actively reflect on what interests them in their counseling practice. Often, researchers have initial ideas about concepts and their relationships that inform potential research questions (Hays & Singh, 2012). Identifying a problem of interest will help the researcher remain focused on the study. Research topics can be found in daily counseling practices. For example, students can look at client issues or characteristics, practices within an agency, or a general social phenomenon of interest. Research questions may be general or particular, descriptive or explanatory, and generated at the beginning of a study or revised throughout fieldwork. Research questions often influence the data collection and sampling methods (Berg & Lune, 2011). Thus, it is important to select a topic and research questions that are suitable given time and financial constraints and accessibility of a setting and population.

What constitutes an important research topic and appropriate research questions? Besides identifying a topic that you would be interested in investigating, students should also consider a topic that will help initiate, revise, or clarify existing counseling theories (Berg & Lune, 2011). To do this, a thorough review of the counseling-related literature is necessary. Madison (2011) provided the following suggestions for developing research questions based on personal interests and a literature review:

- Reflect on what really interests you. Where in your daily personal and professional experiences do you notice missing information about individuals, settings, or social phenomena?

- Review the literature related to your topic of interest. Keep notes about phrases or places that interest you. Consider research in other areas besides counseling. Create an informal yet detailed list from the literature.

- Review your list and combine common phrases and settings to develop research questions. Are there factors that reflect gaps in the literature? Are there factors that could be expanded upon by additional research? Brainstorm possible research questions.

- Look over your list of possible research questions. Are there themes among your research questions? Create broad categories and group similar research questions. Omit research questions that are too similar or overlap. Create a topic sentence or a subject heading for each category.

- Review the broad categories, and then prioritize which research questions you are most interested in and which would be most realistic in a specified time frame.

- Consult with peers about your research questions for appropriateness and clarity (see Box 5.1).

After research questions have been selected, it is important to operationalize terms and concepts. Terms and phrases may have different meanings depending on who is reviewing a research study. For example, consider a qualitative study that is examining professional school counselors' perceptions of school environment factors that facilitate student success. A researcher would want to clearly define *student success* when developing research questions. How will student success be measured or evident? What would

---

**BOX 5.1    Developing your research questions.**

Generate a list of potential research questions and discuss them in small groups. Get feedback on your questions as you discuss the following:

- Do they seem clear?
- What type(s) of questions are you interested in investigating?
- Are the research questions flexible in case changes are made to the research design?
- Are the questions leading, or are they biased in that certain "answers" will be generated that may falsely support what you expect to find?

- Is there evidence of cultural or researcher bias in your research questions?
- How would you define each of the terms and concepts presented in the research questions?
- Are there additional or alternative research questions for the topic you are studying?
- How do you envision your research questions being "answered"? What answers do you hope to find?

© Cengage Learning

---

be considered a *school environment factor*? A clear definition of important terms and concepts will be helpful in data collection and analysis.

## Sample and Site Selection

Once the study's research problem has been established, counseling researchers must decide who should be included in the study. Qualitative researchers typically work with small samples of individuals. In selecting a sample, considerations must be given to defining the boundaries of a case (Hays & Singh, 2012). A case can represent the context to best study the research problem. Cases may involve settings, events, processes, and individuals. Often, the selection of individuals is based on the overall events and processes to be studied. That is, researchers are not typically interested in the sample, per se, but how the sample can help understand particular occurrences in a setting.

One of the strengths of qualitative research is that it allows for increasing the voices of people not typically acknowledged or topics that have been minimally addressed without concern for generalizability. Thus, during sample selection, generalizability is not the goal. The decision of how many individuals to include in a study is typically not made until some data have been collected and analyzed. Because qualitative inquiry is usually an inductive process, it is not necessary to know ahead of time how many participants are required to establish theory or solidify knowledge of a phenomenon. The ideal for counseling researchers is to continue to sample participants in a setting until no new information is present or refutes the findings of previous data, a process known as **saturation**. Unfortunately, researchers may not be able to achieve saturation when access to additional participants is difficult. Also, some topics may not require saturation to reach important conclusions.

For most research designs, selecting a site is a significant part of the research process. For a site to be a realistic option for counseling researchers: (a) entry should be possible; (b) there should be diverse participants or events within the setting to gather rich information; (c) trust among researchers and participants is possible; and (d) trustworthiness, or the study's validity, must be established (Marshall & Rossman, 2011). Selecting a site often involves negotiating entry through formal and informal gatekeepers, such as employers, managers, or principals. It is important to have backup sites in cases where entry becomes impossible.

Often, counseling researchers will have to present a tentative research plan of study before access to a setting may be allowed, especially if the topic is sensitive. It may be necessary to develop both a formal research proposal for any formal gatekeepers—including institutional review boards—as well as a lay summary for other individuals at a site. Madison (2011) and Marshall and Rossman (2011) identified several considerations to include in a research proposal and lay summary:

- State your tentative research questions. What has been written in the literature about the research topic? Why are these questions important to address?
- Describe who you are personally and professionally. Why are you interested in this topic? This setting?
- What do you see as your role in the research process?
- What type and amount of data will be collected? How will data be recorded and managed?
- How will you analyze data? How will participants and other individuals' voices be portrayed in data analysis? In the report?
- What is your timeline for conducting the research?
- How will you maintain an ethical research process?
- If applicable, what are some initial interview questions to be used for the study?
- Are there any data from pilot studies that have helped inform this study?

## The Role of the Researcher and Researcher Bias

Determining the role of the researcher in qualitative research often refers to the degree to which a researcher is involved in the study. This involvement includes the level of participation in the study, degree of deception or how much the researcher's role is revealed to the participants, amount of time spent in the setting, and the duration of the overall study. Often, the intensity of the researcher's role depends on how specific the study's focus is.

Because qualitative inquiry is typically an intensive process, researcher self-care is very important. Researchers should take time away from their studies because of the emotional costs of conducting intense investigations into individuals' lives. Research teams are an excellent resource for self-care, as researchers can discuss their thoughts and feelings with others about the topic or participants as the study progresses.

The role of the researcher is closely related to the concept of researcher bias. Researcher bias refers to how the researcher's worldview and presence in the study influences the research design. It involves any personal or professional perspectives that may positively or negatively affect data collection and analyses (Patton, 2002). Some factors that may influence a study include the researcher's background characteristics (e.g., race/ethnicity, gender, and age), experience and training related to a topic or research site, and personal connections to the topic, participants, and site.

Researcher bias can positively influence a study, such as in the following example. Consider a study in which a counseling researcher seeks to study how adolescents living with mental illness perceive the effectiveness of dialectical behavioral therapy (DBT). The fact that the researcher has extensive training and experience in DBT may be a positive factor in data collection, as the researcher would be able to ask follow-up questions that might relate to techniques used in DBT. Alternatively, a strong knowledge base in DBT might be considered a negative influence in a study if the researcher has a strong preference for DBT and asks questions or codes responses in a manner that makes the data "appear" that participants perceive it as highly effective. Whether researcher bias is considered positive or negative for a particular research design, it is important to include a description of how various researcher factors may have influenced a research study. Trustworthiness, discussed later in this chapter, includes ways negative researcher bias may be minimized to increase the validity of a study. It is essential to understand that this discussion of bias is related primarily to experimental sources of bias, but because the qualitative researcher is a human being acting as an instrument for data collection, one's cultural or power differential biases also need to be kept in check. This is a critical element of any auditing or trustworthiness analyses implemented to ensure the veracity and validity of data and interpretations. It also ensures the appropriate application of social justice and social action.

## Purposive Sampling

To understand sampling issues within qualitative research, it is essential to establish how sampling in qualitative research differs from quantitative research, both in purpose and in method. With quantitative research, the researcher uses probability sampling to make generalizations about the broader population from which the samples were drawn. To accomplish this purpose, researchers select random samples that represent the population from which they were drawn. In contrast, qualitative researchers typically do not engage in probability sampling; instead, they select purposive samples that will maximize their ability to investigate fully the selected research topic. Merriam (2002) makes the following distinction between random sampling and purposive sampling:

> To begin with, since you are not interested in "how much" or "how often," random sampling makes little sense. Instead, since qualitative inquiry seeks to understand the meaning of a phenomenon from the perspectives of the participants, it is important to select a sample from which most can be learned. This is called a purposive or purposeful sample. (p. 12)

Therefore, qualitative researchers attempt to enlist participants who can provide maximum insight and understanding of the topic under investigation (Ary, Jacobs, Sorensen, & Walker, 2013). Polkinghorne (2005) suggested that qualitative researchers avoid using the term *sample* and instead call the process **purposive selection**. He goes on to state that in qualitative research, the unit of analysis is the experience rather than the individual or group itself.

There are several variations of purposive selection. The method of participant selection, as well as the number of participants, varies according to the nature of the research problem and the particular qualitative approach used to study the problem. Although the number of participants included in a qualitative study tends to be smaller than the number included in a quantitative study, sample size can vary from one individual (e.g., case study approach) to several individuals (e.g., phenomenology) and several focus groups (e.g., basic interpretive approach). In addition, Guba and Lincoln (2005) remind us that the primary criterion of sample size involves redundancy of information rather than a specific number of participants; that is, sampling should be terminated when no new information is forthcoming. Several authors (e.g., Ary et al., 2013; Guba & Lincoln, 2005; Polkinghorne, 2005) have described various forms of purposive sampling, including comprehensive sampling; theoretical sampling; snowball, chain, or network sampling; maximum variation sampling; homogeneous sampling; typical case sampling; extreme or deviant sampling; critical case sampling; criterion sampling; and convenience sampling.

### Comprehensive Sampling

*Comprehensive sampling* is feasible only when the number of units is small because every unit is included in the study. For example, if a researcher wanted to study the experiences of families who care for children with a specific, rare disability, such as Klinefelter syndrome, he may want to select all families in a targeted geographic area that meet the criterion.

### Theoretical Sampling

In **theoretical sampling**, the researcher continues to select new participants throughout the research process as the evolving theory emerges. Sampling continues until no new information surfaces, at which point data saturation has occurred. Participants are selected based on the concepts that have theoretical relevance to the evolving theory (Corbin & Strauss, 2007). The process of collecting data, analyzing data, and then selecting additional participants until the description is comprehensive is called **purposive-iterative sampling**. Theoretical sampling may be appropriate for a study that seeks to establish a theory on how counselor trainees select a counseling orientation (e.g., Gestalt, solution-focused, psychodynamic). Participants could include individuals at various points of their training who identify with different theoretical orientations. Data would be collected until a clear understanding has emerged about which factors or processes lead to identification with a particular orientation.

### Snowball, Chain, or Network Sampling

With snowballing, the initially selected participants suggest names of other participants who would be appropriate for the study. This process produces a pool of potential participants. These new participants can, in turn, provide names of other potential participants. *Snowball sampling* is often an appropriate method for sampling participants who are difficult to obtain, such as in the following case. Consider that you want to study gang experiences among young adults of various cultures. Once access has been allowed to gather data from one individual, that individual could connect you with others who might want to tell their stories related to gang membership.

### Maximum Variation Sampling

In some studies, researchers are interested in learning about how a phenomenon is experienced by a divergent group of participants. For example, a researcher may want to know how first-year counseling students experience their initial contact with clients. Using **maximum variation sampling**, the researcher may choose to interview participants who vary in age, race, gender, and other factors. The goal of maximum variation sampling is to explore differences and commonalities across participants, with a particular interest in searching for those who might "think differently" from other participants, thus getting a broad range of perspectives and experiences and constantly look for cases that might dispute present findings.

### Homogeneous Sampling

In contrast to maximum variation sampling, **homogeneous sampling** refers to purposefully selecting participants "from a particular subgroup whose experience is suspected to be somewhat alike; for example, first-year students at a particular college whose parents are non-English speaking" (Polkinghorne, 2005, p. 141). The purpose of homogeneous sampling is to describe the experience of the subgroup in depth. Another example might be examining the experiences of newly immigrated Cuban Americans in career counseling.

### Typical Case Sampling

*Typical case sampling* involves selecting participants whose experience is typical of the one under study. For example, a researcher may want to explore the experiences of college students who reported having negative experiences at a university counseling center. Another example would be investigating the coping strategies of women who have recently experienced a miscarriage.

### Extreme or Deviant Sampling

The purpose of *extreme sampling* or **deviant sampling** is to select participants whose experiences were the most positive or most negative, thereby helping researchers discover the "boundaries of differences within an experience" (Polkinghorne, 2005, p. 141). For example, suppose that you want to evaluate a training seminar on counseling racial/ethnic minorities. You might seek out participants who rated the experience both high (i.e., seminar was extremely helpful) and low (i.e., seminar was not helpful at all) and interview them in depth to understand the boundaries of the experience.

### Critical Case Sampling

Researchers who use **critical case sampling** are looking for experiences that are particularly significant because of their intensity or irregularity. The cases are selected because the researcher believes that they can be used to illustrate a point particularly well. For example, consider a historical analysis of hate crimes against transgender individuals. A researcher may want to select a particular incident that was highly intense (e.g., murder and sexual assault of Brandon Teena, a female-to-male transgender person) and analyze documents and interview participants who were associated with the event in some manner.

### Criterion Sampling

In **criterion sampling**, participants are selected who meet an important, predetermined criterion. For example, a researcher studying the experiences of racial identity development among counselor education students who have taken a multicultural counseling course would select only participants who had completed the course.

### Convenience Sampling

As with quantitative research, samples of convenience are the least desirable types of samples. *Convenience samples* are chosen based on availability or ease of access. Although the process may be expedient, using samples of convenience reduces the credibility of the research investigation. Many of the preceding sampling methods could also be considered convenience samples.

## Data Collection Methods and Data Management

There is no single method of collecting data for qualitative research studies. Instead, the researcher needs to determine what types of data will contribute the most to understanding the phenomenon under investigation. The researcher chooses data sources that are the most likely to inform him or her about the nature of the experience being explored (Polkinghorne, 2005). The three most widely used methods of data collection in qualitative research are interviewing, observation, and document analysis.

### Interviewing

Many qualitative approaches use **interviewing** as the primary method of data collection. Interviews are used to get information about participants' opinions, thoughts, and feelings about the phenomenon under investigation (Ary et al., 2013). They also can be used to verify information collected in other ways, such as through observation or document analysis.

Interviews can be conducted with individuals, dyads, or groups, with most interviews being one to one or dyadic (Polkinghorne, 2005). The degree to which interviews are structured varies, depending on the researcher's purpose. At one end of the spectrum is the **structured interview**, in which the researcher plans all questions in advance. Each participant is asked the same set of questions, often in the same sequence. At the other end of the spectrum is the unstructured interview, in which the questions are prompted by the flow of the interview (Gay, Mills, & Airasian, 2011). An **unstructured interview** can resemble casual conversation with a purpose. Between these two extremes is the **semistructured interview**. Researchers who are using semistructured interviews formulate their questions in advance but may modify the format as the interview progresses (Ary et al., 2013; Erford, 2013). One of the hallmarks of all types of interviews is the use of open-ended questions through which the researcher is interested in gaining a rich account of the participant's experience.

There are several types of interview questions, and the type(s) you ask will depend on how structured your interview is, as well as the type of research questions you are interested in addressing. Patton (2002) outlined six categories of interview questions:

- *Behavior or experience questions.* These questions seek to address specific actions or behaviors of the participants, as well as their reflections on the actions (i.e., experience). With these questions, researchers are trying to gather more information about specific behaviors and experiences rather than understanding *why* they occur.
- *Opinion or value questions.* These questions are focused on understanding *why* certain phenomena occur. Opinion questions involve soliciting individual beliefs, whereas value questions attempt to understand social norms around particular values and beliefs.
- *Feeling questions.* Researchers may use interview questions that obtain information about how participants feel about a phenomenon. The goal with these questions is not to get at the truth or validity of the phenomenon but to identify interviewees' affective reactions to the phenomenon.
- *Knowledge questions.* This type of interview question seeks to understand the amount of knowledge participants have about a phenomenon as well as the origins of their knowledge.
- *Sensory questions.* Researchers may want to increase their insight into how phenomena affect participants' bodily senses. How do they see, hear, taste, smell, or touch in ways that are different when the phenomenon is occurring?
- *Background or demographic questions.* These questions allow researchers to gather concrete information about participants and settings. Responses are often helpful in thoroughly describing the participants, settings, and phenomena.

A common method for conducting individual interviews is Siedman's (2006) three-interview series protocol. Over the course of three interviews, counseling researchers deepen their knowledge of a phenomenon as participants describe the overall context, as well as details related to a phenomenon, and reflect on the meaning of a particular experience. Each interview would begin with an interview prompt outlined by Seidman. Additional interview questions may be asked to gather more information for these prompts.

Consider a study that is investigating high school students' experiences with a recent hate crime against a peer who self-identified as gay. For the first interview, the researcher would seek a focused life history with the students and may ask, "Tell me as much as possible about yourself in relation to the experience of the hate crime." The second interview would involve details of the students' experiences with the hate crime. An interview prompt might be, "Tell me the specific responses you had to the hate crime and the details of those responses." The third interview would involve reflection on the meaning of the hate crime for the participants and setting: "Given what you said about your life in relation to the recent hate crime, how do you understand that hate crime today?"

A specific type of group interview is the **focus group**, which typically consists of 7–12 members who can provide insight about a particular issue. Focus groups are basically group interviews that allow participants to interact with and expand upon the themes and content of other participants' comments. Focus groups are economical and often promote deep exploration of a topic. Nagle and Williams (2013) proposed a five-step model for conducting focus groups: study purpose, methodology, facilitation, analysis, and reporting. Purposes of a focus group study might involve exploration of an issue, determining preferred activities when developing a program, collecting in-depth research data, or evaluating the worth of a program. Focus group methodology involves conceptualizing the study (population, sample size and selection, selecting about five open-ended questions) and logistics (meeting venue, schedule, and myriad details of the encounter). Facilitation is the actual facilitator preparation prior to and implementation during the focus group encounter. Nagle and Williams provided a number of helpful tips for facilitating a focus group. Finally, the focus group member responses are analyzed and the report drafted. As an example, focus groups could be conducted with middle school and high school students to gain understanding about adolescents' outcome expectations with regard to taking higher level math and science courses. Researchers who are using focus groups note the responses of group members as well as interactions within the group itself. Often, two trained members of a research team conduct the focus group: a moderator who leads the interview process and a scribe who records observations of group members' behaviors.

Whether leading group interviews or individual interviews, interviewers need to be skilled in several areas. In many ways, these skills are similar to those held by professional counselors. Interviewers must be excellent listeners who can build rapport and establish a trusting relationship in which participants feel comfortable responding truthfully and openly. Gay et al. (2011, p. 420) suggested the following actions to help interviewers improve communication and facilitate the collection of data:

- Listen more and talk less.
- Follow up on what participants say and ask questions when you don't understand.
- Avoid leading questions; ask open-ended questions.
- Don't interrupt. Learn how to wait.
- Keep participants focused and ask for concrete details.
- Tolerate silence.
- Do not be judgmental about participants' views or beliefs; keep a neutral demeanor. Your purpose is to learn about others' perspectives whether you agree with them or not.
- Don't debate with participants over their responses.

Typically, interviews are audiotaped or videotaped and transcribed afterward. Although some researchers take notes during the interview, taking notes can be distracting and can affect the flow of the interview. Transcription can be tedious, but taping and transcribing help maintain the trustworthiness of the research study.

## Observation

Another form of qualitative data collection is **observation**, in which the researcher watches participants in a natural setting and documents what occurs. Observation frequently takes place over an extended period of time, with the goal of providing a complete description of participants' behavior in a specific environment. The researcher often documents observations in narrative form, describing the particular setting, behaviors, and interactions observed (Ary et al., 2013; Erford, 2013). In many cases, observation is used to supplement and clarify data collected from participant interviews (Polkinghorne, 2005).

The researcher's role as observer can range from that of fully participating in the events or group being studied to that of completely observing without participating at all. Participant observation occurs when the observer becomes part of the situation. When the observation is covert, the researcher becomes part of the group under study without revealing one's role to the group. In other cases, the researcher may actively participate in the group, but the group is aware that the researcher is conducting an investigation. At other times, researchers may act as complete observers, which means that they observe from a distance so that their presence is not noticeable to the participants (Ary et al., 2013).

The researcher needs to take several things into account when selecting methods of observation. First and foremost, it is imperative to protect the rights, dignity, and privacy of the participants under observation. When researchers are associated with a college or university, a proposal documenting plans for collecting data must be submitted to the school's institutional review board (IRB), which is mandated to ensure that research is conducted in a way that protects the rights of human participants.

Ary et al. (2013) described three additional concerns that researchers must keep in mind when making decisions about their degree of participation in collecting observational data. One concern is that of **observer effect**, which refers to the impact of the observer on the participants. When people know they are being watched, they may exhibit different behaviors than they would exhibit otherwise. Another concern is that of **observer expectation**, which occurs when the researcher's knowledge about the participants leads the researcher to expect certain behaviors. For example, a researcher who is studying ways people diagnosed with borderline personality disorder manage stress may have preconceived expectations about how the individuals in the study will respond to stressful situations. A final concern is that of **observer bias**. Observer bias occurs when the observer's personal attitudes and values affect either the observation or the researcher's interpretation of the observation. Observer bias is also an example of researcher bias, described earlier in the chapter.

## Documents

In addition to interviews and observation, documentary evidence can be used as a rich source of data for qualitative researchers. **Documentary evidence** can include written, oral, visual, or cultural artifacts. Merriam (2002) outlined four categories of documentary evidence:

- *Public records* may include documents such as federal reports, agency reports, journals, and various archival records.

- *Personal documents* may include first-person narratives such as journals, autobiographies, home videos, and scrapbooks. Personal documents, which document individual beliefs and perspectives, tend to be more subjective than public records.

- *Physical materials* may include paintings, photographs, and a range of materials that relate to the topic under investigation.
- *Researcher-generated documents* are produced by or for the researcher. For example, a researcher may ask participants to keep a journal for the duration of the study.

Investigators who use documents in their research are responsible for establishing the authenticity of the documents being analyzed. Also, it is important to note whether the document is a primary source, which means that the document was written by someone who has experienced the phenomenon under investigation firsthand. Diaries, autobiographies, and letters are considered primary sources. Secondary sources, which also can be used in qualitative studies, represent secondhand descriptions and are written by people who have not directly experienced the phenomenon.

Interviews, observation, and document analysis represent three of the main types of data collection in qualitative research. Researchers may use a single method of data collection or multiple methods. Effective qualitative research is characterized by carefully selecting the method, or methods, of data collection most likely to yield the greatest amount of trustworthy information about the topic under investigation.

### Data Management: Contact Sheets and Document Summary Forms

Whether you are considering interviewing, observation, or document analysis, data management should begin early in the data collection process. Good data management ensures high-quality accessibility to data, documentation of any analysis, and proper storage and protection of data after a study is complete (Berg & Lune, 2011). Two helpful data management tools during data collection are contact sheets and document summary forms. These have a dual purpose of organizing information about data sources and research settings as well as serving as a source of data in itself to be analyzed.

A **contact sheet** is usually a one-page summary of questions or reflections from a single contact with a case. Contact sheets are used in conjunction with fieldwork to help the researcher reflect between data collections and present salient themes from an interview or observation as well as outline additional questions that need to be addressed in future contacts. Contact sheets should be completed shortly after a specific data collection so that the researcher does not forget helpful information and emerging themes about the research problem.

Miles and Huberman (1994) suggested several facets to include on a contact sheet:

- identifying information about the contact (i.e., date, setting, and method of contact, who or what was the subject of the contact, when contact was made, when contact sheet was completed); this information should appear at the top of the contact sheet
- important issues and themes that either seem salient for the researcher or were most focused on during the contact
- individuals, events, or situations (processes) involved in the setting
- brief responses to interview questions
- new or additional questions to be considered for the next contact.

During a contact, researchers may find themselves collecting various documents. These may include literature such as meeting agendas, newspaper or newsletter articles, brochures, and other public records. Given that there is a potential to collect multiple documents, it is a good idea to organize these documents to prioritize them for data analysis. **Document summary forms** are summary sheets that put a document into context. The format for the summaries can vary depending on what is most helpful for a study; it should contain space to write brief comments summarizing the document, explaining its significance to the overall study or to a specific contact. If a specific document is significant to a particular contact, it may be helpful to attach the document to a contact sheet (Miles & Huberman, 1994).

### Data Management: Data Displays

Another data management tool involves creating and revising **data displays**. The purpose of data displays is to present data in an organized manner to connect it to the various stages of analysis. These displays may involve a table of themes, summaries of codes with corresponding descriptions, or reduced data in later stages of data analysis. Two major families of data displays are matrices and networks. Matrices present data from a case in a row and column table format. Networks involve nodes that connect to each other to show clear relationships between concepts. Researchers should exercise caution and not "count too soon" or reduce data early on in a study. Thus, initial data displays should begin with several details about the participant, setting, and phenomenon and become reduced or refined throughout data analysis.

Data displays may be created for individual data sources or comparison across data sources. Within-case displays present information for a particular case, whereas cross-case displays allow for an increased understanding of a phenomenon across several cases. For example, a counseling researcher may be interested in factors that promote counseling satisfaction among survivors of suicide. A within-case display would present an individual's data about his experience in counseling after surviving a suicide. A cross-case display of the same study might present data from several individuals to better understand common factors that promote counseling satisfaction among the sample. Although qualitative research generally does not have the goal of generalizability, cross-case displays may be helpful to assist researchers describe and explain phenomena thoroughly.

Miles and Huberman (1994) presented several types of data displays that may be used for within- and cross-case displays. To illustrate how each display may be useful in managing data, consider them in the context of a study exploring factors that facilitate racial identity development among counselor trainees:

- *Partially ordered displays.* These displays are useful in exploratory studies with a purpose of describing what is happening in a setting. An example of a partially ordered display for the racial identity study might be a chart that highlights the relationships between classroom dynamics within a multicultural counseling course around the topic of racial identity.
- *Time-ordered displays.* Time-ordered displays are helpful in describing the flow or sequences of events or processes for an individual. For the racial identity study, data describing events that facilitate counselor trainees' racial identity development could be presented.
- *Role-ordered displays.* These graphic displays present information in rows and columns that have been gathered from various individuals in a setting. For instance, data from counselor educators and counselor trainees on their perceptions of the racial identity development process could be presented in a table format.
- *Conceptually ordered displays.* These displays are helpful for managing data in later stages of analysis in a way that brings data that "belong together" conceptually. For example, refined codes that explain racial identity development among counselor trainees could be presented with brief descriptions of events, processes, and individuals' characteristics.

## BOX 5.2    Example of an initial coding.

| Statement | Initial Coding |
|---|---|
| 1 My son, Barry, went through a really tough time about, probably started at the end of fifth grade and went into sixth grade. | 1 MIDDLE-SCHOOL HELL |
| 2 When he was growing up young in school, he was a people pleaser and his teachers loved him to death. | 2 TEACHER'S PET |
| 3 Two boys, in particular, whom he chose to try to emulate, wouldn't, were not very good for him. | 3 BAD INFLUENCES |
| 4 They were very critical of him, they put him down all the time, and he kind of just took that and really kind of internalized it, I think, for a long time. | 4 TWEEN ANGST |
| 5 In that time period, in the fifth grade, early sixth grade, they really just kind of shunned him all together, and so his network as he knew it was gone. | 5 THE LOST BOY |

*Source:* From Saldana, 2013, p. 4.

The reader is encouraged to review Miles and Huberman's classic text (1994) for examples and more information on data displays. Box 5.2 provides a basic example of an initial coding display.

## Trustworthiness

In qualitative research, the soundness of the research is evaluated by its **trustworthiness**. Guba and Lincoln (2005) stated that trustworthiness in qualitative research refers to the investigation's credibility, transferability, dependability, and confirmability. In other words, qualitative researchers seek trustworthiness in terms of truth value, applicability, consistency, and neutrality as opposed to reliability and validity. **Truth value** pertains to the question "How can one establish confidence in the 'truth' of the findings of a particular inquiry for the respondents with which and the context in which the inquiry was carried out?" (p. 290). **Applicability** refers to the extent to which the findings of an inquiry are applicable in other contexts (settings) and with other respondents (participants). **Consistency** pertains to questions about the replication and repetition of themes if the method of inquiry were applied with the same or similar research participants. **Neutrality** pertains to the question asked by many critics of qualitative research: How can one establish that the findings of the research are genuinely a reflection of the participants being studied and not merely a reflection of the researchers' biases, motivations, interests, or perspectives?

Guba and Lincoln (2005) constructed three questions that help determine trustworthiness in qualitative research: (a) Do conclusions of this investigation make sense? (b) Do conclusions sufficiently describe the information received from the participants? and (c) Do conclusions accurately represent the study at hand?

Because most qualitative data are collected and interpreted in a subjective manner, counseling researchers who are engaging in qualitative inquiry are challenged to reflect on how their conclusions "might be wrong" (Maxwell, 2005). In particular, counseling researchers must address specific validity threats to establish the trustworthiness of their study. Validity threats may be a part of all aspects of research design, including data collection methods, data sources, researcher bias, research questions, study goals, and guiding research paradigms.

As Guba and Lincoln (2005) and numerous other qualitative researchers intended, guidelines and specific methods have been established to ensure the trustworthiness of qualitative inquiry and ultimately strengthen the study's credibility, transferability, dependability, and confirmability (Denzin & Lincoln, 2011).

## Credibility

**Credibility** involves demonstrating the "believability" and assurance that conclusions make sense in a qualitative inquiry (Glense, 2010). Guba and Lincoln (2005) offered five major techniques that can be used to help ensure the credibility of findings.

- *Prolonged engagement, persistent observations, and triangulation.* **Prolonged engagement** infers that the researcher invests enough time to establish trust with participants and eventually learn about the culture, climate, and socialization process inherent in human nature and the phenomena under investigation. Whereas "prolonged engagement offers scope, persistent observation provides depth" (Guba & Lincoln, 2005, p. 304). As such, **persistent observation** entails accessing multiple opportunities for the researcher to identify characteristics within various situations that are most relevant to the phenomenon under investigation. As mentioned earlier in this chapter, **triangulation** is the use of multiple and different sources, methods, investigators, and theories to gather information that is pertinent to the study and the participants and that can be used to support assertions and interpretations of the researcher (Ary et al., 2013; Denzin, 2009).

- *Consultation with a peer debriefer* serves the purpose of providing an external check on the inquiry process and researchers' interpretations.

- *Negative case analysis*, or revising hypotheses in hindsight, refers to refining the working hypothesis as more and more information becomes available until the hypothesis accounts for all known cases without any exceptions.

- *Referential adequacy* involves checking preliminary findings and interpretations against archived raw data, previous literature, and existing research to explore alternative explanations for findings as they emerge. This can also lead to searching for rival hypotheses or different interpretations of findings based on existing knowledge regarding the phenomenon at hand. Peer and expert consultants can be used to assist in this process (Creswell, 2012).

- *Member checking.* **Member checking** involves ongoing consultation with participants of the investigation as a means to offer a direct test of the goodness of fit of findings and interpretations as they emerge. This serves as a "direct test of findings and interpretations with the human sources from which they have come" (Guba & Lincoln, 2005, p. 300).

## Transferability

Gay et al. (2011) defined **transferability** as the degree to which the results could be generalized to other contexts and settings. Many naturalists, however, believe that transferability in qualitative research is very different from the concepts of external validity or generalizability (Guba & Lincoln, 2005). Thus, the charge for a qualitative researcher is to "provide only the thick description necessary to enable someone interested in making a transfer to reach a conclusion about whether transfer can be contemplated as a possibility" (p. 316). Therefore, qualitative researchers are encouraged to provide as many details and the widest range of information possible for inclusion in their interpretations of data and final reports of findings. Rich descriptions of the contexts in which interviews and observations take place, details about the process that unfolds throughout each interaction with participants, in-depth descriptions of participants (participant profiles), and the specific steps that researchers take while collecting, interpreting, and reporting the data (reflexive journals or memos) are just a few of the ways that researchers can offer a complete account of the research process.

### Dependability

According to Guba and Lincoln (2005), **dependability** involves the consistency of the results over time and across researchers. Although the dependability of a given study is seemingly inextricably linked with the credibility of the study, qualitative researchers are encouraged to employ steps to establish the dependability of findings that go above and beyond those employed to establish the study's credibility. Consultation with a different or new peer debriefer throughout the analysis and interpretation of data can be a valuable way to add to the dependability of findings. Likewise, the utilization of research teams or multiple researchers who overlap one another or use similar methods of collecting and analyzing the data can enhance the dependability of findings. For example, a counselor educator developed a model for training counselors to train teachers to identify and report suspected child abuse. Both the counselor educator and another qualitative researcher, who was a teacher educator, conducted a study to analyze the model. Although the counselor educator and teacher educator had very different perceptions of the model and the findings, when they synthesized the results of their data analysis, the final product was much more comprehensive and credible. Finally, qualitative researchers are encouraged to employ the services of an auditor who can explore the researchers' reflective journaling throughout the process of data collection and analysis as well as at the end of the final report to ascertain whether or not the results of the investigation are dependable.

### Confirmability

**Confirmability** assumes that the findings of the study were genuinely reflective of the participants' perspectives within the context of their natural environment. As such, confirmability directly addresses whether the researcher's biases and subjectivity interfered with data collection and analysis as well as the researcher's ongoing interpretations and final report. In terms of researcher bias, Creswell (2013) encouraged researchers to clarify their opinions, current life circumstance, and any potential biases or assumptions that might have an impact on the inquiry from the onset and throughout data collection and analysis. Accordingly, it would behoove qualitative researchers to state their perceptions regarding the following issues prior to the initiation of the investigation:

- Discuss their personal and professional motives and reasons for conducting the study at hand.
- Describe any personal or professional affiliations with the participants and/or the phenomena to be investigated.
- State any biases or assumptions that they have about the phenomena at hand.
- Based on their theoretical sensitivity (Glaser, 1978) regarding participants and the phenomena to be explored, describe what they think they might find. What does the researcher expect to find as a result of this investigation?
- Explore how the researchers' initial thoughts, feelings, and behaviors might interfere with the research process.

As discussed earlier in this chapter, the researcher is encouraged to keep an ongoing reflexive journal and audit trail throughout the duration of the investigation so that peer debriefers, peer consultants, and expert consultants can continue to explore how the researchers' biases may or may not interfere with the research process and findings (Merchant, 1997). Peer debriefers, peer consultants, and expert consultants are also encouraged to explore rival or alternative explanations for the researchers' findings. Likewise, researchers are encouraged to review their own reflexive journal and audit trail to explore how their own insights might interfere or contribute to data collection and analysis (Glense, 2010).

# Conclusion

Qualitative approaches are increasingly becoming a part of the counseling profession. Multiple phenomena that affect counseling practice and that have remained largely unexplored as well as the "voices" of understudied populations are well suited for this type of research. In this chapter, various aspects of designing, implementing, and establishing the validity of qualitative research were presented. These included understanding how qualitative research is distinct from quantitative research, identifying the research problem, selecting a population and entering a site, determining the researcher's role, selecting sampling and data collection methods, and establishing trustworthiness. Active self-reflection and peer consultation are extremely important if a counseling researcher decides to use a qualitative approach. Thus, researchers should collaborate with others throughout all phases of a qualitative study to ensure that the study itself and findings are appropriate, meaningful, and ethical for all those involved.

*Now go to the Student Workbook found on cengagebrain.com that accompanies this text for additional application and review activities.*

# Qualitative Research Designs

This chapter provides an overview of types of qualitative research, with a focus on five of the more commonly used research designs in qualitative inquiry: ethnographic, case study, phenomenological, grounded theory, and consensual qualitative research designs. In discussion of each of these designs, steps and strategies are highlighted to illustrate aspects of a specific design. Examples are provided to show how data methods, analyses, and trustworthiness, discussed in Chapter 5, correspond to each research design. It is essential to understand from the very start of this chapter that qualitative models require more depth in content for adequate description of the phenomenon under study and to describe in detail the development of the conceptualization process. Qualitative research is a very time-intensive endeavor.

# Types of Qualitative Research

Several different types of qualitative research, or "strategies of inquiry" (Denzin & Lincoln, 2011), are used in social science research, including ethnographic research, case study method, phenomenological research, grounded theory, participatory action research, historical research, narrative research, and consensual qualitative research. A generic term that is sometimes used to classify these various approaches is **interpretive research** (Gay, Mills, & Airasian, 2011). A brief description of each approach is presented in Table 6.1. In this chapter, the focus is on five

**TABLE 6.1**   Types and descriptions of qualitative research.

| Qualitative Research Approach | Key Characteristics |
|---|---|
| Ethnography | Purpose is to describe the cultural characteristics of a group in its natural setting. Immersion in the site is important. Disciplinary roots are in anthropology. |
| Case Study | Purpose is to address research questions by describing one or more cases, or "bounded systems," in depth. Uses multiple data collection techniques to examine the particular unit of study. Its multidisciplinary roots are in medicine, law, business, education, and social sciences. |
| Phenomenology | Purpose is to determine the meaning, structure, or essence of a particular phenomenon as experienced by an individual or by many individuals. Researchers conduct in-depth interviews with participants to understand the essence of the experience. Disciplinary roots are in philosophy. |
| Grounded Theory | Purpose is to generate theory based on the data collected about a particular phenomenon. Grounded theorists systematically collect data, identify categories found in the data, connect those categories, and use the resulting information to inductively form a theory. Disciplinary roots are in sociology. |
| Historical | Purpose is to systematically examine events that occurred in the past. Its focus is interpretive, and it involves a fluid, dynamic account of past events based on the examination of artifacts and written documents. Disciplinary roots are in history. |
| Narrative | Purpose is to study how different people experience the world around them by asking participants to tell about their lives (personal narratives). The researcher collaboratively constructs a written account about the participant's experiences and the meanings that are attributed to the experiences. Multidisciplinary roots are in literature, history, art, psychology, anthropology, and other fields. |
| Symbolic Interactionism | Purpose is to examine the interpretive processes people use in their interactions. Researchers are interested in common sets of symbols and understandings that provide meaning to people's interactions. Disciplinary roots are in social psychology. |
| Consensual Qualitative Research | Purpose is to conduct in-depth studies of the inner experiences of individuals. This relatively new approach incorporates elements from phenomenology, grounded theory, and other approaches. It involves rigorous methods that allow researchers to examine data and come to a consensus about their meaning (see Hill et al., 2005). |
| Participatory Action Research | Purpose is for the researcher and the participants to elevate critical consciousness and to promote change in the lives of the group or community involved. Researchers and participants collaboratively develop goals and methods, participate in gathering and analyzing data, and then implement results to produce change (see Kidd & Kral, 2005). |

of the more commonly used approaches: ethnographic research, case study research, phenomenological research, grounded theory, and consensual qualitative research.

## Ethnographic Research

Ethnographic research, also referred to as ethnography, is one of the most established and frequently used approaches to qualitative research (Gay et al., 2011). **Ethnography** comes from the Greek word *ethnos*, which refers to "a people" or "cultural group" (Patton, 2002). Ethnographic research, in turn, involves an in-depth study of naturally occurring behavior within a particular cultural group. Ethnography includes both the process of studying a cultural group and the end product of the research (Ary, Jacobs, Sorensen, & Walker, 2013).

### What Is Ethnographic Research?

Ethnographic research has its origins in the field of anthropology and is frequently associated with that discipline. The purpose of ethnographic research is to describe, analyze, and interpret a cultural group's collective patterns of behavior, beliefs, and language (Creswell, 2013). Examples of parameters that may identify a particular cultural group include geography, religion, ethnicity, and shared experiences. For example, parents of children with disabilities may represent a cultural group based on a shared experience. Another example involving a study of a mental health advocacy organization may represent a cultural group based on patterns of behavior, beliefs, and language (see Box 6.1). Ethnographic researchers document people's lives and activities to understand their experiences from their personal perspectives and interpret their behavior as it is shaped by social contexts (Mertens, 2004). Ethnography is oriented toward the study of meaning as structured by a particular cultural group and involves placement, events, and encounters in a more meaningful context (Tedlock, 2011).

Ethnography, in the tradition of anthropology, is characterized by intensive fieldwork (Patton, 2002). Ethnographers spend extensive time at a site, with the amount of time varying from several months to over a year. Ethnographers typically take on the role of **participant observer**, which means that they are participants in the interactions and in the communities that they study (Suzuki, Ahluwalia, Mattis, & Quizo, 2005). Ethnographers typically enter their sites with no a priori hypotheses; instead, hypotheses evolve throughout the course of the fieldwork and data analysis (Ary et al., 2013). While at the sites, ethnographers collect large volumes of material, including field notes, artifacts, audiotapes, and videotapes. In addition, they use multiple data sources and multiple means of data collection. As with other types of qualitative research, ethnographic data collection involves unstructured and semistructured interviews, observation, and archival review.

The primary characteristics of ethnography are depicted in Table 6.2. Many of these characteristics are shared with other qualitative approaches, although some are unique to ethnographic research.

### Conducting Ethnographic Research

In many respects, ethnography represents the most complex of all research methods (Fraenkel, Wallen, & Hyun, 2011). No single method or set of methods can describe the ethnographic research process. However, although the specific methodological procedures selected by ethnographers are often unique to any given research project, there are some common steps that are typically applicable to ethnography (also see Box 6.2). These steps include the following:

1. *Selecting a topic.* As with any research project, topic selection can stem from several sources. Studies may emerge out of a researcher's predetermined interests, out of

## BOX 6.1    Ethnography example: The substance of a support group.

This ethnographic study explored the influence, content, and process of a support group for families of children with mental health needs. The researcher spent two and a half years with the support group to understand its culture and the shared experience of its members.

Using a purposive sampling method (e.g., criterion sampling and critical case sampling), 35 participants were involved in the support group, all of whom were parents of special needs children. The support group held meetings once per month for approximately two hours. The researcher was a participant observer and recorded field notes for 25 support group sessions. After observations and field notes were complete, the researcher conducted 12 semistructured interviews with key informants and stakeholders in the advocacy organization that coordinated the support group.

The researcher analyzed data throughout various points of writing field notes, reviewing interview transcripts, and analyzing other documents generated by the group members. Data analysis was both deductive (i.e., using a priori codes from the literature) and inductive (i.e., existing theory open to revisions based on data). The researcher recorded reflexive notes during data collection. Results described the "culture" of the support group to better understand group content

and process as well as benefits and challenges for the group members. Findings highlighted four major themes of symbols, language, narratives or stories, and practices. Further, the description of the support group provided implications for fostering "cultures of inclusion" among families, children, and caregivers.

The researcher used several strategies to increase the study's trustworthiness:

- *Prolonged engagement* and *persistent observation*, as evidenced by the researcher spending two and a half years in the culture as a participant observer.
- *Triangulation* of data collection methods (i.e., observations with extensive field notes, interviews, and group documents), data sources (participants were of diverse backgrounds), and researchers (assistants were used for consensus coding).
- *Thick description* of the participants and results was provided.
- The researcher kept *reflexive notes* and compared analysis with those of assistants, which are methods for minimizing researcher bias.
- The researcher created an *audit trail*.

*Source:* Mohr, 2003.

## TABLE 6.2    Characteristics of ethnographic research.

Ethnographic research:

- Is conducted in a natural setting
- Involves intimate, face-to-face interactions with participants
- Involves extended time at a site (often a year or more)
- Focuses on a particular cultural group
- Presents an accurate reflection of participants' perspectives and behaviors
- Involves data collection from multiple sources, including interviews, conversations, observations, and documents
- Uses an unstructured approach to data gathering in the early stages so that key issues can emerge gradually through analysis
- Provides a "thick description" (i.e., describing what was seen and heard in great detail)
- Uses local language and terminology to describe behavior
- Does not attempt to eliminate the effects of the researcher

**BOX 6.2    Ethnography example: Client experience of gender in therapeutic relationships: An interpretive ethnography.**

The purpose of this ethnographic study was to understand shared client experiences of gender in therapy. The primary research questions of this study involved understanding how clients interpret how counselor–client gender dynamics influence therapeutic process and outcome.

A criterion sampling method was used to identify participants with at least six therapy sessions with both a female and male counselor. The study included 15 participants (seven female and eight male) ranging in age from 13 to 53 years. Researchers attempted to have minimal influence on the participants' responses by using unstructured, collaborative interviews. The interview process involved five phases in which participants provided interpretations without researcher input as well as clarification of findings throughout the study.

Results indicated six themes related to clients' experiences of gender in therapeutic relationships. These themes involved client–therapist connection, gender differences in therapy style, types of topics discussed based on comfort level with a particular gender, perceptions of counselors' effectiveness based on their gender, and how personality influenced their interpretation of the role of gender in counseling.

Some methods to establish trustworthiness included:

- *Bracketing* of researchers' influence on data collection and analysis.

- Participants with several counseling experiences were selected (*transferability*).

- *Member checking* was established throughout data collection and analysis.

- *Triangulation* of data sources (participants of diverse backgrounds).

- Multiple researchers of different genders, a triangulation method, were used to conduct interviews and consensus code. This served to minimize the effect of the researcher and minimize researcher bias in data analysis.

- *Thick description* of data sources and results are provided.

*Source:* Gehart & Lyle, 2001.

collaborative dialogues with members of the cultural group being studied, or through commissions by institutions that are interested in investigating a particular aspect of community life (Suzuki et al., 2005). It is important for researchers to engage in self-reflection during the process of topic selection. Researchers need to question their motivations for studying a particular topic. Questions such as Why this place? Why this community? Why these people? and What cultural perspectives or biases do I bring to the process? are among those that ethnographers use to guide their decision making.

2. *Accessing and entering a site.* Finding a setting that is conducive to ethnographic research can be a challenging task. Not only is it important for the individuals in the specified cultural group to be open to being observed and/or interviewed, it is also vital that the information gathered is trustworthy. A number of factors may help or hinder the researcher's ability to develop a productive working alliance at a particular site, including one's personal characteristics (e.g., gender, social class, race, and age), issues of difference and power within the community, and the community's openness to "outsiders" (Suzuki et al., 2005). Creswell (2013) recommended identifying a gatekeeper who can provide access to the site and to participants. He also emphasized the need to respect the site, to follow sound ethical practices, to avoid disturbing the site, and to inform all participants of the purpose of the research.

3. *Collecting and managing data.* In this step, the researcher engages in fieldwork to collect extensive data using various procedures. Often, the researcher will begin with broad, descriptive observations and then, after examining the data, become progressively more focused (Ary et al., 2013). Types of data collected include observation, informal conversations, in-depth interviews with informants, focus group interviews, content analysis of documents, and elicitation techniques (e.g., looking at a scrapbook and encouraging the participant to talk about memories) (Creswell, 2013). One way that ethnographic researchers record data is through writing **field notes**.

4. *Analyzing the data.* As with most qualitative research, data analysis begins early and continues until the research project is complete (Ary et al., 2013). The types of analyses vary widely, depending on the goals of the project and the disciplinary training of the researcher. The goal of analysis is to identify the core constructs or deep levels of meaning that stem from the raw data. Interpretation of data should flow directly from the descriptions and the themes inherent in the data (Creswell, 2013). Data are interpreted from the perspective of the population under study, using local language and terminology to describe the phenomenon (Hancock, 2002).

5. *Writing the report.* The report, also called the ethnography, "should be written so that the culture or group is brought to life, making readers feel they understand the people and their way of life" (Ary et al., 2013, p. 447). It is helpful to write early, as the data accumulate, rather than waiting until the project is finished. Weaving together the various sources and domains of cultural information can be a daunting task, and beginning researchers are advised to read other well-written ethnographies prior to writing their own.

### Advantages and Challenges

Ethnographic research has many distinct advantages. An ethnographic approach provides a comprehensive picture of specific cultural groups. It can lead to a deep, rich understanding of human behavior and cultural patterns. It also provides a way for researchers to examine topics that are not easily quantified.

As one might expect, there are several challenges inherent in conducting ethnographic research. First and foremost, the process requires an extensive time commitment on the part of the researcher. Second, ethnography is highly dependent on the researcher's observations and interpretations and consequently is subject to observer bias (Fraenkel et al., 2011). Thus, steps must be taken to enhance the validity of the findings, including such things as *member checking*, which involves returning to the field to check interpretations with the informants. There also is the concern that researchers may not be familiar with the social mores or language of the group being studied, thereby affecting their interpretations of what was said or observed.

One way to address the challenges associated with ethnographic research is by making interpretations and presenting the results reflexively (Creswell, 2013). Ethnographic reflexivity refers to many things, including being aware of one's role in the study in a way that respects the site and the participants, recognizing the need to corroborate and/or verify findings, and presenting results as tentative and open to further questioning (Berg & Lune, 2011; Creswell, 2013).

## Case Study

"Case study" is a term that is often used in conjunction with ethnography and, according to some authors, can be considered a special type of ethnography (Creswell, 2013; LeCompte & Schensul, 2010; Yin, 2009). Although commonalities exist between these two qualitative approaches, there are also some important distinctions. While ethnography examines shared patterns of behavior and beliefs among specific cultural groups, case studies focus on the activities of single entities including individuals, organizations, programs, or specific groups. Although it is acceptable to consider the case study as a special type of ethnographic research, here the case study is presented as a unique approach to qualitative research because of its distinctions.

Creswell (2013) defined a **case study** as "an in-depth exploration of a bounded system (e.g., an activity, event, process, or individuals) based on extensive data collection" (p. 239). A bounded system refers to a system that is separated from others in terms of time, place, or some type of physical boundary. For example, a client who has been abused could be considered a case, but the reasons for child abuse would not, as they do not represent a bounded system. Case studies have been used for developing counseling theories and seem to be a natural research tool for expanding knowledge in the profession. For example, Freud's studies of individuals with psychological issues (e.g., the Rat Man, the Wolf Man, Dora, and Little Hans) represent early examples of case studies. Box 6.3 provides an example of an individual case study of a family caregiver. A case study research example of an organization would be describing the role of professional school counselors in the Parent–Teacher Association (PTA) for elementary school children. A case study research example of an event would be examining the impact of the No Child Left Behind Act on test performance of rural schools.

At times, students confuse case studies with single-subject experiments because both types of research examine single individuals or discrete social units. A primary difference between the two is that single-subject experiments, which are a form of quantitative research, focus on a single behavior or a limited range of behaviors, whereas case studies focus on a wide range of behaviors and the relationship of those behaviors to the participant's environment (Ary et al., 2013). Also, with single-subject experiments, a treatment is usually introduced to determine its effect. With case studies, the researcher seeks to develop an in-depth understanding of the case by examining as many relevant variables as possible. The goal is to provide a thick description of part or all of an individual's life by collecting multiple forms of data. In some studies, the data collected include quantitative, as well as qualitative, information, but the data are not analyzed statistically; instead, they help the researcher tell a story in prose or narrative form (Monette, Sullivan, & DeJong, 2011).

### Types of Cases

As stated earlier, the case in a case study may involve an individual, several individuals (separately or in a group), a program, an organization, or even a particular incident. Cases also may be categorized as intrinsic, instrumental, and collective. A brief summary of each case type follows.

- *Intrinsic case study*. A case may be selected for study because it is unique and "has merit in and of itself" (Creswell, 2013, p. 439). The case is not selected because it represents a particular issue nor is it selected to shed light on an abstract concept or to build theory. Instead, the goal of the case study is to increase understanding of the intrinsic aspects of a particular client, organization, or other entity. For example, a researcher may want to understand an adolescent who has been bullied at school or follow a single mother as she navigates solely providing for her young family.

- *Instrumental case study*. With this type of case study, the researcher is interested in understanding more than just a single case. Unlike intrinsic case studies, instrumental case studies are designed to help the researcher understand some external theoretical question or problem (Hays & Singh, 2012). Case selection is based on the potential for the case to increase understanding of the broader research interest. As

---

### BOX 6.3    Case study example: Family caregiving and the use of formal community support services: A qualitative case study.

This example represents an instrumental case study design in which the experiences of an individual caregiver may be extended to other individuals with similar experiences. A 76-year-old female who was caring for her partner with Alzheimer's disease was interviewed over a three-month period to explore her process of relying on formal support services and subsequently lessening the caregiver role.

The participant was selected using criterion sampling methods after the researcher attended two support group meetings to solicit a case. The researcher used an open-ended interview structure as well as observations of the caregiving environment during each visit to understand the family caregiver's experience with formal support systems. Responses to interview questions influenced interview questions of future visits to the setting. Two formal service providers (i.e., support group provider and day care provider) were also interviewed, with the initial question, "What do you think your service does for family caregivers?"

The article in which the study is presented thoroughly describes the family caregiver's experiences with caregiving and the perceptions of her changing role as a caregiver as her use of formal support services increased. The interview transcripts and field notes were reviewed several times, and 29 codes that closely matched the participant's comments were generated. Further data analysis led to collapsing the codes to 10 categories, which were then

combined to form four general themes. The results of this study were presented in the form of a detailed story of the caregiving transition, beginning with the participant's first experiences with formal support services (i.e., physician and psychiatrist). The participant's story was seated in the description of four general themes (i.e., developing the need for caregiving assistance, sensing community while sustaining caregiving, receiving renewal while being assured of the patient's well-being, and experiencing transitions in the caregiving relationship).

Some examples of the ways that the case study established trustworthiness include the following:

- Use of *persistent observation*, as indicated by the researcher's attendance at support group meetings with a focus that was congruent to the research problem under study.

- *Triangulation* of data sources (participant and two formal support providers) and data collection methods (interviews and observations).

- Strengthening of data analysis with the use of *field notes*.

- Interview questions were developed based on the participant and formal service providers' responses and data analysis, an example of *recursivity*.

- *Thick description* of the case was provided.

*Source:* Winslow, 1998.

---

with the intrinsic case study, the particular case is still examined in depth, but the case is secondary to the external interest that is under investigation. For example, Asmussen and Creswell's (1995) *Campus Response to a Student Gunman* describes a classic, instrumental study in which the case was a particular college campus and the broader research interest was the reaction to campus violence.

- **Collective case studies**. Frequently, researchers will examine multiple cases to increase understanding about phenomena, populations, or states of being. In essence, collective case studies represent an extensive study of several instrumental cases. The specific cases are selected because of their potential to increase understanding about a larger theoretical collection of cases. Kozol's (1991) *Savage Inequalities* is a classic example of a collective case study that describes the extremes of wealth and poverty in America's public schools.

## Conducting Case Studies

Case study designs range in complexity, from illustrative descriptions of single events to extended case studies that trace events involving the same individuals over a period of time (Hancock, 2002). In general, the case study researcher seeks to develop in-depth understanding by collecting multiple forms of data about the case, a process known as "triangulation." The purpose of triangulation is to find support for observations and conclusions from more than one data source (Ary et al., 2013). Researchers employ many methods of data collection, including interviews, testing, and examining personal documents, such as diaries or journals, letters, and photographic or video-graphic material (Berg & Lune, 2011). Depending on the purpose of the study, researchers may want to collect data about the nature of the case, its historical back-ground, other contexts that influence the case (e.g., political, social, and economic), other cases through which the case is recognized and informants through whom the case can be known.

Yin (2009) outlined five steps that can guide the development of a case study research design:

1. *Develop the research questions.* Questions regarding *how* and *why* something occurs are especially appropriate for case study designs.

2. *Identify the propositions for the study.* Propositions are similar to hypotheses and help narrow the focus of the study. They explain why the researcher thinks a particular behavior or relationship will be observed. Often, an examination of relevant literature identifies appropriate theories that can be used to develop propositions. Not all studies, however, will have propositions, particularly if studies are exploratory.

3. *Specify the unit of analysis.* Is the case a specific individual, a program, an orga-nization, or some other bounded system? As stated earlier, studies may include single units or several units (i.e., multiple case studies). Yin (2009) classified single-unit studies as holistic designs and multiple-unit studies as embedded designs.

4. *Establish the logic linking the data to the propositions.* How will the data be used to illuminate the propositions? In particular, how will the data be analyzed? Findings should be organized according to the propositions established earlier.

5. *Explain the criteria for interpreting the findings.* In addition to making plans for data analysis, researchers need to identify ways they will interpret their findings. How will researchers compare their findings to rival propositions?

According to Yin (2009), researchers do not always develop these last two steps (linking data to propositions and explaining criteria for interpreting the findings) as well as the other three steps.

## Benefits and Challenges

A primary goal of case study research is to provide "an ideographic explanation that focuses on an in-depth understanding of a particular case" (Berg & Lune, 2011, p. 241). Each case is particularistic and contextual, with its own issues, contexts, interpretations, and thick descriptions. Case studies can be used to generate hypoth-eses, provide insight to phenomena, refine theory, and suggest possibilities for further investigation (Ary et al., 2013).

One of the criticisms of case study research is that the results are not generalizable. The dynamics that characterize a single individual or social unit are not necessarily

similar to the dynamics of others (Ary et al., 2013). The primary purpose of case study research, however, is to describe, not to generalize. Generalization need not be emphasized in all research. Even so, depending on the study and the selection of the case, findings often can be generalized to some extent in that they can provide understanding about similar individuals, groups, and events (Berg & Lune, 2011).

A second concern that has been raised regarding case study methods, and qualitative research in general, is whether the research is overly influenced by researcher and participant subjectivity (Berg & Lune, 2011). Preconceptions on the part of the researcher can influence decisions about what to pay attention to, what to ignore, and what methods of data collection to use. In addition, the data from case studies contain subjective responses from participants, as evidenced by selective recall and errors in memory (Monette et al., 2011). Collecting data from multiple sources, working with a team of researchers, and maintaining an audit trail are all ways to help ensure that any qualitative study, including the case study, represents sound research. An **audit trail**, which is discussed elsewhere in this chapter, is a way to trace what was done in a study, when, and why (Ary et al., 2013). The trail contains raw data, records of the researcher's decision-making activities, and other materials that make it possible for a third party to evaluate the dependability of the study.

## Phenomenological Research

The purpose of **phenomenological research** is to answer the question, "What is the meaning, structure, and essence of the lived experience of [a particular] phenomenon by an individual or by many individuals?" (Johnson & Christensen, 2012, p. 363). Phenomenology has its roots in philosophy and is associated with the work of German philosopher Edmund Husserl (1859–1938). Phenomenologists attempt to understand individuals' subjective experiences of particular life experiences. Examples of phenomena that may be studied by counseling researchers include the death of a partner, childhood sexual abuse, experiences of first-year counselor educators, coming-out experiences of gays or lesbians, and counselor identity development. Osborne (1990) noted that the intent of phenomenological research is not to test a hypothesis but rather to ask a question and to address the question through data collected by participants who have lived through the particular experience (see Box 6.4).

Several key terms are associated with phenomenology. One such term is the German word *lebenswelt*, which translates to "life-world." **Life-world** refers to a combination of feelings, thoughts, and self-awareness experienced by an individual at any given moment in time (Johnson & Christensen, 2012). Phenomenologists seek to understand an individual's life-world at a deep level and then describe that life-world as it applies to a particular experience. Phenomenologists must empathically enter the lived world of the research participant to gain a true understanding of the meaning of that world from the participant's point of view. In many ways, the role of the phenomenologist is comparable to that of the professional counselor who empathically and nonjudgmentally enters into the world of clients to provide therapeutic help.

Another term associated with phenomenology is **bracketing**, which refers to an intentional process of naming values, biases, and interests of the researcher. Researchers bracket when they set aside their assumptions, beliefs, or feelings about a phenomenon to reflect on how that phenomenon manifests itself in the lived world of the participant (Wertz, 2005). For example, a researcher who is studying the coming-out process of lesbian Latina adolescents would refrain from assuming that the experiences of the adolescents interviewed parallel any previously established identity formation model, such as the classic model described by Sophie (1986). Instead, the researcher would want to

## BOX 6.4     Phenomenology example: Resilience strategies of South Asian women who have survived child sexual abuse.

Using a feminist framework, the purpose of this phenomenology was to understand the essence of resilience strategies of 13 South Asian women who have survived sexual abuse. The research questions were (a) How does a small sample of South Asian women in the United States describe their experiences of child sexual abuse? and (b) What developmental resilience strategies do these survivors report using to cope with child sexual abuse?

Singh (2006) used maximum variation, convenience, and snowball sampling methods that resulted in a culturally diverse sample (i.e., age, education level, socioeconomic status, ability level, sexual identity, geography, religious/spiritual affiliation) with a variety of sexual trauma experiences. Five informants participated in individual interviews (i.e., Siedman's three-interview series protocol) and an independent sample of eight participated in a focus group. Informants completed a demographic sheet; individual interviews were 45–90 minutes long, and the focus group interview lasted approximately 90 minutes.

Data analysis involved the following six-step process:

*Step 1:* horizontalization of the three interviews per informant

*Step 2:* generation of meaning units to create an initial codebook

*Step 3:* further collapsing of data into a structural description of the phenomena under study

*Step 4:* constant comparison as steps 1–3 were repeated for each informant

*Step 5:* identification of general themes and subthemes for each informant who participated in individual interviews and the focus group interview

*Step 6:* reviews of the audit trail

Results indicated two general themes of *South Asian context* and *resilience*, with several subthemes for each of these broad categories. Subthemes for *South Asian context* included *gender*, *family*, *ethnic identity*, and *acculturation*. Subthemes for *resilience* included *sense of hope*, *use of silence*, *social support*, *social advocacy*, and *self-care*. Results indicated a connection between cultural context and use of resilience strategies.

*Trustworthiness* of the study was strengthened through the following processes:

- The researcher maintained a *reflexive journal* throughout the study, and the research team engaged in *bracketing* to minimize any negative impact of researcher bias.

- Informants participated in *member checking* that included reviewing transcripts and emerging themes and subthemes.

- The researcher engaged in *persistent observation* and *prolonged engagement*, as evidenced by extensive periods within the research setting.

- *Triangulation* of data methods (individual interviews and focus group interview) and data sources (multiple informants and use of a research team) was conducted.

- *Constant comparison* methodology was used throughout data analysis.

- Quotes were used to illustrate the results to provide the reader with a *thick description* of the phenomenon.

- The researcher used *peer debriefing* as a method to check biases.

- An *audit trail* was maintained and integrated into data analysis.

*Source:* Singh, 2006.

gain an in-depth understanding of each participant's unique, lived experience. Bracketing occurs as counseling researchers prepare, carry out, and analyze a study as well as when they write the research report. Table 6.3 illustrates some considerations for counseling researchers as they bracket their assumptions (Ahern, 1999).

**TABLE 6.3**   Strategies for bracketing.

Start with a reflective journal to be used throughout a research study. Reflect on the following questions:

- Why are you doing this research? What is your motivation and potential personal and professional gains?
- How might your cultural identity (e.g., race/ethnicity, socioeconomic status, gender) affect the process of gaining access, investigating research questions, and collecting data?
- What are your values and biases related to the research questions?
- What results do you expect to find?
- Are there any potential role conflicts that you expect (e.g., difficult interactions with participants or situations related to the study, gatekeepers who have self-interests that are potentially detrimental to participants)?
- What situations and with which participants do you experience negative feelings? Positive feelings? How might these feelings affect researcher neutrality?
- How can co-researchers and consultants help you maximize your ability to attend to participants' perspectives?
- As you analyze data, are you "looking" for certain codes and themes? How can you be sure to avoid this?
- Are you more involved in the study than you intended? (Have you "gone native"?) How might this be helpful? Harmful?
- How might other ways of gaining access or collecting data be achieved if you experience roadblocks?
- When you write the research report, how much of the findings are your voice rather than the participants' voices? Are you quoting certain participants more?
- Does the literature review support the findings? Are you leaving literature out that contradicts your findings?
- Are you overlooking data that do not "agree" with your assumptions?

© Cengage Learning

In addition to understanding the unique experiences of the individuals in a phenomenological study, researchers also search for commonalities among experiences. The commonality of lived experiences is known as the *essence* of the phenomenon. In other words, there are some universal, core elements of experiences that researchers attempt to determine. For example, grief and sorrow are core elements that are associated with the death of a loved one (Johnson & Christensen, 2012). Searching for the essence of an experience is one of the defining characteristics of phenomenology.

### Conducting Phenomenological Research

Participants, who often are called co-researchers, are selected because they have experienced the phenomenon being studied and are willing to share their thoughts and feelings about it (Ary et al., 2013). The primary method of data collection is the unstructured interview, which may last from one to more than two hours. Also, participants may be interviewed more than once. Ary et al. (2013) indicated that researchers typically interview 10–25 individuals, although the number of participants can vary, depending on the nature of the research (Wertz, 2005).

Interviewers need to be skilled at eliciting information that contains rich descriptions and concrete details. An interviewer may begin by asking the participant, "Please carefully describe your experience with…. " The interviewer needs to be able to listen carefully, prompt when necessary, and encourage participants to elaborate and expand on their descriptions (Ary et al., 2013). Typically, interviews are recorded and then transcribed. Researchers may also ask participants to write about their experiences (Johnson & Christensen, 2012).

Several steps comprise the data analysis process for phenomenological research. First, the researcher (or research team) listens to and transcribes the interviews. As the researcher listens to the tapes and reads the transcriptions, he or she attempts to grasp the participants' expressions and meanings in the broadest context (Wertz, 2005). Next, the researcher differentiates the data into *meaning units* for later analysis. Meaning units are significant statements (words or phrases) that are relevant to the phenomenon being studied. For example, in Morrissette's (2000) phenomenological study of the experiences of rural school counselors, a meaning unit dealing with a school counselor's feelings of isolation was "So I very seldom spend time sitting in the staff room as other teachers might" (p. 202).

After constructing lists of meaning units, the researcher then searches for themes in the data. The goal of this step is to determine the essence for the total group (Johnson & Christensen, 2012). In searching for themes, the researcher continues to maintain an empathic attitude, striving to leave his world behind so as to enter fully into the situations of the participants (Wertz, 2005). In Morrissette's (2000) study of rural school counselors' experiences, themes that emerged included a lack of privacy and anonymity, feelings of isolation, the benefit of professional collaboration and community networking, a lack of community resources, the importance of peer and administrative support, and the opportunity to become well acquainted with students and their families.

Phenomenological research involves a recursive pattern of data collection, interpretation, modification, and further data gathering as researchers and participants interact (Morrissette, 2000). This process often involves "reading between the lines" to grasp the implicit dimensions of the complex experience being investigated. To help ensure validity, data analysis also includes member checking; that is, the researcher asks the participants to review the researcher's interpretations and descriptions of the experience (Johnson & Christensen, 2012).

At the conclusion of the study, the researcher writes a narrative report that includes descriptions of the research question, the participants, methods used to obtain information, the fundamental structure of the participants' experiences, and a discussion of the findings (Johnson & Christensen, 2012). The narrative often contains verbatim descriptions provided by the participants, as well as descriptions of the researcher's method of organizing data (Wertz, 2005). Findings are discussed with regard to their connection with previous research and theory, their practical implications, and their impact on participants. Also included in the narrative report are specific methods used by the researcher to establish the trustworthiness of the study.

### Benefits and Challenges

Phenomenology represents an approach that focuses on faithfully discovering the subjective meanings individuals ascribe to a particular phenomenon. In comparison with other approaches, Wertz (2005) described phenomenology as "more hospitable, accepting and receptive in its reflection on 'the things themselves' and in its care not to impose order on its subject matter" (p. 175). Many of the procedures used in phenomenology, such as in-depth interviews, reflective research journals, naming themes in data, and interpreting within broad contexts, are also used in other qualitative approaches. When used in phenomenological research, however, these approaches must be used in unique ways. In particular, phenomenological research is designed to remain descriptive rather than to test hypotheses.

Perhaps one of the greatest challenges for phenomenological researchers is to remain true to phenomenological principals and procedures. To do so, researchers (a) set aside previous theories, (b) secure descriptive access to the subjective meanings participants ascribe to particular phenomena, (c) analyze the complexities of those meanings by

reflecting on the psychological processes that constitute them, and (d) gain insight about what is essential to those psychological processes (Wertz, 2005).

## Grounded Theory

Unlike the other research approaches described thus far, the purpose of grounded theory research is to generate theory based on the data collected about a particular phenomenon. Creswell (2013) defined **grounded theory** design as a systematic procedure used to generate a theory that explains a process, action, or interaction. Grounded theorists systematically collect data, identify categories found in the data, connect those categories, and use the resulting information to form a theory. The theory that is ultimately produced is "grounded" in data that are collected from participants using qualitative procedures such as interviewing, focus groups, and observation. Box 6.5 provides an example of a grounded theory approach.

Grounded theory has its roots in sociology. The approach was initiated by two sociologists, Glaser and Strauss, in 1967 and was based on the theoretical framework of symbolic interactionism (Fassinger, 2005). As stated earlier in the chapter, symbolic interaction is a process by which individuals interpret their experiences based on interactions with people and their environment. Although Glaser and Strauss diverged in their approaches in the early 1990s, the hallmark of the approach, which is theory generation, remains unchanged. Grounded theory research is a popular approach among many social science disciplines, including psychology, sociology, and counseling (Johnson & Christensen, 2012).

### Key Characteristics of Grounded Theory Research

Grounded theory research does not represent a single investigative process. A qualitative researcher who is using grounded theory would begin with a single research study and collect an extensive amount of data. As data are analyzed, the researcher would develop conditional propositions, which are explored through further data collection. Ultimately, a tentative theory is proposed. The proposed theory is "conceptually dense" in that it presents many conceptual relationships that are stated as propositions relating to a particular situation or context (Ary et al., 2013).

Creswell (2013) outlined six key characteristics of grounded theory research, which can be summarized as follows:

1. *Process approach.* Grounded theory represents a sequence of actions and interactions among people and events pertaining to a particular topic (Corbin & Strauss, 2007). For example, Moore (2005) explored the ways women with disabilities attribute meaning to their lives, experiences, and decisions. Other examples of topics that lend themselves to a process approach include parental practices and student achievement, coping with the death of a spouse, professional counselor identity development, and counselors' conceptualization of privilege and oppression (see Boxes 6.5 and 6.6).

2. *Theoretical sampling.* The researcher intentionally chooses forms of data collection that will yield a rich array of information useful in generating a theory. Sampling is intentional, with a focus on theory generation. The aim of theoretical sampling is to refine ideas, not to increase sample size (Charmaz, 2005). Sampling leads to an emerging design in which data are collected and analyzed immediately. Based on that analysis, the researcher makes decisions about what further data need to be collected. Forms of data collection include observations, conversations, public records, journals, and the researcher's reflections, with personal interviews representing the most common form of data collection.

## BOX 6.5    Grounded theory example: White counselors' conceptualization of privilege and oppression.

This study involved a grounded theory approach to explore white counselors' definitions, attitudes, and experiences toward privilege and oppression issues. Specifically, the research questions were the following: (a) How do White counselors conceptualize privilege and oppression as separate and related constructs? and (b) What experiences do White counselors generally describe concerning privilege and oppression?

A purposive sampling method (i.e., maximum variation sampling and convenience sample) was used to include participants who were identified racially as White with at least a master's degree in counseling and practicing in a counseling setting at the time of the study. The study included eight White counselors who represented diverse cultural identities for age, gender, sexual orientation, and spiritual orientation. In addition to the professional counselors, the research team was considered as participants as they influenced both data collection and analysis.

Data collection methods included semistructured interviews and a participant demographic sheet for each participant. Five of the eight participants were interviewed twice; interviews averaged 45–60 minutes in length. Interview questions were developed to assess participants' definitions and personal and professional experiences with privilege and oppression. Data were analyzed using constant comparison methodology; research team members used open and axial coding (Miles & Huberman, 1994).

A research model was developed based on themes pertaining to the conceptualization of privilege and oppression. The model described how counselors' conceptualization of privilege and oppression is acquired and what factors contribute to their level of awareness of these concepts.

There were several methods used to establish trustworthiness within the study, including the following:

- The research team had established *prolonged engagement* with the participants.

- *Researcher bias* was addressed as the research team discussed their cultural backgrounds, assumptions about the topic, and expectations in data analysis.

- Interview questions were reviewed and revised in a *peer debriefing* process. Peers included a counselor educator and eight doctoral students familiar with qualitative design but not involved in the study.

- *Triangulation* was evidenced in the study as multiple data sources (i.e., participants and research team members) were used to confirm and disconfirm themes.

- Data were concurrently collected and analyzed until the research team reached agreement that data *saturation* was achieved (i.e., data were fully represented by the themes and there was no new data to refute the findings). This process included looking for negative cases, a concept termed **negative case analysis**.

- *Member checking* was used, and participants provided feedback that included reactions to the interview content and process, confirmation that responses were accurate for them, and further elaboration of responses as needed.

- Data from the three participants who had been interviewed once were used to check for new themes related to the research model, a validity check known as *referential adequacy*.

- An *audit trail* of the data was maintained.

*Source:* Hays, Chang, & Dean, 2004.

3. *Constant comparative data analysis.* A hallmark of grounded theory research, constant comparative analysis involves the process of gathering data, sorting it into categories, collecting additional information, and then comparing the new information to the emerging categories. The constant comparative method requires researchers to seek verification for the hypotheses that emerge throughout the data collection process.

---

**BOX 6.6** Grounded theory example: Development of a professional school counselor identity: A grounded theory.

---

The purpose of this grounded theory approach was to understand school counselors' professional identity development process by examining how professional school counselors manage conflict decisions in their roles in schools. Six research questions were addressed: (a) What factors determine the school counseling program? (b) Who is involved in determining the school counseling program? (c) How do professional school counselors make decisions about the school counseling program? (d) What issues of conflict with principals have been dealt with by professional school counselors? (e) What is the decision-making process used by professional school counselors when interacting with principals in professional conflict situations? and (f) In what ways do conflict decisions reflect the role of the professional school counselor?

A purposive sampling method (i.e., homogeneous sampling) was used to include participants who identify as professional school counselors in elementary and middle school settings. The study included 10 professional school counselors who were primarily female with a majority of participants holding licenses and certificates in counseling. The researcher was considered an active participant in the study. Data collection methods included demographic surveys, semistructured individual interviews one-hour in duration, and observations of each participant in the schools. Observations (two to three per participant) were recorded as field notes. Data were analyzed using open, axial, and selective coding as well as memoing (Miles & Huberman, 1994). Final analyses (i.e., selective coding) yielded a grounded theory for the development of professional school counselor identity.

A research model describing the development process emerged during selective coding procedures. Three segments of the model (i.e., context, conditions, and phases) are interrelated to describe how the role of the professional school counselor intersects with activities, services, and events within the school.

Methods used to facilitate the study's trustworthiness included the following:

- The researcher had *persistent observation* with each participant.
- *Triangulation* of methods (e.g., with the use of interviews, survey data, and observations) helped the researcher confirm and disconfirm themes.
- A *peer debriefing process* occurred as multiple faculty members across disciplines reviewed the data collection methods and research questions.

*Source:* Brott & Myers, 1999.

---

4. *Identifying a core category.* After identifying several categories, the researcher identifies a core category that will be used as the basis for developing a theory. The researcher bases this decision on the core category's relationship to other categories, the frequency of its occurrence in the data, and its implications for theory development (Creswell, 2013).

5. *Theory generation.* The theory that is developed in grounded research is an abstract explanation of a process that is grounded in the data. The theory is not expected to have broad applicability or scope; it is not intended to be a "grand" theory (Creswell, 2013). It may be stated as theoretical propositions, which are statements that indicate the relationships among the categories.

6. *Memos.* While researchers are collecting and analyzing data, they also create memos about the data. Memos are notes written throughout the process that express the researchers' ideas about the data and the emerging categories (Creswell, 2013). One purpose of memos is to help researchers move their ideas ahead, thus helping to shape the developing theory. Charmaz (2005) described memo writing as "the intermediate step between data coding and the first draft of the completed analysis" (p. 517).

## Data Collection, Analysis, and Report Writing

As with many qualitative approaches, interviewing is the primary method of data collection in grounded theory research. Interviews, which are typically open ended, provide opportunities for participants to describe the event, experience, or social phenomenon under investigation. Other forms of data that may be used include direct observations, field notes, clinical case notes, historical documents, autobiographies, self-reflective memos, and perspectives from outsiders (Fassinger, 2005).

Data collection and data analysis in grounded theory research are concurrent and continual. As stated earlier, a key characteristic of grounded theory research is the constant comparative method, which "involves the constant interplay between the researcher, the data, and the developing theory" (Johnson & Christensen, 2012, p. 383). Data analysis typically consists of specific coding procedures that were described in detail by Glaser and Strauss (1967) and Corbin and Strauss (2007). The coding procedures can be divided into three types: open coding, axial coding, and selective coding. Although the three types are discussed sequentially as three stages in many grounded theory accounts, they actually occur recursively, as part of the constant comparative method of analysis (Fassinger, 2005). Coding initiates the chain of theory development and continues throughout the grounded theory study.

Open coding, which occurs during the first stages of data analysis, involves examining the initial transcribed data to name and categorize discrete elements in the data. At this stage, transcribed interview statements and other forms of data are analyzed line by line. Important words and phrases are labeled, often using phrases provided by the participants. These labeled phrases are compared with other labeled phrases, thereby helping the researcher determine the concepts that are present in the data.

The next stage in data analysis is axial coding. With axial coding, concepts developed during open coding are examined and organized into categories. Relationships among categories are examined, which may result in the establishment of broader (key) categories and categories that are subsumed under the key categories (Fassinger, 2005). The purpose of examining and prioritizing relationships in this way is to generate theory that fits the lived experiences of the participants.

The final stage of data analysis is selective coding, the goal of which is to create a substantive theory that is grounded in the data. In selective coding, the researcher looks for the main theme that is presented in the data. A core category that integrates all the other categories is selected for the purpose of explaining the participants' experiences. During this stage, the researcher continues to collect and analyze data but with more focus on developing the theory. The researcher continues to recheck existing data to see how the theory matches what has already been collected. The researcher also compares the developing theory with existing processes found in the literature. When no new concepts or categories emerge from the data and when the grounded theory has been validated with the collected data, theoretical saturation is said to have occurred (Johnson & Christensen, 2012). At this point, the researcher is ready to move to the next step, which involves presenting the results.

To illustrate the three types of coding, consider the following research example. A research team is interested in which factors and processes influence relapse prevention for individuals recovering from alcoholism. The research team is investigating this problem to improve existing programming. Data are collected via individual interviews and observations of groups. In analyzing initial interview data, the researchers examine each line closely to identify possible themes or concepts. These might include concepts such as "alcoholic father," "exposure to crime," "recent job loss," "medical illness," "telephone contact with sponsor," and "family support."

These concepts may be conceptualized as open codes. As data collection progresses, researchers, using constant comparison, may identify additional details and note that some data seem to cluster into categories or axial codes. For example, in analyzing a 12-step support group observation, the research team may reach consensus that the open codes "telephone contact with sponsor," "attending 12-step meetings," "positive feedback from group members," and "family involvement in treatment" cluster to form a larger category (i.e., axial code) known as "social support." Further, the researcher may note other axial codes that include "career development," "family history of addiction," and "residential stressors." Knowledge of various axial codes and continued data collection and analyses may reveal patterns and interactions among axial codes, which are called selective codes. These selective codes in conjunction with existing theory and practices may guide program development for individuals recovering from alcohol.

Although there are multiple ways to present the results of grounded theory research, the overarching goal is to describe the theory that was generated from the data. The theory should "offer a coherent, contextualized explanation (versus merely a contextual description) of a phenomenon, and the interrelationships among the constructs undergirding the theory must be articulated" (Fassinger, 2005, p. 162). Typically, a grounded theory report presents the major research question first. Next, the participants are described, as well as the reasons for their selection. Methods of data collection and analysis are discussed, and results are presented in detail. The results section is often lengthy and includes quotations from the participants. The report ends with a description of the theory generated by the data. In some cases, particularly when a phenomenon is being studied for the first time, the generated theory may be put forth as a tentative model or proposition (Fassinger, 2005), recognizing that continued research is needed for substantive theory development.

### Evaluating Grounded Theory Research

Although Guba and Lincoln (2005) established a foundation for evaluating qualitative research in general, there are some specific considerations that should be taken into account when evaluating grounded theory studies. Creswell (2013) cited Glaser and Strauss and Corbin, who outlined criteria for evaluating grounded theory research. To evaluate the theory itself, researchers ask these questions:

- Is there an obvious connection between the categories and the raw data?
- Does the theory provide a useful, relevant conceptual explanation of the process being studied?
- Is the theory modified as conditions change or as additional data are collected?

To evaluate the research process, researchers ask these questions:

- Is the purpose of the theoretical model to conceptualize a process, action, or interaction?
- Is a central phenomenon, or core category, clearly specified?
- Does the theory emerge during the phases of open, axial, and selective coding?
- Does the researcher attempt to show relationships among categories?
- Does the researcher gather extensive data so that the conceptual theory is well developed and grounded in the data?
- Does the study indicate that the researcher validated the theory by comparing it to the data, examining how it supports or refutes existing theories, and/or by checking the theory with the participants?

# Consensual Qualitative Research

**Consensual qualitative research** (**CQR**; Hill, Knox, Thompson, Williams, Hess, & Ladany, 2005; Hill, Thompson, & William, 1997) is an approach that combines grounded theory, phenomenology, and comprehensive process analysis. It comprises components of both constructivist and postpositivist approaches. As a constructivist approach, CQR uses individual participant interviews to understand the phenomenon from participant perspectives. However, the analysis of participant data involves a postpositivist process approach in that research team members use consensus-building procedures to converge upon and form a single reality of the phenomenon under study, rather than proposing that multiple realities exist (Ponterotto, 2005). CQR researchers ordinarily hope to generalize study results to the larger population.

Arriving at a group consensus is the key focus during preliminary categorization, cross-analysis, and audit integration phases. The emphasis is on the use of multiple judges and gaining agreement or consensus among those multiple judges. Judges (research team members) seek a common view of the meaning of the data while respecting the diverse worldviews of the other judges. Judges must have good interpersonal and intrapersonal skills to openly discuss feelings and disagreements. It also helps if the team members like and respect each other.

Researchers are aware of, discuss, and bracket their biases and expectations. It is essential when constructing a CQR report that the authors describe the research team characteristics and biases or worldviews as pertaining to the topic. The team should openly and honestly assess how their biases and expectations may have influenced the study results. CQR views biases as an inevitable aspect of research, rather than an indication of potential problems with interpretation and analysis. Thus, processing biases as a team is encouraged throughout the data collection, analysis, and reporting phases.

CQR also focuses on the equalization of power in all processes; every member of the research team (judges) is to have an equal voice in deliberations. Researchers share power with each other and participants to reduce researcher bias owing to any values or assumptions about what the data mean, by discussing how cultural identities, personal identities, and assumptions about the topic and data can affect interpretations. Training of team members can help equalize power and encourage a culture of self-analysis of biases (Hill et al., 2005).

## Conducting Consensual Qualitative Research

Any topic that can be explored using an interview format is appropriate for CQR. Participants are selected because they are knowledgeable about the topic and can help the researchers draw insights into the phenomenon under study. Hill et al. (2005) recommended interviewing 8–15 participants. CQR usually involves 30- to 60-minute, open-ended, semistructured, taped, face-to-face, or phone interviews. This is done to maintain a degree of consistency across participants, as opposed to the more intensive, longer-term researcher–participant discovery processes discussed previously in other qualitative approaches. Some studies use two interviews, with the follow-up interview designed for greater depth. The entire protocol is administered to each participant. The interview protocol is based on the research literature and researcher self-reflections and changes very little as the research process progresses sequentially from one interviewee to the next. Team members should each have access to the interview transcripts, as well as the audio or videotape of the interview, to better surmise the interviewee's voice tone and inflection.

CQR analysis procedures begin in a fashion similar to other qualitative methodologies: Interview data is collected and summarized, memos are written, and the text of participant comments is organized. However, it is at this point that CQR processes become unique. The next step is the development of categories and domains through consensus among the research team members (i.e., judges). Usually the research team is composed of three to five judges. Each member of the research team reads the interview transcripts. This immersion allows each member to preliminarily identify the themes, categories, and domains they see in the data. The members then meet as a group to discuss their initial observations, debate, and converge on consensus around a group of identifiable domains. Researchers discuss and develop these domains collaboratively, analyzing each other's biases, and reaching group consensus. Next, abstracts of these core domains are constructed (domain abstraction), identifying aspects of the domains previously examined and identified. **Cross-analysis** results from consensus processes as team members look for commonalities as they determine whether categories exist across all, some, or just one or a couple of respondents. Once a final list of categories is derived, the team members return to the data and code all interviews using this set of categories. Cross-analysis results in a list of domains and within-domain categories either found or not found across participant responses. Then these results are further analyzed through an external audit by a secondary research team. The audit team examines the contrived data and categories and communicates back to the primary research team the findings of the audit, making suggestions for changes, revisions, or expansions, as appropriate. After these audit-related adjustments, final category frequencies are tabulated (frequency analysis) and presented in a table format to visually display the results. The categories are then identified as general (all but a few cases), typical (more than half up to general), variant (at least two cases up to typical), and rare (occurring in one or maybe two cases depending on the sample size). Finally, the phenomenon is presented in a written report (Hays & Singh, 2012).

Brief quotes are sometimes used in the research report, although expressing ideas through the "voice" of the participants is minimized. Rather, ideas and concepts are integrated across participants through researcher consensus-building processes. Thus, the combined voice and perspective filtered through the consensual process is heard, rather than individual participant voices and perspectives. Hill et al. (2005) provide an excellent summary of CQR methodology, including a table with more than 40 recommendations for the appropriate use of CQR. Box 6.7 provides a brief example of the use of CQR in counseling research.

# Selecting a Qualitative Research Design for Your Study

Ethnography, case study approaches, phenomenology, grounded theory, and consensual qualitative research represent five of the more commonly selected methods of qualitative inquiry that professional counselors may select. We have provided a general description of each of these approaches to inform the reader of characteristics, benefits, and challenges related to these approaches.

In selecting a research design, readers should be knowledgeable about how these approaches may overlap as well as how they are distinct from one another. To consider which approach is most suitable for a particular study, reflect on the following questions:

- Is the purpose of the study more suitable for a particular approach?
- What data collection methods are appropriate for the qualitative approach you are considering?
- How would the number of participants and type of sample be affected by the various research approaches? Alternatively, how would each approach influence your sampling design?
- What are the benefits and challenges of using various approaches for the research problem you would like to investigate?
- Do you believe that data collection methods affect the approach you would select? That is, do you think that methods drive design or design drives methods?

**BOX 6.7    Consensual qualitative research example: The career decision-making process of Chinese American youth.**

The purpose of this CQR study was to examine the career decision-making process of a sample of eight Chinese American youth negotiating bicultural expectations. Main topics in the interviews included role models, career interests, and people with whom they have discussed their career plans. Initially, the interview data were coded into domains and categories of career decision-making processes by each team member independently. These categories were used to construct a code book. Using the newly constructed code book, each judge then revisited the transcripts using a recursive process to refine the codes in the context of the data. This led to a revision of the code book. Next, the judges independently abstracted the core ideas within the domains, then used consensus-building procedures to arrive at an agreed upon set of core ideas for the career decision-making domains (e.g., identity development, relationships with family, expression of Chinese culture, and family values). Next, cross-analysis was accomplished by "bringing all the transcripts together" (p. 442) and looking at all of the data to construct categories (subdomains). An audit was conducted and the feedback was used to revise and consider or communicate alternative explanations for the original domains (e.g., feelings and concerns about career) and categories derived (i.e., changing or shifting between career interests frequently; having negative feelings such as scared, worried, confused, and pressured as he or she thinks about career-related issues; having difficulties making career decisions; not in a hurry to choose a career; fear of academic failure). Finally, a frequency analysis was conducted, and table results were displayed for each domain/subdomain. Each category was then represented as general, typical, variant, or rare. Interestingly, Okuba et al. (2007) determined all 47 categories across 10 domains to be typical or variant, although they required all eight participants to endorse a category for a label of general, and none for rare, effectively eliminating those two categories from occurring. In general, expectations voiced by the parents of these bicultural youth significantly influenced their career decisions, as did a lack of role models, confusion about self-identity, and confusion about one's ethnic identity.

*Source:* Okubo, Yeh, Lin, Fujita, & Shea, 2007.

- How is data analysis conducted for the qualitative approach you are considering?
- What role do you as the researcher play in each of the approaches?
- How might you establish trustworthiness for a particular approach?

# Conclusion

In sum, there are several types of qualitative research approaches or designs from which to select. The decision becomes more complex as the counseling researcher must consider the issues presented in Chapter 5, such as selecting the research topic and data collection method(s), choosing and accessing various research settings, and deciding the extent of the researcher's role in the qualitative study. Many of the approaches or designs in counseling research have overlapping characteristics as well as marked distinctions that impact the extent to which a phenomenon may be studied. Thus, the reader is encouraged to consult others with experience in qualitative inquiry before selecting a qualitative approach.

*Now go to the Student Workbook found on cengagebrain.com that accompanies this text for additional application and review activities.*

# Quantitative Research Design in Counseling

This chapter provides a brief overview of several types of quantitative research, as well as key concepts related to conducting each type of research and threats to internal and external validity. The primary goal is to provide the requisite information for professional counselors to critically analyze quantitative research in counseling and to be able to transfer that analysis into practice.

Counseling as a profession has made great advances in recent decades. Its progress is due in large part to the research it has produced. To prove its usefulness and effectiveness in the helping professions, professional counselors must continue to conduct research that advances knowledge of human behavior. Although all professional counselors don't become researchers, each must possess the skills to critically analyze research data in an effort to provide the best services possible.

Much of the research in counseling is conducted on large groups of people and involves measurements that can be counted. These types of research studies are often referred to as quantitative methods, which primarily deal with numbers. It assumes that facts and feelings can be separated and that a single reality can be measured. The researcher's role is viewed as more of a detached observer. Basically, through observation and manipulation of variables, quantitative researchers seek to establish relationships between variables to explain the possible causes.

# Internal and External Validity

Before delving into the various types of research design, it is important to discuss the concept of experimental validity. Experimental validity is a pivotal concept in conducting quality quantitative research. Establishing experimental validity is the process of verifying that the research instruments and the results accurately reflect the research question to make correct conclusions and inferences (i.e., generalizability). A research study without validity is rather useless aside from a lesson in what *not* to do. While what follows is a brief introduction to this topic, readers who are interested in an in-depth discussion of validity issues in research are directed to classic books on the topic by Campbell and Stanley (1963) and Cook and Campbell (1979).

**Internal validity** refers to a researcher's ability to determine whether a causal relationship exists between the *independent variable* (i.e., treatment variable) and *dependent variable* (i.e., criterion or outcome variable), rather than because of some *extraneous variable* (i.e., one not related to the experiment). In essence, internal validity describes the level of confidence in which the results of a study are supported by the design or methodology. When examining validity of measurement, the researcher should ask, "Do the scores accurately reflect what the instrument is supposed to measure?" Similarly, internal validity is the extent to which extraneous variables have been controlled or accounted for, to ensure that the inferences or the conclusions drawn from the results of the data are accurate. When it is possible to conclude that extraneous variables caused changes in the dependent variable, internal validity and causal inference are threatened.

**External validity** is also known as generalizability and refers to whether the results of the sample in this particular study can be generalized or applied to a population, group, condition, setting, or other participants. **Population generalizability** is the degree to which the sample is representative of the population of interest on the particular characteristic or variable being studied. **Ecological generalizability** is the degree to which the result of a study can be applied to other settings or conditions. Importantly, if a study's internal validity is limited, then external validity is threatened. Also, external validity is threatened when the observed effects of an independent variable on a dependent variable cannot be guaranteed outside of the experimentally controlled circumstance. This is a valid criticism of laboratory research: Just because someone can make it happen under tightly controlled circumstances in the laboratory, it does not mean that it will happen the same way in the real world.

There are three main types of evidence that researchers may use to determine the internal validity of the study: content-related, criterion-related, and construct-related. **Content-related evidence** asks the question of whether the instrument(s) or sample accurately represents the variable under study. In essence, a researcher who is gathering content-related evidence asks whether the questions used in the instrument adequately assess the variable under study. To ensure content-related validity, researchers should look over the *content* (do the questions or items accurately reflect the definition of the variables and the sample of participants?) and *format* (e.g., clarity, readability, font type and size, and language) of the instrument to be used. Frequently, content experts determine how well an instrument represents a given domain of information or behavior.

**Criterion-related evidence** (i.e., empirical validity) is used to determine validity by comparing the instrument used in the study to another instrument or form of assessment presumed to measure the same variable. Two forms of criterion-related validity are predictive validity and concurrent validity. **Predictive validity** is obtained by administering the instrument and then allowing an elapsed time interval to pass for later comparison with the criterion scores (e.g., aptitude test and end-of-semester grade point average [GPA]). **Concurrent validity** requires administration of the instrument and criterion data at the same point in time (e.g., attitude of students compared to teacher's observations). A correlation coefficient is often used to determine whether a relationship exists between the scores from the two instruments.

**Construct-related evidence** includes a variety of different types of evidence supporting the characteristic being measured. Three common ways to measure construct-related validity includes use of (a) a clearly defined variable, (b) the hypotheses based on theory explaining the variable, and (c) logical and empirically tested hypotheses. While content-, criterion-, and construct-related validity have important applications in research, a more thorough discussion of these concepts can be found in an assessment text (e.g., Erford, 2013). To control for threats to internal and external validity, researchers use various methods of experimental control, which will be explained next. Subsequently, specific threats to internal and external validity will be reviewed.

## Methods of Control in Experimental Research

Planning an experimental study or evaluating the results of a study requires exploring any possible threats to internal and external validity. Any validity threat that may affect the dependent variable, such as comparing group sampling differences, can create problems or discrepancies in the results and necessitate a greater need for control. Experimental research answers two primary questions: (1) Does a relationship exist between the independent variable and a dependent variable? and (2) Is this relationship causal in nature? Accurate answers to these two questions rely on the researcher's ability to maximize the experimental variance caused by the independent variable while minimizing two primary sources of error: (1) systematic error caused by extraneous or confounding variables and (2) random error owing to fluctuations in participants, measurement, or conditions. As a result, researchers must attend to several important experimental control considerations when conducting a quantitative study: (a) maximizing the variability due to the independent variable, (b) controlling confounding (extraneous) variables, (c) minimizing random error, and (d) deciding whether to use control groups.

### Maximizing Variability due to the Independent Variable

After a thorough review of the literature, independent variables are selected because of their perceived potency in influencing the dependent variable, thus creating or controlling experimental variance. This makes the selection of appropriate independent variables critical in experimental research. To enhance the effectiveness of the independent variable, researchers often try to make various levels of the independent variable as different as possible. For example, sometimes researchers use intelligence as an independent variable by measuring and assigning participants to groups of high and low intelligence. When doing so, individuals who are barely above average (e.g., IQ scores of 101–105) are unlikely to be substantively different from individuals who are barely below average (e.g., IQ scores of 95–99). Thus, researchers who want to explore differences due to intelligence are more likely to use groups of participants who vary markedly on this independent variable—for example, establishing a low intelligence group with IQs of less than 85 and a high intelligence group with IQs of greater than 115. Such differentiation allows the effect of the independent variable to be measured. Another example of the applications of an extreme grouping on the independent variable involves sex differences, which can be explored by differentiating between males and females.

### Minimizing Variability due to Extraneous (Confounding) Variables

It is not enough for experimenters to simply strive to maximize the effects of independent variables. Quality research also tends to the chore of minimizing the variability contributed by other variables not selected as independent variables. Variables that contribute unwanted variance are called **extraneous variables** or **confounding variables**. Again, an exhaustive review of the literature is always necessary to identify extraneous variables and control for their unwanted effects on the dependent variable. Researchers typically use four procedures to control for extraneous variables. First, researchers may randomly assign participants to various treatment and control conditions, in effect equalizing the potential error variance contributed by the extraneous variable across all the groups. Random assignment usually randomly distributes error by equalizing participant characteristics, and it has the advantage of controlling for extraneous variables of which the researcher may be unaware. Second, if the researcher is aware of the potential effects of an extraneous variable, he or she can select only participants who are homogeneous on the extraneous variable, thus controlling the effects by holding them constant. For example, if sex is believed to be an extraneous variable in a depression treatment study, the researcher can include only female participants, thus eliminating potential error due to including both males and females. Third, if the researcher is aware of an extraneous variable, the researcher can match participants who are equivalent on the extraneous variable before assigning them to various treatment conditions, thus ensuring equivalence. For example, if intelligence is an extraneous variable, a researcher could assess each participant's IQ score, pair the participants on IQ, and then randomly assign participants from each pair to treatment and control groups. This adds an extra level of precaution or control to traditional random assignment. Finally, an identifiable extraneous variable can be built into the design of the study (i.e., become a "**blocking variable**") to control for its effects. For example, participants could be assessed for IQ and blocked as low, average, and high intelligence. Blocking variables are commonly used in ANOVA designs, in effect becoming an additional identified independent variable.

### Minimizing Random Error

Random error includes unpredictable fluctuations that occur in participants (e.g., distractions, fatigue, and illness), instruments (e.g., scoring errors and lack of appropriate calibration), or experimental or ecological conditions (e.g., the regular room is not available; the room temperature is uncomfortably cold). Random error is one of those banes of the researcher's existence and often difficult to predict and control. Preparation and standardization, however, can usually minimize the influence of random error. Researchers should strive to keep the environment free of distractions, periodically calibrate instruments or check for scorer accuracy, and take extraordinary steps to be sure participants arrive physically and mentally prepared (e.g., well-fed, well-rested). Obviously, researchers will never be 100 percent certain that random error has been eliminated, but appropriate precautions and preparations can diminish these deleterious effects.

### Use of Control Groups

Control groups are commonly used in experimental research because they provide reference groups for comparison with experimental treatment groups. Thus, differences between participants in control or treatment groups can be attributed to the treatment, intervention, event, or some other independent variable under study. Researchers ordinarily use either no-treatment (waitlist) control groups or placebo control groups. No-treatment control group participants receive no treatment at all, whereas treatment group participants receive the experimental treatment (e.g., intervention or drug). Frequently, no-treatment control group participants are referred to as "wait-list" participants because they were the individuals selected from the list of possible participants required to wait until the treatment's effectiveness was established before being given the treatment. In contrast, **placebo control group** participants are exposed to a "treatment" unrelated to the experimental treatment and not expected to alter the participants' performance on the dependent variable. Placebos include sugar pills that are substituted for an experimental depression drug or a "personal growth group" that is substituted for a depression treatment group. In each case, neither the sugar pill nor the personal growth group is expected to alter the participants' levels of depression, but researchers sometimes find that some participants react to these nontreatments in a way that does affect the dependent variable. In other words, some participants taking a sugar pill or participating in a personal growth group may report feeling less depressed, but it may just be from all the attention they are getting. The participant may believe he or she is helping the researcher to get better results by inflating scores, or perhaps the participant just wants to please someone he or she perceives as being in an evaluative or powerful position. **Treatment-as-usual** conditions are becoming more commonly used in outcome literature. Usually, clients do not "wait" or take a "placebo" in real life, and even if they do, it is probably better to compare an experimental treatment with some previously existing treatment that the client would have received if the client showed up for counseling services. The treatment-as-usual condition is a control condition in which the participants receive what they usually would have received if they had come for counseling. *Treatment as usual* is often described in empirical articles as "supportive counseling" or "case management services."

Regardless of the methods employed to exercise experimental control, it is essential to understand that, ironically, exercising more control over the variables in the research tends to decrease the generalizability or external validity of the results. This is because practitioners in the field seldom have the kind of tight control that researchers have, and so they cannot replicate the treatment in such a standardized format. Thus, there are trade-offs between internal and external validity when conducting an experimental study. Regardless of the trade-offs, researchers should be aware that threats to both internal and external validity exist. These threats will be explained next.

# Controlling for Specific Threats to Internal Validity

Generally speaking, there are four ways to minimize threats to validity: (a) standardize the conditions in which the study occurs, (b) know the characteristics of the participants in the study, (c) know the details of the study (i.e., where, when, and the extraneous events that may occur), and (d) plan and choose a suitable design. Nevertheless, there are more specific ways in which researchers can minimize or control threats to internal validity in an experiment. These include randomization, holding variables constant, building the variable into the design, matching, participants as their own control, and analysis of covariance.

Randomization or **random sampling** is the process of drawing a research sample in which each member of a population has an equal chance of being selected (random selection). Random selection reduces sampling biases and increases generalizability of the results to the larger population (external validity). Statistically speaking, some statisticians suggest having at least 15 participants to a cell in a factorial design and 10 participants for each variable in a multiple regression. This is only a guideline suggestion, and a more precise method is a power analysis. (For more in-depth statistical information, see Anderson, Tatum, & Black [2006].)

Another randomization process is *random assignment*, which is usually done after the research participants are selected to determine which participants will have a certain value of the independent variable. Random assignment is essentially the process of assigning individuals or groups to different treatment conditions to maximize the probability that participant characteristics are matched between the experimental groups, thus controlling for confounding variables (e.g., internal validity). **Matching** refers to the technique of equating groups on one or more variables with the result of each member of one group having a direct counterpart in another group. Random assignment can be accomplished through the use of a table of random numbers.

Participants as their own control often occurs in single-subject experimental design (see Chapter 8) or in some pretest–posttest designs. This option provides high internal validity because participants serve as their own controls; the results, however, are extremely low with respect to external validity. Single-subject studies increase external validity through the process of replication and extension (e.g., repeating the study in different settings, with different participants, etc.).

Analysis of covariance (see Chapter 16) tests the main and interaction effects of categorical variables on a continuous dependent variable, controlling for the effects of other selected continuous variables that covary with the dependent variable. The control variable is called the covariate. The main purpose of the analysis of covariance is statistical control of variability when experimental control cannot be used. It is a statistical method for reducing experimental error or for removing the effect of an extraneous variable.

# Threats to Internal Validity

Several threats to internal validity are possible: selection (subject characteristics), history, maturation, mortality, instrumentation, testing, location, implementation, experimental bias (attitudinal effect), and regression.

## Selection

**Selection** is the manner in which participants are chosen to participate in a study and the manner in which they are assigned to groups. **Participant characteristics** are those individual factors that may account for an observed effect, such as age, gender, critical thinking, or ability. Differences that may be present between the groups prior to the study will continue throughout the study and may result in a treatment effect when no true experimental effect is present. For example, a researcher might be interested in the effectiveness of a particular counseling intervention. The researcher gives the intervention to group A and compares the results of a brief symptom checklist with individuals from group B who received no treatment. Analysis of the data reveals a significant difference between group A and group B supporting the effectiveness of the intervention. However, if the researcher failed to control some of the participant characteristics, it may be difficult to determine whether individual differences of group members led to the outcome of the study rather than the intervention. This happens frequently when researchers use two intact groups for the treatment and control conditions, rather than randomly assigning participants to the two conditions. Randomization (i.e., random sampling and random assignment) can reduce the possibility of effects due to participant characteristics, as can participant matching at the outset of the study through the use of a pretest to determine preexisting similarities on the dependent variable.

### History

**History** refers to confounding events outside of the research study that can alter or affect participants' performance, such as experiential environmental events. For example, professional counselors who are studying college student anxiety may have discovered different trends in anxiety level directly after the September 11, 2001, attack on the World Trade Center, or a study of depression in participants could be affected by a publicized suicide. As it is often impossible to make everyone's experience identical except for the independent variable(s), using randomization procedures can often minimize this risk, ensuring that outside events that occur in one group are also likely to occur in the other. Thus, considering our example and the use of randomization, it would be likely that students affected by 9/11 would be equally distributed among experimental and control groups, and subsequent differences could be attributed to experimental conditions. Likewise, if participants were randomly assigned, a publicized suicide would likely affect the dependent variables of both groups equally. A time-series design can also help detect the influence of a historical event, although it will not control for the effects of an event.

### Maturation

**Maturation** refers to the natural process of aging and development over time or short-term physiological or psychological effects. Maturation can play a major role in longitudinal studies and when studying children. For example, researchers may be interested in the process by which counselor trainees develop ethical decision-making skills. If researchers investigated this phenomenon from a participant's first graduate course through his or her internship, some maturation would be expected to occur. Short-term effects are generally related to facets such as fatigue, hunger, or boredom. As is the case with history, control of maturation can be addressed through subject matching or randomization.

### Mortality

**Mortality** (i.e., attrition) refers to the possibility of a differential effect due to those participants who drop out during the study versus if the participants had stayed in the study. Human participants' research is regulated by standing bodies (i.e., institutional review boards) that review proposals for potential ethical dilemmas. According to standard review board policies, all research participants must have the right to withdraw from the study at any point without penalty. Thus, it is difficult for researchers to control mortality. Pretesting of participants often allows researchers to determine if those who later drop out of a study differ in important ways from those who remain. Mortality is particularly problematic in longitudinal studies, as the sample that the researcher ends up with may differ substantially from the sample selected at the study's onset. Again, pretesting is the best control for mortality. Mortality is also a big problem in treatment efficacy studies. For example, if 50 participants begin treatment for depression and only 25 are left at the conclusion of the study, the results may indicate that the depression treatment was very effective for those who stayed in the study until the conclusion, but primarily because those for whom the treatment was not working left the study! Thus, researchers often do "intent to treat" analyses in addition to "completer" analyses.

### Instrumentation

Another threat to validity is **instrumentation** or changes in the measurement device(s) used during the course of the study. Changes in scores may be related to the instrument differences rather than the independent variable. Thus, reliability of instrument scores is important. *Reliability* refers to the consistency of the scores obtained for each individual from one administration of a test or instrument to another. Consistency of scores is affected by any changes in **data collector characteristics**, **data collector bias** (e.g., unintentional bias of data collector and changes in the accuracy of the scorer over time), or **instrument decay** (e.g., changes in instruments over time). To control for the threat of instrumentation, it is recommended that pretests and posttests be identical and that measurement procedures and measurement devices do not change over time. This is also a prime reason why researchers are strongly encouraged to use instruments that yield highly reliable scores. Many studies do not yield true differences because of faulty instrumentation (e.g., unreliable scores stemming from selected tests or rating scales and uncalibrated devices).

### Testing

**Testing** refers to the practice effect of participants who are exposed to the intervention or test on multiple occasions (i.e., test–retest). Chances are that participants will perform better the second time merely due to practice or memory of the items. Some instruments (e.g., *Wide Range Achievement Test, 4th Edition* [WRAT-4], Wilkinson & Robertson, 2006) have alternate forms to control for this effect. In lieu of alternate forms of an instrument, control group studies are recommended. In addition, some researchers administer the test only once, whereas others design the test to minimize practice effects.

### Location

**Location** may affect the accuracy of scores if differences exist for the place of testing and the data-collection process (e.g., testing site). Although attention to such details may seem overly stringent, factors such as lighting, noise, or comfortable seating can affect a person's ability to concentrate. Thus, it is important to ensure that the environment is the same across conditions. For example, it is not difficult to imagine that one group of students who are taking their SATs while sitting on the floor in a dimly lit room with distracting noises may differ somewhat from another group of students taking their SATs while sitting in comfortable chairs at tables in a well-lit, quiet room.

### Implementation

**Implementation** refers to variations in the way that the intervention is introduced or conducted, which may affect the results of the study. Single-subject researchers place a high degree of emphasis on implementation. Most journals that publish single-subject research (e.g., *Journal of Applied Behavior Analysis*) require manuscript authors to report interrater reliability data. Thus, single-subject researchers must ensure that procedures are implemented with a high degree of integrity. Although quantitative research studies do not typically contain data related to the integrity of implementation, researchers are required to report their procedures in a stepwise fashion.

### Experimental Bias

**Experimental bias** refers to the researchers' possible bias toward the expected or hypothesized results, a violation of the objectivity required in experimental research. Control of this threat to validity can be addressed by using an experimenter who is unaware of the anticipated results (e.g., double-blind study) to administer the intervention(s) or treatment. Similarly, **attitudinal effect** refers to the possible perception by either group that they may be receiving special attention, which may affect the results of the study. **Double-blind studies** address both researcher bias and attitudinal effect. For example, if researchers were interested in the effect of a drug on the hyperactivity of children, they could avoid experimental bias by using research assistants who were not privy to the identity of the experimental or control group members. The assistants could be instructed to give an unmarked pill to each participant each day and to record data relative to the participant's behavior. Only the researchers would know if the treatments were actual medications or **placebos** (i.e., a condition or drug that should have no effect, such as a sugar pill). The participants would not know if they were assigned to the experimental or control conditions either. Thus, neither the researcher's bias nor the attitudinal effect of participants could influence the outcome of the study.

### Statistical Regression

**Statistical regression**, or regression to the mean, refers to the tendency for participants with extreme scores (very high or very low) to score more toward the mean on subsequent testing. For example, if a participant received an IQ test score of 130 (e.g., two standard deviations above the mean, Very Superior, "gifted"), the odds that this participant's score will be lower on subsequent tests are much greater than the odds of increasing the score. This is simply a statistical phenomenon readily observed when working with participants who were selected for their extreme performance or characteristics (e.g., gifted students, depressed patients, intellectually delayed adults, hyperactive children). Use of control groups or the collection of multiple baselines can help minimize the effects of statistical regression. For example, it is common practice for pediatricians and psychiatrists to administer a behavior rating scale to parents or teachers of supposed hyperactive children, determine elevated scores on hyperactivity scales, prescribe stimulant medication, re-administer the rating scales several weeks later, see that the scores on the hyperactivity scales have dropped closer to normal, and proclaim the treatment a success. Unfortunately, such a process does not account for the effects of statistical regression. The physician does not know how much of the improvement in scores is due to the medication and how much is due to statistical regression. Collecting multiple baselines corrects for this problem. Likewise, it is normal for a group of very depressed clients to become less depressed on average over the course of a study because of statistical regression alone. Using a control group helps determine how much of the "improvement" is due to the treatment and how much is due to statistical regression because statistical regression is about the only thing the control group will experience. That is, any improvement in the control group is due to statistical regression, whereas any improvement in the treatment group is due to statistical regression *plus* treatment effects. Therefore, if the treatment group scored much higher (or much lower) than the control group, one knows the treatment actually accounted for the difference. In summary, Table 7.1 provides some helpful ways to control for threats to internal validity.

| TABLE 7.1 | Controlling for threats to internal validity. |
|---|---|
| **Threat to Internal Validity** | **Possible Ways to Control Threat** |
| Selection | Random selection, random assignment |
| History | Random selection, random assignment |
| Maturation | Subject matching, randomization |
| Mortality | Subject matching and omission |
| Testing | Control group |
| Instrumentation | Consistency and reliability |
| Experimenter Bias | Double-blind study |
| Statistical Regression | Omit extreme scores, randomization |

© Cengage Learning

## Threats to External Validity

External validity determines to what extent the results of a study represent or apply to other situations (i.e., generalize beyond the current study). There are generally three threats to external validity: (1) reactive arrangements (e.g., placebo effect, Hawthorne effect, demand characteristics, and evaluation apprehension); (2) order effects (or carry-over effects); and (3) treatment interaction effects.

### Reactivity Arrangements

**Reactivity** involves participants behaving (reacting) in certain ways because they have knowledge that they are being observed or experimented on. A number of types of reactivity have been identified, including the placebo effect, Hawthorne effect, Pygmalion effect, evaluation apprehension, and demand characteristics. **Placebo effects** are those occasions when participants in a study act according to expectations derived from inadvertent cues to the anticipated results of the study. For example, in pharmaceutical studies, control participants are given a sugar pill instead of the experimental drug to counterbalance the act of actually taking the pill. Amazingly, it is not unusual for about 20 percent of the participants who are taking the placebo to report a substantial reduction in symptoms. It is assumed that these participants are responding in accord with what they believe the experimenter wants them to report. Conducting a **blind study** reduces the possibility of this threat by ensuring that participants are not aware of anticipated outcomes.

The **Hawthorne effect** refers to changes in performance by the mere presence of others; that is, participants in an anxiety study may become less anxious just because of the attention they receive from researchers. Having a control group (i.e., a group of participants not exposed to treatment) can be one method of controlling for the Hawthorne effect.

**Demand characteristics** are environmental cues or statements that let participants know about the purpose of the study or what actions, behaviors, or outcomes are expected of participants. As a result of these insights, participants may react in accordance with those expectancies.

The **Pygmalion effect**, sometimes called experimenter expectancy, occurs when the experimenter acts in ways that bias the study without necessarily affecting the participant directly, or when the experimenter unintentionally provides cues (demand characteristics) to let participants know what is expected of them. Thus, when a well-intentioned researcher tells clients that he or she knows they will feel much better after participating in the treatment phase of the study, the researcher is setting forth an expectancy statement that could influence participant responses.

Finally, **evaluation apprehension** occurs when participants act in ways they believe will help them avoid the negative evaluations of the researcher, observers, or other

| TABLE 7.2 | Controlling for threats to external validity. |
|---|---|
| **Threat to External Validity** | **Possible Ways to Control Threat** |
| Demand Characteristics | Blind study, control group |
| Hawthorne Effect | Control group |
| Order Effects | Counterbalancing treatment order, multiple groups |
| Treatment Interaction Effects | Subject matching, naturalistic observation |

© Cengage Learning

participants. Evaluation apprehension results from an eagerness to please (reactivity) and some facets of social desirability. For example, a lethargic, monotonic teacher may completely change her teaching style on a day she is observed by her supervisor, acting in accord with the manner she believes the supervisor wishes to see.

Reactivity is generally best controlled by using (a) single-blind or double-blind methodology, (b) unobtrusive measures so participants do not know they are being observed, or, when all else fails, (c) deception. Also, note that some consider reactivity to threaten both internal and external validity because experimenter bias can affect both the validity of the study (internal validity) and generalizability of findings to the general population (external validity).

### Order Effects

The term **order effects** (or carryover effects) refers to treatment effects derived from the order in which treatment is administered rather than from the treatment itself. This is a common problem in within-subjects designs or in single-subject research in which participants are exposed to more than one treatment. Counterbalancing the order of treatments sometimes helps to counteract order effects, but the primary problem is that generalizability of results from the sample to the general population is often not possible unless the population is also exposed to the multiple treatments (and in the most effective order).

### Treatment Interaction Effects

**Treatment interaction effects** refer to the potential for a treatment protocol to have an effect based on the characteristics of the participant rather than on the group as a whole. This is known as an interaction effect of treatment and selection and is confounded because the characteristics of the selected participants may make them respond to treatment in a way that nonparticipants may not. For example, study participants are always "volunteers," and nonvolunteers may respond differently. Also, results of a study of girls may not be readily generalizable to boys. Another type of interaction pertains to treatment and testing. Here, the administration of a pretest may sensitize the participant to the study's purpose, thus changing the participant's reactions to the treatment condition. Consequently, unless individuals in the population are also exposed to and sensitized by the pretest, the results from the sample may not generalize to the population. Table 7.2 provides a summary listing of ways to control for threats to external validity.

## Sampling

As discussed briefly in Chapter 2, sampling decisions are critically important in research because the type of sampling helps to control for threats to internal and external validity. At this point, we will take a look at some sampling methods, including convenience sampling, simple random sampling, stratified random sampling, cluster sampling, and multistage sampling. Then we will explore sampling bias and how to minimize the effects of such bias.

## Convenience Sampling

Convenience sampling involves gathering participants who are available and willing to participate. The degree of generalizability of a convenience sample to the population under study is often questionable, and so reporting demographic characteristics of the sample is critical to determining similarities to a given population of interest. If you are a school counselor conducting a study and ask permission to use the students in your school whose parents sign a consent form, you are using a convenience sample: students can easily access who volunteer to participate.

## Simple Random Sampling

Whenever possible, researchers use simple random sampling to randomly select a portion of the population to comprise the sample. This is different from random assignment, which involves randomly assigning selected participants (such as from any of these sampling methods) to the various treatment conditions (if any). Randomization is a hallmark of experimental designs, and so problems with sampling procedures limit the usefulness of the resulting data from a research project. In simple random sampling, every participant from the population has an equal chance of being selected into the sample. Also, selection of one participant must not affect the selection of any other participant. In true experimental research designs, researchers strive to use simple random sampling to obtain a representative sample from the population and then assign these sample participants to various treatment conditions using some randomizing procedure.

## Stratified Random Sampling

Stratified random sampling is used when the researcher wants to ensure that certain characteristics of participants are reflected in the final sample in the same proportion that they occur in the population. These characteristics are called strata. For example, if 14 percent of a given population is African American, and 86 percent is White, the researcher will separate the population by race and then randomly select 14 percent of the sample from the African American population pool and 86 percent of the sample from the White population pool. This ensures that the study's sample reflects the population on the stratum of race. Commonly used strata are sex, age, socioeconomics, race, ethnicity, educational level, and area of residence.

## Cluster Sampling

Cluster sampling requires the researcher to (randomly or conveniently) select units (clusters) of participants (e.g., several classes of counseling students) and then either randomly select individual participants or select all participants from the cluster. Of course, using random cluster sampling followed by randomized individual participant selection will lead to better representation and generalizability. Because clusters tend to be more homogeneous, larger numbers of clusters enhance demographic strata diversity.

## Multistage Sampling

Multistage sampling is frequently used in large-scale surveys in which initial stratified random samples of larger entities (e.g., states and counties) are followed by simple random samples of smaller entities (e.g., residences and communities) and sometime then even further by simple random sampling of individual participants within the smaller entity. Thus, this procedure uses both randomization and stratification to minimize sampling bias.

## Sample Size and Bias

Random selection and stratification are meant to minimize or eliminate bias, but another consideration in minimizing bias is the size of the sample. Sample sizes are often determined by the research design and nature of the analyses selected. A general rule is that the larger the sample size, the greater the statistical power (i.e., probability of rejecting the null hypothesis when the alternative is true or the likelihood of detecting an effect when the effect is truly present). Although this is an oversimplification of rigorous guidelines, professional counselors can follow the general rule that the larger the sample and more representative the sample is of the population under study, the greater the power and the better the study—as long as high-quality randomized sampling procedures were used.

Determining the appropriate sample size can be a complicated process. First, researchers must consider the magnitude of difference (i.e., effect size) necessary to determine statistical significance. Although a thorough understanding of statistics is necessary to fully comprehend the calculation of effect sizes, a beginning researcher could follow Cohen's (1988) classification of effect sizes into small, medium, and large (see Chapter 4). A majority of researchers in counseling are satisfied with medium effect sizes.

The second significant factor when determining sample size is the statistical power desired. Although not carved in stone, an accepted standard in research is a power level of .80, which means that researchers are willing to accept a 20 percent probability that they will fail to detect a true effect through their research procedures. See Chapter 16 for a more detailed discussion of effect size and statistical power.

When researchers determine their effect size and power level, they can then use various statistical tables to determine the appropriate sample size for their methodology. Many researchers, however, now rely on computer programs such as *Statistical Power Analysis* by Borenstein and Cohen (1988) to determine appropriate sample size. As the Internet continues to evolve, counseling researchers can turn more to online sources for sample size determination as well.

# Types of Research Designs

As a professional counselor, you may or may not ever create your own research projects. But regardless of setting, it is exceedingly important that you provide your clients with the best practice approaches available to you. For you to be able to make these types of decisions, you will need a basic understanding of research design. There are various types of quantitative research designs: experimental research, quasi-experimental research, nonexperimental research, survey research, correlational studies, causal-comparative studies, single-case research, meta-analysis, and action-based research (Figure 7.1).

Most quantitative designs can be classified into two major categories: experimental or nonexperimental research. Experimental research ordinarily includes true experimental, quasi-experimental, and single-case designs. In **true experimental designs**, which can be used to make cause–effect determinations, researchers introduce treatments to participants and observe if any changes in behavior occur. A form of experimental design is the **single-case design**, in which researchers manipulate variables or introduce a treatment to one participant or group over time and intently study its effects. **Quasi-experimental designs**

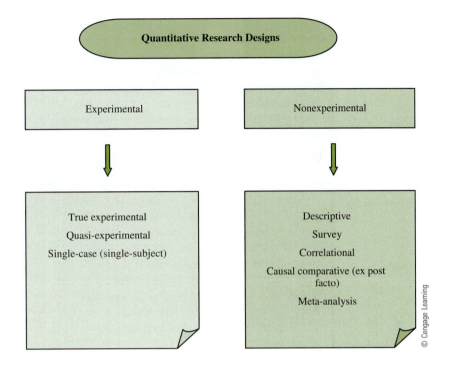

© Cengage Learning

**Figure 7.1**

Quantitative research designs.

are similar to true experimental designs but do not use random assignment as a means of control, thus limiting their ability to infer cause and effect. Each of these designs will be explored in greater detail later in the chapter.

**Nonexperimental designs**, which are used to describe participant characteristics or behaviors, do not involve the application of any treatment to participants; usually the participants just answer questions or complete protocols. Often, nonexperimental studies may be called **descriptive studies** or **survey research**. Descriptive studies merely describe an existing phenomenon by using numbers to characterize individuals or groups. Survey researchers administer questionnaires or interview participants to collect data. Researchers who are using **correlational designs** (e.g., administer several rating scales or questionnaires and correlate the scores) merely look at the degree and direction of the relationship between variables. Another form of nonexperimental study is the causal-comparative study. **Causal-comparative studies** (i.e., **ex post facto studies**) observe and describe some current condition, but rather than introduce treatments, researchers look to the past to try to identify possible causes. **Meta-analysis** is a statistical procedure for examining the results of several to numerous research studies on the same topic and determining the congruence and divergence of outcome data. Each of these designs will be described in greater detail throughout the remainder of this chapter.

## Designs Commonly Used in Human Development

Human development researchers frequently identify research design procedures as cross-sectional, longitudinal, and cross-sequential (i.e., cohort sequential). **Cross-sectional designs** compare groups of participants of different ages at the same point in time. Cross-sectional studies are quick and economical but subject to cohort effects (e.g., generational effects), in which the differences in results between age groups may be because of the differences in shared experiences rather than to increasing age. For example, if a researcher wanted to study intelligence using a cross-sectional design, the researcher would administer an IQ test to groups of 5-, 10-, 15-, 20-, 25-, and 30-year-olds at the same time and compare the differences between or among age groups.

Longitudinal designs evaluate changes in participants over an extended period of time, often years or decades. Longitudinal studies are expensive to conduct and potentially experience contamination because of repeated testing or exposure to the dependent variable, and because of mortality. In addition, generalizability of longitudinal results to other generations not represented in the sample may be limited. For example, if a researcher wanted to study intelligence using a longitudinal design, the researcher would administer an IQ test to a group of 5-year-olds and then re-administer the test to the same group of participants when they become 10, 15, 20, 25, and 30 years old, and compare the differences between or among age groups.

Cross-sequential designs, also called cohort-sequential designs, comprise combinations of cross-sectional and longitudinal designs by assessing participants from two or more age groups (usually generations apart) at more than one point in time. The primary advantage of a cross-sequential design is that it allows compensation for both cohort effects and generalizability of results. For example, if a researcher wanted to study intelligence using a cross-sequential design, the researcher would administer an IQ test to a group of 5-year-olds and another group of 20-year-olds and then re-administer the test to the same groups every five years for a 15-year period (or more) and compare the differences between and among groups. Likewise, a previous study that assessed the same group of 5-year-olds at five-year intervals 30 years ago could be replicated on a present day sample of 5-year-olds assessed at five-year intervals.

## Experimental Research Designs

By now, most readers have some experience with research as an experimental procedure. Whether conducting experiments in high school or undergraduate science classes or required to read about experiments in introductory psychology courses, the reader probably knows that experimental designs allow a researcher to make more direct causal conclusions through the establishment of different treatments or the manipulation of some variable. The treatment(s) or intervention(s) manipulated is identified as the independent variable, whereas the scores or results of the treatment are considered the dependent variable (e.g., criterion or outcome variable). Some variables that may be manipulated include treatment methods for depression, teaching methods, or student learning methods. The experiment usually includes two groups of participants, identified as the experimental group (e.g., receives treatment) and a control group (e.g., receives no treatment) or comparison group.

### Considerations in Experimental Research Designs

In general, experimental research designs are classified as group designs and single-subject designs. (Single-subject research designs will be mentioned briefly later in this chapter, but covered in detail in Chapter 8.) Group designs are further categorized as between-groups designs, within-subjects designs, and mixed-group designs. Between-groups designs are popular in experimental studies because they allow participants to be separated into groups according to some characteristic or intended treatment (independent variable) so that their performances on a dependent variable can be compared. The classic between-groups design involves participants being randomly assigned to either a treatment or control group (e.g., medication versus placebo, respectively), conducting the experiment by administering the treatment over some period of time and then finally measuring the participants' performance on some outcome measure (dependent variable). Usually employing some statistical procedure, the researcher determines whether the participants in the treatment group differed from the participants in the control group—thus the term *between-groups* design (i.e., determining a difference between the treatment group and control group participants).

A **within-subjects design** exposes the same group of participants to several levels of a treatment (independent variable), measuring their performances on the dependent variable after receiving each level of treatment and comparing their average group performance between the various levels of treatment. For example, each participant may be pretested, then assessed again after taking a placebo for two weeks, and finally tested again after receiving the experimental medication for two weeks. By employing statistical procedures, the researcher then attempts to determine whether any change occurred between the pretesting observation and postplacebo observation, or between the postplacebo observation and posttreatment observation administered to each participant within the subject group—thus the term *within-subjects design* (i.e., determining the differences occurring within participants due to treatment). Within-subjects designs have two advantages over between-groups designs. First, within-subjects designs require fewer participants because each participant is exposed to multiple conditions. Second, within-subjects designs offer better control of individual differences (i.e., possible across group differences are eliminated) because the same individuals are used for all conditions, thus causing the results to be more powerful.

**Mixed-group designs**, also called **split-plot designs**, combine between-groups and within-subject designs into a single study, usually by implementing two independent variables, one being a between-groups variable and the other a within-subjects variable. For example, if it is hypothesized that males and females may have different reactions to the experimental drugs, males and females may be split into two different groups (sex being a between-groups variable) and each group then pretested, exposed to a placebo, assessed a second time, then exposed to the experimental drug (treatment being a within-groups variable), and assessed a third time. More sophisticated statistical analysis is required for mixed-group designs, but the question is similar: Is there a difference between or within groups?

## Weak Experimental Designs

There are various group designs in experimental research, each with advantages and disadvantages. Some weaker experimental designs, called nonexperimental designs by some, include the one-shot case study, the one-group pretest–posttest design, and the static-group comparison design. Table 7.3 presents a visual comparison of these weaker experimental designs. The **one-shot case study** involves a single group that is exposed to a treatment with a subsequent observation of the dependent variable. This method offers little control of the variable and does not allow comparison of treatment results. Usually, a one-shot case study is conducted after some event has occurred unexpectedly and only a convenience sample is available. Because no control is possible over the sample or event, no causal inference is possible. The **one-group pretest–posttest design** observes (pretest) a single group prior to treatment and after exposure to treatment (posttest). This design allows the researcher to know whether there was an effect, but lack of participant randomization or a control group means other threats to internal validity may also explain the results (e.g., history, maturation,

**TABLE 7.3**  Weak experimental group research designs.

| | | | | |
|---|---|---|---|---|
| One-Shot Case Study | | | X | O |
| One-Group Pretest–Posttest | O | X | O | |
| Static-Group Comparison | | $X_1$ | O | |
| | | $X_2$ | O | |

*Note:* O = observation of the dependent variable; X = treatment condition; $X_1$ and $X_2$ = variations of the treatment condition.
© Cengage Learning

instrument decay, data collector characteristics, data collector bias, testing, statistical regression, attitude of participants, and implementation). The **static-group comparison design** uses two existing groups (but participants were not randomly assigned) that are exposed to different treatments for comparison. In this design, no pretesting is conducted. This design offers more control over history, maturation, testing, and regression threats than either the one-shot case study or one-group pretest–posttest design, but it tends to be more vulnerable to mortality and location and differential subject characteristics. Each of these three designs suffers from major flaws of experimental control and therefore has limited usefulness when a researcher wants to establish cause and effect or to generalize results to other populations.

### True Experimental Designs

True experimental designs use the tool of random assignment to control for all sources of internal validity and allow research to legitimately infer causation. **Random assignment** refers to each participant having an equal chance of being assigned to any of the experimental or control groups. Of course, this differs from **random selection**, which is the possibility of every member of a population having an equal chance of being selected to be a member of the sample (e.g., using a table of random numbers). Random assignment is used to eliminate or minimize variance due to extraneous variables (e.g., an uncontrolled variable). An extraneous variable may threaten the validity of a study by providing an alternate explanation for the effect of an experiment, thus interfering with making direct cause-and-effect explanations. An experimental study should attempt to make the groups as equivalent as possible and minimize any characteristic of individuals that might affect or alter the outcome of the study.

Four types of true experimental research designs are the randomized posttest-only control group design, randomized pretest–posttest control group design, randomized Solomon four-group design, and random assignment with matching design. Table 7.4 diagrammatically represents these designs.

| **TABLE 7.4** True experimental research group designs. |
|---|

| | | | | |
|---|---|---|---|---|
| *Randomized Posttest-Only Control Group* | | | | |
| Treatment Group | R | $X_1$ | O | |
| Control Group | R | $X_0$ | O | |
| *Randomized Pretest–Posttest Control Group* | | | | |
| Treatment Group | R | O | $X_1$ | O |
| *Randomized Solomon Four-Group Design* | | | | |
| Treatment Group | R | O | $X_1$ | O |
| Control Group | R | O | $X_0$ | O |
| Treatment Group | R | | $X_1$ | O |
| Control Group | R | | $X_0$ | O |
| *Random Assignment Posttest-Only Control Design with Matching Participants* | | | | |
| Treatment Group | $R_m$ | $X_1$ | O | |
| Control Group | $R_m$ | $X_0$ | O | |
| *Random Assignment Pretest–Posttest Control Design with Matching Participants* | | | | |
| Treatment Group | O | $R_m$ | $X_1$ | O |
| Control Group | O | $R_m$ | $X_0$ | O |

*Note:* R = random assignment; X, $X_1$, or $X_2$ = treatment; $X_0$ = control; O = observation of the dependent variable; Rm = randomly assigned matched participants.

© Cengage Learning

Randomized posttest-only control group design involves random assignment of participants into two groups: one group receives no treatment (i.e., control group) and one group receives the treatment (i.e., experimental group). After conclusion of the experiment, members of each group are assessed relative to their performance on the dependent variable. It is assumed that randomization makes the two groups equivalent, thus making a pretest unnecessary. For example, professional counselors may want to know the effect of a psychoeducational group (e.g., the experimental condition) on stress reduction of participants. In using a posttest-only control group design, the professional counselors would randomly assign clients to either a waiting list (i.e., control group) or to the experimental condition. At the conclusion of the group, the professional counselors could measure stress levels in both the control and experimental groups. As one may already see, it could be important to know the stress levels of participants prior to beginning the experiment to understand the true effects of the psychoeducational group. But randomized assignment is meant to minimize initial group differences, although additional assessment may be required to tell if this was actually accomplished.

The randomized pretest–posttest control group design involves randomly assigning participants into two groups (i.e., control group and treatment group), with both receiving the pretest, then subjecting each to their level of treatment, and finally administering a posttest. This method allows the researcher to check for the accuracy of random assignment. Using our previous example of the psychoeducational group, professional counselors would administer a stress scale to all participants prior to beginning treatment and after the group ended. Thus, researchers would have more confidence in the results of their analyses because they would know if the treatment actually increased or decreased scores on the stress scale as compared to the control group. Using the pretest in this design, however, may result in an interaction between testing and treatment. Thus, other designs may be even more appropriate.

The randomized Solomon four-group design reduces the pretest effect of the previous design by having participants randomly assigned to four groups. In this design, two groups (control A and treatment group A) receive pretests and two groups do not (control B and treatment group B). Thus, researchers who are studying the effect of the psychoeducational group as just discussed would be able to determine the effects of the intervention and rule out any interaction between pretest measurement and treatment. Basically, the randomized Solomon four-group design is a combination of the randomized posttest-only control group and pretest–posttest control group designs.

Another experimental design, random assignment with matching design, attempts to increase the equivalency of groups of participants by matching individuals on certain variables (e.g., sex and race). The members of each matched pair are then randomly assigned to an experimental or control group. Random assignment with matching can be accomplished using the posttest-only control or the pretest–posttest group control design, the latter being more common.

## Quasi-Experimental Research Designs

Quasi-experimental research designs are similar to experimental research designs with the exception that quasi-experimental research does not use random assignment to control internal validity but rather relies on other techniques for control. Sometimes in research studies a control group may not be available or the experimenter cannot control the random assignment of participants because the independent variable may be organismic (e.g., sex and race), meaning that only a **comparison study** is possible between the two nonrandomized groups. Also, sometimes only one group may be available for study, or only intact or preexisting groups must be used, disallowing random assignments.

In each of these instances, the inability to randomly assign participants prohibits the use of an experimental design, thus often relegating the researcher to a quasi-experimental design. At least five types of quasi-experimental designs exist: matching-only designs, counterbalanced designs, time-series designs, factorial designs, and nonequivalent control group designs.

The **matching-only design** is similar to the experimental matching designs (Table 7.4) in that it uses intact groups of matched participants on a particular variable, but it does not use random assignment. Matching should not be construed as a substitute for random assignment in that matching controls for only the variables being matched.

**Counterbalanced designs** can use two or more groups, but each group is exposed to all of the treatments and in a different order. Note that no randomization or matched groupings are attempted. The treatments are rotated (i.e., counterbalanced) to compensate for potential errors due to ordering effects. Each group's scores are then averaged together to provide the degree of effectiveness of the various treatments. This design controls for participant characteristics but may lead to multiple-treatment interference. See Table 7.5 for an example of a counterbalanced design.

**Time-series designs** make numerous measurements or observations over a period of time prior to and after treatment (e.g., O O O X O O O). When using these designs, some possible threats to internal validity are the effects of history, instrumentation, testing (practice effect), and pretest–treatment interaction. **Factorial designs** allow the researcher to study additional variables and/or the interaction of an independent variable with one or more other variables, thus extending the number of relationships that can be investigated. One of the most popular quasi-experimental designs is the **nonequivalent control group design**, in which the treatment group is given the treatment in between the pretest and posttest, whereas the control group is not. Note that neither group is subjected to participant randomization or matching. In conclusion, quasi-experimental designs give up some experimental control but can lead researchers to infer some degree of causality, which of course should be followed up by more powerful true experimental designs in future studies.

Suppose a counselor wants to study whether a new counseling treatment (cause) reduces the effects (effect) of post-traumatic stress disorder (PTSD) in clients over a period of six months. To conduct this study, the researchers need to find a large sample of people with PTSD. To obtain participants, they might call professional counselors in the region seeking nominations of clients, advertise in the local newspapers, and write to other medical schools looking for possible candidates to be participants. To obtain their samples, the researchers contact each one of the people nominated by professional counselors or medical centers and all the people who reply to the advertisement in the newspaper. But as soon as a potential participant chooses (self-selects) to participate in a study, then one of the conditions of a true or pure experiment is compromised. Participants who volunteer to participate in a study are not necessarily the same as participants who are already in a setting and reassigned to an experimental or control group. In other words, there is something about being a volunteer in a study that may affect the results.

| **TABLE 7.5** | Three-treatment counterbalance design. | | | | |
|---|---|---|---|---|---|
| Group I | $X_1$ | O | $X_2$ | O | $X_3$ | O |
| Group II | $X_2$ | O | $X_3$ | O | $X_1$ | O |
| Group III | $X_3$ | O | $X_1$ | O | $X_2$ | O |

*Note:* $X_1$, $X_2$, or $X_3$ = various forms of treatment; O = observation of the dependent variable.

© Cengage Learning

There are many other kinds of compromises that can affect the results of the study at this point. Perhaps the researchers paid the participants to participate. That is a trade-off that could turn an experimental design into a quasi-experimental design. Consider a study where the researchers want to investigate the extent to which a set of classroom instructional materials (cause) designed to make classroom interactions more humane and less threatening actually produces that effect (effect). In this example, the researchers cannot easily randomly assign the students in the classrooms to the experimental and control groups. That would disrupt the rest of the business of the school. They must, in this example, accept the intact nature of the classrooms as a trade-off or compromise in this study. Good researchers are cognizant of these design compromises and write them into their research report for other researchers to note. It is essential to be clear about the limitations of any study because any one of them can affect the results and how they are applied either in future research or even in practice.

Now, if the study were of cattle on a farm, then the herd could be divided into different groups without the taint of volunteering. The cattle do not already exist in a social structure like a teacher's class that cannot be divided up into two or more groups of participants without disrupting that social structure in other important ways. It is at this point that one would label the study of clients with PTSD or the study of the instructional materials as quasi-experimental designs because they do not meet all the strict criteria of an experimental design. In fact, it is often impossible in the human science fields to meet all the requirements of an experimental method, so we accept the quasi-experimental method and write the research report acknowledging the necessary compromises the researcher had to make to obtain the best possible data to study the effects of the new treatment on PTSD, or the instructional materials on classroom climate. Of experimental and quasi-experimental designs, the latter dominates in the quantitative studies literature in the human sciences.

## Nonexperimental Research Designs

Nonexperimental research does not manipulate any variables or test hypotheses; rather, it merely obtains data to determine specific characteristics of a group or to describe a phenomenon (e.g., descriptive study or case study). This method is used in a high percentage of counseling studies and is also useful for investigating educational issues. A descriptive study is conducted with a large number of individuals via mail, telephone, computer, or in person. When questions are asked in person, this is called an interview. One type of descriptive study is survey research. Survey research is conducted to describe the characteristics of a population by selecting a representative sample of respondents for the research. Two characteristic types of surveys are cross-sectional and longitudinal. In a cross-sectional survey, researchers obtain data from a sample drawn from a predetermined population (e.g., all high school counselors). In a longitudinal survey, however, researchers collect data at different points in time to study any changes that occur. There are three types of longitudinal surveys: trend study, cohort study, and panel study. A **trend study** is used to survey different samples from a population whose members may change over time. Thus, the same population is studied using different random samples from that population. A **cohort study** includes members of a particular population who do not change over the course of the survey (e.g., if a researcher wanted to study competency, a list of all master counselors who graduated from a specific university would be obtained and a sample chosen from this cohort). A **panel study** includes the same sample of individuals surveyed at different times.

Survey research can be a difficult process, largely because we, as a society, are inundated with surveys from all walks of life. As an example, you may notice that many restaurants have comment cards on the tables for customers to complete. Also, retail stores may offer an incentive if you complete a questionnaire on their web site. Both these examples are marketing research efforts that use a survey design. How often do you fill out these research requests? Chances are that you ignore them to some degree. If you completed each request, you may never get anything else accomplished! Thus, one of the main challenges of conducting research in counseling that uses survey design is to get individuals to buy into the research and complete the instrument. Failure to obtain an adequate sample leads to nonresponse bias. **Nonresponse bias** occurs when the participants who respond to the survey differ in characteristics from those who do not respond. In general, the lower the response rate the greater the threat of nonresponse bias. To counteract nonresponse bias, survey researchers take great measures to motivate potential respondents using incentives and multiple follow-ups and reminders. In the end, survey researchers must determine that those who choose not to respond are equivalent to those who did respond—a time-consuming and procedurally daunting task given that nonresponders usually do not respond because they do not wish to participate.

The first step in getting participants to buy into your project is the cover letter. Survey researchers send a letter along with the survey requesting participation and identifying information about the researcher, the purpose of the survey, potential benefits and drawbacks to participation, and the importance of the participant's cooperation. Informed consent (i.e., agreement to participate) is important for any research effort. In some cases, researchers include an informed consent form for participants to sign. The informed consent form should thoroughly provide participants with the necessary information to make an informed decision whether to participate in the study. The informed consent form should include identification of and qualifications of the researchers, the purpose of the study, how the research is to be conducted, and if there may be any possible risk, discomforts, or benefits. With survey research, however, informed consent is often implied by the participant's completion of the survey.

Another important aspect of conducting survey research is choosing the appropriate instrument(s). The most common instrument is the questionnaire (completed by the participant) or interview schedule (verbally administered by the researcher). Appearance and format of the questionnaire should be visually appealing, precisely written, and easily understood by the participant. Closed-ended questions offer multiple-choice answers and can be easily used, scored, and coded for statistical analysis. Open-ended questions allow for more detailed information but are often hard to analyze and interpret. It is important to pilot test any instruments and check the format of the questionnaires through administration to a small sample of trusted individuals, such as fellow students or colleagues.

Because individuals may hesitate to complete surveys, the data-collection methods chosen for this type of research are critical. There are several ways to do this: (a) direct administration to a group, (b) mail surveys (or e-mailed surveys), (c) telephone interviews, or (d) face-to-face interviews. Direct administration is used when the researcher has access to the members of a particular group at the same time. This method ordinarily provides a high rate of responses, is generally low cost, and allows explanation of the research to participants prior to participation. Mailed surveys are sent to each individual via the mail with a request for completion and return by a designated date. They have the added benefit of allowing access to individuals who may be harder to reach in person or via telephone. The disadvantage of this method, however, is that it offers little control and less opportunity to encourage participation. Nonresponse rates and nonreturn rates may be high, depending on the sample surveyed.

Thanks to advanced methods of technology, an innovative means of conducting surveys is through the Internet or e-mailed surveys. Rather than sending surveys via postal delivery, e-mail surveys are sent electronically. E-mailed surveys have the added advantage of allowing mass e-mails at low or no costs. Disadvantages of the e-mail method are difficulty determining the accuracy of sampling and potential nonresponse bias. Gaining access to a group of e-mail addresses relative to respondents with certain characteristics can be difficult. In addition, researchers must consider the fact that although the world is advancing technologically, many people do not have computers or access to e-mail. Thus, randomization of the sample procedures can be affected to some degree.

For researchers who are interested in collecting data via the Internet, web sites are now available that assist in creating surveys. Some Internet companies maintain large databases and will allow researchers access to existing data for a fee. Before you use Internet databases, however, it is important to verify that these sites are regulated and abide by the human subjects ethical research guidelines.

Telephone surveys offer a little more control over standardizing questioning procedures and can be conducted fairly quickly. The disadvantages of telephone surveys can include long-distance costs, lack of access to some samples (i.e., those without phones), and the inability to visually observe participants. Face-to-face interviews offer many advantages and possibly the most effective means of enlisting cooperation from participants. Some advantages of interviews are that they allow rapport building, question clarifications, follow-up questions, and place less burden on the literacy skills of the participant.

Ekstrom, Elmore, Schafer, Trotter, and Webster (2004) provided an excellent example of the use of survey research to examine the means by which and the degree to which professional school counselors performed various assessment and evaluation activities in an effort to develop assessment competencies for the school counseling profession. The researchers reviewed state assessment training requirements, state-mandated performance expectations, and state department of education expectations for assessment practices of professional school counselors. Based on their review of materials, the researchers discovered 39 program development and assessment-related activities that were used as the basis of the survey.

As is the case with many surveys, participants were asked to rate their level of engagement in the identified activities (i.e., 3 = often, 2 = occasionally, and 1 = seldom or never). The researchers sent surveys to a random sample of 600 professional school counselors who were members of the American School Counselors Association (ASCA). Ekstrom et al. (2004) clearly understood the need to obtain buy-in from participants, evidenced by their inclusion of a cover letter signed by the ASCA president that described the importance of the survey. Although the researchers made efforts to ensure a high response rate, only 179 school counselors responded to the survey (a 30 percent return rate). Of these respondents, only 161 indicated that they worked as professional school counselors (a 27 percent yield).

Based on the results of the survey, Ekstrom et al. (2004, p. 27) reported the following nine assessment activities in which professional school counselors often engage:

- Referring students to other professionals, when appropriate, for additional assessment/appraisal (98 percent)
- Interpreting scores from tests/assessments and using the information in counseling (91 percent)
- Reading about and being aware of ethical issues in assessment (86 percent)
- Reading about and being aware of current issues involving multicultural assessment, the assessment of students with disabilities and other special needs, and the assessment of language minorities (84 percent)
- Synthesizing and integrating test and nontest data to make decisions about individuals (84 percent)

- Reading a variety of professional literature on topics such as use of testing and assessment in school *counseling*, school *counseling* research, and career *counseling* research (84 percent)
- Communicating and interpreting test/assessment information to parents (81 percent)
- Communicating and interpreting test/assessment information to teachers, school administrators, and other professionals (80 percent)
- Helping teachers use assessments and assessment information (80 percent)

As another example, a researcher might be interested in how professional counselors view their preparation for practice with children who have attention-deficit/hyperactivity disorder (ADHD). He would send a questionnaire to a sample of practicing counselors to find out how well the institution where they earned their professional degree prepared them to work with children diagnosed with ADHD. His goal may be to design a professional development experience for professional counselors that will help them develop greater skill in this area now that they are in practice. From the resulting data, the researcher will learn in what areas the greatest number of professional counselors feel prepared and underprepared, and he can then begin to design the professional development program. You have likely been a participant in one survey or another, either in a formal study or a telephone interview or even a brief questionnaire about your satisfaction with a product you purchased, such as an automobile. The findings of survey research are treated with some power. All media outlets like to report the results of surveys because we tend to treat them as barometers for self-comparison. When we hear that 42 percent of the population trusts the national government, we tend to compare ourselves with that number. Survey results are, however, only descriptive of the time in which they are produced. In other words, they are quite limited to the time and contexts in which the data were collected.

## Correlational Research Designs

The correlational research design, sometimes referred to as **associational research**, is used to investigate the relationship among two or more variables without attempting to manipulate them. The purpose of a correlational study is to determine relationships between variables or to use these relationships to make predictions (e.g., linear regression). Correlational research is usually conducted to help explain human behaviors or to predict likely outcomes. Explanatory studies seek to clarify or understand the relationship among variables pertaining to important phenomena. Prediction studies can be used to determine another variable based on the known magnitude of one variable in a correlational relationship.

Researchers who use correlational designs seek to describe the direction and degree to which two or more variables are related through the use of a correlation coefficient. A correlational coefficient ranges between .00 and 1.00 in both the positive and negative directions. Correlation coefficients closer to .00 indicate a weaker to no relationship. Correlation coefficients closer to 1.00 indicate a stronger relationship between variables (see Chapter 17). A positive correlation indicates that high scores on one variable are associated with high scores on the other variable or that low scores on one variable are associated with low scores on the other variable. Most people have been directly affected by correlational research. For example, you may have taken the Graduate Record Exam (GRE) as part of the admission requirement for a graduate program of study. The reason this examination is used is that it was hypothesized that GRE scores would have a positive correlation with subsequent grades in graduate school (i.e., GPA). In other words, those students who perform well on the GRE should perform well in graduate school.

The predictor variable is the variable used to make the prediction, whereas the criterion variable is the variable upon which the prediction is made. By the way, while a positive relationship between GRE scores and GPA scores exists, many believe that the relationship is not strong enough to warrant an admission decision solely based on student GRE scores. Thus, counseling programs use a range of information to make admissions decisions.

A negative correlation indicates a contradictory (i.e., inverse) relationship, with low scores on one variable being associated with high scores on the other variable or vice versa. For example, one may be able to identify a negative correlation between the number of course-related reading assignments during the semester and the amount of time dedicated to leisure activities. Although I am attempting to add some humor to this discussion of correlational research, the implications of such a negative correlation can be vast (e.g., increased stress levels, less physical exercise, increased weight, increased relationship problems). Hopefully, through this example, one can see the importance of identifying the relationships between or among variables.

Readers, however, should be cautioned that correlational studies do not indicate any cause and effect relationship among variables (i.e., correlation is *not* causation), merely the magnitude (how strong) or the direction (positive or negative) of the relationships. Thus, one cannot say that the number of reading assignments received will cause one to gain weight, but one may be able to see a relationship between these two events. A correlation score above $+.40$ or below $-.40$ usually indicates a fairly strong relationship that researchers may want to further investigate using an experimental design.

As an example of correlational research, a counseling researcher may be interested in the relationship between a personality characteristic, such as "strength of faith" and a measure of "fear of dying," both measured with standardized questionnaires that each yield a score. The researcher cannot alter either variable—strength of faith or fear of dying—and so might simply want to understand the relationship between the participants' strength of faith and its relationship to their fear of dying. The researcher might, based on previous research, hope to see a negative correlation between these two variables (e.g., as strength of faith increases, the fear of dying decreases). There is most certainly a relationship, but without intervening in some way, the researcher cannot discern whether it is cause and effect. It is just a relationship of two variables that occur together. Correlations are very useful in helping researchers understand how various aspects of the participants' lives relate to other aspects of interest. But in and of themselves, correlational studies are not as confirming as experimental and quasi-experimental designs, which seek to isolate the relationship as cause and effect, and determine the effectiveness of interventions.

## Causal-Comparative Research Designs

Causal-comparative designs are used to determine the possible causes or the consequences of differences between groups of people or individuals (e.g., ethnicity, gender, and race). In this type of research, variables reflecting group differences cannot be manipulated or have not been manipulated in the study, or some ethical considerations prevent such manipulation. Causal-comparative designs describe both the effect(s) and the alleged causes(s) of the differences between existing groups and thus are sometimes referred to as *ex post facto*, meaning "after the fact" in Latin.

Causal-comparative designs are a type of associational research, similar to correlational research, as both describe conditions that already exist or have already occurred. While correlational studies compare two or more quantitative variables or scores for each subject and present data using scatterplots or correlation coefficients, causal-comparative studies compare two or more groups of participants with at least one categorical variable (e.g., group membership). Most data results are presented as averages or cross-break tables (i.e., a table that shows all combinations of two or more categorical variables and portrays the relationship, if any, between the variables).

The advantage of a causal-comparative design is apparent when attempting to study the link between cigarette smoking and health, for example. It would be unethical to introduce cigarettes to healthy individuals to see the results on health, not to mention that it may take a long time for any effects to be observable. Thus, researchers may begin by noting the differences in previously collected data on existing smokers and non-smokers to look for possible causes, or consequences, of the health differences.

Although helpful in some cases, the causal-comparative design has its disadvantages: mainly, threats to internal validity (e.g., lack of randomization and inability to manipulate independent variables) as a result of the lack of control over the variables. This lack of control limits the researcher's ability to state conclusively whether a particular factor is a cause or a result of the behavior observed. The observed differences may be an actual effect, or it may be a cause rather than an effect, or there may be some third unidentified factor that can account for the cause or effect.

For example, Wilson (1999) discovered that African Americans ($n = 3,852$) and European Americans ($n = 13,124$) with disabilities are equally likely to use vocational rehabilitation (VR) services. Using a causal-comparative design, Wilson examined archives of VR clients and compared acceptance rates for services by race to reach this conclusion. Then in a more specific analysis Capella (2002) also used a causal-comparative design to examine acceptance rates for VR services between participants of different racial backgrounds. In two samples of 10,000 participants (sample 1 = severe disabilities and sample 2 = nonsevere disabilities), Capella found that African Americans were significantly less likely to be accepted for VR services than European Americans among the severe disability group. This result, however, was not found for the nonsevere disability group. Through similar research, Capella found that African Americans and Native Americans were significantly less likely to successfully obtain employment than European Americans. Although Capella did not provide any treatment to the samples in an experimental sense, the results of the analyses are still very relevant and important to individuals who are providing counseling services to people of varying ability levels, because these results indicate that when attempting to provide VR services to an African American client with a severe disability, a concerted effort would be placed on employment.

## Single-Case Research Designs

An interesting form of experimental research design useful to practicing professional counselors is the **single-subject research design** or **single-case research design**, which involves an intensive study of a single individual or sometimes a single group over time after exposure to a treatment or intervention (see Chapter 8 for an in-depth discussion of single-subject methodology). To measure what changes occur, a **baseline** (e.g., the state of the individual or group prior to intervention or treatment) must first be established. A line graph is most frequently used to show the participant's changes over time. The dependent variable is displayed on the vertical axis, which may represent the scores of students learning to read. The horizontal axis usually indicates the passage of time. The **condition lines** indicate that the condition has changed, and the **data points** represent the data collected at various times during the study. Figure 7.2 provides a diagram of a commonly used single-case design.

Many types of single-subject designs exist, including the A-B design, A-B-A design, A-B-A-B design, B-A-B design, A-B-C-B design, and the multiple-baseline design. The **A-B design** introduces a treatment or intervention with the same participant acting as

**Figure 7.2**

Simple phase change.

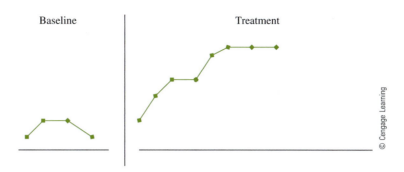

Baseline     Treatment

© Cengage Learning

his or her own control. The *A* represents the baseline period or pretreatment phase where no treatment is introduced. The *B* represents the introduction of the treatment intervention or condition. The participant is usually then observed for a specific number of responses or behaviors. One of the disadvantages of using the A-B design is that it does not control for various threats to internal validity, such as extraneous variables. Using the **A-B-A design** may minimize this threat. This design merely adds another baseline period and thus adds stronger evidence for the treatment's effectiveness. This design, however, contains a disadvantage to the participant in that it leaves the participant without the treatment condition, which may have been ineffective. For this reason, researchers may choose to implement the **A-B-A-B design**, which involves two baseline periods and two treatment periods. Once the baseline is established, the treatment is introduced. This is followed by another baseline during which the treatment is withdrawn, and then finally the treatment is again introduced. This pattern of response provides strong evidence that the treatment, rather than other extraneous variables, was responsible for the changes in the participant.

The **B-A-B design** involves introducing the treatment first and then taking a baseline, followed by reintroduction of the treatment. This design is used most frequently when researchers cannot wait to establish a baseline due to the client's disturbing or severe behavior. This design can also be used if the participant has never shown or lacks the behavior under investigation or when an intervention is already ongoing. The **A-B-C-B design** introduces a variation of the intervention in the B condition to control for any differences in treatment protocol that may affect participant responses.

The *multiple-baseline designs* are used when it is impossible or unethical to withdraw treatment or return to a baseline. This design can be used to collect data on several participants on a single behavior or to measure a participant's behavior in more than one different setting. Multiple-baseline designs collect several baseline behaviors for one participant during the same period and setting. The researcher then systematically introduces the treatment at different times for each behavior the participant displayed. This requires that the treatments being introduced are independent of each other. It can be assumed that if behavior changes in each case after treatment was applied, then it was the treatment that caused the change. Again, various single-subject research designs will be explored in far more detail in Chapter 8. In this era of accountability and managed care, single-case research designs are particularly helpful to professional counselors striving to document outcomes.

## Meta-Analysis

**Meta-analysis** refers to a statistical procedure developed by Glass (1976) that combines the results of several similar studies on a specific topic or area of research. The researcher takes an average of the results of selected studies on the same topic to get an overall index of outcome or relationships. There are certain requirements in conducting a meta-analysis. Most commonly, researchers examine the *effect size* (see Chapters 4 and 16) by using the standard deviation as a way of quantifying the difference between two groups (e.g., the ratio of the difference between the means to the standard deviation) or examining correlation coefficients across studies. The obvious disadvantage of a meta-analysis is that a poorly designed study is weighted as much as a well-designed study, possibly skewing the results of the final analysis. As an example of a meta-analysis, Gonzalez et al. (2004) examined 19 research studies on rational emotive behavioral therapy (REBT) with children and adolescents. Based on the meta-analysis, the largest mean effect size was related to the treatment of disruptive behavior, meaning that REBT may be most effectively used when dealing with this population of students. Although the findings related to the effects of REBT were important for the treatment of children and adolescents, an interesting discovery was that nonmental health professionals using REBT had a greater impact on children and adolescents than mental health practitioners. Rongione, Erford, and Broglie (2011), Erford, Erford et al. (2011), and Erford et al. (2013) conducted several meta-analyses demonstrating that counseling was effective in the treatment of substance use in school-aged children, depression in school-aged children, and bulimia, respectively, generally resulting in medium effect sizes at termination and follow-up.

# Conclusion

Research is a critical component of effective counseling practice. Ethically, professional counselors should take a best-practice approach to their work. One way to accomplish this is through the use of empirical data. Quantitative research designs provide professional counselors with relevant group data for the populations served. Although many readers may not ever produce new research, understanding and interpreting quantitative data are critical skills for every professional counselor to possess. In an effort to hone those skills, experimental research methods (i.e., true experimental, quasi-experimental, and single-case designs) in comparison with nonexperimental research methods (i.e., descriptive, survey, correlation, causal-comparative, and meta-analysis) were discussed within the context of counseling. Although this review of quantitative methods is limited in scope, readers should have a basic understanding of threats to internal validity (i.e., selection, history, maturation, mortality, testing, instrumentation, experimenter bias, and statistical regression), external validity (i.e., reactivity arrangements [placebo effect, Hawthorne effect, demand characteristics, Pygmalion effect, and evaluation apprehension], order effects, and treatment interaction effects), and methods of control in experimental design (i.e., maximizing variability due to the independent variable, minimizing variability due to extraneous variables, minimizing random error, and use of control groups).

*Now go to the Student Workbook found on cengagebrain.com that accompanies this text for additional application and review activities.*

# Practical Counseling Research Approaches: Using Action Research and Single-Subject Research Designs

## CHAPTER 8

Many counseling students and professional counselors alike have difficulty viewing themselves as researchers, and students often fail to see the relevance of a research course to their applied area of practice. As professional counselors, it is increasingly important to become scientists in one's approach to clinical practice. The primary reason that a scientific approach to counseling is important is the increased demands for measurement of outcomes. In other words, there is an emphasis on the ability of professional counselors, regardless of setting, to determine whether the counseling process is effective. For those professional counselors who practice in a managed care setting, outcome evaluation is of the utmost importance. Understanding and evaluating the effectiveness of our work, however, is important in any of the counseling disciplines (e.g., student affairs, marriage and family, rehabilitation, school, mental health, community, substance abuse, career, college counseling).

This chapter provides a brief overview of two practical approaches counselors are increasingly using: action research and *single-subject research design* (SSRD). More than ever, professional counselors are being required to demonstrate the effectiveness of counseling interventions. Because professional counselors often work with individuals, between-groups studies are not usually possible. Fortunately, action research and SSRDs are easy to use and demonstrate effectiveness quite readily. Other chapters in this text focus on the means by which professional counselors can use the results of group design research studies for practical application purposes. This chapter focuses on the means by which professional counselors can incorporate research methodology in the evaluation of their own work.

# Action Research

Professional counselors who are using **action research** focus on obtaining information that will change conditions in a particular setting or situation. Typically, action research is designed and conducted by educators, practitioners, or researchers who analyze the data to improve their own area of practice. Action research is used quite often in the classroom or school setting and has many advantages. First, most professionals or groups of professionals can conduct action research with minimal training. Second, action research can assist in developing more effective means of performing job responsibilities through identification of problems and issues affecting work performance today. An added benefit of action research is that it can assist professionals to be more competent and effective. Finally, action research can also create a sense of community and collaboration in working together to address and improve a specific situation.

Mills (2014) identified two types of action research: practical and participatory. **Practical action research** focuses on the application aspect of conducting a study in the classroom, school, or community. It is usually informative, and its primary purpose is to improve practice in the short term in a particular setting. **Participatory action research** (i.e., collaborative research) is similar in nature to the practical action researcher. Participatory action research has an additional focus of involving individuals and groups from diverse backgrounds to empower and bring about social change. Table 8.1 reviews the steps ordinarily considered when developing an action research plan. Gay, Mills, & Airasian (2011) stated that action research is meant to apply the scientific method to solve practical problems. Action research can be easily adapted to clinical and school settings and can be adapted to accommodate wide ranges in available limits of time and resources.

As an example of action research in a school setting, Zinck and Littrell (2000) examined the effectiveness of group counseling with at-risk girls. The researchers examined five questions in their study: Does group counseling effectively decrease problem severity for at-risk students? Does progress toward goal attainment endure beyond termination?

| **TABLE 8.1** | Steps to developing an action research plan. |
| --- | --- |

1. *Identify and clarify the research question.* The main focus of this step should be to make improvements in practice or troubleshoot and correct existing problems.

2. *Gather data.* In action research, the data are gathered using only a specific or particular group of individuals, so that the sample and population are identical. Using more than one method of gathering data (e.g., triangulation) is suggested to provide a more thorough picture of the situation.

3. *Analyze and interpret data.* Any of the aforementioned methodologies may be used to collect and analyze the data.

4. *Create an action plan.* One of the main goals of action research is to understand and improve practice in applicable settings. The way to accomplish this goal is to plan and create the steps necessary to alter or improve the situation. The action plan should support and validate the data gathered.

5. *Evaluation and reflection.* Once an action plan is created, the next step is to critically and periodically evaluate the plan's effectiveness. Evaluation can be accomplished by validation through testing the claims of improvements in practice (e.g., Do the action plan changes implemented produce the desired outcomes?). Self-evaluation of participants can also be used as a tool for reflection and validity.

© Cengage Learning

Do students notice other changes in themselves related to what they learned in group counseling? How do students evaluate group characteristics? Is group counseling an efficient use of counselor time? Zinck and Littrell included 35 high school–aged, adolescent girls who participated in one of four small groups. Many of the participants were involved in high-risk relationships (e.g., with friends, boyfriends, family members, and/or gangs). The participants were at risk for dropping out of school, running away, criminal activity, pregnancy, abuse, and exploitation. Based on the results of the study, Zinck and Littrell concluded that group counseling was effective in promoting individual change. The participants reported significant reductions in problem severity at the end of the group sessions. In addition, the participants reported positive changes in their attitudes and in their relationships with other people.

Mills (2014) indicated that the tools and procedures of qualitative research are particularly well suited to action research because researchers are trying to form a theory about the problem under study, which is an inductive process, and because tight experimental control and randomization are not ordinarily possible. Of particular help are observation strategies (i.e., active participant, privileged active, and passive observation), field notes, informal ethnographic interviews, structured formal interviews, focus groups, e-mail interviews, questionnaires, and recordings (which can be transcribed using Dragon Dictate or Siri for an iPhone). Technological innovations like Wikis, blogs, and Skype can also be helpful.

Action research has usefulness for professional counselors regardless of work setting as long as the professional counselor is interested in improving practice effectiveness. Integration of the procedural aspects of action research will be demonstrated in the following sections through a case example of an action research study.

# An Example Action Research Study

## Introduction: Identifying and Clarifying the Action Research Question

Giraffton Middle School has a problem. The students say school is "boring," and the teachers say the students are "unmotivated." The children seem to do fairly well on teacher-created tests and quizzes, but the school was labeled "at risk" because of low test scores on the state-mandated tests. The students, in general, seem to have the ability, but they are unfocused, rarely seem engaged with the school process, and frequently do not complete their homework. The teachers say that this is the case with 2–20 percent of their students, depending on the class, and this has been an ongoing issue for the students at this school. Teachers at the high school say that many of the Giraffton students are "not ready for ninth grade." In addition, many students tend to drop out when they turn 16 years old. Those who graduate often have no clear postsecondary plans. For these young people, their aspirations are limited to remaining in the area and working in the local factories or in small local businesses. Although this doesn't trouble everyone, the Giraffton teachers are concerned that many of the students are not working to their full potential and are capable of doing much more.

Giraffton is located in an older suburban area of the large southern city of Zooville. In this school, there are few major behavioral or attendance problems. There is a cadre of highly involved parents, primarily of the middle to upper socioeconomic status and European American. The student body is fairly diverse: 20 percent of students are on free or reduced lunch, 68 percent are European American, 22 percent African American, 8 percent Hispanic American, and 2 percent are other. There are two full-time professional school counselors (both females, one African American, one European American) and a school social worker and school psychologist, each of whom is there one day a week. The principal, a white female, has been the primary administrator at this school for five years. The two vice principals (an African American male and a European American male) have been in the school division for 15 and 10 years, respectively, and have been at Giraffton the past five years also. As is true of many schools in this division, most of the teachers are white females (70 percent).

The professional school counselors are actively engaged in implementing the *National Model for School Counseling Programs* espoused by the American School Counselor Association (ASCA, 2012). Although they use many of the suggested approaches for data collection and analysis, and school-wide change and advocacy, they feel that there would be some additional and sizable benefits from conducting an action research study. Both have advocated that this action research study should target implementation and evaluation of a systemic program to address this significant issue of social-emotional engagement in student learning.

Toward this end, the principal, assistant principals, professional school counselors, several parents, and a number of teachers met one late summer morning to discuss the possibility of designing a research study that would focus on this challenge. During the meeting, many ideas were put forth, and a good deal of frustration was evident. Toward the end of the meeting, one of the professional school counselors suggested that they design an action research study. She explained that action research is conducted primarily to solve a problem or to address a particular issue. This type of design uses ongoing data collection and ongoing adjustments to original plans, as well as summative data collection and evaluation. She added that this type of design can use both qualitative and quantitative approaches and that both written and oral information as well as numbers could be used to make decisions about the success of any plan they might implement. In an uncharacteristic show of her intense interest in research, she added that generalizability is not an issue in an action research project and that internal reliability or the control of extraneous factors is only an important issue when determining the cause of desired changes.

## Gather Data

The attendees agreed that an action research/participatory design best fit the mission and culture of their school, appropriately involved the research participants in design and in the evaluation, and was the best way to address this challenge. They decided that their first step was to gather information from a needs assessment, which will involve inventories of interests, emotional, behavioral, and cognitive engagement, assessment of teacher practices, parental influences on motivation and aspirations, and ongoing peer pressures, both positive and negative. Focus groups will also be used to collect narrative information about the perceptions of the various participant groups (e.g., teachers, parents, students, community members, and ninth-grade teachers from the high school).

## Analyze and Interpret Data

A month later, after administering the assessments, conducting focus groups, compiling the data, and involving a local university counselor educator in the process, the work group concluded that programmatic and systemic issues are apparent at several levels. In general, many parents, especially those less involved with the school, felt disconnected from Giraffton and the teaching and learning that went on there. Part of their concern seemed to center on the presence of an uninviting secretary/receptionist at the front desk and the exclusionary school practices around drop-in visits. It was also noted that the office area and entrance were "dreary," "dark," and "like entering a cellar." A large number of parents also said that the teachers seemed to tell them what to do with their children, rather than trying to understand their situations and circumstances. They felt judged and "looked down upon," rather than valued and welcome. The above quoted information (and much more) was collected through use of open-ended questions.

Assessments showed that students were not emotionally or cognitively engaged in the learning process. On further analysis, it became clear that students believed that their input wasn't valued, the course content didn't seem meaningful, and they didn't know whom to go to for help when the homework became difficult. Those students, whose parents weren't free to pick them up late from school or bring them early, didn't feel connected to the activities of the school. They were constrained by the bus schedule and couldn't attend the after-school clubs or the before-school service meetings.

Many teachers believed they were pressured by the testing and accountability system of their district, that they had no creative input to the teaching process, that they were constantly being evaluated, and that the students didn't want to be there and didn't want to learn. They felt it was the student's choice whether they were going to do what was required. If they didn't complete homework, then they should just earn the lower grades. This in turn seemed to lead to more and more disengagement by these students and their parents.

The principal was understandably concerned about the upcoming test results, as their school had not made the "passing mark" the year before and was on "probation." As she said, "This year really matters." The vice principals felt that they were so involved in dealing with small disputes and disagreements among students that they rarely had time to connect to other students on a more personal level. The assistant principals said they sometimes felt like a "police officer" and found themselves beginning to act the part. The two professional school counselors felt overworked but believed that the initial investment in this action research project would be the best possible approach to developing a shared and individual sense of engagement. They were, however, concerned about faculty, student, and parent commitment and participation.

The university consultant understood the many issues involved and agreed with many of the observations. He felt the important thing was to start small, use appropriate motivation approaches, conduct ongoing evaluation, and perhaps focus on some of the underlying processes and school culture.

## Create an Action Plan

The overall aim of the action research project was to implement and evaluate interventions that will increase test scores through student engagement and positive teaching and parental involvement. After some discussion and analysis, an action plan of five goals with associated strategies was created.

1. Students: Increase student engagement in learning.

   STRATEGIES:

   a. Encourage students to work in groups, get each other's phone/cell numbers.
   b. Provide group process time for learning content within each classroom.
   c. Provide small groups for study skills and test-taking skills.
   d. Provide student-to-student tutoring.
   e. Provide more out-of-area field trips that will connect learning to the world of work.
   f. Design and deliver classroom guidance lessons on educational/career development.
   g. Bring in role models and community mentors.

2. Students: Increase student before and after-school involvement in school activities.

   STRATEGIES:

   a. Provide an activities bus that leaves the school 90 minutes after the after-school buses.
   b. Allow middle school students to take the elementary school busses to Giraffton if behavior is appropriate and if they are involved in an activity.

3. Teachers: Increase teacher commitment to engaging students in the learning process.

   STRATEGIES:

   a. Provide in-services on student engagement.
   b. Provide observational feedback to teachers.
   c. Allow time for teachers to process and share their experiences.
   d. Provide diversity training and experiences.

4. Parents: Increase parental involvement in school activities and student engagement.

   STRATEGIES:

   a. Allow parents to ride busses into school to "visit."
   b. Have a heart-to-heart with the receptionist, followed by more stringent performance evaluations, if necessary.
   c. Have pairs of teachers and other staff members visit families at work or home.
   d. Provide dinner (soup and bread) and babysitting for all evening school or parent activities.
   e. Have evening school or parent activities at reasonable times.
   f. Have early morning "coffees" for parents who cannot make evening activities.
   g. Provide parent sessions on how to engage their child in learning.

5. School: Increase inviting atmosphere of school.

   STRATEGIES:

   a. Have contests for design of the entrance to school and have students complete the project.
   b. Petition local businesses for supplies and as "sponsors."

## Evaluation and Reflection

Eight primary directions for evaluation were identified:

1. Conduct focus groups every nine weeks of parents, teachers, and students by grade level regarding sense of engagement and involvement. Use qualitative data to assess change in perceived engagement and reasons for this, according to the various groups.

2. Use measures of student engagement, completed at the beginning of the year (done as part of the needs assessment), mid-year, and end of year. Quantitatively measure and analyze the change in average levels of student engagement in learning (behavioral, cognitive, and emotional).

3. Tally ongoing use of busses, parent attendance, use of babysitting services, and so on. Chart changes over time. If babysitting and transportation to parent functions are not increasing levels of parent participation, assess the reasons for this. Have research assistants conduct follow-up phone calls to a random sample of those parents who didn't come.

4. Have observers assess engagement of students in lesson content through process groups at least once each nine weeks. Have these observations done by trained research assistants.

5. For each group on study skills and so forth, check knowledge of skills after group completion. Use a posttest-only "knowledge" assessment. Check on students' ability to transfer skills to the classroom. Use classroom observations conducted by classroom teachers. Follow up as needed until the skills are learned.

6. After field trips and units of classroom guidance lessons on educational and career development, have students complete projects (fine arts or performing arts projects that display their learning). Display these prominently throughout the school. Assess application of higher-order thinking and processing skills and levels of engagement during the process of project completion.

7. Involve mentors in the school activities and have them periodically and informally assess the levels of engagement of their mentees.

8. The major outcome measures will include end-of-year levels of student engagement, parental participation, teacher use of new teaching approaches, and end-of-year test scores.

The initial goals of the advisory group were revisited every nine weeks. The information from focus groups, the measures of student engagement, tallies of participation, classroom observations, knowledge assessments, observations of skill acquisition and project engagement, and teaching assessments indicated that some changes needed to be made in the assignment of projects. For example, some classrooms were making better use of this technique than others, and it was clear that the teachers who were less involved in student projects based on field trips were those who had the least-engaged students. These results led the advisory group to increase the level of teacher training and to use a co-teaching approach to the projects. In this way, the formative data were used to redirect some of the focus in one particular aspect of the study.

The study undertaken at Giraffton Middle School is typical of action research approaches. Multiple sources of data are used to inform the approaches taken to address real-life issues at a specific location and with a specific, unique group of individuals. Sometimes these studies can lead to similar projects in other locations. More important, although the results and the interventions are quite "usable" for the particular population, they are not as "generalizable" as some other research designs.

# History and Issues in Single-Subject Research Designs

The counseling profession has placed an increasing emphasis on single-subject methodology in recent years. This trend is evidenced by the accreditation requirements for single-subject information in research-related coursework by the Council for the Accreditation of Counseling and Related Educational Programs (CACREP, 2009). Although the counseling profession is just beginning to incorporate this practical method of research, SSRD has a long history in behavioral psychology and applied behavioral analysis. In 1949, the Boulder Conference for the Experimental Analysis of Behavior was held to help develop a model for the solidification of scientific design and research (Kennedy, 2005). The scientist–practitioner model emerged as a result of the conference solidifying an agreement that clinical training should be a fusion of science and practice. Prior to the 1940s, much, if not all, of psychological research was based on the uncontrolled, individual case study (e.g., Freud's Frau Emmy). Although these types of case studies proved interesting and helped in the development of theoretical foundations of personality, they lacked the rigor and sound methodology to be useful in practice. Part of the reason for problems inherent in early individual case studies was that practitioners were not yet introduced to the scientific method, and therapy was more art than science. Today, however, because of the fusion between science and practice, case studies maintain a useful place in counseling literature.

## Professional Counselors Within the Scientific Model

The scientist–practitioner model, as it stands today, has three primary foci. First, professional counselors will be consumers of research findings (e.g., journals, research papers, and presentations). Second, professional counselors will be evaluators of their interventions and accountable through empirical validation. Third, professional counselors should *produce* their own authentic research (Hayes, Barlow, & Nelson-Gray, 1999).

Like the counseling profession today, however, not all members of the Boulder Conference were in direct favor of the marriage between science and practice. Some members believed that traditional and statistical research is not appropriate or applicable for professional counselors and that science is more concerned with the establishment of laws and boundaries rather than the application of those individual laws.

The majority of Boulder Conference members decided to combine the two ideologies and form the scientist–practitioner model. These members decided that there was a demand for students with an interest and background in these two areas. It was agreed that effective practice needed to be more research based and not based solely on the concept of common sense. A marriage between the worlds of science and practice would promote the desire for researchers to investigate problems that were commonly found in the field of practice, as well as fund practice-relevant research. As a result of the efforts of the members of the Boulder Conference, practitioners in behavioral psychology began to emulate the scientist–practitioner philosophy (Hayes et al., 1999). Today, professional counselors are doing much the same. With regard to research, professional counselors now have three distinct roles: consumers, evaluators, and producers.

### Consumers

Like the members of the Boulder Conference, professional counselors today are more interested in **clinical significance** than statistical significance. It only makes sense that professional counselors would be interested in what they may possibly use within the scope of their training. A typical complaint from professional counselors in the field is that large-group designs have such tight control over variables that it is difficult to apply the research results to clinical practice. Although trends found in large-group studies have significance, research results fail to apply to the individual who falls outside the scope of the sample and the population mean. As consumers of research, counselors need results that apply to these individuals and take the severity of their needs into account.

### Evaluators

Professional counselors often have a different set of practical concerns than those related in the discussion sections of large-group research articles (e.g., concerns about the size of case loads in their respective agencies). One practical concern of professional counselors is the effectiveness of their program. Professional counselors are often charged with evaluating aspects of program operation, such as cost efficiency, time effectiveness, or quality customer service.

Along with a different set of practical concerns for professional counselors comes a variety of ethical dilemmas. For example, academics often place value on true experimental designs using a control group to evaluate difference. As described in Chapter 7, the control group is a designated group in which an intervention or treatment is withheld. Although a control group makes sense from a research perspective, it is not best practice to withhold treatment from an individual. Some professional counselors might consider withholding treatment to be unethical. Professional counselors focus on the well-being of the individual and will not necessarily adhere to a rigid treatment protocol, especially if that protocol does not appear to correlate with clinically significant gains. In the absence of progress, professional counselors are more likely to change or vary the treatment strategy.

Thus, a schism still exists between the worlds of academia and counseling practice. Current marketplace trends (e.g., accreditation and managed care), however, are forcing the world of practice (e.g., public schools, hospitals, community agencies, and institutions of higher education) to integrate accepted research strategies and to implement empirically based methods.

### Producers

Although the trend has been to build a bridge between academia and the world of practice, professional counselors still use more nontraditional methods of field research that (a) allow a focus on individual clients, (b) foster the ability to observe a single participant or small number of participants, and (c) allow observation of those individuals over an extended period of time (Kennedy, 2005). Because the purpose of this chapter is to help prepare professional counselors to evaluate the outcomes of practice, considerable time will be spent introducing single-subject methodology. Before beginning that process, however, it is necessary to shed some more light on the context of SSRD development.

## The Experimental Analysis of Behavior

B. F. Skinner was the forerunner in the establishment of what we have come to know as single-subject case methodology. Skinner's (1956) original research focused on the **behavioral processes** of an individual organism, concentrating on the order of consequences and how those may affect the observed behavior. Although Skinner's work may not be popular with all professional counselors, it is clear that the behavioral terminology that has emanated from his research has been accepted in the counseling lexicon (e.g., antecedent, discrimination, punishment, reinforcement).

B. F. Skinner was first interested in studying the rates of frequency of behavior with regard to performance. He chose studying frequency, because he could observe the baseline, or the normal rate of behavior, prior to introducing the intervention or treatment phase. Because Skinner collected baseline data, he was able to see the effectiveness of each intervention being introduced. Skinner's research methodology was focused on the examination of either one participant or a small sample (group) of participants, an additional precursor to modern single-case design. As a result, Skinner was able to see the given effects of the experiment in the population immediately rather than having to generalize the results of a group-design experiment from a sample to a population. As a result of Skinner's continuous work, SSRD later became synonymous with research using operant conditioning.

## Applied Behavior Analysis

During the 1950s and 1960s, single-case research became more commonly used, and by the early 1960s, an *applied* area of research was becoming more frequent. The academic community began to see the use of applied methodologies in the education and special education setting, community counseling, outpatient treatment, and psychiatric hospital settings. In response to the expansion of experimental analysis of behavior to applied areas, this type of research became known as applied behavior analysis (Baer, Wolf, & Risley, 1968). By 1970, applied behavior analysis was used in measuring behaviors related to child rearing, education, crime, and psychiatric disorders (Kazdin, 1982).

As a result, single-case designs have become a methodological tool for researchers and practitioners alike that helps examine the question "What treatment, and by who, is most effective for this individual with that specific problem, and under which set of circumstances?" (Paul, 1967, p. 111). Since the Boulder Conference, researchers in the field of applied behavior analysis have established the precedent for using single-subject case design to help answer our questions about the effectiveness of therapeutic intervention (Heppner, Kivlighan, & Wampold, 2008).

## The Data-Based Problem Solver Model

Counseling is a complex process, and understanding the effectiveness of an intervention can be a difficult task because of numerous intervening variables. Thus, it is important for professional counselors to approach each client from a scientific perspective and to choose interventions based on the empirical evidence available relative to the identified problem. The data-based problem solver (DBPS) model was developed as an extension of the scientist–practitioner model (see Table 8.2 for an overview of DBPS). While the scientist–practitioner model provides an overarching philosophy to guide the training of professional counselors, the DBPS provides a clear structure for bridging the gap between academia and the world of practice (Eaves, Emens, & Sheperis, 2008). The DBPS model is divided into four different phases: problem identification, problem analysis, problem solution, and problem evaluation.

In the first phase, **problem identification**, professional counselors are required to formulate appropriate research questions relative to identifying the client's problems.

**TABLE 8.2**  Comparison of the traditional research model, clinical practice, and the DBPS model by phase.

| Traditional Research | Phase of DBPS Model | Clinical Practice |
| --- | --- | --- |
| Research Question | Phase I<br>Problem identification (PI) | Referral problem |
| Pilot Studies | Phase II | Assessment |
| Defining Research Question | Problem analysis (PA) | Defining a problem |
| Formulating a Hypothesis | | Formatting goals and objectives |
| Methodology of Research | Phase III<br>Problem solution (PS) | Development of an intervention |
| Empirical Evaluation | Phase IV | Empirical evaluation |
| Data-Based Conclusions | Problem evaluation (PE) | Data-based conclusions |

In the problem identification stage, professional counselors complete a review of theory and databases, review of literature, and seek consultation. In the second phase of the DBPS, researchers are concerned with three areas of **problem analysis**: pilot studies, definition of research questions, and formation of hypotheses. Practicing counselors who are working in the problem analysis phase, however, would be more concerned with assessment, definition of the problem, and the formation of goals and objectives. In the third phase of the DBPS, researchers and professional counselors are focused on developing the **problem solution**. Professional counselors, however, are concerned with the development of an intervention, whereas researchers are primarily focused on the development of research methodology. The fourth phase of the DBPS is **problem evaluation**. In this final phase, researchers and professional counselors are seeking the same two common goals: empirical evaluation and data-based conclusions (Eaves et al., 2008).

Even though the scientist–practitioner model and the DBPS model are used in training programs in psychology and counseling, Crane and Hafen (2002) claimed that neither model has adequate empirical support. In an effort to validate the DBPS for professional counselor training, Eaves et al. (2008) examined the effects of DBPS counseling on 55 participants. The researchers in this case trained professional counselors to use the DBPS over five sessions. Eaves et al. discovered a significant reduction in self-report symptomology across all participants, thus supporting the use of the model in training professional counselors. The results of the research provide support for continued use of the model. Reduced symptomology is a key outcome for managed care organizations. It appears that the DBPS model provides professional counselors with a guide for accurately defining problems, developing effective interventions, and systematically collecting data (Noell & Witt, 1998; Wakefield & Kirk, 1996).

# Research Design

Although Chapter 7 contains an overview of group research designs and quantitative methods, it is important to briefly summarize some of the discussion here in an effort to delineate the differences between SSRD and traditional quantitative methods (Table 8.3). As behavioral psychology began to adopt SSRD methods in the 1940s, other researchers in psychology began to espouse nomothetic approaches toward comparing data produced by experimental procedures applied to individuals in different research conditions (i.e., experimental and control groups). As we saw in Chapter 7, between-groups designs often compare the differences in the responses of one group to the treatment, or lack thereof, with those of another group in which participants have been randomly assigned. While in SSRD, or sometimes called single-case or time-series

**TABLE 8.3**  Comparison of group and single-subject research designs.

| Group Designs | Single-Subject Research Designs |
| --- | --- |
| Compare differences within and between experimental conditions. Participants have been randomly assigned. | Compare different experimental conditions presented to the same participants of a group over time. |
| Requires a large number of homogeneous participants. | Permits experimental analysis with a single participant or a small number of participants. |
| Requires the use of differential and inferential statistics to evaluate the results. | Relies on visual inspection of the data on a graph to describe the meaningfulness of results. |

© Cengage Learning

design, inferences are made about the type of intervention by comparing different treatment conditions presented to the same participants of a group over time.

Between-groups designs (see Chapter 7 for a detailed discussion) are perhaps the most traditional and widely used of the research designs. These models can address a broad range of questions and can compare two or more groups in terms of their effects on target behaviors. Large-group designs require numerous amounts of homogeneous participants who are assigned randomly (e.g., to treatment and control conditions) and require the use of differential and inferential statistics to evaluate the results.

SSRDs are appealing to professional counselors for various, yet primarily practical, reasons. SSRDs permit experimental analysis with single clients or participants, which tend to be the focus of most interventions. Single-case design is often referred to as time series design because it allows for the study of an individual across repeated observations before, during, and following the introduction of an intervention. Single-case design may be considered more user friendly. This model of research primarily relies on visual inspection of the data on a graph rather than statistical procedures to describe the meaningfulness of results. SSRDs can also be used to compliment between-groups designs and as another tool for research.

## Benefits of Single-Subject Research Designs

As professional counselors become producers of research, it is important that methodology fits into the world of practice. Perhaps the most strenuous task of any research model is the computation and interpretation of statistics. In SSRD, however, data can be quickly and easily evaluated without the use of complicated statistics. Because single-case designs are small by nature, encompassing individual participants or small groups, collecting data is often fairly inexpensive. As mentioned previously, both private and public agencies are being held more accountable for the effectiveness of individualized treatment interventions. Overall, SSRD is a low-cost, time-efficient research approach that allows professional counselors to be accountable for their practice decisions.

## Features of Single-Subject Research Designs

Now that the benefits of SSRD for professional counselors have been presented, we can examine the distinct characteristics that define SSRDs. The first characteristic is the *repeated* measurement of the target behavior over a period of time. The measurement process begins with a *well-established baseline* phase or treatment measure of the observed target behavior. The baseline data have to show *stability* before conditions change (i.e., before an intervention is introduced). In other words, we need to know that the behavior we see without any treatment is consistent and representative of the client's normal state of operation. This is essential because when interventions are introduced, one should be able to observe and link changes in the stable pattern of behavior to the intervention (e.g., causation). In single-case designs, professional counselors introduce one change at a time, which may change from baseline to treatment or vice versa. Finally, perhaps the most important aspect of the particular features of SSRD is the need for replication. Replication is the introduction of the same intervention across the same individual or across other individuals to show that the effects of the treatment were not coincidental.

## Misconceptions About Single-Subject Research Designs

There is a misconception that an SSRD is the same thing as the case-study approach commonly used in psychology prior to the 1940s; this is not so. As stated earlier, the case-study approach is characterized by unsystematic observations and subjective measures, whereas an SSRD requires systematic observations (e.g., establishment of reliability through interobserver agreement and behavioral observations that are objective and quantifiable). Another fallacy is that SSRD is only used to observe behavior-modification techniques. Even though SSRD has its roots in behavior modification, it is applicable to a wide variety of counseling settings and presenting issues. Another common misconception among researchers is the belief that SSRD provides a flawless alternative to between-groups designs. Like any other type of research design, SSRD has limitations. In the next section, we discuss methods of observation and assessment within SSRD and the relative limitations resulting from this process.

# Methods of Observation and Assessment

Because practical research approaches is the focus of this chapter, SSRD is discussed within the context of the DBPS model. As part of the problem identification phase within the DBPS, professional counselors must identify a target behavior. To derive reliable measures of the target behavior, it is important to define the behavior in concrete and observable terms. For example, if you work with young children, teachers and parents often report concerns about children who are "hyperactive." As you may have already guessed, the term *hyperactive* is somewhat ambiguous and difficult to measure reliably. To help these children, one may identify several target behaviors representative of hyperactivity. In one case, we may wish to measure out-of-seat behavior as a component of hyperactivity. To reliably measure out-of-seat-behavior, we operationally define it as "any time the student's bottom loses contact with his/her assigned seat." With this operational definition, other professional counselors or teachers would be able to see the target behavior and measure it consistently.

An operational definition provides the professional counselor with clear, concise, and concrete parameters to measure the target behaviors, while maintaining the integrity of the design. Researchers who are using SSRD often incorporate multiple observers into the research process. By doing so, a degree of reliability or interobserver agreement (IOA) can be calculated based on the level of agreement among observers. For example, assume that a child named Kijuan is exhibiting a high degree of out-of-seat behavior in a classroom. The professional counselor who is working with Kijuan could ask another professional counselor to review the operational definition and the two counselors could collect data simultaneously over several 15-minute periods. They could then compare data to see how much their individual observations of the target behavior agreed. The higher the level of agreement, the more trust they could have in their observations.

Thus, the operational definition is a key element in SSRD. The operational definition should pass two different yet practical examinations: the "stranger test" and "dead-man test." The stranger test requires that the operational definition be clear, concise, and free of any confusing language such that a complete stranger could reliably conduct the observations. The dead-man test prohibits the inclusion of target behaviors that could be completed only by someone who is deceased. While this test may seem silly, one sometimes witnesses parents and teachers telling children to sit still and to not move a muscle. In contrast to developing interventions for these unreasonable behavioral expectations, behaviors could be targeted such as inappropriate vocalization, self-injurious behavior, or out-of-seat behavior.

## Direct Observation

There are two types of direct observations: nonsystematic and systematic. **Nonsystematic observation** can be approached through one of two components: narrative recording and contingency analysis. *Narrative recording* is a process by which a professional counselor records all observed behaviors as if writing a script for a play (e.g., "and Bobby then marched over to the shelves and pushed the books out of place").

Through narrative recording, professional counselors can track behaviors of current concern and/or identify behaviors that may be of importance in the future. It is important to note that narrative recording requires the professional counselor to record behaviors without filtering or censoring content. Although some observed behaviors may have little or no intensity at the time of data collection, it is possible that the recorded observations may serve as an antecedent to more pronounced actions. Identifying clear antecedents to a behavior helps professional counselors to formulate more effective treatment interventions. Because narrative recording does not require a high degree of training, this is found to be a common homework assignment for teachers and parents.

The second type of nonsystematic recording is sequence or *contingency analysis* (A-B-C-F). In **sequence analysis** one visualizes this as a chain of events where there is an (A) antecedent, (B) behavior, (C) consequence, and possible (F) function (see Table 8.4 for an example). By observing behaviors in this fashion, one can better understand and form hypotheses about functional relationships. Alberto and Troutman (2004) claimed that a functional relationship exists when systematic changes in the independent variable can be attributed to the dependent variable. In other words, if one suspects that Kijuan is increasing his out-of-seat behavior to get attention, one can demonstrate the functional relationship by manipulating the amount of attention he receives and consequently decreasing his out-of-seat behavior. Narrative recording can be a useful tool for professional counselors to identify potential behaviors for systematic observations and to develop possible interventions.

The second type of direct observation is **systematic observation**, of which there are eight subtypes. The first subtype of systematic observation is **event recording**, which involves counting the frequency of occurrences of the observed behavior(s) within a designated observation period (e.g., days, hours, minutes). Event recording is very useful when working with discrete behaviors, or behaviors that have a clear beginning and end. Some examples of discrete behaviors may be children who bang their heads, counting the amount of correctly spelled words, picture naming, or correct coin selection. Event recording is reported as a rate instead of a frequency. Rate is the "total number of occurrences" ($O_T$) divided by the "total number of minutes" ($M_T$) of observation (i.e., Rate = $O_T/M_T$).

Another form of recording is called event recording of discriminated operants. This style of recording is used to record behaviors that are most often seen in the presence of clear antecedents. When using this type of recording, it is important that measures are

| **TABLE 8.4**   A-B-C narrative observation format. | |
|---|---|
| A (Antecedent) | A counselor asks a client to do some therapeutic homework on logging number of times he or she washes hands. |
| B (Behavior) | Client pouts (i.e., speaks in short sentences and complains about the task). |
| C (Consequence) | Counselor tells client, "Let's find another task that is more suitable for you." |
| F (Function) | Client sought to escape task. |

elicited as percentages, not rates, because the antecedents are not constant (e.g., a child not complying with the request of a parent). This is often shown in an equation:

$$\text{Percentage of occurrence} = \frac{\text{Total \# of occurrences of target behavior}}{\text{Total \# of opportunities}} \times 100$$

A third way one may record observations systematically is using the *finite response class*. This class of recording involves taking multifaceted behaviors and compiling them into simpler components that can be more easily observed and measured. Some of these behaviors may be very simple, such as a child who has a self-injurious behavior (Kennedy, 2005): (1) Child begins to take deep breaths; (2) child walks to a safe area of the room; (3) child sits on the floor; (4) child places his hands in his lap; and (5) child continues activity with zero head-banging.

The fourth subtype of systematic observation is **duration recording**, which can be frustrating to researchers because it estimates the average time that has elapsed from the beginning to the end of the behavior. Observers, however, may disagree on when the actual behavior started and ended; this establishes the credence for two types of coding under duration recording. The first method of duration recording can be reported as a *true duration*, or percentage, which is expressed as follows:

$$\text{True duration (TD)} = \frac{\text{Total time engaged in the behavior (TTB)}}{\text{Total time of the observation period (TTO)}} \times 100$$

or (TD = [TTB/TTO] × 100). This can also be shown as an *average duration* (AD), which is simply expressed by dividing the "total time engaged in the behavior" by the "total time of the observation period" (AD = TTB/TTO).

**Latency recording** measures the elapsed time between the occurrence of the signal (discriminative stimulus) and the beginning of the behavior. Kennedy (2005, p. 102) reported that an advantage of latency recording is that "it provides an index of the temporal relation between one event and another." He also cited limitations to the process in that some of the responses in latency recording require consecutive ascertainment and the use of a time-assisting apparatus (e.g., stopwatch). Like duration recording, latency can be demonstrated as a percentage and as an average. One expresses average latency (AL) by dividing the "total time to start behavior" by the "number of occurrences of behavior" (AL = TT/OCC). When expressing true latency (TL), one divides the "total time to start the behavior" by the "number of occurrences of behavior" times 100 (i.e., TL = [TT/OCC] × 100).

The sixth subset of systematic observation is **interval recording**. Kazdin (1982) reported that interval recording is based on observations recorded in a unit of time rather than on discrete response units. With interval recording, researchers often use time periods of 15–30 minutes as standard observation times. Short intervals of time, such as 10–15 seconds, are subdivided from the larger portion. The behavior of the client is observed during each interval.

When using interval recording, a professional counselor observes the client in 10- to 15-second periods (Figure 8.1). Target behaviors are counted if they occur at any point in the interval as opposed to individual occurrences, sometimes resulting in an overrepresentation of frequency of behavior. If the target behavior is continuous (e.g., talking, walking about the classroom, and not keeping hands to self), each consecutive interval is counted as containing an occurrence of the target behavior.

There are two types of interval recording: partial-interval recording and whole-interval recording. Partial-interval recording dictates that an interval is checked any time that a target behavior is observed throughout the time of that interval. This, however, can lead to an overestimation of an occurrence of a behavior. Whole interval recording occurs when a behavior is observed for the entire period of the interval; this can tend to underestimate the occurrence of a behavior. Formulaically, this is shown as "percent of intervals" (%*I*) equals the "number of intervals of occurrences" (#IO$_{cc}$) divided by the "total number of intervals observed" (#IO$_{bs}$) multiplied by 100 (i.e., %I = [#IO$_{cc}$/#IO$_{bs}$] × 100).

**Figure 8.1**

Interval recording form.

| Behavior | 10" | 20" | 30" | 40" | 50" | 60" |
|---|---|---|---|---|---|---|
| Antecedent | D<br>C<br>T | D<br>C<br>T | D<br>C<br>T | D<br>C<br>T | D<br>C<br>T | D<br>C<br>T |
| Targets | OT<br>OS<br>IV | OT<br>OS<br>IV | OT<br>OS<br>IV | OT<br>OS<br>IV | OT<br>OS<br>IV | OT<br>OS<br>IV |
| Consequences | E/A<br>TP<br>TN<br>PP<br>PN | E/A<br>TP<br>TN<br>PP<br>PN | E/A<br>TP<br>TN<br>PP<br>PN | E/A<br>TP<br>TN<br>PP<br>PN | E/A<br>TP<br>TN<br>PP<br>PN | E/A<br>TP<br>TN<br>PP<br>PN |

© Cengage Learning

*Note:* Operational Definitions:

*Antecedents*

D:  Demand—Instruction given to complete educational work or an assignment.
C:  Command—Behavioral instruction (e.g., "Sit down," "Be quiet," "Go to your desk," "Stop talking," "Look at me").
T: Transition—Moving from one location to another in the classroom or school. Switching from one assignment to another.

*Target Behaviors*

OT: Off-task—Student's eyes are not directed toward the teacher during lecture/instruction or the assignment for more than 5 seconds.
OS: Out-of-seat—Student's bottom breaks contact with the seat/floor for more than 5 seconds.
IV: Inappropriate vocalizations—Student talks to teacher without permission; student talks to peers without permission; student argues with teacher or peers; student makes noises (e.g., whistling, howling, humming, clicking sounds, etc.).

*Consequences*

E/A: Escape/Avoidance—Student is allowed to refrain from working on or completing the assignment; teacher takes the assignment away; teacher does not make the student comply (follow through or complete) with a command.
Teacher Attention:
        TP: Teacher Positive Attention—Smiles, praise statements, proximity following appropriate behavior, physical touch for appropriate behavior.
        TN:  Teacher Negative Attention—Frowns, reprimands, redirections, interruptions, proximity following problem behavior, physical touch for problem behavior.
Peer Attention:
        PP:  Peer Positive Attention—Smiles, praises, proximity, and physical touch for appropriate behavior.
        PN:  Peer Negative Attention—Frowns, put-downs, name calling, proximity following problem behavior, physical touch following problem behavior (e.g., pushing, hitting, kicking, touching).

**Calculation of Performance of Behavior** :
1.  OT:                            _____ / 6 × 100 = _____  % of the intervals
2.  OS:                            _____ / 6 × 100 = _____  % of the intervals
3.  IV:                            _____ / 6 × 100 = _____  % of the intervals
Total Disruptive Behavior:      _____ / 18 × 100 = ____ % of the intervals

**Momentary time sampling** occurs when the observer records occurrences of the target behavior in the beginning or final portion of the interval period (i.e., only part or a moment of the interval is observed from its entirety). Kennedy (2005) called the portion of the nonobservational period, the *wait* period, and the observational portion, *record*. For instance, if a researcher was observing for 20 seconds, the first 10 seconds may be the wait period and the latter 10 the record portion. This is often referred to as **spot checking**. This cuts down on "drift" that may occur between observers. As a result, momentary time sampling tends to be more accurate than partial- or whole-interval recording by creating a balance between over- and underestimation. One of the major difficulties of this design can arise when independent observers make their observations at the same time.

Finally, in the **review of permanent products**, instead of directly observing a behavior, one measures or evaluates the product of the behavior. This type of observational process is often used in academic settings. For instance, instead of observing a child completing a spelling worksheet, we can collect the worksheet at the end of the work period and review the number of words attempted in contrast to those spelled correctly. Because permanent product data are displayed in absolute numbers instead of ratios of events and timelines, it is easier to visually interpret. This subtype has excellent reliability and few problems with reactivity. Permanent product is displayed as "percent correct" equals the "number of correct responses" (#Cor) divided by the "number of opportunities" (#Opp) multiplied by 100 (i.e., % = [#Cor/#Opp] × 100).

**Reliability of observations** is the key to accuracy in all the subtypes of systematic observations. It is of the utmost importance that the observations are clear, concrete, and concisely defined (i.e., pass the stranger and dead-man tests). Reliability is simply being able to quantitatively establish the degree in which behaviors, tasks, or other measures are being recorded consistently (Kennedy, 2005). As discussed earlier, reliability in SSRD is calculated as IOA. In calculating IOA, one attempts to decipher the degree to which two independent observers, looking at the same behavior at the same time, record the same event. Minimum accepted reliability rate for SSRD is considered to be 80 percent agreement. IOA is expressed as follows:

$$IOA = \frac{\text{\# of intervals of agreement}}{\text{Total \# of intervals}} \times 100$$

Professional counselors should remember that effectiveness or outcome data can only be proven accurate to the extent that it can be shown to be consistently studied over time (i.e., valid and reliable). For example, when collecting observation data, if one observer records fewer instances of aggressive behavior for a client on a particular day than another observer, then it is difficult to measure the true outcome of any interventions. By implementing IOA procedures, professional counselors minimize any biases that may occur from individual observation.

One of the largest threats to reliability is reactivity to the presence of the observer. Observers should avoid disrupting the environment and, if possible, allow time for habituation within the setting (i.e., visit the environment a couple of times to allow the participants to grow accustomed to the observer). It is also important to ask parents, teachers, or other adults not to inform children or adolescents of the purpose of the professional counselor's presence.

## Self-Monitoring

Professional counselors are usually familiar with the self-monitoring process. Self-monitoring is the ability of the participant to notice and record the number of occurrences of their selected target behavior as they occur throughout a designated time period. Forms can be devised to assess for intensity, duration, and frequency of behavior. Self-rating scales and diaries are self-monitoring devices.

Self-monitoring assessments can be used with a wide range of clientele, can measure behaviors that are not necessarily directly observable, and can help a participant manage behavior and productivity. It should be noted that participants are not always compliant when asked to monitor their own behavior. Thus, it is necessary to examine some common reasons for noncompliance. If a professional counselor fails to explain the purpose of the exercise in understandable terms, the participant may see little relevance to the self-monitoring or fail to grasp its significance to their therapeutic goals. Also, participants may lack the requisite skills or training to accurately self-monitor. Thus, to increase the reliability of the self-monitoring process, professional counselors should provide proper training, positive reinforcement for accurate self-monitoring, and have the participant monitor only one behavior at a time.

# Single-Subject Research Designs

Participants invest time, money, and energy into counseling, and they want to feel better as a result of the process. Thus, professional counselors should develop a process by which they can measure outcomes. Error, however, is a component in any form of measurement. SSRD is designed to reduce the number of errors a professional counselor makes by continuously evaluating interventions and conducting measurements over a designated amount of time. This assessment of variables (e.g., behaviors, interventions, and study habits) is known as **time-series methodology** (Hayes et al., 1999). In other words, professional counselors establish the reliability and validity of their interventions and the respective results by observing target behaviors, establishing baseline data, and replicating results of the intervention over a period of time.

## Why Is It Called Time Series?

Time-series measurements are those taken repeatedly over the course of a designated time period (Sheperis, Doggett, & Henington, 2006). Professional counselors who are using SSRD employ systematic and repeated measurement of target behaviors to ensure the accuracy of their outcome evaluations. Without taking the necessary repetitive measures, a professional counselor is unable to determine who improved and by how much. Without a systematic measurement process, there is a greater degree of subjectivity in the evaluation of outcomes. As is the case with experimental methods, in SSRD it is important to standardize measurement procedures (i.e., time of the assessment, observer, and setting). Any change in measurement procedures can make it difficult to determine the source of variability in the data. The primary benefit of SSRD for professional counselors, however, is that it is time and cost effective. If measures are taken *too* frequently, they may become cumbersome, time consuming, and cancel out the related benefits.

In SSRD, professional counselors visually analyze data (i.e., inspect the data on a graph) related to target behaviors for changes in level, trend, and variability across baseline and the various phases of treatment (Creswell, 2012). Each observation session represents an individual data point that could be derived from any of the various recording procedures described in this chapter (i.e., event, duration, intensity, latency, or interval recording procedures; Sheperis et al., 2006). Derived data points are grouped together in a phase to form a series of data points where each datum is assessed relative to those that precede and follow it. The number of data points contained within each phase is determined by the amount of stability in the data. In some cases, however, one data point may be used per phase as long as each phase is replicated at least one time.

Figure 8.2 represents a hypothetical research project in which the professional counselor was attempting to increase the number of positive esteem statements spoken by the participant (i.e., increase positive self-talk statements). This case is used to represent level, trend, and variability across phase changes. At least three data points are needed to evaluate the level, trend, and variability in the data. *Level* refers to the average of the data points. In this case, the baseline level was 0, and the treatment phase was 3.5. *Trend* refers to the direction of change in the data points from the beginning to the end of the series. In Figure 8.2, there is a clear trend toward increased positive esteem statements during the treatment and follow-up phases. The variability refers to the spread of data points in relation to level and trend. With regard to baseline data, it is important to have a low degree of variability, or conversely, to obtain stability in the data before implementing an intervention. In the hypothetical research project, there is clear stability in that no positive esteem statements were spoken during the baseline phase. Professional counselors should note that variability and stability are inversely related, and so more data points may be needed, depending on the amount of variability in the data.

In SSRD, professional counselors study the effects of intervention by visually inspecting the data across phases. Change (i.e., variability), however, can occur across (i.e., between) two phases or within a single phase. When within-phase variability occurs, it is often due to extraneous variables and/or measurement error. However, when between-phase variability occurs (i.e., variability occurring between two separate phases), it can be attributed to treatment/intervention implementation. Professional counselors should remember that greater within-phase variability (e.g., during the baseline phase) necessitates even greater between-phase variability to demonstrate success of an intervention. In Figure 8.2, there is stability in the baseline data and a clear change in level and

**Figure 8.2**

Simple phase change SSRD.

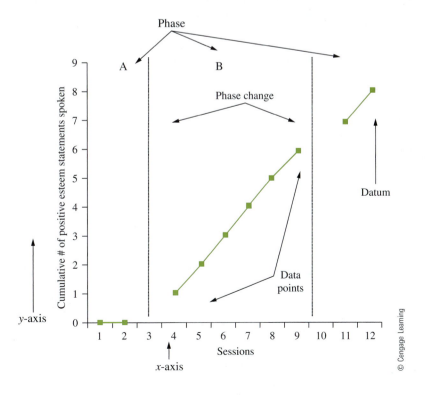

© Cengage Learning

trend between baseline, treatment, and follow-up phases, indicating the efficacy of the intervention.

As in other research designs, professional counselors using SSRD need to concretely and objectively define the target behaviors and the components of treatment so they may be measured and replicated. Greater specificity in the identification of target behaviors and intervention protocols enhances the ability to identify effective and ineffective components of the counseling process.

## Procedural and Treatment Integrity

Two components of SSRD that may be more applicable to researchers than professional counselors are procedural and treatment integrity. These components have become standard requirements for published research. If professional counselors are interested in publishing the results of their work, procedural and treatment integrity should be observed for a minimum of 25 percent of the sessions. Although bias may play a role in the collection of integrity data, the minimum accepted level of treatment and procedural integrity agreement is 80 percent. These percentages can be demonstrated by using checklists and direct observations.

For example, when discussing various procedures for training parents to implement time-out procedures with children, it would be important to develop a checklist of the steps in time-out. Professional counselors conducting the training would then monitor the parents' use of the procedures and ensure that they were implemented with at least 80 percent accuracy.

## Stability

**Stability** refers to the index of within-subject (intrasubject) variability. Stability has been reached when extraneous variability and/or measurement error has been sufficiently limited or cleared so as to enable a legitimate statement regarding the effects of the independent variable at its expected strength. It is important to note that data collected during the baseline phase can contain an identifiable trend but still be considered stable. It is feasible to predict less stability during the baseline phase when a large treatment effect is expected, immediate treatment changes are expected, treatment is suspected to reduce variability, and the pretreatment phase is opposite to the treatment phase.

### When Stabilization of the Data Is Not Reached

In some cases, data may not stabilize during the baseline phase. In these instances, it is important to analyze the sources of variability. The professional counselor should start with minimizing measurement variability such as observer drift, reactivity, and/or extraneous variability. One method for assessing stability is to divide a particular phase ($P$) in half ($P1 + P2$); calculate the overall phase mean ($M_P$) and means for each half ($M_{P1}$, $M_{P2}$); calculate the difference between the overall and divided means ($[M_P - M_{P1}]$ & $[M_P - M_{P2}]$); and then divide by the total mean ($[M_P - M_{P1}]/M_P$ & $[M_P - M_{P2}]/M_P$). To show stability, the results should express a 15 percent (.15) difference or less. A second way to examine stability is to determine whether 80–90 percent of the data points fall within a 15 percent range of the phase mean.

## Replication

*Replication* is one of the most fundamental aspects of SSRD. Professional counselors can use replication in SSRD to evaluate internal validity and external validity. In SSRD, internal validity represents the degree to which the observed effects are due to the treatment/intervention. By replicating the effects of an intervention in a single case, the professional counselor can have more confidence that the effects are not due to chance. While internal validity is related to a single case, external validity in SSRD is the degree to which observed effects are likely to generalize to other clients. Although SSRD does not involve large sample sizes, there are occasions where more than one participant is used in the research process. Thus, some degree of external validity can be achieved through the replication of therapeutic effects across different clients. For example, a professional counselor could examine outcome data for clients who are experiencing moderate depression as measured by a self-report scale. In this case, the professional counselor could select an SSRD to systematically collect data and implement interventions across time (i.e., phases). If the professional counselor can demonstrate similar changes in trend and level across phases for each participant, there is evidence for the generalizability of the intervention.

When evaluating outcomes using SSRD, professional counselors should attend to three threats to internal validity (i.e., extraneous events, instrumentation shift, and effects of time). Although professional counselors would like to attribute any reductions in symptoms or increases in appropriate behavior to the therapeutic process, it is possible that coincidental or extraneous events could have affected the outcome. For example, if a client was experiencing anxiety from financial problems and inherited a great deal of money during the course of the treatment, reduction of anxiety symptoms could not be attributed to treatment alone. Second, before attributing therapeutic gains to an intervention, counselors should be sure that instrumentation shifts did not occur and that measurement procedures remained unaltered. Finally, professional counselors should consider the possibility that changes in level or trend (a) could be due to time alone (i.e., did the participant simply get older and mature?), (b) are related to a practice effect with regard to instrumentation or procedures, (c) or were due to a regression toward the mean. Through replication of effects, however, professional counselors can increase their confidence in the validity of their results.

# Within-Series Elements

As discussed earlier in this chapter, SSRD is a process by which professional counselors can evaluate the effectiveness of their practice across time and in distinct phases. Because within-series elements allow professional counselors to study changes in a single measure or set of measures over the course of time, they are the basic building blocks for all other variations within SSRD methodology. The A-B design, A-B-A-B design, interaction element, and changing criterion design are the most common forms of within-series SSRD (Sheperis et al., 2006). The most basic within-series design is the A-B design (i.e., simple phase change).

### Simple Phase Change (A-B Designs)

Often denoted as an A-B design, a **simple phase change** (Figure 8.2) is used to answer two simple questions: "Is treatment effective?" and "Does one treatment work more convincingly than another?" In simple phase change, like many other SSRDs, A denotes the baseline phase and B denotes the treatment or intervention phase. Professional counselors will hope to see a change in level, trend, or variability due to the introduction of the treatment. A professional counselor can determine the significance of data changes in simple phase change by determining which changes (a) have the greatest magnitude, (b) are closely associated in time with that of the phase change, and (c) show consistency throughout the phase.

Doggett, Edwards, Moore, Tingstrom, and Wilczynski (2001) used the A-B-A-B design to demonstrate the effects of peer attention on disruptive behavior. In this study, the researchers placed a target student with peers who were likely to pay attention to his disruptive behavior during each A phase. In contrast, a target student was seated away from peers who would observe the problem behavior during each B phase. Although one might be able to guess that the incidence of problem behavior was high in each A phase and low in each B phase, it is important to be able to verify this outcome empirically. Professional counselors can use the A-B-A-B design to generate confidence in their assessment procedures, treatment procedures, and subsequent outcomes.

### Benefits of Within-Series Designs

With most of the within-series designs, professional counselors can draw causal inferences between an intervention and changes in behavioral data. Within-series designs can even provide evidence of the effectiveness of an intervention with minimal changes in a treatment phase. In cases where behaviors are known to be rather resistant to change without treatment, professional counselors can draw causal inferences by collecting lengthy and consistent baseline data. In these cases, even small changes during the treatment phase can be powerful. If professional counselors choose to be consumers of research data rather than producers, they can still develop confidence in their interventions by reviewing controlled studies that show their treatment of choice to be beneficial. Thus, whether one ever chooses to evaluate the outcomes of one's own work or not, one can approach counseling efforts with more confidence through developing an understanding of these designs.

### Establishing the First Phase—Baseline A

As indicated through the emphasis on stability of data, the *baseline* phase is a critical component in evaluating outcomes relative to the therapeutic process. If a professional counselor is not objective in the problem identification phase, then evaluation of change can only be subjective. Thus, professional counselors should visually inspect the level and trend in their baseline data to ensure stability prior to implementing interventions. Regardless of phase, trend should be level or opposite of treatment effect.

### Phase II—Treatment Phase B

After a stable baseline is established, professional counselors who are using a within-series design next move to phase B (i.e., the treatment phase). Data relative to the intervention are gathered during this phase. A range of possible interventions exist for most presenting problems. Because some interventions are more intrusive than others, it is important that professional counselors attempt to institute the least-intrusive intervention that can be of reasonable benefit to the client. In some cases, it is important to obtain therapeutic gains as fast as possible (e.g., when the client has self-injurious behavior). In these cases, professional counselors might choose to implement interventions that are more intrusive. Professional counselors may also implement more intrusive interventions, however, when it is difficult to correctly identify aspects of treatment that are critical to success. Regardless of the level of intrusiveness, professional counselors are required to consider the best interest of the client. Thus, if no treatment effects are evident, the professional counselor should revise the protocol or try another approach.

In the case of ineffective treatments in a within-series design, the failed intervention becomes another baseline phase. The design is then changed to an A-B-C, where phase C is the additional treatment phase. If symptoms deteriorate during a treatment phase, treatment should be stopped to determine whether symptoms improve, stabilize, or continue to deteriorate. In contrast, if the client shows improvement during the treatment phase, the professional counselor should focus on evaluation of the treatment components and attempt to replicate the results with the identified client across time, across settings, and with other individuals who display similar behaviors.

### Withdrawal

In any treatment situation, the possibility exists that a client will drop out of treatment (i.e., withdrawal). Withdrawal from treatment can occur naturally (e.g., the client may move away, decide not to participate in treatment any longer due to deleterious effects, or may discontinue due to positive effects of treatment). In SSRD, however, professional counselors can be purposeful in planning a withdrawal phase (e.g., a **reversal design**, or A-B-A-B). In a reversal design, baseline data are collected in the initial phase A, followed by the treatment phase B. In the second A phase, instead of collecting baseline data, the treatment is removed and changes relative to the removal of the treatment are recorded. If behaviors in the withdrawal phase resemble those of the baseline phase, treatment can be considered successful. Through a return to baseline in the second A phase, professional counselors can infer that the changes are due to the removal of treatment. Because professional counselors have an obligation to do no harm, the treatment phase is reintroduced as a second phase B. Aside from attempting to replicate the therapeutic gains in the first B phase, professional counselors using an A-B-A-B design can increase internal validity by demonstrating an opposite pattern in trend and variability between the A and B phases.

Professional counselors are often concerned about the ethical ramifications of removing a treatment that is showing positive effects in the first B phase. However, it is essential to understand that counseling is a time-limited process and treatment will conclude at some point. It is important to be able to predict what will happen when treatment is removed. Removal of treatment in the second B phase can be a short experiment and should serve to promote the independence of the client. Alberto and Troutman (2004), however, caution that there are particular times that a reversal design may not be appropriate. For example, it would be inappropriate to remove an intervention that is eliciting positive results and reducing harm to an individual (e.g., when working successfully with people who are demonstrating self-injurious behaviors). Because information cannot be unlearned, professional counselors should avoid the use of a withdrawal design when addressing academic issues. Thus, with academic issues, it would be difficult to demonstrate a return to baseline once an intervention is removed.

As data-based problem solvers, professional counselors should strive to demonstrate cause-and-effect relationships and to carefully evaluate efforts that fail to provide positive results. Success in counseling often benefits from a positive correlation between level of treatment and level of symptomology. Although professional counselors can elucidate a treatment–effect relationship in an A-B design, more confidence in results is derived from an increase in experimental control (e.g., when there is a removal of treatment, a return to baseline, and clear treatment effect in the second B phase).

## A-B-C Design (Interaction Element)

Although it is ideal to choose an intervention based on empirical evidence, there are times when a professional counselor must evaluate the benefits of one or more components of treatment over another. The A-B-C (i.e., **interaction element**) SSRD provides professional counselors with a method for evaluating the benefits of one component of treatment in interaction with another. The two components in an A-B-C design are measured against the data in the baseline phase. Moore, Tingstrom, Doggett, and Carlyon (2001) used an interaction element design to investigate the requisite components of a token economy in a residential facility for children. The researchers found a significant reduction in the number of daily trips to seclusion and significant improvement in total points earned by combining the two components of treatment. As part of their study, Moore et al. examined the relationship between the number of tokens earned by three children and the resulting trips to seclusion. Because the researchers were evaluating components of an existing token economy, they considered data relative to behavior in the unaltered token economy the A phase (i.e., baseline). The first modification of the token economy (i.e., phase B) involved redefining rules for earning tokens to make them more concrete. In the next phase, the researchers continued the use of the new rules and changed the schedule of reinforcement from once per day (baseline) to four times per day (C). Thus, both treatment components were necessary to improve the target behaviors.

## Changing-Criterion Designs

A **changing-criterion design** emulates (in design) an A-B simple phase change in that there is a baseline and only one treatment implemented. During the treatment phases, however, the criterion for success is gradually increased. By using a changing criterion design, a professional counselor can evaluate the level of intervention necessary to achieve the therapeutic goals. For example, Fox and Rubinoff (1979) were interested in methods for reducing caffeine consumption. In their study, if participants were able to reduce the amount of caffeine intake to a predetermined criterion level, they were rewarded monetarily. But if participants did not meet the criterion, they did not get the reward. Fox and Rubinoff were able to demonstrate that individuals will continually change behaviors each time a criterion is lowered if the reward for changing is adequate.

Likewise, DeLuca and Holborn (1992) used a change in criterion design to help promote exercise among obese boys. In an effort to discover the degree to which the participants would exercise to receive prizes, the researchers established varying criteria across phases with regard to the amount of bicycle pedaling required for reward. During each treatment phase, the amount of pedaling (i.e., the criterion) was increased to earn more points. The participants increased their pedaling output each time the criterion was raised. Thus, professional counselors can see that increasing desired behaviors or decreasing undesirable behaviors can be accomplished in a stepwise fashion when using a changing-criterion design.

Professional counselors should keep a few things in mind when using a changing-criterion design. Remember that a change in level and variability from baseline to the intervention phase increases the confidence in any SSRD. To achieve this goal, begin by setting the criterion reasonably high to help establish greater significance. Like other SSRDs, the more criterion shifts that show causation, the higher the validity.

## Parametric Designs

Parametric designs are similar to changing-criterion designs, but treatment results are compared with other phase designs rather than a specific criterion. In a parametric design (e.g., A-B-B1-B2-B3), each phase progresses along the lines of a continuum. This particular design is often found when studying the effects of medication on participants. Murray and Kollins (2000) studied the effects of methylphenidate (Ritalin®) on a math student. The researchers were interested in evaluating the interaction of several components: (1) the number of math problems solved by the participant, (2) the effects of positive reinforcement in comparison to placebo, and (3) the effects of methylphenidate. Although it may seem logical that the amount of positive reinforcement had an effect on the number of math problems solved in this research, professional counselors should be interested in the notion that dose-response of the counseling intervention was more important than that of psychotropic intervention. In other parametric studies, researchers often increase dosage of medications to achieve the desired results.

# Between-Series Elements

Professional counselors use within-series designs to evaluate treatment outcomes, with regard to a specific behavior, over the course of real time (i.e., behaviors were recorded as they occurred). Professional counselors, however, are often interested in evaluating the results of treatment across settings. Between-series designs allow professional counselors to group target behaviors by condition (i.e., setting).

One of the most common between-series designs is the **alternating treatment design** (ATD). According to Barlow and Hayes (1979), the ATD is used to measure more than one treatment method on a single dependent variable (Figure 8.3). Like other SSRDs, the ATD was originally used in behavioral analysis. The ATD, however,

**Figure 8.3**

Alternating treatment design.

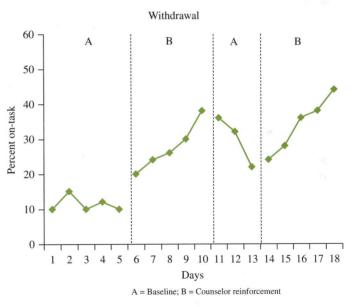

A = Baseline; B = Counselor reinforcement

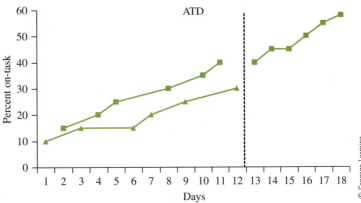

can be useful in a wide range of counseling settings. For instance, professional counselors could use an ATD to measure the differences between rote instruction and small-group discussion on retention of material in a psychoeducational parenting class.

Kennedy and Souza (1995) used a modified version of an ATD to reduce the amount of eye poking with an individual with various disabilities. The researcher established a baseline and introduced two interventions in an effort to evaluate the best method for reducing the child's self-injurious behavior. When working with these types of presenting problems, it is even more important for professional counselors to consistently evaluate the benefits of treatment. Thus, Kennedy and Souza modified their ATD so that the baseline extended into the second treatment phase in an effort to continue comparisons of the independent variables and baseline. In this case, the researchers were able to effectively compare two varying treatments (i.e., independent variable) to the child's eye poking (i.e., dependent variable).

# Combined Elements

Although each of the SSRDs has its place in the evaluation of counseling outcomes, professional counselors often need to evaluate the effectiveness of an intervention on multiple targets (i.e., dependent variables) at different points in time. In other words, professional counselors may want to know the effectiveness of their interventions across behaviors, settings, or people. In quantitative approaches, a researcher might choose a split-plot analysis of variance to evaluate differences within and between subjects (see Chapter 7). In SSRD, professional counselors can accomplish the same goal with very few participants. One of the most common SSRDs used to accomplish this task is the multiple baseline.

## Multiple Baseline

A **multiple-baseline** design is simply two or more replicated simple phase changes, duplicated across two or more series categorized by time, setting, participant, or any combination thereof (Table 8.5). Multiple-baseline designs are beneficial when a researcher wants to provide an internal validity check on a simple phase change. In multiple-baseline designs, phase changes occur at different points in real time and follow first phases of different lengths. Behavior change is seen in the interrupted series before phase changes occur in the noninterrupted series. Professional counselors can answer several questions using a multiple-baseline design: Does an intervention work? Does one intervention work better than another given that both are effective to some degree? Considering two interventions, does either work and does one work better than the other? Which components of an intervention make it effective? What is the optimal level of intervention?

| TABLE 8.5    Steps in multiple-baseline design. |
| --- |
| Multiple targets are selected and baselines started simultaneously. |
| Treatment is administered to one target while the rest remain in baseline. |
| Treatment is administered to second target; first target continues treatment; remainder of targets stay in baseline. |
| Pattern continues until all targets receive treatment. |

*Source:* Adapted from data by Furlong, Lovelace and Lovelace (2000).

An advantage of the multiple-baseline design is the numerous comparisons that can be made throughout the design (see Figure 8.4 for the following comparisons). Comparisons can be made within the simple phase change that occurs within the first series (1 versus 2). The second and third comparisons can be made between the baselines of the first with the baselines of the next two series (1 versus 3 and 1 versus 5, respectively). The fourth comparison can be made in the simple phase change of the second series (3 versus 4). The fifth comparison is made between phase change in the second series and the baseline in the

**Figure 8.4**

Multiple-baseline SSRD.

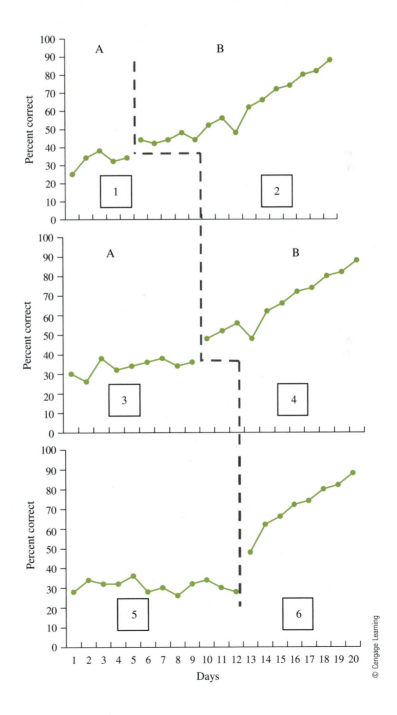

third series (3 versus 5). Finally, the sixth comparison is made in the simple phase change in the third series (5 versus 6).

Sterling-Turner, Watson, and Moore (2002) used a multiple-baseline design to investigate the impact of direct and indirect consultation methods on treatment integrity and treatment outcomes. In this study, the researchers trained teachers to use behavior modification methods on children who were disruptive (e.g., displayed episodes of self-injurious behavior and inappropriate vocalizations). The researchers found a significant difference in the degree to which the teachers implemented the behavioral techniques correctly and the degree to which disruptive behaviors were reduced when consultation was direct. By examining the effects of direct versus indirect training across consultees in staggered phases, the evidence was overwhelmingly in support of direct methods.

# Case Example: Identifying Problem Behavior

The following case is presented in an effort to demonstrate the importance of establishing baseline data in all SSRD research and implementation of a simple A-B design. While the case example involves problem behavior in a classroom setting, the process applies to myriad identified problems across diverse settings. Prior to developing any intervention, a professional counselor must fully implement the problem identification phase of the DBPS and develop a true understanding of the target behaviors.

In this case, Juan's teacher, Mrs. Jones, referred Juan for mental health services to determine environmental variables associated with problem behaviors Juan exhibited in the classroom. These behaviors included noncompliance (e.g., failure to initiate instruction given by teacher) and aggression (e.g., hitting and kicking). In accordance with the DBPS, work with Juan began in the problem identification phase. As part of the problem identification phase, we wanted to gain a better understanding of Juan's behavior. Thus, we used a semistructured interview (i.e., *Functional Assessment Informant Record for Teachers; FAIR-T*) to gain the following information: (a) description of the target behaviors of concern, (b) identification of physical and environmental factors predictive of the target behaviors, and (c) identification of factors potentially maintaining the problem behaviors.

As part of the *FAIR-T*, Ms. Jones reported two main problem behaviors: noncompliance and aggression. Jones rated all of Juan's problem behaviors as very unmanageable as well as very disruptive and as having occurred the entire school year. According to Jones, Juan was noncompliant and aggressive more than 13 times per day. Jones stated that Juan engaged in noncompliance during difficult tasks, when a request had been made to stop or begin a new activity, and when Juan's requests had been denied. Jones stated that aggression tended to occur during transition times and during unstructured activities. Reported consequences for noncompliance included escape or avoidance of presented tasks or instruction and teacher attention (i.e., in the form of peer verbal and physical retaliation, redirections, interruptions, reprimands, and reasoning). Reported consequences for aggression toward peers included peer attention (i.e., in the form of peer verbal and physical retaliation) and teacher attention (i.e., in verbal or physical form, redirections, interruptions, reprimands, and reasoning).

## Targeted Behaviors

1. Noncompliance—failure to initiate administered command (behavioral instruction) or demand (academic instruction)
2. Verbal aggression—yelling/screaming at peers, cursing
3. Physical aggression—hitting/pushing/kicking peers, throwing objects

## Direct Observation: Frequency Data

Juan was observed on three separate occasions at different times of the day from April 29 to May 12. Ten-minute, 10-second, partial-interval recording was used to assess the frequency of noncompliance and aggression. Juan was observed on April 29 from 10:30 to 11:00 A.M. in Jones's classroom during center time. Juan was observed to be noncompliant 10 percent of the intervals observed, verbally aggressive 12 percent of the intervals observed, and physically aggressive 10 percent of the intervals observed (Figure 8.5).

Juan was observed on May 5 from 10:00 to 10:30 A.M. in Jones's classroom during center time. Juan was observed to be noncompliant 17 percent of the intervals observed, verbally aggressive 8 percent of the intervals observed, and physically aggressive 5 percent of the intervals observed.

Juan was observed on May 12 from 10:50 to 11:20 A.M. in Jones's classroom during quiet time at the table before going outside. Juan was observed to be noncompliant 10 percent of the intervals observed, verbally aggressive 8 percent of the intervals observed, and physically aggressive 3 percent of the intervals observed.

Frequency data were also collected on the occurrence of noncompliance with demands (e.g., academic instructions) and commands (e.g., behavioral instructions). Juan was observed on April 29 to be noncompliant with 86 percent of the instructions administered by Jones from 10:30 to 11:00 A.M. Juan was observed to be noncompliant with 77 percent of the instructions administered by Jones from 10:00 to 10:30 A.M. on May 5. Juan was observed on May 12 to be noncompliant with 86 percent of the instructions administered by Jones from 10:50 to 11:20 A.M. (Figure 8.6).

**Figure 8.5**

Inappropriate behavior.

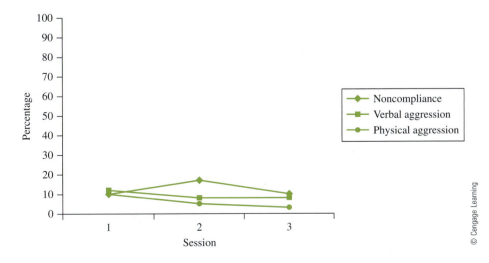

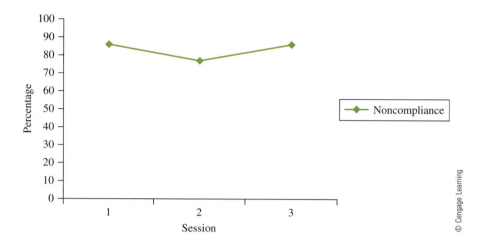

**Figure 8.6**

Noncompliance.

## Direct Observation: A-B-C Data

In addition to direct observation of the frequency of Juan's inappropriate behaviors, direct observation of antecedent-behavior-consequence (A-B-C) analyses were also conducted by a professional counselor from April 29 to May 12. A series of observations indicated that Juan's behaviors resulted in escape from or avoidance of tasks or instructions and negative peer and teacher attention. Direct classroom observations indicated that Juan received escape from or avoidance of instruction approximately 74 percent of the times he exhibited noncompliance, and received teacher attention approximately 17 percent of the times he exhibited noncompliance. A-B-C analysis indicated that Juan received peer attention approximately 65 percent of the times he exhibited verbal aggression toward peers and received teacher attention approximately 18 percent of the times he exhibited verbal aggression toward peers. A-B-C analysis indicated that Juan received peer attention approximately 82 percent of the times he exhibited physical aggression toward peers and received teacher attention approximately 27 percent of the times he exhibited physical aggression toward peers.

In terms of antecedents, A-B-C analysis indicated that Juan is most likely to engage in noncompliance when a command (e.g., "Sit down") has been placed on him. According to A-B-C analysis, Juan is likely to engage in noncompliance in a less-structured environment. A-B-C analysis also indicated that Juan is more likely to engage in noncompliance when issued a behavioral instruction as opposed to an academic instruction. According to the results of A-B-C analysis, Juan is likely to engage in both verbal and physical aggression during unstructured times, such as center time.

Based on the A-B-C analysis, the probable maintaining variable for noncompliance was escape. Analysis of antecedents indicated that noncompliance occurred after administration of behavioral instructions—both low- and high-probability instructions. The primary maintaining variable for aggression, based on the A-B-C analysis summary, appeared to be peer attention in the form of verbal and physical retaliation and crying. Analysis of antecedents indicated that aggression occurred during unstructured times and was maintained by peer attention.

## Hypotheses

1. Based on A-B-C analysis, the probable maintaining variable for noncompliance appeared to be escape.

2. Based on A-B-C analysis, the probable maintaining variable for verbal aggression appeared to be peer attention in the form of peer verbal and physical reaction.

3. Based on A-B-C analysis, the probable maintaining variable for physical aggression appeared to be peer attention in the form of peer verbal and physical reaction.

Although the interpretations should not be considered conclusive or representative of the actual function of these target behaviors because of the limited number of observations and the limited settings of observations, it is clear that understanding the problem is a key element in designing an effective intervention. In this case, Juan did not want to complete tasks that were assigned to him and didn't like to hear "no" from his teacher. Juan became disruptive in an attempt to escape the assigned activities and to gain access to things he wanted. As often happens, parents and teachers get frustrated with children's behavior and surrender to it. In this case, Juan's behavior was further fueled by the attention he received from peers and the negative attention he received from the teacher. Thus, changing Juan's behavior meant learning to ignore some of the disruptive behavior and making sure that Juan completed all assigned tasks. Although this sounds simplistic, it takes a concerted effort and direct feedback to implement behavior change properly. Without appropriate assessment of the functions of Juan's behavior, interventions might have increased the disruptive behavior. From this point on, the professional counselor can monitor the baseline phase and then implement a behavior-management strategy (e.g., time-out, token economy, and response cost) using one of the SSRDs mentioned earlier.

# Conclusion

Action research and SSRD are viable alternatives to large-group research methods in evaluating outcomes in counseling. Professional counselors are scientists and practitioners capable of consuming and producing research. As scientists, professional counselors should embrace an empirical approach to their therapeutic efforts. Through SSRD, professional counselors can track changes in client behaviors, evaluate the effectiveness of one treatment over another, evaluate the effectiveness of one treatment with several different clients, determine the level of intervention necessary, and determine when clients cease to gain benefit from the therapeutic process. In considering the benefits of SSRD, it only makes sense that the counseling profession is beginning to embrace this practical approach to validating treatment outcomes. Although limits exist in any research method, SSRD provides professional counselors with the tools for making sound clinical judgments.

*Now go to the Student Workbook found on cengagebrain.com that accompanies this text for additional application and review activities.*

# Needs Assessment

CHAPTER **9**

When planning for programs and services, professional counselors must assess the needs of target populations. This chapter reviews data-driven and perceptions-based approaches to assessing client needs, which contribute to program development and eventual program evaluation and outcome research.

Needs assessment helps to answer the question "What are the needs of those being served?" In answering this question, a needs assessment fulfills two primary purposes. First, different subpopulations or stakeholder groups may have very different needs or, at least, different perceptions of those needs. Subpopulations may include clients, families, students, parents, teachers, community organizations, local businesses, or numerous other entities. Subpopulations may also include smaller partitionings of these larger groups; for example, males and females receiving a group counseling intervention; White, African American, Asian American, Hispanic American, and Native American racial groups in school achievement; or low-, middle-, and upper-class socioeconomic groupings in a community services program. Second, a needs assessment helps in the determination of a program's priorities. All programs are limited by funding and services, so no program can meet the needs of an entire population. Needs assessments identify needs, quantify needs, and allow professional counselors to prioritize needs within the scope of program resources and objectives. In other words, a needs assessment provides a link between the current (or perceived current) condition of program participants and the expected condition if program goals are fully implemented, thus allowing professional counselors to efficiently use resources to establish a trajectory of intended progress so that participants will reach those goals.

Erford (2015) discussed two primary methods for assessing needs: data-driven needs assessment and perceptions-based needs assessment. Each of these methods will be discussed further. But first, some attention must be given to systemic planning for the needs assessment, particularly through the use of an advisory or steering committee. Then the discussion of needs assessment will be followed by a brief review of how to write program objectives.

# Planning for a Needs Assessment: The Advisory Committee

Advisory committees can be invaluable sounding boards when properly constituted, motivated, and implemented. An advisory committee is ordinarily constituted of representatives of the primary stakeholder groups served by the program. In an agency or community counseling program, a professional counselor may seek representation from former clients who have used the services, other agencies that collaborate with the program, area employers who refer to or otherwise have a stake in the program, administrators who supervise or fund the agency (publicly or through private grants), and citizens from the community. A School Counseling Program Advisory Committee may be constituted from stakeholder groups such as students, teachers, parents, administrators, local employers, and citizen members. Regardless of the committee's constitution, the most important factors in the selection of members are competence and influence. The professional counselor should invite members who are interested in and knowledgeable of the program and able to understand and provide insights into program goals, implementation, and evaluation. More important, members do not need to be experts in these processes but just be able to understand and contribute diverse perspectives and points of reference so that the program will reflect the diverse constituencies it is designed to serve. The potential for influence that members bring to the committee is perhaps the most important consideration.

Often professional counselors who are administering programs are under the control and auspices of administrators or supervisors who control budgets and other resources. Selecting particularly influential parents, businesspersons, or citizens can help provide motivated, engaged advocates who are ready to act on a program's behalf. Everyone has observed instances when someone who was advocating on their own behalf was marginally effective because of a perceived "self-serving" motive. Advisory committee members are often perceived as several steps removed from day-to-day program operations and are therefore often perceived to be more objective in their opinions and points of view. Often, business or community leaders may carry with them a certain stature or level of respect, giving their opinions greater weight by administrators and decision makers. In all honesty, sometimes they may have political or social connections that give them influence or access that the professional counselor could only dream of! Properly selected and motivated advisory committee members can make all the difference in selling a successful, worthy program, particularly when funding is tight.

It is frequently a good idea to invite administrators (e.g., principal, supervisor, and funding source) who oversee the program to become a member of the advisory committee. This allows administrators to see firsthand how a program is planned and evaluated, and it gives the professional counselor and other committee members firsthand access and opportunities to influence the administrator regarding program effectiveness. Each member of the advisory committee must be chosen purposefully and serves as a conduit to various constituencies to both receive and provide information regarding the program.

Convening the advisory committee is generally the responsibility of the professional counselor who ordinarily chairs the committee. It is a good idea to make the committee meeting open to anyone who would like to attend, and it is often valuable to invite those individuals who actually implement the program so that they can receive and give input firsthand. The advisory committee has several primary responsibilities and can either undertake these responsibilities from the ground level or ask the professional counselor to delegate, collect summaries, and facilitate dissemination of information on their behalf. Efficiency is the key, and most advisory committees deal primarily with the "big picture" rather than the details. Primarily, advisory committees help design and review the results of the needs assessment, suggest program goals and objectives, suggest program priorities, and review accountability data. Some committee members even help locate and solicit internal and external funding for programs.

# Data-Driven Needs Assessment

**Data-driven needs assessment** deals with real needs that are identified through analysis of program data. *Data driven* most often refers to information derived through the administration of tests or other standardized and objective sources of information. It is the (mostly) objective nature of how the data are derived, which differentiates these from perceptions-based data, which is, by definition, "biased" by the respondents' points of view or perspectives. Although data-driven analysis can be very helpful in clinical and agency settings, it is currently used most prominently in educational settings. For example, large-scale school-testing programs generate a huge amount of student achievement data on an annual basis, and testing corporations provide individual schools with summaries of these results. For years, this kind of achievement information was provided in an aggregated format, meaning that all of the scores were lumped together to provide the educators with average performances for all students in a given grade on each subject area tested. The "total grade" line in Table 9.1 provides an example of an aggregated

**TABLE 9.1**   Aggregated and disaggregated achievement test results from a large-scale reading achievement test for a school's eighth-grade reading performance.

| | *n* | NPR | % in Quartile | | | |
| --- | --- | --- | --- | --- | --- | --- |
| | | | Q1 | Q2 | Q3 | Q4 |
| Total Grade | 300 | 50 | 21 | 29 | 28 | 22 |
| Male | 144 | 43 | 20 | 34 | 27 | 19 |
| Female | 156 | 57 | 12 | 29 | 30 | 29 |
| White | 24 | 70 | 0 | 23 | 39 | 37 |
| Black | 93 | 36 | 30 | 52 | 14 | 5 |
| Hispanic | 24 | 42 | 28 | 50 | 22 | 0 |
| Asian | 159 | 58 | 9 | 30 | 33 | 28 |
| Low SES | 144 | 27 | 39 | 40 | 20 | 2 |
| Non–Low SES | 156 | 71 | 5 | 24 | 36 | 35 |
| English Primary Language | 10 | 38 | 0 | 70 | 30 | 0 |
| English Second Language | 290 | 51 | 19 | 30 | 27 | 24 |
| Special Education | 30 | 25 | 60 | 20 | 20 | 0 |
| Non–Special Education | 270 | 58 | 11 | 31 | 32 | 26 |

*Note: n* = number of students in sample; NPR = national percentile rank; "% in Quartile" means the percentage of the sample that performed in a given quartile.

© Cengage Learning

score report. Although this type of summary information can be helpful to understand how the average members of a group perform, it does little to help understand the strengths and weaknesses of subpopulations of the entire group.

The implementation of legislation and school reform movements around the world, and particularly those advocated by the Education Trust (see www.edtrust.org), have led educators to determine whether subgroups of students (e.g., gender, socioeconomic, and racial) are performing to equivalent degrees and, if not, whether these students are given equal access to rigorous curricula, funding, specialized services, and so on. This kind of information, known as **disaggregated data**, is far more helpful in the decision-making process because it allows the identification of programmatic strengths and weaknesses and the determination of equity in subgroup performance. Although proficiency in understanding and using disaggregated data relies on a comprehensive knowledge of **norm-referenced** and **criterion-referenced** score interpretation (see Erford, 2013), the use of percentile ranks helps individuals understand the basics of score meanings and differences between scores of various subpopulations.

In Table 9.1, the average national percentile rank (NPR) for the population of 300 eighth-grade students on the reading test was 50, meaning that on a line of 100 eighth-grade students, with the first being the least-proficient reader and the 100th being the most-proficient reader, the average reader in the eighth-grade at that middle school stood at the 50th position in the line. The 50th position is the exact middle of the distribution, so one could easily conclude that the population of eighth-grade students is average. Indeed, looking at the percentages of individuals falling within each quartile, one could easily conclude that the population of eighth-grade students is reasonably normal (e.g., the mean NPR of the total grade population is 50, and about 25 percent of the population falls in each of the quartiles). When data are aggregated in such a manner, few additional conclusions can be surmised. If one is able to disaggregate the data and analyze subgroup performances, however, interesting conclusions emerge.

*Disaggregation* means that total group scores have been broken down into specific sub-population scores so that differences between and among subgroups can be analyzed. Most publishers of large-scale tests now provide disaggregated score reports upon request. Note in Table 9.1 that reading performance has been disaggregated by sex, race, socioeconomics, English proficiency, and special education status. Note also that slight to significant differences can be observed in every facet of these disaggregated results: Females outperformed males by nearly 10 percentile rank places; Whites and Asians outperformed Blacks and Hispanics; students from middle and upper socioeconomic status (SES) strata outperformed students from the lower SES stratum; English-proficient students outperformed nonproficient English-speaking students, and students identified as needing special education services were outperformed by those students who were in the regular education curriculum.

In an example from clinical practice, Table 9.2 provides baseline and end-of-treatment change data from the Beck Depression Inventory, 2nd edition (BDI-II; Beck, Steer, & Brown, 1996) for a group of 25 clients seen for a standardized treatment regimen of counseling only (e.g., no medication). Analyzing the aggregated data, one would conclude that the 25 clients began with an average BDI-II score of 25 (moderate to severe levels of depressive symptoms) and finished the standardized treatment regimen with an average BDI-II score of 15 (mild to moderate levels of depression)—an average raw score change of 10 points. Statistically and practically, these data show that the treatment regimen was successful in reducing the symptoms of depression for the group. A question that often arises in the treatment outcome literature, however, is whether a differential effect of the treatment based on certain client characteristics (e.g., sex, race, and SES) was present. Disaggregating the total sample data in Table 9.2, one observes that some differences do appear to exist with regard to the effectiveness of the treatment on certain subgroups. For example, females appear to have reported a higher level of symptom expression at the beginning of the study and experienced twice the level of symptom relief when compared to males at the completion of the study (i.e., change of 13 raw score points for females versus a change of 6 for males). Likewise, African American clients reported higher levels of symptoms at baseline than Whites and experienced nearly two and a half times the degree of symptom relief (i.e., a change of 17.5 raw score points for Blacks versus a change of 7 raw score points for Whites).

**TABLE 9.2**   Aggregated and disaggregated data of 25 clients treated for depression with an eight-week standardized individual counseling protocol on the *BDI-II* (raw score).

|  | *n* | *BDI-II* **Baseline (A)** | $\Delta$ *BDI-II* **(8 Sessions) (B)** | *BDI-II* |
| --- | --- | --- | --- | --- |
| Change (A-B) | | | | |
| Total Sample | 25 | 25 | 15 | 10 |
| Males | 10 | 21 | 15 | 6 |
| Females | 15 | 28 | 15 | 13 |
| White | 18 | 23 | 16 | 7 |
| Black | 7 | 30 | 12.5 | 17.5 |
| Low SES | 10 | 25 | 19 | 6 |
| Non–Low SES | 15 | 25 | 12.3 | 12.7 |

($\Delta$ = change in)

© Cengage Learning

Finally, low SES and non–low SES (i.e., middle- and upper-class) clients reported identical levels of symptoms at baseline but experienced only half the degree of symptom relief at termination (i.e., a change of 6 raw score points for low SES clients versus a change of 12.7 for non–low SES clients). Such observations, based on disaggregated data, can help professional counselors make future decisions about treatment efficacy for prospective clients and determine whether all clients are benefiting equitably from an otherwise effective approach or program. Of course, such "eyeballing" observations are less accurate than well-controlled experimental studies, but the point is that existing data, or easy-to-collect data, can be helpful in determining population needs and equitable treatment.

One can easily see how disaggregation of data-driven analyses can lead to social action and social justice initiatives and improve client or student access, opportunity, and achievement. Differences can be determined through statistical means or simply by noting gaps in performance. Observing gaps in performances provides objective (not perception-based) evidence of differing results, thus identifying needs to be addressed. When such needs are identified, professional counselors and advisory committees can begin the process of addressing the needs through well-written objectives, interventions, and programmatic initiatives. However, it all starts with data—hence the term *data driven*. Data provide the impetus for responsive initiatives and program improvements.

# Perception-Based Needs Assessment

Perceptions of primary stakeholder groups often focus a program's direction. **Perception-based needs assessment** is a more traditional and familiar approach than the data-driven model just discussed, primarily because most citizens are familiar with surveys and accustomed to (perhaps even expectant of) being asked for their perspectives, wants, and needs. Such needs assessments ask the consumers of the counseling services for help in prioritizing needs and directing a program's focus. When planning for a perceptions-based needs assessment, a professional counselor and advisory committee should consider the questions of who, what, when, and how.

## Whose Needs Should Be Assessed?

*Who is assessed* depends on who the professional counselor considers to be stakeholders. Common stakeholder groups may include other professional counselors, clients, students, parents, local business people, educators, local agencies, funding sources, and so forth. In schools, professional school counselors have ready access to students, teachers, and parents, and these groups can often provide helpful insights into school-based needs. In the clinic, clients (and their parents if a client is a minor) could be assessed at intake, and the professional counselor and advisory committee members could attempt to identify community (public or private) agencies and local businesses willing to provide an assessment of community need. In general, it is considered good practice to assess the needs of several stakeholder groups so that the results can be *triangulated* (i.e., compared across groups) to arrive at needs that have widespread applications. This is not to say that a specific need that is targeted by one stakeholder group cannot be the focus of intervention, only that with limited time and funding, most programs aim at accomplishing objectives that are seen as important by many constituencies. This helps to balance the potential influence of one more powerful constituency over another. For example, the priority of a funding source (or principal or agency administrator) may in some ways be mitigated by evidence from clients and local employers (or students, parents, and teachers) that other concerns are of greater importance. Triangulation helps to confirm and balance a program's emphases.

## When Should Needs Be Assessed?

In the past, some organizations assessed programmatic needs annually. Unfortunately, a needs assessment can be costly in terms of time and money, so the collection of needs assessment data should be a planned activity that considers cost and benefit. In any event, a needs assessment should be designed to be brief and efficient, allowing for the collection of essential data over a short period of time that is able to be quickly compiled and analyzed so that it can be used to plan program initiatives. The best estimate of how frequently to conduct a needs assessment in agencies, clinics, or other nonschool venues is about every three to six years, or when the professional counselor is considering major programmatic changes and wants some perception-based data to guide program focus.

Fortunately, information is available about school-based needs assessment and much of this can be transferred to nonschool counseling programs. Erford, Moore-Thomas, & Wallace (2010) suggested that adoption of the American School Counselor Association's (ASCA) *National Standards* (Campbell & Dahir, 1997) and *National Model* (ASCA, 2012) lend themselves to a six-year continuous needs assessment and accountability cycle in which professional school counselors divide the academic, career, and personal-social standards. This effectively means that programmatic needs related to academic standards are assessed half in year 1 and half in year 4, career needs half in years 2 and 5, and personal-social needs half in years 3 and 6. Alternatively, years 1 and 2 could be dedicated to the academic standards, years 3 and 4 to the career standards, and years 5 and 6 to the personal-social domain. Thus, every six years the entire comprehensive developmental school counseling program will be assessed for need and accountability (Erford, Moore-Thomas, et al., 2010).

Sometimes funding; priorities at the local, state, or national levels; or historical events may lead to dramatic program shifts. Although professional counselors must maintain flexibility and responsiveness in program implementation, such shifts must be the result of real changes in client needs, not historical artifacts, blips, or whims that will be here today and gone tomorrow.

## What Needs Should Be Assessed?

What should be measured by needs assessments is a source of some disagreement within the counseling profession. Some argue for **comprehensive assessments** that collect demographic information and evaluate multiple facets of a counseling program, including services offered, topics of interest addressed, and goals/objectives pursued. There is no argument that such a comprehensive format can yield valuable information about a program, particularly when one considers the potential for disaggregating the results by respondent demographics to better focus on the needs of specific subpopulations. Comprehensive needs assessments, however, are very time consuming for professional counselors to design and analyze and for consumers to respond to. Time-consuming assessments frequently result in low response rates by consumers, and a poor sample diminishes the meaningfulness of the results.

Erford (2015) suggested that focused needs assessments were a more efficient manner of collecting consumer input. **Focused assessments** are usually short, one-page surveys that assess a specific topic of concern. These topics represent the smaller facets that comprise the comprehensive program. Examples of focused, specific topic needs

**Figure 9.1**

A needs assessment focused on stress management.

Name: _____

Below is a series of statements about stress and how you manage it. Respond to each statement by placing a check mark in the appropriate column.

| | Almost Never | Sometimes | Often | Almost Always | I need help with this. | |
|---|---|---|---|---|---|---|
| | | | | | Yes | No |
| 1.  I obsess or can't stop thinking about some things. | | | | | | |
| 2.  I think negative thoughts about myself or others. | | | | | | |
| 3.  Some of my muscles are tense. | | | | | | |
| 4.  I hyperventilate or breathe too fast. | | | | | | |
| 5.  I visualize negative images of myself or others. | | | | | | |
| 6.  I feel stressed out. | | | | | | |
| 7.  I have trouble dealing with "difficult people." | | | | | | |
| 8.  I have poor organizational skills. | | | | | | |
| 9.  I have poor time management skills. | | | | | | |
| 10.  I have behavior problems that cause me stress. | | | | | | |
| 11.  I have difficulty being assertive with people. | | | | | | |
| 12.  I am anxious or nervous. | | | | | | |
| 13.  I have poor nutritional habits. | | | | | | |
| 14.  I have poor exercise habits. | | | | | | |
| 15.  I have difficulty identifying stressors in my life. | | | | | | |

assessments include social skills, academic skills (e.g., study skills, test preparation, and homework), mental disorders (e.g., depression, anxiety, or just about any disorder that is the focus of clinical intervention), career awareness and development, parenting or family issues, rehabilitation issues, substance abuse, and so on. Focused needs assessments have the advantage of providing coverage of an important area of service that will help establish priorities and be easily converted into goals and objectives for program development and modification. Figure 9.1 shows an example of a focused needs assessment on the topic of stress management that can be used with adolescents and adults to plan for a developmental or clinical intervention program.

## How Should Needs Be Assessed?

How needs should be assessed concerns two primary issues: the method of collection and how to interpret and report the results. The method used for assessing needs has important practical implications. First, the professional counselor should determine whether to use an informal or formal method. An informal assessment has the advantages of speed and access. **Informal assessments** use available sources of information familiar to the professional counselor and can be completed very quickly, often in a matter of hours or days. Because the process is informal, however, it lacks procedural safeguards such as standardization and objectivity, which results in an inability to replicate the evidence. Thus, what evidence and conclusions the professional counselor uncovers one week may be very different from the evidence and conclusions derived the next week.

Formal methods for conducting a needs assessment have these and other procedural safeguards and are more likely to generate replicable results over various periods of time and perhaps even with different samples. At least seven methods are commonly used for collecting evidence of need: surveys (including questionnaires and inventories), interviews, review of existing records, use of outside consultants, systematic program evaluation, program statistics, and site observations. Each of these has advantages and disadvantages, but surveys have emerged as the most popular method by far (see Erford, 2015, for a concise summary of these methods), which will be the focus of the remainder of this section.

**Surveys** are used to measure opinions, attitudes, and behaviors, and they have the advantage of being able to generate a tremendous amount of useful perception-based data over a relatively short period of time and inexpensively. Surveys should be limited to a single page and require only one to three minutes to fill out. Time is a very important factor in return rate of surveys, although meaningfulness/relevance and method of collection are just as important. So to motivate respondents to complete a survey, professional counselors must design surveys to be quick, provide an excellent rationale for why it is essential for the respondent to complete the survey, and arrange for the collection of the survey using procedures that will boost the response rate. Usually, response rates for mailed or electronic surveys are less than 20 percent—too low to be of much scientific value. Thus, whenever possible, professional counselors should administer surveys using a "captured audience" technique. Thus, having clients complete a needs assessment at intake, professional counselors during a conference or workshop, parents at "parents night," teachers at a faculty meeting, or students during a guidance lesson are all likely to result in high response rates. As long as these samples are representative of the populations you want to assess, you should receive meaningful results for your intended purposes.

When designing a survey, the professional counselor needs to consider many design issues. Key among these concerns is the scale's content and scaling method. Early on in scale development, the professional counselor must determine whether to use open-ended questions, closed-ended questions, or a combination of both. Of course, each has advantages and disadvantages. Usually, open-ended questions are easier to design and reveal broad-ranging information, sometimes giving the professional counselor valuable perspectives not previously considered. On the other hand, responses to open-ended questions are often more difficult to categorize, interpret, and translate into programmatic goals and objectives. Closed-ended questions limit the responses of stakeholders, but they are much simpler to categorize, analyze, explain, and translate into program objectives.

Content of a needs assessment should include important demographic information of the person completing the form (and characteristics of clients they may represent) and questions related to the topic being assessed. Concurrent with question development, professional counselors must address the issue of response format. A number of response formats have become popular in survey research, including yes/no (or sometimes), multiscale formats (e.g., almost never, sometimes, frequently, almost always), Likert-type scales (e.g., very dissatisfied, dissatisfied, satisfied, very satisfied), and even the familiar true/false or multiple-choice formats. Referring back to Figure 9.1, notice the single-page format, wording of the questions, and scaling method used.

Finally, the professional counselor must consider how best to analyze or interpret and report the survey results. Depending on the **scale of measurement** used (i.e., nominal, ordinal, and interval), survey results can be analyzed using the statistical procedures discussed later in this book. Table 9.3 contains responses for the focused stress management needs assessment presented in Figure 9.1.

Attention to the design issues of a needs assessment just discussed leads to efficient and meaningful tabulation and interpretation procedures. Notice how client responses in Table 9.3 have been both tallied and computed (i.e., mathematically summarized). Tallying involves a process for counting, for example, the number of clients who may benefit from intervention. Notice that the needs assessment (Figure 9.1) was designed with the query "I need help with this" and a yes/no response for each item. A simple tally of client responses to this query is summarized in Table 9.3 and is extremely helpful in assessing a client's motivation to pursue counseling interventions. In this case, the professional counselor was interested in determining how many of the clients who were completing the needs assessment thought the problem was significant enough to warrant intervention. The efficiency of this process is obvious: If a lot of clients indicate they are willing to address a number of the problems listed, the professional counselor has a core of individuals for a small group counseling intervention or large group education session. For example, note that 10 or more clients indicated "yes" to items 1, 2, 3, 5, 6, 7, 8, 9, 11, 12, 13, and 14. By cross-referencing the individual needs assessment responses, a professional counselor may be able to determine that a core group of clients share the same core issues—so many that a group counseling intervention may be the best way to intervene. Alternatively, six or fewer clients identified items 4, 10, and 15 as problematic;

**TABLE 9.3**  Data from the stress management needs assessment ($n = 30$).

| | AN(0) | S(1) | O(2) | AA(3) | Yes | No | Ave(rank) |
|---|---|---|---|---|---|---|---|
| 1. I obsess or can't stop thinking about some things. | 4(0) | 8(8) | 12(24) | 6(18) | 18 | 12 | 1.60(7) |
| 2. I think negative thoughts about myself or others. | 2(0) | 9(9) | 13(26) | 6(18) | 16 | 14 | 1.77(5) |
| 3. Some of my muscles are tense. | 5(0) | 12(12) | 9(18) | 4(12) | 14 | 16 | 1.40(10) |
| 4. I hyperventilate or breathe too fast. | 21(0) | 4(4) | 5(10) | 0(0) | 6 | 24 | 0.47(14) |
| 5. I visualize negative images of myself or others. | 5(0) | 8(8) | 14(28) | 3(9) | 19 | 11 | 1.50(8.5) |
| 6. I feel stressed out. | 0(0) | 8(8) | 16(32) | 6(18) | 25 | 5 | 1.93(1) |
| 7. I have trouble dealing with "difficult people." | 10(0) | 8(8) | 12(24) | 0(0) | 13 | 17 | 1.07(12) |
| 8. I have poor organizational skills. | 7(0) | 10(10) | 11(22) | 2(6) | 10 | 20 | 1.27(11) |
| 9. I have poor time-management skills. | 3(0) | 7(7) | 12(24) | 8(24) | 18 | 12 | 1.83(2.5) |
| 10. I have behavior problems that cause me stress. | 15(0) | 8(8) | 6(12) | 1(3) | 5 | 25 | 0.77(13) |
| 11. I have difficulty being assertive with people. | 5(0) | 6(6) | 9(18) | 10(30) | 20 | 10 | 1.80(4) |
| 12. I am anxious or nervous. | 3(0) | 6(6) | 14(28) | 7(21) | 17 | 13 | 1.83(2.5) |
| 13. I have poor nutritional habits. | 6(0) | 7(7) | 9(18) | 8(24) | 15 | 15 | 1.63(6) |
| 14. I have poor exercise habits. | 6(0) | 10(10) | 7(14) | 7(21) | 15 | 15 | 1.50(8.5) |
| 15. I have difficulty identifying stressors in my life. | 22(0) | 4(4) | 3(6) | 1(3) | 3 | 27 | 0.43(15) |

*Note*: Almost Never (AN) = 0; Sometimes (S) = 1; Often (O) = 2; Almost Always (AA) = 3. The number of clients responding (tally) is entered first in each column, followed by the tally multiplied by the numeric response equivalent—for example, item 1 under the AA(3) column reads 6(18), meaning that 6 clients responded "Almost Always," and this tally was multiplied by 3, resulting in a product of 18.

thus, an individualized approach with these clients may be suggested, or these problems may even subside after addressing other more pressing needs. If the professional counselor who is administering the needs assessment is a school counselor, he or she may conclude that a critical mass of students responding to the assessment was obtained to address many of the problems through classroom guidance lessons aimed at the developmental needs of all adolescent students.

Computations of needs assessment responses are a simple way of showing how important a given problem is within context or even how necessary a particular service or intervention is. Usually, these computations involve presenting a mean for each item and then rank-ordering each in terms of the item's importance. This is best accomplished by assigning a number value to each response category and averaging all responses for a given item. For example, in Table 9.3, assume that the response categories are assigned the following values: Almost Never = 0, Sometimes = 1, Often = 2, and Almost Always = 3. For item 1, "I obsess or can't stop thinking about some things," simply add all client response values and divide by the number of responses. Therefore, of the 30 clients who completed the needs assessment, four clients marked "Almost Never" ($4 \times 0 = 0$), eight clients marked "Sometimes" ($8 \times 1 = 8$), 12 clients marked "Often" ($12 \times 2 = 24$), and six clients marked "Almost Always" ($6 \times 3 = 18$). Next, simply add up the points ($0 + 8 + 24 + 18 = 50$), and divide by the number of client responses ($50 \div 30 = 1.60$) to compute the average frequency rating. Finally, the items can be rank-ordered from "most important" (1) to "least important" (15) to give the professional counselor some idea of the relative importance of responses to each item. According to the data in Table 9.3, item number 6 ("I feel stressed out") received the highest mean rating ($M = 1.93$) and, therefore, was ranked 1st (i.e., the highest rank). Not surprisingly, the item was also identified by 25 of the 30 respondents as a problem they would like to receive help with, the highest number for any of the items. Likewise, item number 15 ("I have difficulty identifying stressors in my life") received the lowest mean rating ($M = 0.43$) and was ranked 15th (i.e., the lowest rank). Again, not surprisingly, the item was identified by only 3 of the 30 respondents as a problem they would like help with, the lowest number for any of the items.

Notice that the use of a mean within descriptive statistics assumes an interval or ratio scale. Technically, this scale is an ordinal scale (designed to look like an interval scale), and so the computation of a mean of this sort, although commonly used in practice, is somewhat nebulous (e.g., What does a 1.60 really mean if the response choices are not equidistant?). Still, it does offer a reasonable estimate of the average frequency of a behavior or an issue's importance within the context of the other issues under study. Thus, an item's importance in absolute terms is not knowable, but it is understandable relative to other item means. The use of additional descriptive statistics obtained through SPSS, as well as parametric and nonparametric statistical tests useful in the analysis and interpretation of data from a needs assessment, will be presented in the remaining chapters of this book.

# Converting Needs to Program Goals (Standards) and Objectives

A correctly designed needs assessment will directly translate into **program goals** (or standards) and objectives. The terms *goals* and *standards* will be treated as synonyms in the discussion that follows, and the term **goal** will be used as the preferred term. (*Standard* is the term of preference in education because it refers to some principle against which performance is compared and judged.) Goals are usually written in language not

**Figure 9.2**

An example of an aggregation model using goals and objectives.

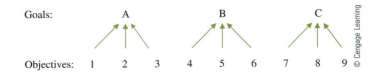

Goals:    A    B    C

Objectives:    1    2    3    4    5    6    7    8    9

© Cengage Learning

amenable to direct measurement and verification because goals lack specific measurable language. This is where objectives come in. By definition, objectives are written in language that makes them amenable to direct measurement. How to specifically word objectives to accomplish direct measurement will be described below. For now, it is essential to understand that objectives (specific content) must align precisely with goals (general content). When the alignment is precise, objectives provide the direct evidence of progress, which helps professional counselors to conclude that program goals are being met. So a given goal may have a couple or even several dozen objectives attached to it. The extent to which these goals and objectives are aligned and the objectives met provides the evidence that a goal (or standard) is met or achieved. This process is referred to as aggregation (Erford, Moore-Thomas, et al., 2010) and is displayed in Figure 9.2. In this figure, objectives 1, 2, and 3 are aligned with Goal A; objectives 4, 5, and 6 are aligned with Goal B; and objectives 7, 8, and 9 are aligned with Goal C. In this example, if the professional counselor can demonstrate that objectives 1–3 have been met, then one can reasonably conclude that Goal A has been met. Likewise, if objectives 4–6 have not been met, one can reasonably conclude that Goal B has not been met. The interpretation, however, is a bit more complicated when some objectives aligned with a given goal are met, whereas others are unmet—for example, if objectives 7 and 8 are met and objective 9 is not met. In this case, the professional counselor can, at most, conclude that Goal C was only partially met.

Practically speaking, when translating needs into program goals, the professional counselor initially must prioritize the needs in order of importance while balancing the needs in relationship to a program's existing components. The tallying, computing, and triangulation strategies mentioned in the preceding sections can be helpful methods for establishing this prioritization and balance.

Second, the needs must be translated into new program goals (or standards) or matched with existing program goals. In the school counseling profession, the ASCA has specified nine standards that form the core of a comprehensive developmental school counseling program, called the *ASCA National Standards* (Campbell & Dahir, 1997). Many school systems have adopted the *ASCA National Standards*, whereas others use previously developed state and local standards.

Third and finally, the goals are operationalized through development of learning objectives. Erford (2010) suggested the ABCD model for writing a learning objective: (A) audience, (B) behavior, (C) conditions, and (D) description of the expected performance criterion. *Audience* refers to the people who are affected by the objective. The audience could be clients, students, parents, teachers, agency counselors, and so on. Often, objectives begin with "The client will …" to define the intended audience. *Behavior* refers to what the audience will be expected to do, think, or feel. Generally, the behavior consists of a descriptive verb (e.g., "The client will *reduce* his level of depression"). *Conditions* provide the context within which the behavior will occur—for example, a test or worksheet, role play, observation, or some activity that is structured and standardized so as to be replicable (e.g., "The client will reduce his level of depression as demonstrated *through multiple administrations of the Beck Depression Inventory— 2nd Edition [BDI-II]*"). *Description* of the expected performance criterion refers to the level of performance or proficiency the audience must attain for the objective to be met. On a teacher-made exam, this may involve the percentage correct needed to pass

**TABLE 9.4** Data from a social skills needs assessment (*n* = 20) for a brief self-check activity on peer relationships.

| | AN(0) | S(1) | O(2) | AA(3) | Ave(rank) | | Yes | No |
|---|---|---|---|---|---|---|---|---|
| 1. I am teased by peers. | 7(0) | 7( ) | 4( ) | 2( ) | | This is a problem for me. | 5 | 15 |
| 2. I am bullied by peers. | 8(0) | 7( ) | 3( ) | 2( ) | | This is a problem for me. | 5 | 15 |
| 3. Peers show me respect. | 3(0) | 5( ) | 6( ) | 6( ) | | This is a problem for me. | 9 | 11 |
| 4. I have trouble making friends. | 10(0) | 6( ) | 3( ) | 1( ) | | This is a problem for me. | 4 | 16 |
| 5. I have trouble keeping friends. | 11(0) | 6( ) | 2( ) | 1( ) | | This is a problem for me. | 4 | 16 |

*Note*: Almost Never (AN) = 0; Sometimes (S) = 1; Often (O) = 2; Almost Always (AA) = 3. The number of students responding (tally) is entered first in each column.

© Cengage Learning

(e.g., 70 percent or 80 percent), although within a group of people, this could be 80 percent of couples having two or fewer arguments per day (as operationally defined, of course). In this continuing example, the addition of D completes the learning objective by making it observable and measurable. The completed example objective now reads, "The client will reduce his level of depression by 25 percent over a four-week treatment period as demonstrated through the raw score of multiple administrations of the Beck Depression Inventory—2nd Edition [BDI-II]."

Goals and objectives are a critical aspect of program planning and evaluation. Professional counselors are well advised to pay close attention to the transformation of needs assessment data and results to the formulation of goals and objectives. Well-written goals and objectives that are closely aligned with program needs and outcomes markedly simplify the program evaluation process and yield very meaningful results that will lead to continuous program improvement. To demonstrate, a potential goal from the needs assessment shown in Figure 9.1 might be "To reduce clients' levels of stress." A possible objective stemming from this goal and related to item 3 (i.e., "Some of my muscles are tense") might be "After participating in a series of group counseling sessions focusing on progressive muscle relaxation training, 80 percent of the clients will report a 25 percent decrease in perceived muscle tension as measured using the subjective units of distress scale (SUDS)." Again, notice how the objective designates the audience (A), the stated behavior (B), how the behavior will be measured (C), and the level of expected performance (D) (Erford, 2010). As a culminating exercise, see the small item set contained in Table 9.4, compute the means for each item, rank them in order of priority, and construct a learning objective and strategy for how you will address the three most important issues.

# Conclusion

Careful planning is a hallmark of effective programs. Professional counselors must periodically assess the needs of target populations to ensure that program activities align with stated goals and objectives. Ordinarily, professional counselors assess needs using data-driven or perception-based procedures. Data-driven procedures use existing data to identify overall effectiveness and gaps in performance between or among various subpopulations. These data then drive changes in program emphasis and resource allocation. Perception-based procedures ordinarily involve surveying or interviewing key stakeholder groups to determine their perceptions of program components. Triangulation of perceptions across stakeholder groups helps identify key areas for program improvement and resource allocation. Key questions of who, when, what, and how must be determined for needs assessment results to be useful. Of course, needs assessments are not an end in themselves. Once results are analyzed, professional counselors convert identified areas of need into program goals and objectives, which then feed the program evaluation cycle.

*Now go to the Student Workbook found on cengagebrain.com that accompanies this text for additional application and review activities.*

# Program Evaluation and Accountability

*A*ccountability and *reform* are catchwords in today's sociopolitical environment. Professional counselors in education, community agencies, colleges and universities, and the private sector are continually challenged to demonstrate necessity, effectiveness, and efficiency of counseling services they provide. This chapter provides an overview of counseling program evaluation and accountability with an emphasis on a practical framework for conducting counselor-implemented program evaluations for improving counseling services and for providing accountability to stakeholders.

# Accountability in Counseling

Professional counselors in the 21st century are faced with many professional challenges. Community agency and mental health counselors must navigate the increasingly complex world of managed behavioral health care and compete for scarce program funding. In the era of the No Child Left Behind Act (U.S. Congress, 2001), professional school counselors have experienced increasing demands to demonstrate their effectiveness and necessity in the education sector. Accountability has therefore become a central concern among today's counseling professionals. In addition to excellent counseling skills, today's professional counselors must also have strong evaluation skills to demonstrate the impact and effectiveness of their counseling services. In many ways, program evaluation procedures parallel the counseling process with clients. Professional counselors routinely assess and gather information from clients to guide their counseling interventions. Feedback from clients becomes central in the helping process as a means for modifying or adapting techniques and interventions. Similarly, counseling program evaluation involves a systematic collection of information about a program or a program component to determine its effectiveness, efficiency, and benefit for the clients served. Counseling program evaluation may therefore be viewed as a type of action research used for assessing the provision and outcome of counseling services.

As a profession, counseling often relies on external funding and financial support for the provision of services. For example, school counselor positions are typically funded through local, state, and federal education monies and grants. During times of fiscal crisis or economic hardship, school counseling positions may be vulnerable to elimination. Similarly, mental health and community counseling agencies are often funded through grants, donations, and third-party payers and may be at risk during budgetary cutbacks and downsizing of social programs. Private practice counselors also often rely on managed care companies and insurance providers for payment. Thus, accountability has become a very tangible concern for practicing counselors. Professional counselors must be aware of the demands and expectations for accountability to their specific stakeholders and have the tools for providing program outcome reports.

## Mental Health Counseling Accountability

Perhaps one of the biggest influences on the livelihood of today's mental health counselors involves the advent of rigorous managed care in mental health services. In a study of the impact of managed care on mental health counseling practice, Danzinger and Welfel (2001) found that mental health counselors are often providers for one or more managed care organizations and that managed care organizations have substantially impacted counseling practice. Mental health counselors generally have negative views about the impact of managed care on their ability to provide quality mental health counseling, particularly because of pressures to demonstrate outcomes and provide cost-effective counseling services (Scheid, 2003). Some professional counselors have even sought to avoid working with managed care organizations by counseling primarily with self-pay clientele and using sliding fee scales.

In today's mental health marketplace, professional counselors who do work with managed care organizations are often expected to maintain detailed records regarding treatment interventions and outcomes of counseling sessions (Jackson & Daughhetee, 2015). Furthermore, managed care organizations sometimes require that professional counselors use interventions from a prescribed list of evidence-based practices (EBPs) and empirically supported treatments (ESTs). Clearly, managed care organizations compel today's mental health counselors to evaluate and document the effectiveness of their services. Loesch (2001) even suggested that the historical avoidance of such evaluations by mental health counselors actually helped lead to the development of the rigorous standards now used by many managed care organizations. Ultimately, to thrive in today's managed care environment, mental health counselors must proactively demonstrate the effectiveness of their treatments and programs.

## School Counseling Accountability

Professional school counselors have also experienced increased accountability demands, especially to demonstrate the effectiveness of comprehensive school counseling programs. Recent education reform, particularly the No Child Left Behind and Reach for the Top acts, has increased the scrutiny of educational programming, particularly targeting the outcomes of educational practices on student achievement. Accountability efforts in school counseling are evolving to meet the pressures for accountability in public schooling. In fact, evaluation and accountability are featured prominently in the American School Counselor Association's (2012) *ASCA National Model*. Professional school counselors have regularly been connected with education reform measures (Erford, 2015), yet they have not frequently been held to the same accountability standards as others in education. Recently, school counseling visionaries have promoted a new professional identity for school counselors, which emphasizes leadership, advocacy, and utilizes comprehensive school counseling programs to ensure the academic success of all students. With a heightened professional visibility, professional school counselors are poised to use accountability data as a means for student advocacy. Ultimately, accountability of comprehensive school counseling programs serves to help students and strengthens the professional identity of professional school counselors.

The **ASCA** (2012) **National Model** highlights three main categories of accountability data for use by professional school counselors to advocate for program effectiveness and impact. *Use-of-time analysis* refers to tallies of actual services provided and numbers of stakeholders impacted by the professional school counselor's services. *Evaluation and improvement* assessment addresses performance appraisals and competency evaluation related to services provided by the school counselor. Finally, a *results report* refers to the outcomes of programs and interventions provided in the comprehensive school counseling program. Erford (2015) also emphasized the use of outcome evaluation and EBPs in school counseling accountability. Using a program evaluation framework, professional school counselors can systematically gather accountability information by identifying program needs, developing or modifying programs, and assessing program outcomes. In addition, state education standards and the new Common Core Standards are changing the way professional school counselors deliver and assess services to students by helping to ensure that all students are college and career ready and able to access educational opportunities and achievement. Today's professional school counselors are thus becoming proactively involved in providing accountability for the effectiveness of their school counseling programs.

## The Relationship Between Accountability and Program Evaluation

Because they are frequently discussed together in the counseling literature, the terminology regarding accountability and counseling program evaluation has sometimes been imprecise, and at times the terms have been used interchangeably or as subcategories of each other. Erford (2015) indicated that such misunderstandings of accountability and program evaluation concepts might be preventing counselors from engaging in regular evaluation activities. It may be helpful to consider counseling program evaluation as independent of accountability. Again, *counseling program evaluation* refers to the ongoing use of evaluation principles by professional counselors to assess and improve the effectiveness and impact of their programs and services. Thus, counseling program evaluations should be part of routine counseling practice even in the absence of accountability pressures. When called upon to provide evidence of program effectiveness, however, evaluation data may play a significant role in providing accountability to stakeholders. *Counseling accountability* refers to "providing specific information to stakeholders and other supervising authorities about the effectiveness and efficiency of counseling services" (Astramovich & Coker, 2007). Accountability is therefore the *process* of providing program evaluation information to stakeholders. Ultimately, effective accountability in counseling relies upon the skills of professional counselors in program evaluation methods.

This chapter provides an overview of counseling program evaluation to help you begin developing evaluation skills for your professional practice. We first explore the background of program evaluation and provide definitions of key concepts. Then we review the use of program evaluation in counseling and discuss challenges to counselor-implemented evaluations. Next the Accountability Bridge model of counseling program evaluation is presented, and case studies of its use are provided. Finally, you will be asked to assess your current readiness to evaluate your counseling services and make plans to further your professional development in evaluation skills.

# Examples of Counselors Experiencing Program Evaluation Demands

Before exploring the process of counseling program evaluation, consider the following scenarios of professional counselors experiencing firsthand the need for strong evaluation skills.

## Mental Health Counseling Agency Scenario

Holly works as a licensed professional counselor at a mental health counseling agency in Dallas, Texas. The agency provides counseling and referral services to people who are living in poverty and homeless families. Holly has spent three years developing and implementing an outreach program designed to help homeless families receive needed counseling services. The program was originally funded through a city mental health services grant. Recently, the community agency director told Holly that the funding for the program and her position with the agency are in jeopardy because many constituents in the city government have questioned the effectiveness and need for this program.

## School Counseling Scenario

Steve has worked for six years as a professional school counselor at an elementary school in rural northern Nevada. The entire school district serves 300 students K–12. Steve has recently received word from the superintendent that all nonteaching staff and paraprofessional positions are on the school board's agenda to be cut from next year's budget because of a fiscal shortfall. Steve and the district's secondary school counselor, Judith, have been asked to develop a presentation about the counseling needs of students and the effectiveness of school counseling in the district. Unless compelling evidence is presented to the school board, next year students will no longer receive school counseling services, and Steve and Judith will need to look for other school counseling positions.

### College Counseling Scenario

Martha is in her first year as a counselor at a university counseling clinic in Alabama. The student body is ethnically diverse, with a 50 percent minority student population, but Martha is concerned that only about 20 percent of the clients served at the clinic are minority students. She wonders what factors may be preventing minority students from seeking services at the clinic and what can be done to ensure that the campus counseling clinic serves all students at the university.

### Questions to Consider

Each of these scenarios reflects the need for professional counselors to have strong evaluation and research skills to provide accountability and to evaluate the impact and effectiveness of counseling programs and services. For each of these scenarios, answer the following questions:

1. What would you do first?
2. Whose help would you enlist?
3. What information would you need to gather?
4. How would you gather the information you need?
5. How would you analyze your information?
6. To whom would you communicate your findings?
7. What format and venue would you use to present your findings?
8. How would you use information to modify, refine, or create new counseling services and programs?
9. What are some challenges you might encounter while attempting to conduct a program evaluation?

To be proactive in meeting accountability demands, professional counselors must have a foundational understanding of evaluation concepts and be competent in practical, counselor-specific methods of program evaluation. Successful professional counselors in today's sociopolitical climate are not only skilled clinicians but also those who can document the worth and merit of their programs and utilize evaluation methods for improving their counseling services.

# Purpose and Benefits of Program Evaluation in Counseling

Program evaluations may be undertaken for a variety of reasons, but the primary goal of counseling program evaluations is to provide useful information to the practitioner about the effectiveness and impact of counseling services. Program evaluations can help professional counselors determine the extent to which clients are being helped by interventions and can help identify the most effective interventions for the client populations served. Program evaluations may also be used as an advocacy tool in counseling when practitioners use their findings to determine program impact on larger sociopolitical concerns of clientele. Finally, counseling program evaluations can provide essential feedback for consideration in the development or modification of counseling programs and services.

## Counseling Program Evaluation Questions

In the counseling field, program evaluations are generally guided by questions about the effectiveness and impact of counseling programs and interventions. For instance, a community counseling agency may want to determine the long-term impact and effectiveness of a weekly family support group, or a professional school counselor may want to know how a study skills seminar impacts student achievement. In general, evaluation questions address four main programmatic categories: needs, contexts, operations, and outcomes. More specifically, counseling program evaluations may help practitioners answer the following questions:

- To what extent are clients being helped?
- What methods, interventions, and programs are most helpful for clients?
- How satisfied are clients with the services received?
- What are the long-term effects of counseling programs and services?
- What impact do the services and programs make on the larger social system?
- What are the most effective uses of program staff?
- How well are program objectives being met?

Because counseling program evaluation is considered a dynamic, cyclical process, questions addressed during one program evaluation process may clarify some information while generating new questions for further evaluation.

## Benefits of Counseling Program Evaluation

As discussed earlier, EBPs and ESTs have significantly affected mental health counseling services, yet not all effective counseling practices may be identified through typical EBP and EST research (Hutchinson & Razzano, 2005). In fact, program evaluations may help highlight effective and new counseling practices that are not yet supported in the EST literature. Practitioners who implement action research and evaluation as a method for strengthening the research base of the counseling profession also may provide crucial information about the effectiveness of new programs and interventions, particularly before the interventions have received enough attention to warrant large-scale research. Thus, in addition to meeting accountability demands, professional counselors can promote innovative programs and treatment methods by evaluating and reporting results of such interventions to stakeholders.

Another benefit of regular counseling program evaluation involves strengthening the professional identity of counselors. In the mental health field, a variety of service providers compete to provide mental health care to clients. Professional counselors, psychologists, psychiatrists, and social workers all provide mental health services, yet historically professional counselors may have not held the same prestige as other mental health providers. As a result, professional counselors may experience difficulty when seeking positions in mental health or government agencies. They also may be prevented from participating in managed care organization preferred provider lists or be compensated at a lower rate than comparable mental health providers. Professional school counselors likewise face professional identity concerns, particularly related to the roles and functions of counselors in the school setting. For all professional counselors, the ability to evaluate and document the impact and effectiveness of counseling interventions and services may be seen as a critical step necessary for enhancing the professional identity of professional counselors and the counseling profession as a whole.

# Important Evaluation Terms

Like many specialized aspects within the discipline of research, program evaluation has a specialized language. Professional counselors who learn and understand this language will be well positioned to function effectively. The purpose of this section is to introduce some commonly used evaluation terms. *Accountability* involves demonstrating responsibility for one's actions (Erford, 2015), usually by providing evidence of efficient services or evaluation of program effectiveness. Accountable professional counselors seek to understand the effects of their interventions and take responsibility for their actions. Accountability should always be based on evidence. Evidence is any information or data helpful in a decision-making or judgment process. These data can be derived using quantitative or qualitative methods. Typical sources of evidence include standardized or counselor-made tests, surveys, questionnaires, interviews, focus groups, external judges, portfolios, self-assessments, actual performances, and work samples.

Related to accountability is evaluation, which is the measurement of worth based on the evidence collected (Erford, 2015). Evaluation of program effectiveness is usually described as formative or summative. Formative evaluation is a way of gathering information about program implementation and effectiveness during the course of the program. One facet of formative evaluation is a determination of whether the program is being implemented properly. Another facet involves whether the program outcomes are progressing as planned and objectives are being met. Often, program implementation includes milestones or benchmarks en route to full implementation. These milestones not only indicate which facets of a program have been implemented but also the expected levels of progress the participants should be achieving. If participants are not meeting expectations at these points in program implementation, formative evaluation allows for midcourse adjustments or modifications to be made for the program to meets its objectives. Formative evaluation is very cost effective when implementing large-scale, expensive programs where a lot is riding on effective outcomes. In such cases, when professional counselors know halfway through a treatment regimen that the desired results are not being obtained, it is good practice to take corrective action to reach the desired outcomes.

Summative evaluation is an end-of-program evaluation, and it is very frequently performed, sometimes even mandated, by funding agencies or administrators. The primary purpose of summative evaluation is the determination of whether and to what degree program objectives and outcomes have been met; in other words, did the program accomplish what it set out to accomplish? Usually, summative evaluation is pursued to determine whether a program should be continued, but outcome results often can be helpful in making program modifications prior to beginning a new cycle of program implementation (e.g., the next academic year, the next group counseling experience, and the next client treated) (Erford, 2015).

*Stakeholders* are individuals to whom the professional counselor is responsible: anyone who may benefit from, is involved in, or interested in the program. Stakeholders may include clients, students, participants, parents, educators, other professional counselors, community leaders, taxpayers (if a program is publicly funded), employers, or other researchers/evaluators. Stakeholders are frequently interested if the activities undertaken are cost-effective, or effective at all. Tangentially related to cost-effectiveness is value-added assessment. **Value-added assessment** seeks to determine and document what a program adds to what participants already possess. For example, if students participate in a conflict resolution curriculum, it is reasonable to expect that they will demonstrate measurable gains as a result of their participation (i.e., did gains outweigh the cost of spending valuable time and scarce resources in the endeavor?). Thus, a professional counselor will establish expected attitudinal, knowledge, and skill objectives and collect a baseline (i.e., pretest) measurement prior to program implementation and then collect an end-of-program measurement (posttest). If the posttest results are significantly higher than baseline results, the program is determined to have "added value" to the participants' attitudes, knowledge, and/or skills in resolving conflicts (Erford, 2015).

# Challenges to Implementing Counseling Program Evaluations

Despite the clear benefit and need for conducting program evaluations, professional counselors have historically avoided evaluation and research activities. Such hesitance by professional counselors to implement evaluations may be attributed in part to the widely discussed research–practice gap in counseling (Loesch, 2001). Indeed, the counseling professions have been criticized for artificially dichotomizing research activities and counseling practices to the extent that professional counselors rarely read research and generally avoid conducting their own evaluation and research activities (Sexton, Whiston, Bleuer, & Walz, 1997). With their already overextended work schedules, many professional counselors find it virtually impossible to allocate time to evaluation activities.

Another challenge of professional counselors who are engaging in regular program evaluation practices involves the minimal training in research and evaluation methods that most professional counselors receive during their graduate training. Counselor education programs frequently only require a single course in research methods. In addition, the existing curriculum in counselor education has little room for expanded coursework in research and evaluation methods, as many programs already require 60 credit hours of coursework. Thus, many professional counselors are methodologically unprepared for the demands for accountability and evaluation.

A final reason for professional counselors' reluctance to evaluate their services involves a lack of practical models for professional counselors to implement. Historically, professional counselors have had few accessible models to guide their own development and implementation of program evaluations. Some models emphasize the use of independent evaluators (e.g., Benkofski & Heppner, 1999) to carry out counseling program evaluations. Further complicating the matter is that many program evaluation models were developed for large-scale evaluations and may be unfeasible for professional counselors to undertake on their own. Erford (2015) indicated that existing models of program evaluation needed to be adapted to meet the needs of the counseling profession. Therefore, counseling-specific models of evaluation like the one presented in this chapter may help provide a needed framework for the increased use of evaluations by professional counselors.

Although several challenges exist to professional counselors' use of program evaluation methods, recent studies have suggested that professional counselors do have interest in conducting evaluations but believe they lack the specific skills necessary to do so (e.g., Astramovich, Coker, & Hoskins, 2005). Overall, it appears that one remedy to the traditional avoidance of program evaluation and research by professional counselors involves training professional counselors in evaluation-specific methods and providing them with frequent opportunities for practice during their graduate training and professional careers.

# The Accountability Bridge Counseling Program Evaluation Model

The Accountability Bridge Counseling Program Evaluation Model (Figure 10.1) was developed to help provide a practical framework for professional counselors in conducting evaluations of their programs and services. A key purpose of this model is to help professional counselors assess if their program goals are being met and their clientele are being optimally served. The Accountability Bridge model organizes the evaluation process into two repeating cycles that form a continuous feedback loop. The **counseling context evaluation cycle** emphasizes the ecological or systemic factors that contribute to the success of counseling services. Ecological perspectives in evaluation are not only concerned with the outcomes of programs but also aim to build and strengthen collaborative relationships with stakeholders (Perkins, Born, Raines, & Galka, 2005). Information gathered during the context evaluation cycle directly influences the planning, development, delivery, and assessment of counseling services.

The **counseling program evaluation cycle** therefore emphasizes the actual implementation of counseling services and outcome evaluations of impact. Accountability to stakeholders essentially forms a "bridge" between the context and counseling program evaluation cycles. Outcome data are provided to stakeholders, and feedback about program impact and effectiveness are gathered. The evaluation cycle then repeats, forming a dynamic process of continual program improvement, refinement, and assessment based on the evolving needs of clients served.

## Counseling Context Evaluation Cycle

The effects of counseling services on the larger system of stakeholders and the environment within which counseling programs are provided forms the emphasis of the **counseling context evaluation cycle**. In this phase of program evaluation, professional

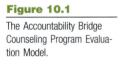

**Figure 10.1**

The Accountability Bridge Counseling Program Evaluation Model.

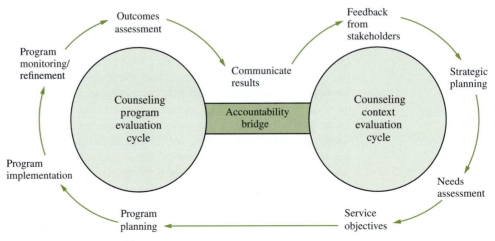

© Cengage Learning

counselors actively seek feedback and suggestions from stakeholders about the impact of counseling services to develop strategic plans for services that meet the needs of clients. Information gathered during the context evaluation cycle provides a foundation for professional counselors in developing programs and services for populations served.

## 1. Feedback From Stakeholders

**Stakeholders** are those individuals and organizations with a vested personal or financial interest in the success of counseling services. In the mental health setting, stakeholders may include clients served, funding entities, administrators, staff, advisory boards, community members, and referral sources. Stakeholders of school counseling programs can include students, parents, teachers, administrators, school boards, funding agencies, and the local, state, and federal governments. Professional counselors should routinely seek feedback from the variety of stakeholders who are interested in the outcomes of their services and programs. This information can play a key role in the alignment of counseling programs and services with the goals of stakeholders. Obtaining multiple perspectives from various stakeholders helps ensure that all individuals and groups have the opportunity for input. The viability of counseling services is maintained and strengthened when stakeholders experience opportunities to shape services provided to clients.

## 2. Strategic Planning

Feedback from stakeholders can help provide key information in the **strategic planning** stage of the context evaluation. For example, stakeholders' input about a substance abuse aftercare program at a community agency can help the agency counselors and administrators develop goals and plans for effective service delivery. Part of the strategic planning process involves examining organizational structures and the mission and goals of the organization in meeting the needs of clients and stakeholders. Decisions about program emphasis, as well as use of staff and financial resources, are considered during the strategic planning phase. The result of strategic planning should be a clear philosophy and mission that will help guide the development of client programs and professional counselor practices.

## 3. Needs Assessment

An essential step in the context evaluation cycle involves identifying specific needs of clients and stakeholders in the outcomes of counseling services. **Needs assessments**, therefore, can provide important information that will help shape and guide the provision of counseling programs and services. Needs assessments of stakeholders can help programs and professional counselors stay focused on providing optimal outcomes of counseling for the population served. Needs assessments should obtain the perspectives of multiple stakeholders and should be focused on gathering specific information necessary for developing counseling programs and services. Ultimately, needs assessments can offer insight into the concerns of various stakeholders and can help professional counselors prioritize and focus the goals of their counseling programs. Because needs assessments serve a central role in the program evaluation process, a more detailed discussion of their development is provided in Chapter 9.

## 4. Program Objectives

Information from needs assessments, stakeholder feedback, and strategic plans help professional counselors develop specific goals and objectives of counseling programs. Without the development of clear goals and objectives, professional counselors may experience difficulty when evaluating the outcomes and impact of services (Erford, 2010). Professional counselors may find it useful to consider two forms of program objectives discussed by Royse, Thyer, Padgett, and Logan (2001). Process objectives are considered benchmarks or competencies needed to achieve long-term goals. For instance, a process objective in a school counseling program might be to increase the use of career information systems by high-school students. Outcome objectives refer to more specific and immediate steps toward meeting goals—for example, providing regular career information system workshops to sophomore students so that by the end of the academic year, 80 percent of sophomores will have a working knowledge of the school's computerized career information system. A single process objective may yield multiple outcome objectives for counseling programs. Thus, process objectives can help professional counselors to conceptualize more specific outcome objectives that can in turn be measured and assessed to determine the effectiveness and impact of counseling services. Erford (2010) promoted use of the ABCD model for constructing learning objectives: A = Audience, B = Behavior, C = Conditions, and D = Description of the expected performance criterion. For example, "After completing a worksheet listing 10 scenarios of cooperative group behaviors, 75 percent of fifth-grade students will be able to recognize one cooperative group behavior in each scenario" (p. 222).

## Counseling Program Evaluation Cycle

The counseling program evaluation cycle draws upon information obtained during the counseling context cycle to help professional counselors plan, implement, monitor, and assess the outcomes of individual and group counseling, guidance services, and counseling programs. This phase of the evaluation process focuses specifically on the array of services provided by the professional counselor and the effectiveness and impact of those interventions and programs. Before proceeding with the steps of this cycle, professional counselors should give consideration to what sort of counseling outcomes they expect to assess and the ways in which the impact and effectiveness of services and interventions will be measured.

### 1. Program Planning

During the program planning stage, professional counselors identify appropriate counseling interventions and programs that can be implemented to meet the needs of their client populations. Needs assessment results as well as program objectives of the larger organization can guide professional counselors in developing specific counseling methods and activities. Furthermore, during the program planning stage, professional counselors should consider additional factors that may influence their provision of counseling services including staff and facility resources and any special program materials or requests.

A critical part of the program planning stage involves identifying methods for measuring program outcomes. Professional counselors can help ensure that program objectives are being met by developing results-based interventions with specific outcome criteria that can be assessed for effectiveness and impact (Lapan, 2001). For example, during the program planning phase, a college counseling clinic that is implementing a substance abuse recovery program for undergraduates should identify methods for assessing client progress throughout the program. Multiple outcome measures should be identified to strengthen the validity of the results. Professional counselors can easily administer a variety of outcome measurement tools and strategies including pre/post instruments, performance indicators, and client checklists (Gysbers & Henderson, 2012). In the school setting, outcome data may be drawn from a variety of sources including assessment instruments, observations, school databases, and interviews of students, parents, and teachers. In mental health and community agencies, professional counselors can measure client progress through standardized brief measures of progress including symptom inventories and behavior checklists and goal attainment scaling. Outcome data may also be collected through surveys, qualitative interviews, and documents or artifacts related to client progress. After outcome measures have been identified, professional counselors should plan when assessments and data will be collected and who will be responsible for administering and gathering the information.

## 2. Program Implementation

Once programs and interventions have been planned and outcome measures have been identified, counseling services are implemented. During the initial stages of program implementation, professional counselors need to consider if the planned programs and interventions are functional based on the professional counselors' actual practice. Professional counselors should therefore determine in the initial stages of service delivery if changes must be made before programs are fully implemented. More specifically, feedback from clients during the initial stages of program implementation can help professional counselors improve the outcomes of their interventions.

## 3. Program Monitoring and Refinement

As counseling services become fully implemented, professional counselors will need to monitor the progress of interventions and programs and make modifications based on client feedback and improvement. Program monitoring and refinement may also be initiated based on the professional counselor's own assessments and observations as well as the administrator's observations and feedback. A main purpose of program monitoring is to determine if program objectives are being addressed through counseling services. Emphasizing the attainment of treatment or program goals will assist professional counselors in identifying successful outcomes during the outcome assessment stage.

## 4. Outcome Assessment

The final stage of the counseling program evaluation cycle involves using outcome assessments to determine whether counseling objectives have been met and whether treatments and programs have been successful. During the outcome assessment phase, professional counselors collect final data identified during the program planning stage. Next, professional counselors analyze all data sources and draw conclusions about intervention and program effectiveness. To help professional counselors stay focused on completing the outcome assessment, Gysbers and Henderson (2012) stressed that all outcome data should be interpreted immediately following interventions and programs.

To assess the outcomes of programs and to draw conclusions about treatment success, professional counselors will need to analyze outcome data collected throughout the counseling program evaluation cycle. Careful planning during the program planning stage of the counseling program evaluation cycle will facilitate the professional counselor's success at collecting and analyzing outcome data. Professional counselors should carefully select analysis methods that are appropriate for the type of data being examined. Quantitative data will often be explored through descriptive statistics including percentages, means and standard deviations, medians, and modes. More advanced quantitative analysis may involve parametric and nonparametric procedures such as chi-square tests, *t*-tests, correlations, and analysis of variance. Qualitative data should be explored with appropriate qualitative analysis procedures, including thematic coding and categorizing data. After completing the data analysis, professional counselors should have the information necessary to draw conclusions about program effectiveness.

Analyzing outcome assessment data can be facilitated through a variety of widely available computer software programs, such as *SPSS*, *Excel*, and *R-stat*. In particular, spreadsheet software allows for easy data entry and computation of descriptive statistics. Furthermore, spreadsheets may be used to create charts and graphs of outcome results that may later be used in evaluation reports and presentations. Professional counselors with little background or practice using current spreadsheet programs should consider continuing education training workshops to learn about the variety of functions and capabilities of the software. Finally, when working with outcome data, professional counselors may need to actively seek assistance from supervisors and peers with more advanced knowledge in managing datasets and using spreadsheets for analysis.

## The Accountability Bridge

The last step in the evaluation cycle involves communicating outcome data and program results to stakeholders. Astramovich and Coker (2007) conceptualized this process as the Accountability Bridge, whereby counseling program outcome data are provided to stakeholders as a means of program accountability. Accountability therefore bridges the actual counseling practice with the context in which counseling services are provided. Rather than thinking of accountability as a defensive action for maintaining positions and funding of counseling services, accountability may better be thought of as a proactive measure that strengthens the professional identity of the counselor in the larger sociopolitical environment. Therefore, professional counselors should not wait until stakeholders demand accountability but should regularly provide them with program evaluation results and seek their feedback to continually improve counseling services.

The main step in the accountability process involves providing presentations or evaluation reports to stakeholders. To maximize the impact of the accountability information, reports and presentations should be targeted for specific stakeholder populations. Therefore, professional counselors should determine whether an accountability report or presentation should focus more on statistics or if case studies or personal narratives will be more appropriate for their audience. For instance, a school counseling outcomes presentation to parents might focus on personal experiences and changes of students, whereas a similar presentation to administrators and the school board might emphasize statistical findings. Counseling program evaluation presentations and reports should include the following elements (Gysbers & Henderson, 2012):

1. an introduction defining the purposes and goals of programs and of the evaluation
2. a description of programs and services
3. a discussion of the evaluation design and data analysis procedures
4. a presentation of the evaluation results
5. a discussion of the findings and recommendations

Furthermore, during professional presentations of program outcomes, professional counselors should also add a sixth section to the presentation that includes a question and answer segment for members of the audience.

With the dissemination of program outcomes to stakeholders, the context program evaluation cycle reoccurs and the entire program evaluation process begins anew. Counseling program evaluation may therefore be considered a dynamic and evolving process of continual program refinement and development based on multiple sources of data and stakeholder input.

# A Case Study of Counseling Program Evaluation

## Needs Assessment

Matthew, a counselor at Desert Hills High School, wanted to ensure that incoming freshmen were on track for a successful high school experience. At the beginning of the fall semester, Matthew implemented a needs assessment to clarify problems and concerns of incoming freshmen. In addition, Matthew hoped that information from the needs assessment would help focus the implementation of current services for freshmen students. In creating the needs assessment, Matthew specifically wanted to identify freshmen's biggest concerns or potential roadblocks to a successful high school experience. The needs assessment survey would offer valuable data that were not currently available in existing data archives. Matthew wanted to create an instrument that would address students' concerns while offering ease of item response through a ranking system. Matthew also intended to keep the instrument to one page so that it could be completed and collected in the same setting.

After informal classroom observations and interviews, Matthew worked with other professional school counselors to create the instrument. The needs assessment survey included the following items to be ranked by order of importance for students: graduation requirements, classroom success, study skills, credits/grade status, making up lost credit, organization, career awareness, coping with stress, and peer pressure. In addition, Matthew asked students to rank-order their knowledge of the same topics. The needs assessment survey was administered to 100 ninth-grade students during their health class. Students were given verbal and written directions for completing the needs assessment survey. The four most important topics that students wanted to learn about were graduation requirements, credits/grade status, organization skills, and making up lost credit. These items were also the four topics that students stated they knew about the least.

## Service Objectives

From the information gathered, Matthew, along with a school counseling advisory committee, retooled their current service objectives to focus on the current needs expressed by the ninth-grade students. The objectives needed to be specific and measurable. In addition, the objectives would hopefully help guide the program planning for the current school year. The first objective was to make sure that students knew their professional school counselor and the services provided by the school counseling program. The second objective that the advisory committee settled on was to improve student knowledge in graduation requirements, credits/grade status, organization skills, and making up lost credit. Developing a curriculum to address these needs would commence during the fall semester. The third objective was to offer a ninth-grade student seminar to address the concerns and questions of all freshmen.

## Program Planning

A ninth-grade student seminar was created by Matthew and refined by the advisory committee. Based on information from the needs assessment survey, the new freshman seminar would last eight weeks during the fall semester and include a different topic each week. The topics of discussion included: know your counselor, the "ABC's" of school success, graduation requirements, diplomas, GPA concerns, new algebra requirement, proficiency exams, summer school, and grade status.

After the curriculum was created, the next step was to develop and identify measures of the seminar impact. Perception data collected through a pretest/posttest measure design was chosen. The pretest/posttest data gathered would help determine the outcomes, including information regarding the impact and effectiveness of the seminar. Because Matthew and the advisory committee were interested in perception data related specifically to the developed curriculum, Matthew chose to create a pretest/posttest rather than try to find a preexisting instrument.

## Program Implementation

Before beginning the ninth-grade student seminar, pretest data were collected. Ninth-grade students were asked the following questions on a pretest questionnaire:

1. What is your counselor's name?
2. How many credits do you need to earn a regular diploma?
3. What math class must you pass to earn a regular diploma?
4. What three areas are tested on the state proficiency exams?
5. How many credits must you earn to become a sophomore?

Matthew collected their responses to be later compared with posttest results. The ninth-grade student seminar was implemented during the first quarter of the fall semester. All ninth-grade students at Desert Hills High School participated.

## Program Monitoring and Refinement

Because Matthew was the only professional school counselor implementing the seminar, it was easier to monitor and ensure that all students were offered the developed curriculum in the same way. During the process, Matthew kept a log of his personal observations of what worked well and what he would like to improve upon in the future. Examples from his log included "Students seem to really like today's activity" and "Next time, maybe I should try a computerized presentation to go with the handout." This log of qualitative data would help Matthew remember details about the experience when refining the program for the following year.

## Outcome Assessment

After eight weeks, Matthew had students complete the posttest survey. The posttest asked the same questions as the pretest survey. The hope was that students' perceptions of their knowledge would have increased after the seminar. The pretest/posttest data that Matthew collected could now be assessed. The ninth-grade student seminar pretest/posttest results are as follows:

1. What is your counselor's name?
   Pretest—18 percent correct          Posttest—93 percent correct

2. How many credits do you need to earn a regular diploma?
   Pretest—25 percent correct          Posttest—94 percent correct

3. What math class must you pass to earn a regular diploma?
   Pretest—35 percent correct          Posttest—74 percent correct

4. What three areas are tested on the state proficiency exams?
   Pretest—5 percent identified all three      Posttest—73 percent identified all three

5. How many credits must you earn to become a sophomore?
   Pretest—10 percent correct          Posttest—89 percent correct

By examining the change in the pretest/posttest answers, Matthew and the advisory committee were able to consider the seminar a success at increasing students' knowledge in the five areas assessed. In addition, the three main objectives set forth by the committee had also been accomplished. To offer the ninth-grade student seminar in subsequent years, Matthew and the advisory committee needed support from the school board and parents.

## Communication of Results

Matthew created a letter to be sent home to parents of ninth-grade students. The letter included basic information about the seminar, the topic areas covered, and suggestions of how parents could reinforce the information with their children. Next, Matthew developed a presentation for the December school board meeting. The presentation included results from the needs assessment survey, committee objectives, curriculum areas, and pre/post survey results. During the school board presentation, school board members were given a one-page handout on which they could write down any comments regarding the following:

1. Use of needs assessment
2. Objectives/curriculum
3. Pretest/posttest data
4. Overall impression of seminar importance

This information was then collected and returned to Matthew during the January meeting along with a unanimous vote in support of offering the seminar on a continuous basis.

## Strategic Planning

During the advisory committee's annual spring strategic planning meeting, Matthew shared feedback from his personal log, parents, and the school board. The information was used to enhance the existing curriculum and revise the pretest/posttest instrument for use in the future. One stakeholder suggestion that was implemented involved changing the pretest/posttest instrument so that it contained eight questions that reflected the main seminar curriculum areas. Based on the success of the freshman seminar, the school counseling advisory committee made plans to develop another fall seminar for seniors that would focus on concerns of students nearing graduation.

# Assessing and Developing Your Program Evaluation Skills

Becoming proficient in counseling program evaluation may be conceptualized from a developmental perspective. Much like learning counseling skills, the development of program evaluation competence can be considered a process that involves the practice and application of evaluation principles along with regular feedback and supervision to refine and enhance your skills. To help you identify strengths and weaknesses in your current program evaluation skills, rate your ability in the evaluation activities listed in Table 10.1.

Integrating program evaluation practice and skill development into your counselor training can help prepare you to effectively evaluate your counseling services once you begin professional practice. Trevisan (2002) indicated that, in addition to didactic presentations and relevant readings, counselor program evaluation training should involve hands-on experience in evaluation activities. Initially, simulated evaluation activities in class may help you become familiar with evaluation concepts and methods. Using "real world" situations of counselor settings, small groups can work to develop ideas and procedures for conducting appropriate counseling evaluations. Small evaluation projects can also be incorporated into the counseling curriculum to facilitate the development of skills. During practicum and internship experiences, program evaluation activities can be practiced in field settings.

**TABLE 10.1**   Checklist of program evaluation skills.

Directions: Please circle the number for each item that indicates your current level of skill on each task according to the following key:

1 = My current skill level is *totally lacking/absent.*
2 = My current skill level *needs a LOT of improvement.*
3 = My current skill level *needs SOME improvement.*
4 = My current skill level is *adequate.*
5 = My current skill level is *high.*

| | Current Ability | | | | |
| | None/ Absent | Needs a Lot of Improvement | Needs Some Improvement | Adequate | High |
|---|---|---|---|---|---|
| 1. Conducting needs assessments | 1 | 2 | 3 | 4 | 5 |
| 2. Analyzing needs assessment data | 1 | 2 | 3 | 4 | 5 |
| 3. Developing/modifying programs based on needs assessment results | 1 | 2 | 3 | 4 | 5 |
| 4. Identifying program components to be evaluated | 1 | 2 | 3 | 4 | 5 |
| 5. Identifying appropriate outcome measures for program components | 1 | 2 | 3 | 4 | 5 |
| 6. Collecting data for evaluation purposes | 1 | 2 | 3 | 4 | 5 |
| 7. Analyzing data to evaluate program impact and outcomes | 1 | 2 | 3 | 4 | 5 |
| 8. Utilizing data analysis computer software | 1 | 2 | 3 | 4 | 5 |
| 9. Utilizing outcome data to modify program components | 1 | 2 | 3 | 4 | 5 |
| 10. Communicating the results of evaluations to stakeholders | 1 | 2 | 3 | 4 | 5 |
| 11. Utilizing stakeholder feedback to modify program components | 1 | 2 | 3 | 4 | 5 |
| 12. Developing questionnaires/surveys | 1 | 2 | 3 | 4 | 5 |

© Cengage Learning

Once you have completed your graduate counseling training, continuing education on program evaluation and research skills can help you refine and broaden your evaluation and research skills and help you stay current with evaluation methodology. Attending professional conferences, such as those sponsored by the American Counseling Association, the American School Counselor Association, and the American Mental Health Counselors Association, among others, can provide you with opportunities to expand your knowledge base on evaluation-related topics. Furthermore, taking continuing education coursework offered through universities can help you further develop your research and evaluation skills beyond what you receive in your graduate training. Courses such as descriptive and inferential statistics, quantitative research methods, qualitative research methods, and evaluation methods can help build your foundation and confidence in conducting program evaluations. In addition, becoming proficient with software programs including spreadsheets and presentation creators can help you analyze program data and develop professional presentations and reports. Finally, continuing education programs sponsored by community colleges and universities may offer workshops and training series designed to help you learn the functions and applications of popular software programs.

# Conclusion

Professional counselors in the 21st century face significant demands to demonstrate successful program outcomes and efficient counseling services. Program evaluations can help counselors monitor the effectiveness and impact of their services and help them to provide critical accountability information to stakeholders. Counseling program evaluation may therefore be considered as a type of action research in which counselors use evaluation principles to assess and improve the effectiveness and impact of their programs and services. The counseling program evaluation model presented in this chapter emphasizes two primary cycles involved in the evaluation of programs and interventions. The *counseling context evaluation cycle* involves gathering information from stakeholders, organizational strategic planning, conducting needs assessments, and identifying program objectives. *The counseling program evaluation cycle* is based on information gathered from the context evaluation and includes program planning, implementation, monitoring, and outcome assessment. Providing accountability information to stakeholders may be viewed as forming a bridge between the two evaluation cycles. Professional presentations and reports on counseling program outcomes and impacts can provide accountability to stakeholders and help counselors market their counseling services. Overall, counseling program evaluation involves a dynamic and ongoing process of program development and refinement based on client needs and stakeholder input.

The increased application of counseling program evaluation by practitioners may be one of the most significant developments currently occurring in the counseling professions. In fact, Astramovich and Coker (2007) suggested that program evaluation is an evolving standard of practice in counseling. Successful counselors in the 21st century will be those who have both clinical expertise and the ability to evaluate and document the outcomes of their counseling programs and services. As the counseling profession grows, and services are expanded to meet the needs of increasingly diverse client populations, program evaluations will ultimately help practitioners and stakeholders identify and develop the most effective counseling services available to clients.

*Now go to the Student Workbook found on cengagebrain.com that accompanies this text for additional application and review activities.*

# SECTION III
# Collecting and Analyzing Data in Counseling Research and Evaluation

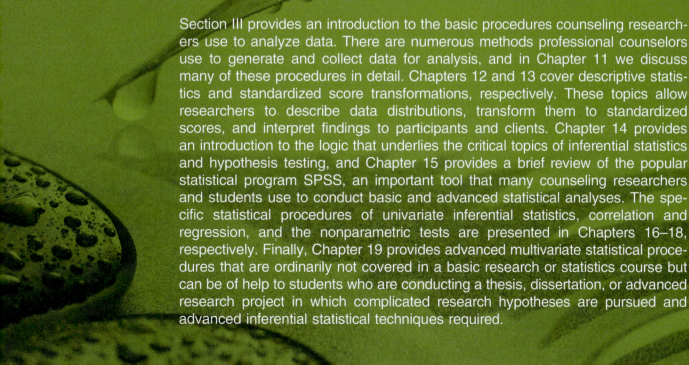

Section III provides an introduction to the basic procedures counseling researchers use to analyze data. There are numerous methods professional counselors use to generate and collect data for analysis, and in Chapter 11 we discuss many of these procedures in detail. Chapters 12 and 13 cover descriptive statistics and standardized score transformations, respectively. These topics allow researchers to describe data distributions, transform them to standardized scores, and interpret findings to participants and clients. Chapter 14 provides an introduction to the logic that underlies the critical topics of inferential statistics and hypothesis testing, and Chapter 15 provides a brief review of the popular statistical program SPSS, an important tool that many counseling researchers and students use to conduct basic and advanced statistical analyses. The specific statistical procedures of univariate inferential statistics, correlation and regression, and the nonparametric tests are presented in Chapters 16–18, respectively. Finally, Chapter 19 provides advanced multivariate statistical procedures that are ordinarily not covered in a basic research or statistics course but can be of help to students who are conducting a thesis, dissertation, or advanced research project in which complicated research hypotheses are pursued and advanced inferential statistical techniques required.

# Collecting Data

## CHAPTER 11

T his chapter familiarizes the professional counselor with methods commonly used to collect data. Professional counselors frequently collect data using measurement instruments composed of nominal-, ordinal-, interval-, or ratio-scale items. Design of items for data collection usually takes one of the following types: open ended, forced choice, ranking, checklist, binary option, Likert scale, Guttman scale, or semantic differential scale. Methods for collecting data usually involve interviews, observations, written questionnaires, surveys, rating scales, program records, standardized or counselor-made tests, performance indicators, and products or portfolios.

# What Is Measurement?

**Measurement** involves assigning numbers to characteristics of an individual so that the numbers accurately describe the presence, amount, or degree of the characteristic the individual possesses. As one can imagine, this can become an incredibly complex endeavor when dealing with the more abstract constructs that comprise human nature. In counseling or any field within the social sciences, individual differences are of great interest. Clients have many characteristics or attributes that help professional counselors understand the nature of presenting problems, strengths or resiliency factors, and the likelihood of success of different therapeutic approaches. Measurements of these characteristics give professional counselors a time- and cost-efficient method of discovering the best way to help clients and students.

Unfortunately, the measurement of psychological characteristics, such as intelligence, personality, or interests, is a bit more difficult, and therefore less precise, than the measurement of physical characteristics such as height and weight. The physical realm has conventions of measurement that are widely used, accepted, and very accurate. For example, when measuring one's height during a physical examination, nurses generally use standardized instrumentation and procedures, and the scale of measurement is always in feet/inches (or meters/centimeters). Note that the method, instrument, and scale are agreed on and commonly used. Measurement of psychological characteristics is somewhat more challenging because the instrumentation (e.g., observation, test, rating scale, and interview), although frequently standardized, must be accomplished using a scaling procedure that is not always as precise as one might hope and is often quite subjective. Wouldn't it be nice to measure depression or substance abuse with the accuracy of a tape measure?

## Scales of Measurement

Important to one's understanding of measurement are the concepts of discrete and continuous scales. **Discrete scales** leave little to no room for disagreement. Male and female are arguably the only two categories possible on the variable sex, making it a discrete variable. It would not be meaningful to refer to someone as both male and female or something else (Note: granted, there are some exceptions, such as individuals with sex-related genetic anomalies). Politicians on a candidate slate (i.e., Washington, Adams, or Jefferson), parental education (i.e., less than a high school graduate, high school graduate, some college, or college graduate), and residential area (i.e., population <2,500 or population ≥2,500) are other examples of discrete variables. By definition, individuals must belong to only one category at any given time.

**Continuous scales** are used to measure variables that, theoretically, can be divided to provide a more precise measurement of some psychological characteristic. Some examples of continuous scales include Likert-type scales (e.g., multiple response format used to assess perception, usually with no middle point, such as very dissatisfied, dissatisfied, satisfied, or very satisfied), frequency estimates (e.g., almost never, sometimes, frequently, or almost always), and even a thermometer or ruler. Thus, any characteristic measured using a continuous scale is referred to as a continuous variable (e.g., hyperactivity, intelligence, math achievement, or anxiety).

An important caveat regarding continuous scales warrants mention here. Measurements of psychological constructs are best thought of as approximations or estimates rather than precise measurements. Thus, if a client's parent is completing the *Disruptive Behavior Rating Scale* (Erford & Clark, 2011) and is asked to respond to the prompt "Argues," it is quite possible that none of the response choices (0 = Rarely/Hardly Ever, 1 = Occasionally, 2 = Frequently, or 3 = Most of the Time) perfectly reflects the frequency of the observed behavior. The parent is simply asked, "Circle the appropriate number to indicate how often …" Thus, the parent may choose 3 (most of the time) because even though the child doesn't argue "most of the time," he does argue more often than "frequently." The point is, *all continuous variables have some measurement error.* This is why standardization is so essential to measurement procedures. Without standardization, professional counselors would use assessment tools any way they want, and the results would be inconsistent, inaccurate, and downright dangerous!

The presence or absence of certain properties defines the type of measurement scale one is using. These properties include identification, order in terms of magnitude, equivalent intervals, and an absolute zero point. *Identification* means that the number or score identifies or names the individual or group of scores. *Order of magnitude* refers to how much of a characteristic a client may have and the ability of the professional counselor to rank these magnitudes in some ascending or descending manner. Some clients or students can be more depressed, intelligent, or angry than others, but one cannot have more gender, race, or religious affiliation (e.g., Islam, Hindu, Jewish, or Catholic) than another. Thus, magnitude applies to some scaling methods but not others. The concept of *equal intervals* means that the mathematical distance between the numbers must be accurately reflected in the distances between scale descriptors. On an intelligence, aptitude, or achievement test, this is sometimes accomplished by scaling each answer as correct (1 point) or incorrect (0 points). Simply stated, a 0 is the absence of correctness, and a 1 is the presence of correctness. When 20 equally weighted items comprise the test, one may conclude that someone with a higher score had more correct answers, thus indicating greater mastery of what was being tested. It becomes a bit more complicated when scales use the descriptors 0 = Almost Never, 1 = Sometimes, 2 = Frequently, 3 = Almost Always. In this case, the burden is on the test developer (and test interpreter) to demonstrate that the distance between responses 0 (Almost Never) and 1 (Sometimes) is the same as between responses 1 (Sometimes) and 2 (Frequently). An *absolute zero point* is the designated score on some scales indicating the total absence of some characteristic. For example, for the question "How many alcoholic drinks did you have last week?", the client's response scale would have an absolute zero point to indicate the total absence of alcoholic drinks. For most psychological constructs, it is difficult to create a scale with an absolute zero point. What would someone who has absolutely no intelligence, shyness, or anxiety be like? Table 11.1 shows how these four measurement properties combine to form the four types of measurement scales: nominal, ordinal, interval, and ratio. Note how the more sophisticated scaling methods include all the characteristics of the less-sophisticated methods.

## Types of Scales

A helpful, specific way to describe variables used in the social sciences uses the acronym NOIR to identify four types of scaling methods: *N*ominal, *O*rdinal, *I*nterval, and *R*atio. Later in this book, we will learn that different statistical procedures apply to different types of variable scaling methods.

**TABLE 11.1** Classifying scales of measurement by properties.

| Scale Property | Type of Scale | | | |
| --- | --- | --- | --- | --- |
| | Nominal | Ordinal | Interval | Ratio |
| Identify | Yes | Yes | Yes | Yes |
| Order According to Magnitude | No | Yes | Yes | Yes |
| Equivalent Intervals | No | No | Yes | Yes |
| An Absolute Zero Point | No | No | No | Yes |

© Cengage Learning

## Nominal Scales

**Nominal scales** are the simplest type of scale to understand and use, although their usefulness is quite limited. Nominal scales simply classify or categorize a client characteristic into nonordered, exhaustive, and mutually exclusive categories; that is, the categories cover all possible choices, cannot be ordered in a meaningful way, and do not overlap in any way. Notice that nominal scales have only the property of identification listed in Table 11.1. They merely provide labels to describe a participant characteristic. Sex is one of the most commonly used examples of a nominal scale because female (coded 1 or F) is a completely separate category from male (coded 2 or M). Notice that the 1 and 2 are arbitrarily defined because being designated a male or female has nothing to do with "better than" or "higher than" in a quantitative sense, just "different than." Males coded as a "2" and females coded as a "1" does *not* mean that males have twice as much of the characteristic under study than females. The numbers or other coded letters are simply substituted for categories or names. *Male* and *female* are simply descriptors used to "name" the categories under study—hence the term *nominal scale*. Individual assessment items often employ a nominal scaling method (e.g., Are you under the care of a psychiatrist?: yes or no; Have you ever used an illegal substance?: yes or no), and the numbers on race cars or athletes' uniforms are nominal; they simply name (identify) the race car or athlete but provide no other information. Player number "22" is not twice as valuable as player number "11." Here are some other examples of nominal scales:

**Sex**

___ 1. Male

___ 2. Female

**Marital Status**

___ 1. Single (never married)

___ 2. Married

___ 3. Divorced

___ 4. Separated

___ 5. Widowed/Widower

**U.S. Geographic Area of Residence**

___ 1. Northeast

___ 2. South

___ 3. North central

___ 4. West

Because nominal scales have no magnitudes, equivalent intervals, or absolute zero point, few mathematical operations can be performed on the results. Reporting a mean (i.e., average score) or median (i.e., middle score) is not possible; only the mode (i.e., most frequently occurring score) has some relevance. Investigators usually simply report the frequency with which these response categories occur for a variable (frequency count) or use these frequencies to determine a proportion of frequency. Such examinee characteristics provide essential information to test developers and test users because standardization samples almost always reflect demographic characteristics (i.e., sex, area of residence, marital status, race/ethnicity, and geographic area of the country).

Interestingly, the DSM-5 (APA, 2013) diagnostic nosological system uses a nominal scaling system. The coded numbers are simply used to name or designate a diagnostic category (i.e., 303.00 means Alcohol Intoxication and 312.82 means Conduct Disorder, Adolescent-Onset Type). As just mentioned, you cannot add, subtract, multiply, or divide nominal codes; thus, one *cannot* average the two example codes just given to arrive at a diagnosis of "307.91—Inebriated Delinquent!"

### Ordinal Scales

Similar to nominal scales, **ordinal scales** display named categories, but these categorical choices also fall in an ordered sequence. Thus, it is possible to conclude that clients in one category have more or less of some characteristic than clients in another category. In other words, ordinal scales allow individuals to be ranked according to magnitude or some degree of quality or frequency. High school class rank is an example of an ordinal scale. The differences between the ranks of students 1 (highest) and 2 (2nd highest) are not necessarily equivalent to the difference between the ranks of students 2 and 3 (3rd highest); that is, the categories are not equal interval. In such a case, these top three ranked students may have grade point averages of 4.00, 3.95, and 3.94, respectively. Likewise, when running a race, the winner may beat the second-place finisher by one-tenth of a second while the rest of the runners are seconds behind, but the race results are still reported as 1st, 2nd, 3rd, 4th, and so on. One can easily see from these examples that the ranks do not accurately reflect the actual differences in scores, just that there is a difference, and the order of the individuals that obtain those different scores. Developers of behavioral, clinical, and personality rating scales frequently employ ordinal scales. Here are some examples

From the Achenbach System of Empirically Based Assessment (ASEBA) (Achenbach & Rescorla, 2001)

0 = Not True (as far as you know)

1 = Somewhat or Sometimes True

2 = Very True or Often True

From the Conners 3 (CRS-R; Conners, 2007)

0 = Not True At All (Never, Seldom)

1 = Just a Little True (Occasionally)

2 = Pretty Much True (Often, Quite a Bit)

3 = Very Much True (Very Often, Very Frequent)

From the Reynold's Adolescent Depression Scale, 2nd edition (RADS-2; Reynolds, 2002)

1 = Almost Never

2 = Hardly Ever

3 = Sometimes

4 = Most of the Time

A typical Likert-type scale

0 = Strongly Disagree

1 = Disagree

2 = Agree

3 = Strongly Agree

Notice that in each example an order of increasing magnitude or frequency is evident, but there is no evidence to conclude that someone getting a 2 has twice as much of the characteristic as someone getting a 1, and so forth. The numbers assigned do not accurately reflect the magnitude of the client's characteristic (i.e., it is not equal interval). This lack of precision gives the test developer some flexibility when choosing descriptors. As a result of these inaccuracies, however, mathematical operations that use ordinal scales are very limited, theoretically speaking. However, this does not stop most researchers or test developers, who treat ordinal scales as though the scales have the scaling property of equal intervals. One can certainly (albeit inappropriately) add, subtract, multiply, and divide ordinal data, and even compute means and standard deviations, but inaccuracies occur because of the nonequivalence (lack of equal intervals) issue. Thus, caution should always be exercised when interpreting instruments that involve norms based on ordinal scales. Determining medians, ranges, interquartile, or semi-interquartile ranges are very appropriate descriptive techniques for ordinal data. Interestingly, as raw scores from multiple ordinal items (10, 15, and 20 items) are summed, the resulting distribution usually behaves more like an interval scale, and researchers and test developers rely on this phenomenon.

Also, *please* observe how each of the preceding example scales has a descriptor attached to each rating point. Such a practice enhances precision and accuracy. Unfortunately, many scales used in research continue to violate this commonsense rule. When stating, "I feel that no one cares about me," it is far more accurate and interpretable to receive a response of "3" to the choices on the RADS-2 descriptors than on the scale 1 = Almost Never to 4 = Most of the Time. In the latter case, the clinician is left wondering what a response of 2 or 3 really means. The precision of the RADS-2 response choices allows the clinician to understand that a 2 means something close to "I hardly ever feel that no one cares about me" and a 3 means something close to "I sometimes feel that no one cares about me." When making decisions about people's lives, a little bit more accuracy can make a huge difference!

### Interval Scales

**Interval scales** have ordered response categories, and the magnitude between each category choice is of an equal interval. Thus, the difference between response choices 1, 2, 3, 4, and 5 accurately reflect the same distance between the magnitudes of the categories assigned to them. Interval scales, however, do not have an absolute zero point, so no absolute comparisons can be made; that is, one still cannot say that someone with a score of 4 has four times as much extraversion, anxiety, or math achievement as someone with a score of 1.

Examples of instruments using interval scales include thermometers and many standardized intelligence and achievement tests. The Celsius and Fahrenheit scales are both interval in nature. The Celsius thermometer requires the same amount of heat to raise the temperature one degree, whether it is from 0°C to 1°C or from 21°C to 22°C. Likewise, on an intelligence test (i.e., Wechsler Adult Intelligence Scale—4th edition, Wechsler, 2008; Stanford-Binet Intelligence Scale—5th Edition, Roid, 2003; Slosson Intelligence Scale—Primary, Erford, Vitali, & Slosson, 1999) or an achievement test (Woodcock-Johnson: Tests of Achievement—3rd edition, Woodcock, Mather, & McGrew, 2001; Wide-Range Achievement Test—4th edition, Wilkinson & Robertson, 2006), the standard scores are based on a normal curve and frequently viewed as being an interval scale. Notice that the absence of an absolute zero point disallows absolute comparisons, so an individual with an IQ score of 150 cannot accurately be said to be twice as intelligent as an individual with an IQ score of 75.

### Ratio Scale

The **ratio scale** is ordered, equal interval, and has an absolute zero point; thus, any mathematical operation can be applied to ratio data. Notice from the examples just given that just because a scale has a zero point does not make that point an "absolute zero point." Absolute zero means the total absence of quantity of the characteristic being measured, such as being totally out of water or gas. Being out of energy, inspiration, or motivation are misnomers and better described through ordinal or interval scaling methods because even though one may feel that way, these characteristics are never truly absent (assuming one is still alive, of course).

Professional counselors rarely encounter standardized instruments created using ratio scales in clinical practice because so few human characteristics can be totally depleted or absent. Examples of ratio scales include the Kelvin scale of temperature and just about any physical measure (e.g., length or weight) or frequency tally (e.g., number of times a behavior was observed). The Kelvin thermometer starts at absolute zero (0°K is the theoretical estimate for the temperature at which all cellular activity ceases and is equivalent to –273.16°C). In the physical measurement realm, a client who is six feet tall is twice as tall as a client who is three feet tall. During a frequency tally, a kindergarten student who left her seat or work area 12 times without permission during the observation period did so far more frequently than her tablemates, none of whom got up a single time. A couple who argued only four times this week appears to have improved markedly over the 16 arguments the week before. Generally, if one is interested in the relative size, density, weight, frequency, or speed of an individual or object, one is most likely to use a ratio scale.

# Constructing Questions for Data Collection

A great deal of thought should go into how data will be scored and entered for analysis long before the researcher heads to the field to collect the data. Experienced researchers know to select or design data-collection instruments so that participant responses can be readily coded, entered, and analyzed. For example, many researchers studying hyperactivity will select published rating scales (e.g., Conners 3 [Conners, 2007], Disruptive Behavior Rating Scale—2nd edition—Teacher Version [DBRS-II-T; Erford & Clark, 2011]). A sample of DBRS-II items is provided in Figure 11.1. Notice how the format of the DBRS lends itself to easy quantification of participant responses: 0 = Rarely/Hardly Ever, 1 = Occasionally, 2 = Frequently, and 3 = Most of the Time. This ease of quantification is one of the primary reasons that rating scales are so commonly used in counseling research.

Once the research data have been collected, professional counselors next must code it and enter it into a computerized database, such as SPSS, Excel, or R-stat. Note that most of the data derived from the DBRS in Figure 11.1 is already in a quantifiable format and ready to go into a database. But not all data are derived so easily. Often, demographic variables are collected to aid in the description of the sample and allow for subsequent analyses based on participant characteristics. Coding these and other types of variables takes some extra care and consideration.

Frequently, researchers must describe the characteristics of the sample participants, such as participant's sex (i.e., male or female), age, race (e.g., white, African American, Hispanic American, Asian American, or Native American), education (e.g., less than a high school education, high school graduate, some college study, or college graduate), marital status, and so forth. As explained in the preceding section on scaling and

**Figure 11.1**

The DBRS-II.

**Disruptive Behavior Rating Scale – Teacher Version (DBRS-II-T)**

Student's Name: _____ Age: _____ Teacher's Name: _____

INSTRUCTIONS: Please circle the appropriate number below to indicate how often the student displays each of the following behaviors. Respond to all statements.

KEY:     0 means the student **rarely or hardly ever** displays the behavior.

1 means the student **occasionally** displays the behavior.

2 means the student **frequently** displays the behavior.

3 means the student displays the behavior **most of the time**.

| | | | | |
|---|---|---|---|---|
| 1. Has difficulty concentrating on tasks in a group | 0 | 1 | 2 | 3 |
| 2. Easily embarrassed | 0 | 1 | 2 | 3 |
| 3. Calls out unexpectedly | 0 | 1 | 2 | 3 |
| 4. Skips school (truant) | 0 | 1 | 2 | 3 |
| 5. Stubborn | 0 | 1 | 2 | 3 |
| 6. Fidgety | 0 | 1 | 2 | 3 |
| 7. Perfectionistic | 0 | 1 | 2 | 3 |
| 8. Has difficulty sitting still | 0 | 1 | 2 | 3 |
| 9. Worries | 0 | 1 | 2 | 3 |
| 10. Finds it hard to await turn in group situation | 0 | 1 | 2 | 3 |
| 11. Fearful | 0 | 1 | 2 | 3 |
| 12. Refuses to comply with the commands of authority figures | 0 | 1 | 2 | 3 |
| 13. Restless, squirmy | 0 | 1 | 2 | 3 |
| 14. Finds it hard to play quietly | 0 | 1 | 2 | 3 |
| 15. Easily distracted by sights and sounds | 0 | 1 | 2 | 3 |
| 16. Steals | 0 | 1 | 2 | 3 |
| 17. Has difficulty organizing work | 0 | 1 | 2 | 3 |
| 18. Gets into physical fights with other kids | 0 | 1 | 2 | 3 |
| 19. Throws temper tantrums | 0 | 1 | 2 | 3 |
| 20. Uses obscene language | 0 | 1 | 2 | 3 |
| 21. Unhappy | 0 | 1 | 2 | 3 |
| 22. Has difficulty following simple instructions | 0 | 1 | 2 | 3 |
| 23. Destroys the possessions of others | 0 | 1 | 2 | 3 |
| 24. Misplaces items needed for activities | 0 | 1 | 2 | 3 |
| 25. Talks too much | 0 | 1 | 2 | 3 |
| 26. Does not cooperate with others | 0 | 1 | 2 | 3 |
| 27. Nervous | 0 | 1 | 2 | 3 |
| 28. Resentful | 0 | 1 | 2 | 3 |
| 29. Short attention span | 0 | 1 | 2 | 3 |
| 30. Tells lies | 0 | 1 | 2 | 3 |
| 31. Does not finish activities undertaken | 0 | 1 | 2 | 3 |
| 32. Is physically cruel to people or animals | 0 | 1 | 2 | 3 |
| 33. Argues | 0 | 1 | 2 | 3 |
| 34. Lonely | 0 | 1 | 2 | 3 |
| 35. Looks for revenge when feeling picked on | 0 | 1 | 2 | 3 |

measurement, each of these variables can be readily quantified to facilitate data-coding procedures and then analyzed using descriptive statistical techniques, many of which are described in Chapter 12. Subsequent analyses using these coded demographic variables may include inferential techniques to answer interesting and important research questions. For example, using the DBRS and basic demographic information, many questions can be pursued: Is there a significant difference between males and females on scales of hyperactivity, distractibility, or oppositional behavior? Is there a significant relationship between age and behavior? How many factors underlie the 35 items of the DBRS? Is there a difference in behavior between children whose parents are married or divorced? Is childhood behavior related to marital stress? Does one's behavior as a child predict career decisiveness and salience? Many interesting questions can be answered with data sets.

Of course, not all data are derived from already existing instruments. Frequently counseling researchers must develop questions to address specific areas of inquiry. When designing instruments, researchers typically rely on items of the following types: open ended, forced choice, ranking, checklist, binary, Likert-type, Guttman, or semantic differential.

## Open-Ended Items

Open-ended items provide a question or incomplete sentence stem that cannot be answered yes or no or with a single-word response. Likewise, no specific answers are provided for the participant to choose among. Rather, open-ended items are designed to generate extended responses that are not biased by a researcher's preconceived notions of what participant response should or might be. Participants analyze the question or stem and construct a response that is meaningful. Qualitative research and program evaluation studies frequently use open-ended questions because these questions yield thick, rich descriptions and narratives from the participants' own perspectives. Unfortunately, coding and analyzing responses to open-ended questions is often challenging. Also, open-ended questions are frequently skipped by participants who lack motivation because of the extra effort required. Here are some examples of open-ended questions:

- What additional comments or concerns would you like to express?
- How was the program most helpful to you?
- What were the strengths of the program?
- What suggestions do you offer for improving the program?

## Forced-Choice Items

Forced-choice items are quite popular in testing. Most forced-choice questions are some permutation of a multiple-choice question format. Multiple-choice items provide a question or stem of a question/statement along with several possible answers. Participants are instructed to choose the correct or best answer from among the given response choices. The categories of forced-choice items are often meant to be exhaustive. Forced-choice items are easy to code and analyze. Here are some examples of forced-choice items:

- What is your sex? 1. Male, 2. Female
- What is your marital status? 1. Single, never married, 2. Married, 3. Divorced, 4. Separated, 5. Widowed.
- Who is the father of psychoanalytic theory? 1. Skinner, 2. Bandura, 3. Rogers, 4. Freud.

# Ranking Items

Ranking items require participants to rank order a number of provided choices. Ordinarily, three to four answer choices provide for optimal ranking. Although ranking items are easy for participants to respond to, they are difficult to statistically analyze, often because participants do not always rank all of the given choices, thus creating "missing data." But perhaps the greatest limitation of ranking items is that ranked data require the use of nonparametric or descriptive statistics, not the more powerful parametric statistical techniques (e.g., $t$-test and Pearson $r$). Here are some examples of ranking items:

1. Rank the following types of potato chip flavors according to how much you would like to eat them (1–4, with 1 = Most Preferred and 4 = Least Preferred). Please use each number only once, and use all four numbers.

    _____ Plain    _____ Salt & Vinegar    _____ Barbecue    _____ Cheddar

2. Rank the following genres of novels according to how much you would enjoy reading them (1–4; 1 = Most Preferred, 4 = Least Preferred). Please use each number only once, and use all four numbers.

    _____ Horror    _____ Mystery    _____ Science Fiction    _____ Adventure

# Checklist Items

Checklist items list response choices so that participants can mark the response choice that applies. Sometimes participants are asked to check their favorite or the "best" choice; other times they may be asked to check all that apply. Of course, the more items the participant is allowed to check, the more complicated data analysis and interpretation become. Here are some examples of checklist items:

1. Check (√) your favorite type(s) of potato chips. Check all that apply:

    _____ Plain    _____ Salt & Vinegar    _____ Barbecue    _____ Baked
    _____ Cheddar

2. Check (√) your favorite genre(s) of novel.

    _____ Horror    _____ Mystery    _____ Science Fiction    _____ Adventure

# Binary Option Items

Binary option items provide only two, mutually exclusive answer choices for each question or prompt (e.g., yes/no, agree/disagree, true/false, and satisfied/dissatisfied). This two-choice response format simplifies statistical analysis and interpretation but restricts participant responses to an "all or none" dimension. Attitudes or preferences are rarely so easily categorized, leading to inherent response error owing to the lack of response sensitivity. Here are some examples of binary option items:

1. I work hard in school. Yes _____ No _____

2. I usually do my homework. True _____ False _____

3. I enjoy school. Agree _____ Disagree _____

4. How satisfied are you with the quality of your teacher. Satisfied _____ Dissatisfied _____

## Likert-Type Scale Items

**Likert-type scale items** assess a participant's attitude or preference using a question or stem accompanied by an order of response choices (e.g., Strongly Disagree, Disagree, Agree, or Strongly Agree). The classic Likert scale did not have a neutral middle choice (e.g., Undecided, Neutral, Neither Disagree nor Agree), but researchers frequently add a middle choice (thus the term, Likert-type item). Usually researchers do not provide a numerical rating with the verbal description but add one during coding or data input to allow quantification of response choices (0 = Strongly Disagree, 1 = Disagree, etc.). There is some disagreement over the optimal number of response choices to offer, but four or five answer choices tend to provide optimal score reliability. It is also essential that every point on the response continuum be labeled:

| Strongly Disagree | Disagree | Agree | Strongly Agree |
|:---:|:---:|:---:|:---:|
| _____ | _____ | _____ | _____ |

*not*

| Strongly Disagree | | | Strongly Agree |
|:---:|:---:|:---:|:---:|
| _____ | _____ | _____ | _____ |

Here is an example of a Likert-type scaled item:

Rate each of the following questions along the following continuum of agreement.

| Strongly Disagree | Disagree | Undecided | Agree | Strongly Agree |
|:---:|:---:|:---:|:---:|:---:|
| _____ | _____ | _____ | _____ | _____ |

**1.** Professional counselors provide an effective service to the public.

**2.** Research is my favorite course.

**3.** Likert scales are an efficient way of assessing participant attitudes.

## Guttman-Type Items

**Guttman-type items** (also called cumulative items) provide a series of items on a continuum linked in a manner such that a participant's response to one item in the series indicates approval of all choices below the indicated level. To be analyzed, these data must be coded in a sequence (e.g., 1, 2, 3, or 4, according to the item number selected) rather than each item coded separately. As such, Guttman-type items are somewhat complex to code, analyze, and interpret. Here is an example of a Guttman-type item:

**1.** The amount of alcohol consumed by the average undergraduate exceeds 13 drink-equivalents per week.          _____ Agree _____ Disagree

**2.** The amount of alcohol consumed by the average undergraduate exceeds 9 drink-equivalents per week.          _____ Agree _____ Disagree

**3.** The amount of alcohol consumed by the average undergraduate exceeds 5 drink-equivalents per week.          _____ Agree _____ Disagree

**4.** The amount of alcohol consumed by the average undergraduate exceeds 1 drink-equivalent per week.          _____ Agree _____ Disagree

A commonly used alternative to Guttman-type items is a single item with the continuum choices offered as mutually exclusive multiple-choice responses:

**1.** The amount of alcohol consumed by the average undergraduate _____ drink-equivalents per week.
   a. exceeds 13
   b. is between 9 and 13
   c. is between 5 and 8
   d. is less than 5

## Semantic Differential Scale Items

**Semantic differential scale items** use bipolar adjectives comprising the activity pairs (e.g., active-passive or fast-slow), evaluative pairs (e.g., good-bad or dirty-clean), or potency pairs (e.g., large-small or hot-cold). In quantitative research, evaluative pairs are most common. To avoid a response set bias, it is good practice to periodically alternate the poles of the positively and negatively connoted words. Notice that the examples here use five choices to enhance score reliability, although many researchers design items with between five and nine choices. Also, notice that only the bipolar end points are labeled, inevitably leading to diminished precision over exactly what a rating of 2, 3, or 4 really means. Semantic differential scale items are relatively simple to code, analyze, and interpret. Here is an example of a semantic differential scale item:

**1.** Graduate school is:

| Horrible | 1 | 2 | 3 | 4 | 5 | Awesome |
| Challenging | 1 | 2 | 3 | 4 | 5 | Easy |
| Valuable | 1 | 2 | 3 | 4 | 5 | Worthless |
| Expensive | 1 | 2 | 3 | 4 | 5 | Inexpensive |

# Methods of Collecting Data

There are probably as many ways of measuring phenomena and collecting data as there are research questions—virtually limitless. In counseling research, most data are collected via interviews, observations, questionnaires, surveys and rating scales, program records, standardized or counselor-made tests, performance indicators, and products or portfolios.

## Interviews

Interviews of key personnel can be sources of detailed, meaningful information. These interviews can be structured, semi-structured, or unstructured. Structured interviews present interviewees with a formal sequence of questions, and little variation in administration is allowed. Every interviewee pretty much gets asked the same questions in the same order, thus providing a pattern of data that can be more easily coded, quantified, and analyzed, and, as a result, are used more frequently in quantitative studies. Unstructured formats provide a basic set of questions but allow for deeper exploration of participant responses.

As a result, unstructured interviews are commonly used in qualitative studies. Semi-structured interviews provide a mid-ground, presenting a set of structured questions but allowing participants to expand upon and explore more diverse possible responses. When using an interview as a data-collection technique, multiple respondents are ordinarily required for conclusions or patterns to emerge. While phone interviews are certainly less costly and more convenient for both the researcher and participants, it is easier to motivate participants in face-to-face interviews, and face-to-face meetings generally yield more detailed data. Researchers must take precautions to minimize bias during an interview and give special attention to the development of interview questions. It is good practice to field test interview questions before beginning data collection to be sure participants will readily grasp the meaning of the questions and provide meaningful responses.

## Observations

Observations can be informal or formal (e.g., structured). Informal observations ordinarily yield anecdotal data as researchers scan the environment and make notes on what is observed. As a result, different observers may come away with different reports or perspectives of the same observation target. Formal or structured observations collect specific types of data, for specified periods, using predetermined procedures. Such a structured approach tends to minimize bias and results in different observers recording similar data. The process of observations is very familiar to professional counselors as all counselors-in-training will be observed, either live or via video. In research, observation tends to be time intensive and expensive but yields rich perspectives of participants in naturalistic settings. Observation is commonly used in qualitative studies.

## Questionnaires, Surveys, and Rating Scales

Written **questionnaires**, *surveys*, and **rating scales** are usually paper-and-pencil instruments, although the Internet is allowing for more convenient electronic administration. These methods typically involve the researcher asking many open- and/or closed-ended questions. Technically, surveys ask participants for their perceptions about the topics under study, whereas questionnaires and rating scales typically ask for more factual responses. Nonresponse bias is frequently problematic with this data collection method. **Nonresponse bias** occurs when participants do not complete or return the instrument. A second concern is that a certain level of literacy is required to understand and complete the instruments. It is good practice to keep the questions simple and closed-ended, giving the opportunity for participants to expand upon a response if needed.

## Program Records

**Program records** can be helpful sources of evaluation data and are usually easy to locate because they are generated by organizational bureaucracies. Indeed, it is excellent practice to construct organizational databases to maintain, store, and retrieve valuable programmatic data. This makes everyone's work easier when it comes to evaluation! Likewise, paper archives should consistently be organized to facilitate record retrieval. Perhaps the most important information professional counselors should keep includes previous and newly generated outcome study reports and previous program improvement documents. These data sources help programs chart trajectories of program initiatives and document what has been done to address past suggestions for improvement.

## Standardized or Counselor-Made Tests

Standardized and counselor-made tests provide objective sources of measurable participant performance. Standardized tests measure achievement, intelligence, anxiety, substance use, hyperactivity, career interests, and many other behaviors. Publishers of psychological tests are a good source of commercially available products, and *Mental Measurements Yearbook* provides independent, critical reviews of many of these products. On the other hand, professional counselors can design and develop tests to measure behaviors and characteristics they would like to study. These tests can be constructed using methods similar to how teachers design tests to measure academic achievement.

## Performance Indicators

Performance indicators include any data that can be generated to represent how a participant performs on a given task or perceives how he or she performed a given task. For example, a student's grade point average (GPA) or classroom grade is a performance indicator. Daily work behaviors (e.g., attendance, times out of seat without permission, or number of times washing one's hands) and attitudes (e.g., social self-efficacy and attitude toward school) are also performance indicators.

## Products and Portfolios

Products and portfolios involve real-life examples of performance that an evaluator can study and evaluate. A product is anything created by a participant representing a program goal (e.g., artwork, composition, or poster). A portfolio is a collection of products that can be evaluated to determine the quality of an individual's performance.

# Proceeding to Data Analysis: A Case Example

Once the data have been coded, the researcher is ready to enter the data into a computerized database and then "clean" the data. Data entry and checking procedures using the SPSS Data Editor functions are reviewed in Chapter 15. Using a computerized program such as SPSS, Excel, or R-stat makes raw data entry, error checking, and analysis incredibly simple.

Figure 11.2 provides a survey protocol that demonstrates the types of items and data sources covered in this chapter. Figure 11.3 provides a sample data set for 20 participants aligned with the survey protocol. The reader is encouraged to study and critique the wording and scaling methodology of each item and then enter the data into an SPSS Data Editor File (note that lettered response choices are transformed alphanumerically, so A = 1, B = 2, C = 3, D = 4, etc.), develop some interesting research questions, and run some preliminary descriptive or correlation analyses. Here are some examples:

1. What is the mean and standard deviation of the depression and anxiety scale responses for the sample (Q14 & Q15, respectively)?

2. What were the frequencies of responses for each answer choice for Q1 and Q2?

3. What is the correlation between GPA (Q3) and depression (Q14)? GPA (Q3) and anxiety (Q15)?

**Figure 11.2**

A sample survey.

1. What is your sex? (circle one)
   a. Male
   b. Female

2. What is your primary race? (circle one)
   a. White
   b. African American
   c. Hispanic American
   d. Asian American
   e. Native American
   f. Other

3. What is your current graduate grade point average? _____

4. What is your current marital status? (circle only one)
   a. Single, never married
   b. Married
   c. Divorced
   d. Separated
   e. Widowed

5. What is your current age (in years)? _____

6. What is your favorite type of TV show? (circle only one)
   a. Sitcoms
   b. Sports
   c. News
   d. Movies

7. What is/are your favorite snack(s)? (circle all that apply)
   a. Chips
   b. Popcorn
   c. Pretzels
   d. Fruit
   e. Nuts

8. Rank order the following list of snacks according to your preferences (rank 1–5, and be sure to rank each item; 1 = favorite, 5 = least favorite).
   _____ Chips _____ Popcorn _____ Pretzels _____ Fruit _____ Nuts

9. On average, I usually study and read schoolwork more than _____ hours per week. (circle the single best)
   a. Not at all
   b. 1
   c. 5
   d. 10
   e. 15
   f. 20

*(Continued)*

**Figure 11.2**
(*continued*)

For items 10–13, circle the answer choice that most closely indicates your level of agreement with the statement.

10. Graduate school is too hard.
    a. Strongly disagree
    b. Disagree
    c. Agree
    d. Strongly agree

11. I am satisfied with my current GPA.
    a. Strongly disagree
    b. Disagree
    c. Agree
    d. Strongly agree

12. I am happy with my life.
    a. Strongly disagree
    b. Disagree
    c. Agree
    d. Strongly agree

13. I am under a lot of stress.
    a. Strongly disagree
    b. Disagree
    c. Agree
    d. Strongly agree

14. What was your score on the standardized depression scale?

15. What was your score on the standardized anxiety scale?

16. I enjoy graduate school.
    a. Yes
    b. No

17. I work hard in graduate school.
    a. Yes
    b. No

For items 18–21, circle the answer choice (1–5) that most closely indicates your attitude toward the following question. Graduate school is:

| 18. Relaxing | 1 | 2 | 3 | 4 | 5 | Stressful |
| 19. Depressing | 1 | 2 | 3 | 4 | 5 | Uplifting |
| 20. Challenging | 1 | 2 | 3 | 4 | 5 | Easy |
| 21. Worthless | 1 | 2 | 3 | 4 | 5 | Valuable |

22. What suggestions do you have for improving this survey?

**Figure 11.3**

Sample survey database.

| | Q1 | Q2 | Q3 | Q4 | Q5 | Q6 | Q7A | Q7B | Q7C | Q7D | Q7E |
|---|---|---|---|---|---|---|---|---|---|---|---|
| 1 | 1.00 | 1.00 | 3.64 | 1.00 | 23.00 | 2.00 | 1.00 | 1.00 | 1.00 | .00 | 1.00 |
| 2 | 1.00 | 1.00 | 3.48 | 4.00 | 29.00 | 2.00 | 1.00 | 1.00 | 1.00 | 1.00 | 1.00 |
| 3 | 2.00 | 2.00 | 4.00 | 2.00 | 25.00 | 3.00 | .00 | 1.00 | 1.00 | 1.00 | .00 |
| 4 | 2.00 | 1.00 | 3.91 | 2.00 | 27.00 | 4.00 | 1.00 | 1.00 | 1.00 | 1.00 | .00 |
| 5 | 2.00 | 1.00 | 3.71 | 2.00 | 23.00 | 1.00 | 1.00 | 1.00 | 1.00 | 1.00 | 1.00 |
| 6 | 1.00 | 1.00 | 3.85 | 2.00 | 29.00 | 4.00 | 1.00 | .00 | .00 | .00 | .00 |
| 7 | 2.00 | 1.00 | 3.76 | 1.00 | 21.00 | 2.00 | .00 | 1.00 | 1.00 | 1.00 | 1.00 |
| 8 | 2.00 | 4.00 | 3.80 | 1.00 | 22.00 | 1.00 | .00 | 1.00 | .00 | 1.00 | .00 |
| 9 | 2.00 | 3.00 | 3.87 | 2.00 | 35.00 | 3.00 | .00 | 1.00 | .00 | 1.00 | .00 |
| 10 | 1.00 | 1.00 | 3.85 | 1.00 | 21.00 | 2.00 | 1.00 | .00 | .00 | 1.00 | .00 |
| 11 | 2.00 | 1.00 | 3.61 | 2.00 | 28.00 | 4.00 | .00 | 1.00 | 1.00 | 1.00 | .00 |
| 12 | 2.00 | 1.00 | 3.72 | 2.00 | 24.00 | 1.00 | 1.00 | 1.00 | 1.00 | 1.00 | 1.00 |
| 13 | 1.00 | 1.00 | 3.82 | 1.00 | 28.00 | 2.00 | 1.00 | 1.00 | .00 | .00 | .00 |
| 14 | 2.00 | 1.00 | 3.61 | 5.00 | 38.00 | 3.00 | .00 | 1.00 | 1.00 | .00 | .00 |
| 15 | 2.00 | 1.00 | 3.25 | 2.00 | 25.00 | 1.00 | .00 | .00 | 1.00 | 1.00 | .00 |
| 16 | 2.00 | 1.00 | 3.42 | 2.00 | 26.00 | 4.00 | .00 | 1.00 | 1.00 | .00 | .00 |
| 17 | 1.00 | 1.00 | 3.10 | 3.00 | 32.00 | 2.00 | 1.00 | 1.00 | 1.00 | .00 | 1.00 |
| 18 | 1.00 | 1.00 | 3.81 | 1.00 | 22.00 | 1.00 | 1.00 | 1.00 | .00 | .00 | .00 |
| 19 | 2.00 | 2.00 | 3.96 | 1.00 | 23.00 | 1.00 | .00 | .00 | 1.00 | 1.00 | .00 |
| 20 | 2.00 | 2.00 | 3.97 | 1.00 | 24.00 | 1.00 | 1.00 | 1.00 | .00 | 1.00 | .00 |

| | Q8A | Q8B | Q8C | Q8D | Q8E | Q9 | Q10 | Q11 | Q12 | Q13 | Q14 |
|---|---|---|---|---|---|---|---|---|---|---|---|
| 1 | 1.00 | 2.00 | 4.00 | 5.00 | 3.00 | 4.00 | 3.00 | 1.00 | 3.00 | 3.00 | 10.00 |
| 2 | 1.00 | 3.00 | 4.00 | 5.00 | 2.00 | 2.00 | 3.00 | 1.00 | 3.00 | 2.00 | 13.00 |
| 3 | 5.00 | 3.00 | 1.00 | 2.00 | 4.00 | 5.00 | 1.00 | 4.00 | 4.00 | 1.00 | 6.00 |
| 4 | 1.00 | 4.00 | 2.00 | 3.00 | 5.00 | 4.00 | 2.00 | 4.00 | 2.00 | 1.00 | 16.00 |
| 5 | 1.00 | 5.00 | 4.00 | 2.00 | 3.00 | 5.00 | 2.00 | 3.00 | 4.00 | 4.00 | 3.00 |
| 6 | 1.00 | 4.00 | 3.00 | 5.00 | 2.00 | 4.00 | 4.00 | 3.00 | 4.00 | 4.00 | 8.00 |
| 7 | 5.00 | 2.00 | 3.00 | 1.00 | 4.00 | 4.00 | 3.00 | 3.00 | 2.00 | 2.00 | 14.00 |
| 8 | 5.00 | 2.00 | 4.00 | 1.00 | 3.00 | 3.00 | 4.00 | 3.00 | 4.00 | 3.00 | 8.00 |
| 9 | 4.00 | 2.00 | 3.00 | 1.00 | 5.00 | 5.00 | 4.00 | 3.00 | 2.00 | 2.00 | 18.00 |
| 10 | 1.00 | 5.00 | 4.00 | 2.00 | 3.00 | 5.00 | 4.00 | 3.00 | 1.00 | 2.00 | 15.00 |
| 11 | 5.00 | 2.00 | 3.00 | 1.00 | 4.00 | 5.00 | 3.00 | 2.00 | 4.00 | 4.00 | 7.00 |
| 12 | 3.00 | 4.00 | 1.00 | 2.00 | 5.00 | 4.00 | 4.00 | 3.00 | 2.00 | 2.00 | 14.00 |
| 13 | 1.00 | 2.00 | 3.00 | 5.00 | 4.00 | 4.00 | 4.00 | 4.00 | 3.00 | 3.00 | 12.00 |
| 14 | 3.00 | 1.00 | 2.00 | 5.00 | 4.00 | 5.00 | 2.00 | 3.00 | 2.00 | 3.00 | 10.00 |
| 15 | 4.00 | 5.00 | 1.00 | 2.00 | 3.00 | 5.00 | 3.00 | 1.00 | 4.00 | 3.00 | 12.00 |
| 16 | 4.00 | 1.00 | 2.00 | 3.00 | 5.00 | 4.00 | 2.00 | 2.00 | 1.00 | 1.00 | 20.00 |
| 17 | 3.00 | 2.00 | 4.00 | 5.00 | 1.00 | 1.00 | 3.00 | 1.00 | 2.00 | 2.00 | 18.00 |
| 18 | 1.00 | 2.00 | 4.00 | 5.00 | 3.00 | 5.00 | 4.00 | 4.00 | 2.00 | 2.00 | 13.00 |
| 19 | 4.00 | 3.00 | 1.00 | 2.00 | 5.00 | 5.00 | 1.00 | 4.00 | 4.00 | 4.00 | 9.00 |
| 20 | 1.00 | 2.00 | 4.00 | 3.00 | 5.00 | 6.00 | 1.00 | 4.00 | 1.00 | 1.00 | 14.00 |

| | Q15 | Q16 | Q17 | Q18 | Q19 | Q20 | Q21 |
|---|---|---|---|---|---|---|---|
| 1 | 7.00 | 1.00 | 1.00 | 3.00 | 5.00 | 2.00 | 4.00 |
| 2 | 6.00 | 1.00 | 2.00 | 2.00 | 4.00 | 3.00 | 3.00 |
| 3 | 16.00 | 1.00 | 1.00 | 3.00 | 5.00 | 2.00 | 5.00 |
| 4 | 20.00 | 1.00 | 1.00 | 4.00 | 5.00 | 1.00 | 5.00 |
| 5 | 2.00 | 1.00 | 1.00 | 4.00 | 4.00 | 1.00 | 4.00 |
| 6 | .00 | 1.00 | 1.00 | 5.00 | 3.00 | 2.00 | 5.00 |
| 7 | 10.00 | 1.00 | 2.00 | 3.00 | 4.00 | 1.00 | 4.00 |
| 8 | 6.00 | 1.00 | 1.00 | 4.00 | 4.00 | 2.00 | 5.00 |
| 9 | 12.00 | 1.00 | 1.00 | 5.00 | 5.00 | 3.00 | 5.00 |
| 10 | 14.00 | 1.00 | 1.00 | 5.00 | 5.00 | 3.00 | 5.00 |
| 11 | .00 | 1.00 | 1.00 | 4.00 | 3.00 | 3.00 | 4.00 |
| 12 | 8.00 | 1.00 | 1.00 | 3.00 | 5.00 | 2.00 | 5.00 |
| 13 | 8.00 | 1.00 | 1.00 | 3.00 | 5.00 | 1.00 | 5.00 |
| 14 | 16.00 | 1.00 | 2.00 | 2.00 | 3.00 | 2.00 | 5.00 |
| 15 | 7.00 | 2.00 | 2.00 | 3.00 | 4.00 | 3.00 | 3.00 |
| 16 | 16.00 | 1.00 | 2.00 | 4.00 | 5.00 | 3.00 | 4.00 |
| 17 | 4.00 | 2.00 | 2.00 | 2.00 | 2.00 | 3.00 | 4.00 |
| 18 | 8.00 | 1.00 | 1.00 | 5.00 | 5.00 | 1.00 | 5.00 |
| 19 | 2.00 | 1.00 | 1.00 | 5.00 | 5.00 | 1.00 | 4.00 |
| 20 | 18.00 | 1.00 | 1.00 | 5.00 | 4.00 | 1.00 | 5.00 |

As you read this book, please feel free to enter the provided databases into an SPSS Data Editor file and perform the analyses via computer, receiving aid from instructors and peers as needed. Remember, perfect practice makes perfect!

# Conclusion

Collecting meaningful data is essential to conducting meaningful research. Measurement of the dependent variable becomes critical to this end and involves assigning numeric values to determine the presence, amount, or degree of some participant characteristic. Scales of measurement can be described as discrete or continuous, or, more commonly, as nominal ordinal, interval, or ratio. Nominal scales use numbers to identify categorical data (e.g., male or female). Ordinal scales both identify categories and order them in some meaningful context (e.g., first place, second place, etc.). Interval scales order response choices, while also ensuring that intervals between response choices are equivalent (e.g., the Celsius temperature scale). Ratio scales ensure equivalence between intervals but also provide an absolute zero point (e.g., height, beginning at 0 inches).

Researchers frequently need to construct items or questions for data collection. Open-ended items provide a question or stem that cannot be answered with a yes or no response. Forced-choice items provide a question or stem along with several possible answer choices. Ranking items require participants to rank order a number of provided choices. Checklist items list response choices so that participants can mark all response choices that apply. Binary option items provide only two, mutually exclusive answer choices for each question or prompt. Likert-type items assess a participant's attitude or preference using a question or stem accompanied by an order of response choices. Guttman-type items provide a series of items on a continuum linked in such a manner that a participant's response to one item in the series indicates approval of all choices below the indicated level. Semantic differential items use bipolar adjectives composed of activity pairs, evaluative pairs, or potency pairs.

Collection of data is ordinarily accomplished through a variety of potential methods. Interviews present questions to participants whose responses are recorded and categorized for analysis. Observations yield behavioral data from informal or formal situations, with formal procedures providing more reliable information. Questionnaires, surveys, and rating scales differ slightly from each other but share in common a standardized set of open- or closed-ended questions administered ordinarily via paper and pencil. Program records are existing sources of archived data that can be analyzed and summarized. Standardized tests measure a wide variety of participant characteristics, including achievement, intelligence, personality, attitudes, behaviors, and aptitudes, and commercially available tests usually come with previously reported evidence of score reliability and validity. Performance indicators are data generated to represent how participants performed on a given task (e.g., GPA, attendance, or attitude toward school). Products and portfolios provide real-life examples of performance. Ordinarily, a product is a single piece of evidence, and a portfolio is a collection of products. Once quantitative data have been collected, it is ordinarily submitted for statistical analysis and used to answer the questions that originally led to its collection. This process composes the remaining chapters of this book.

*Now go to the Student Workbook found on cengagebrain.com that accompanies this text for additional application and review activities.*

# Describing Data

## CHAPTER 12

This chapter familiarizes the professional counselor with the basic statistical concepts and computations commonly used to describe data. Distributions of scores are commonly displayed in frequency distributions, or graphed using a histogram, frequency polygon, box-and-whisker plot, or stem-and-leaf plot. More commonly, distributions of scores are analyzed statistically. Measures of central tendency (i.e., mean, median, and mode) mathematically describe the middle of a distribution of scores, whereas measures of variability (i.e., standard deviation, range, and semi-interquartile range) mathematically describe the distribution away from the middle. Related to variability, kurtosis (i.e., mesokurtic, leptokurtic, and platykurtic) indicates the general shape of a (more or less) normally distributed curve, whereas skewness (skewed left and skewed right) describes distributions in which an abundance of scores are located at either end of the distribution.

# Why Statistics Are Essential in Counseling

A basic understanding of statistical concepts is essential in any field of human study, especially when professional counselors are trying to measure human characteristics as complex and diverse as depression, intelligence, and family cohesion. When a professional counselor interacts with and observes a client or student, the process of assessment begins. Data are flowing in through the professional counselor's senses and being analyzed through various processes, both intuitive and logical. How the counselor organizes and makes judgments about the data is one of the functional characteristics of counseling, which includes clinical orientation, experience, and the objectivity of the data. Usually the data are not collected systematically, so two different professional counselors may obtain very different data from the same client. Likewise, the data are often analyzed through very different processes, so two professional counselors will often interpret the data in different manners. Measurement and statistics allow all mental health practitioners to use a common language to describe data and interpret it in consistent and meaningful ways. In a manner of speaking, statistics is a sort of language in which professional counselors must become fluent. Statistics help professional counselors to understand and communicate complex information to clients, students, and other professionals.

In terms of understanding data, statistics serve three primary purposes. First, statistics help to describe and summarize data in meaningful ways. To the trained eye and keen mathematical mind, a listing of 20 test scores may yield a wealth of information at first glance. However, most will understand far better what the scores mean when they are grouped or put in some display that helps to describe what is observed. Graphical displays (i.e., histograms and scatterplots) or common statistics (i.e., mean and standard deviation), reviewed later in this chapter, aid in this understanding and communication. These are examples of what is termed *descriptive statistics*, because they help professional counselors to describe and understand data. This is the topic of the current chapter. Statistics is a branch of mathematics, and so a basic understanding of mathematical processes and principles is essential. Second, statistics help to understand relationships between scores of different individuals (interpersonal differences) or within different scores for the same individual (intrapersonal differences). In Chapter 17, the concepts of correlation and regression will be examined. **Correlation statistics** reveal how strongly two sets of scores are related. This is essential knowledge because in the field of counseling, facets of personality or other personal characteristics or behaviors often appear in concert (i.e., are related). Knowing how depressed someone is can help a professional counselor relate other behaviors or characteristics, such as likelihood of suicidal ideation or substance abuse. When using standardized assessments, reliability and validity of scores are often discussed using correlation coefficients, and so an understanding of the concept of correlation becomes a critical element in both assessment and research.

Finally, statistics can be used with quantitative research methodologies to help draw conclusions or make inferences to support or disconfirm hypotheses. *Inferential statistics* allow researchers to study a sample of participants using scientific methodologies to reach conclusions that may generalize to larger populations. Studies that use inferential statistics help professional counselors predict human behaviors and reach likely conclusions (within a reasonable band of error). For example, inferential studies help professional counselors know characteristics of children from divorced families and what strategies and procedures are helpful in promoting adjustment to the family and school environments. Likewise, researchers can help determine the primary causes of conflict among couples and interventions most likely to facilitate resolution of these conflicts and promote good couples communication. The field of counseling is based on a wealth of social science research, and statistics play a huge part in determining what is and is not known about human characteristics (and the degree of confidence one can have about what is known!).

Fortunately, computers and specialized software such as SPSS, Excel (by Microsoft), and R (see http://www.r-project.org/) perform these routine computations at incredible speed. Nonetheless, professional counselors need to understand the concepts, formulas, and computations that comprise the incredibly useful statistical techniques presented throughout the rest of this book.

# Commonly Used Statistical Symbols

Table 12.1 displays and defines the symbols commonly used in statistics and measurement. The purpose of these symbols is to serve as a shorthand method of communicating statistical meanings and mathematical equation building. Each symbol describes an important part of a formula or characteristic of a test score. As you progress through this book, many of these symbols will become more familiar but take a few minutes now to scan the symbols and meanings and commit as many to memory as possible; it is a good idea to flag this page for easy reference. This will help you to quickly locate this table, which from this point on becomes more difficult to locate depending on how desperately you need the information contained in it.

| **TABLE 12.1** | Common statistical and measurement symbols. |
|---|---|
| $X$ | Raw score on variable $X$ |
| $x$ | Deviation score ($X - M_x$) for a raw score on variable $X$ |
| $\Sigma$ | Sum of (Greek letter Sigma); means to add up everything that comes after |
| $Y$ | Raw score on variable $Y$ |
| $y$ | Deviation score ($Y - M_y$) for a raw score on variable $Y$ |
| $M, \bar{X}$ | Mean |
| $SD, S$ | Standard deviation of the sample |
| $S^2, s^2$ | Variance of the sample |
| $N$ | Number of participants in a sample |

*(Continued)*

| TABLE 12.1 | *continued* |
|---|---|
| $n$ | Number of participants in a subsample |
| $f$ | Frequency |
| $cf$ | Cumulative frequency |
| P, %ile | Percentile |
| IQ | Intelligence quotient (deviation IQ); mean of 100 and standard deviation of 15 (or 16, depending on the test) |
| $r$ | Pearson correlation coefficient |
| $r^2$ | Coefficient of determination |
| $r_s$, $\rho$ | Spearman rank-order correlation coefficient |
| $r_{bis}$ | Biserial correlation coefficient |
| $r_{pb}$ | Point-biserial correlation coefficient |
| $r_{tt}$ | Test-retest reliability coefficient |
| $r_{ic}$ | Internal consistency coefficient |
| $r_{ab}$ | Alternate-forms reliability coefficient |
| $r_{xy}$ | Validity coefficient |
| $R$ | Coefficient of multiple regression |
| $IR$ | Interquartile range |
| $Q$ | Semi-interquartile range |
| $Q_1$ | First quartile score (25th percentile) |
| $Q_3$ | Third quartile score (75th percentile) |
| $p$ | Probability or proportion |
| SEM | Standard error of measurement (also written as $SE_m$, $SE_{meas}$, $S_m$, $s_m$, $s_{meas}$, or $s_{err}$) |
| $SE_{est}$ | Standard error of estimate (also $SE_E$) |
| $\Sigma X$ | Sum of raw scores for the X variable |
| SS, $\Sigma X^2$ | Sum of squares of raw scores for the X variable |
| $\Sigma Y$ | Sum of raw scores for the Y variable |
| $\Sigma Y^2$ | Sum of squares of raw scores for the Y variable |
| $\Sigma xy$ | Sum of the cross products of deviation scores for variables X and Y |
| $z$ | $z$ score; mean of 0 and standard deviation of 1 |
| $T$ | T score; mean of 50 and standard deviation of 10 |
| CEEB | College Entrance Examination Board score (SAT); mean of 500 and standard deviation of 100 |
| $t$ | $t$-test |
| $\Phi$ | Phi coefficient |
| $\chi^2$ | Chi square |
| a | regression equation intercept constant |
| b | regression equation slope constant |
| c | constant determined through multiple regression |
| $F$ | Fisher's F ANOVA test statistic |
| $Mdn$ | Median |
| $\sqrt{\phantom{x}}$ | Square root |
| SS | Standard Score |
| AD | Average Deviation |
| NSS | Normalized Standard Score |
| % | Percentage |
| $SE_m$ | Standard error of the mean (also written as $S_m$, $s_m$) |

# Describing Distributions of Scores

Understanding data is in many ways like detective work. A detective collects clues (scores), organizes them in a meaningful way (description), and finally draws conclusions (score interpretation or inferences based on a score). Of course, the process is frequently more complicated than this because sometimes the conclusions are based on faulty clues or are tentative, pending the collection of further confirmatory evidence. Importantly, notice that a clue (raw score) in isolation is often not very meaningful, but when it is related to other scores, more meaning can be constructed. This section addresses the process of organizing and describing the scores. Generally, this is accomplished through the construction of a frequency distribution or graph (e.g., histogram, bar graph, frequency polygon, curve, stem-and-leaf plot, and box-and-whisker plot). Later in the chapter, measures of central tendency (i.e., mean, median, and mode) and dispersion (e.g., range and standard deviation) will be discussed.

## Frequency Distributions

**Frequency distributions** allow researchers to quickly view the frequency with which each score occurs in a distribution; there are two types: simple and grouped. A **simple frequency distribution** lists every score and the number of times it occurs, generally from the highest score to lowest score. Table 12.2 shows a distribution of 20 participant scores on measures of depression and substance use. The depression score has been designated variable $X$ and the substance use variable $Y$. The reasons for these variable designations will make more sense as the chapter progresses.

| **TABLE 12.2** Student scores on depression and substance use. | | |
|:---:|:---:|:---:|
| **Student ID Number** | **Depression Score (X)** | **Substance Use Score (Y)** |
| 01 | 10 | 7 |
| 02 | 13 | 6 |
| 03 | 6 | 16 |
| 04 | 16 | 20 |
| 05 | 3 | 2 |
| 06 | 8 | 0 |
| 07 | 14 | 10 |
| 08 | 8 | 6 |
| 09 | 18 | 12 |
| 10 | 15 | 14 |
| 11 | 7 | 0 |
| 12 | 14 | 8 |
| 13 | 12 | 8 |
| 14 | 10 | 16 |
| 15 | 12 | 7 |
| 16 | 20 | 16 |
| 17 | 18 | 4 |
| 18 | 13 | 8 |
| 19 | 9 | 2 |
| 20 | 14 | 18 |

**TABLE 12.3**    Simple frequency distribution for the depression score.

| Midterm Score | Tallies | Frequency (f) | Cumulative f | Cumulative % |
|:---:|:---:|:---:|:---:|:---:|
| 20 | I | 1 | 20 | 100 |
| 18 | II | 2 | 19 | 95 |
| 16 | I | 1 | 17 | 85 |
| 15 | I | 1 | 16 | 80 |
| 14 | III | 3 | 15 | 75 |
| 13 | II | 2 | 12 | 60 |
| 12 | II | 2 | 10 | 50 |
| 10 | II | 2 | 8 | 40 |
| 09 | I | 1 | 6 | 30 |
| 08 | II | 2 | 5 | 25 |
| 07 | I | 1 | 3 | 15 |
| 06 | I | 1 | 2 | 10 |
| 03 | I | 1 | 1 | 5 |

© Cengage Learning

A simple frequency distribution of scores on the depression scale is found in Table 12.3. Notice that in the first column, the scores are listed in descending order (20 down to 3), the second column presents a tally marking system, and the third column provides the frequency that each score occurs (it always matches the tallies in the second column). Two additional columns are provided that will commonly appear on a computerized statistical printout, such as SPSS. The fourth column presents what is called the cumulative frequency. Cumulative frequency is simply the cumulative tally of a given score, usually starting from the lowest score and working to the highest score. In the midterm column, the cumulative frequency for a score of 7 is 3 because there are three scores at 7 and below. The fifth column provides the cumulative percentage. This value indicates the percentage of scores that fall at or below the value of interest. Using the score of 7 again, the cumulative percentage is 15 percent because 3 of the 20 scores (15 percent) fall at or below a score of 7. The highest score will always have a cumulative percentage value of 100 percent.

**Grouped frequency distributions** are similar to the simple frequency distribution, except that instead of reporting every score obtained, the scores are grouped into convenient class intervals (i.e., a lot of scores are collapsed into fewer groupings of scores). Grouped frequency distributions provide a meaningful graph of scores and allow computation of some statistics with greater ease. Of course, with the widespread use of computers, the latter reason is a less pressing concern. It is important to realize that when using a grouped frequency distribution, one loses some precision while gaining some advantages in understanding the visual summary. In Table 12.4, the depression scores

**TABLE 12.4**    Grouped frequency distribution for the depression test scores.

| Class Interval | Midpoint | F | Cumulative f | Cumulative % |
|:---:|:---:|:---:|:---:|:---:|
| 18–20 | 19 | 3 | 20 | 100 |
| 15–17 | 16 | 2 | 17 | 85 |
| 12–14 | 13 | 7 | 15 | 75 |
| 09–11 | 10 | 3 | 8 | 40 |
| 06–08 | 07 | 4 | 5 | 25 |
| 03–05 | 04 | 1 | 1 | 5 |

© Cengage Learning

presented in Table 12.3 have been grouped into class intervals. The process for establishing the groupings or classes can be simplified if one thinks first about how the final visual display should look. What is the range of scores (lowest to highest scores), and how many categories make sense. These are decisions and choices that the researcher must make, and there are no hard and fast rules. In general, however, it is best to establish groupings with an integer at the center of the interval (meaning the classes frequently are made up of an odd number of score values) and use enough intervals to allow the spread of the scores to be displayed. Too few intervals give the appearance that most people received the same result, and too many intervals lead to little understanding. Generally, establishing five to eight categories is a good rule of thumb.

Using the depression scores it is easy to see that the scores ranged from 3 to 20 (a range of 18 possible test scores: $20 - 3 + 1 = 18$). For simplicity sake, in this instance, it makes sense to group the scores into six intervals of three points each. This allows for a display of not too many or too few intervals. Perhaps most important, intervals have an odd number of potential scores, meaning that an integer can comprise the center of each interval class (because although not essential, it is usually easier for people to understand whole numbers). Simply start at the lowest value (3) and group the scores by threes until the highest value is reached (i.e., 3–5, 6–8, 9–11, 12–14, 15–17, 18–20). Then fill in the rest of the table the same way as for the simple frequency distribution. If the scores are amenable to some sort of criterion-referenced interpretive scheme, then all the better. An example of displaying a summary grouping of scores might be according to the course grading policy (i.e., $93-100 = A$; $90-92 = A-$; $88-89 = B+$; etc.). However, note that this strategy leads to an unequal number of possible scores in each class interval. For example, the A range is composed of eight possible scores and the A– range three possible scores. Thus, one should not be surprised when a class receives more A's than A–'s. Such a system simplifies and complicates interpretation at the same time. Ah, statistics!

## Graphing Frequency Distributions

"A picture is worth a thousand words." Although many people can extract meaning from a table of numbers, nearly all understand data to some extent when they see it presented graphically. Distributions of scores are usually displayed using bar graphs, histograms, frequency polygons, smoothed curves, stem-and-leaf plots, or box-and-whisker plots. Each will be introduced in turn.

### Bar Graphs

We have already discussed discrete and continuous variables. **Bar graphs** look a lot like histograms, but one will notice that the bars on a bar graph never touch each other, whereas the bars on a histogram do. This is because bar graphs are a method for visually displaying discrete variables (e.g., sex or religious affiliation), whereas histograms are used to display continuous variables. Basically, any nominal variable can be appropriately displayed on a bar graph. This is because the categories of a nominal scale are discrete and never touch or overlap; males and females are different categories, as are candidates running for an elected position. Usually, a bar graph places the categories of the nominal scale on the horizontal axis (also called the *x*-axis or abscissa), and the frequency of occurrence on the vertical axis (also called the *y*-axis or ordinate). Figure 12.1 shows two examples of bar graphs. Professional counselors frequently use bar graphs when displaying demographic or other characteristics that are nominal in nature.

**Figure 12.1**

Two examples of bar graphs.

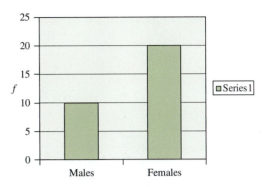

(a) Bar graph displaying participants' sex.

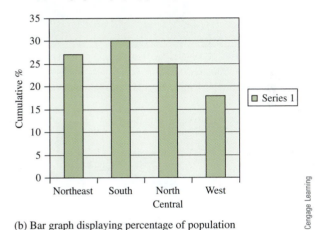

(b) Bar graph displaying percentage of population
from each geographic region of the United States.

© Cengage Learning

## Histograms

Histograms are similar to bar graphs in appearance, but you will immediately notice that the categories are actually continuous and, therefore, touch adjacent values. **Histograms** are used to visually display ordinal, interval, or ratio data and thus are more useful when summarizing test scores and most other variables used in research. As can be seen in Figure 12.2, histograms also usually display the measured scores along the horizontal axis and frequencies along a vertical axis. Again, for the grouped frequency distribution, each interval of scores is positioned on the horizontal axis with the inclusive values indicated by two vertical lines at the extreme limits for each value (i.e., in the depression example: 2.5–5.4, 5.5–8.4, 8.5–11.4, etc.). The height of the graph is proportional to the frequency of each score. In some ways, a histogram resembles a set of building blocks with each individual's score representing a single block. These blocks are stacked one on top of the other in a given response category to represent the total distribution of scores. Figure 12.2 shows the histograms for both the simple and grouped frequency distributions of depression scores presented earlier in Tables 12.3 and 12.4, respectively.

## Frequency Polygons

A **frequency polygon** is also used to visually display continuous variables. A polygon is a many-sided figure. It is basically the same as a histogram, except instead of using bars rising from the horizontal baseline, a single point above the midpoint of the interval is

**Figure 12.2**

Two examples of histograms.

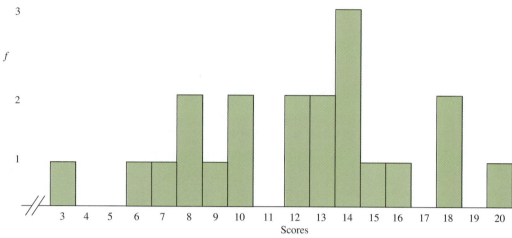

(a) Histogram displaying simple frequencies of the midterm scores.

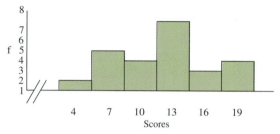

(b) Histogram displaying group frequencies of the midterm scores.

© Cengage Learning

provided. In classic graphing fashion, this point represents both the score value (i.e., class interval) and the frequency of occurrence for each value. Once these points have been charted, straight lines are drawn from point to point until all the points are connected. Finally, a straight line is drawn from the farthest point at each end of the graph down to the baseline to indicate where the scores end.

Figure 12.3 displays the frequency polygon for the depression frequency distribution. Notice that the frequency polygon is interpreted to mean the same as the histograms; it just has a different, more angular look.

### Stem-and-Leaf Plots

Basically, **stem-and-leaf plots** are histograms turned on their sides. The frequency of a given range of scores is represented by the length of each row. A decided advantage of a stem-and-leaf plot over a histogram, however, is that the actual numerical values provided can be used to reconstruct the scores comprising the database. Figure 12.4 is a stem-and-leaf plot for the depression scores broken into five raw score point intervals (i.e., 0–4 [stem = 0], 5–9 [stem = 0*], 10–14 [stem = 1], 15–19 [stem = 1*], 20–24 [stem = 2]). The column at the far left is referred to as the stem (i.e., a class interval), and the lengths of scores projecting to the right are referred to as the leaves. Thus, the stem-and-leaf plot provides a general shape of the distribution, much as the histogram, but with more

**Figure 12.3**

Example of a frequency polygon displaying frequencies of the depression scores.

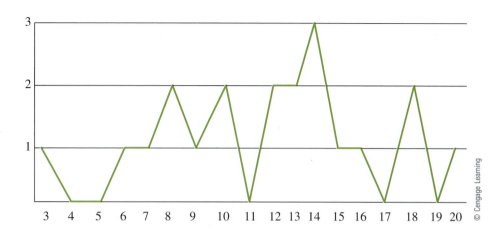

**Figure 12.4**

Stem-and-leaf plot of the depression scale scores.

```
0   3
0*  67889
1   02233444
1*  5688
2   0
```

precision because it accurately identifies the raw scores comprising the distribution. One can easily construct a stem-and-leaf plot by hand using the following steps:

1. Enter the stem digits in the left column vertically in order from lowest to highest or highest to lowest.
2. Either draw a vertical line to the right of the stem column or leave a space.
3. Enter each score in the row corresponding to the appropriate stem digit, forming the leaves.
4. Order the digits within each leaf from lowest to highest moving from left to right.

### Box-and-Whisker Plots

A **box-and-whisker plot** (sometimes shortened to boxplot) is useful for displaying trends in data. To construct a box-and-whisker plot, you have to know the lowest score, highest score, median score, first quartile demarcation ($Q_1$), and third quartile demarcation ($Q_3$). (We will discuss computing quartiles in Chapter 13.) SPSS can construct box-and-whisker plots as selected output. See Figure 12.5 for a box-and-whisker plot of the depression score data. Notice that the box begins at 8.25 ($Q_1$) and ends at 14.75 ($Q_3$). Notice also that the center line through the box falls at 12.5 ($Q_2$, the median). The "whiskers" are the lines protruding from the box all the way down to the lowest score (3) and to the highest score (20). The primary advantage of the box-and-whisker plot is the visual display of potential skewing, similar to several other graphical displays just reviewed. Finally, notice that 50 percent of the distribution's scores fall within the box, 25 percent below the box, and 25 percent above the box.

**Figure 12.5**

Box-and-whisker plot for the depression scale scores.

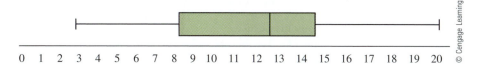

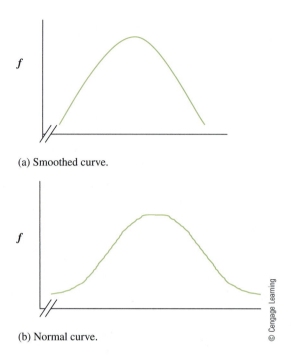

(a) Smoothed curve.

(b) Normal curve.

© Cengage Learning

### Curves

As an extension of the frequency polygon, many score distributions are represented as curves, particularly if the number of participants is large, such as in a standardization sample. Curves start as frequency polygons but undergo a smoothing process and so the data are displayed not as sharp peaks and valleys but as a smooth progression between values. Figure 12.6 shows the smoothed curve for the depression frequency polygon presented earlier. **Curve smoothing** is a common procedure but should be undertaken carefully because it involves a number of interpolations (e.g., guessing within the bounds of what is known). Thus, caution is warranted when using an estimation technique like smoothing because it introduces another source of potential error. On the other hand, the reason measurement specialists use smoothing is to correct for what is believed to be sample measurement error; that is, the measurements yielded by the sample under study may not reflect the data that would have been obtained if a larger, more representative sample (or the entire population) had been assessed. Curves are frequently described by using the following characteristics: mean (central tendency), standard deviation (a measure of dispersion), skew, and kurtosis. The mean is the mathematical average, or "balance point," of a distribution of scores. The standard deviation is the dispersion or spread of scores around the mean. Skew describes the symmetry of a curve, and kurtosis the "peakedness" of a curve (i.e., how quickly the curve rises and falls). Each of these curve characteristics (central tendency, dispersion, skewness, and kurtosis) will be described in greater detail in the following sections.

# Measures of Central Tendency

Various measures of **central tendency** are meant to give an idea of what the center or middle of a distribution looks like. It is (usually) the single score that is most representative or typical of the entire set of scores. Three measures of central tendency are important to understand: mode, median, and mean. When viewing a normal curve, the mean median and mode are at the exact middle of the distribution.

## Mode

The **mode** is the most frequently occurring score in a set of scores. It is also the only measure of central tendency that can be used with nominal data. It is a simple concept, easily recognized during a visual scan of a frequency distribution or graph because it is the highest point on a curve, histogram, or frequency polygon. The mode of the depression scores in Table 12.3 (see also Figure 12.2a) is 14 because it occurs three times; no other score occurs more than twice. If two scores simultaneously occur most frequently, the distribution is called *bimodal*. For example, if a 21st client responded to the depression scale and received a score of 13, then a bimodal distribution would occur (13, 14). Likewise, if one score of 14 was eliminated from the original list, the distribution would be *multimodal* because the scores 8, 10, 12, 13, 14, and 18 would each occur twice. By the way, if every score in a distribution occurs only once, it is referred to as a *rectangular* distribution and has no mode.

When using a grouped frequency distribution, the mode is the midpoint of the most frequently occurring class interval. From Table 12.4 (and Figure 12.2b), it can be seen that the class interval 12–14 contained seven scores. Thus, 13 is the mode of the grouped distribution because it is the midpoint of the interval. The mode is rarely reported as a measure of central tendency but may be of interest when decision makers are interested in knowing what score the most examinees obtained.

## Median

The **median** is defined as the middlemost score, the value below and above which 50 percent of the cases fall. The median, by definition, also becomes the 50th percentile rank. To determine the median, first line up all scores in order from lowest to highest, then determine the number of scores, and finally locate the middle score in the rank order. As an example, take the following set of IQ scores: 86, 131, 101, 125, 111, 79, 75, 95, 88, 106, and 119. To find the median (*Mdn*), align the scores in order by magnitude: 75, 79, 86, 88, 95, 101, 106, 111, 119, 125, and 131. If you have an odd number of scores, the median is easier to find because you just divide the number of scores by 2 and round up. In this example, there are 11 scores, so the median score is the sixth score from either end ($11 \div 2 = 5.5$, which rounds up to 6). Thus, 101 is the median score.

Finding the median is only a bit more complicated if there are an even number of scores. Take the depression exam score distribution that comprises 20 scores. When arranged in order from lowest to highest, the midterm score distribution looks like this:

$$3, 6, 7, 8, 8, 9, 10, 10, 12, 12 \quad 13, 13, 14, 14, 14, 15, 16, 18, 18, 20$$

$$\uparrow$$

$$Mdn = 12.5$$

Dividing the number of scores by 2 ($20 \div 2 = 10$) means that the 10th score from each end is the median. *But* there are two 10th scores, depending on which end you count in from. This means there are two middlemost scores. Now if both scores are the same, the answer is simple because the median is equal to that number. If the two middlemost numbers are different, however, you must average them to get the median score. In the case of the preceding depression score distribution, the two middlemost scores are 12 and 13, so the median score is 12.5 ($12 + 13 = 25$; $25 \div 2 = 12.5$). The median is always at the middle of a distribution of scores. Take a moment to determine the median of the substance use score distribution from Table 12.2. Did you get 8? There are actually three scores of 8 in the substance use distribution holding the places 10, 11, and 12 in a 20-score distribution. Because score numbers 10 and 11 are the same (i.e., 8), determining the median is simple.

Median scores are commonly used when it is suspected that outliers (i.e., extreme scores) may "skew" a distribution (see the discussion of skewness following). Medians are less likely to be pulled in the direction of the skew than the mean. Medians are also the preferred measure of central tendency for "truncated" distributions. Truncation occurs when scores are cut off at a certain point, even though some individuals may have attained either higher or lower scores. Tests on which a lot of participants get the highest (or lowest) possible score would be examples of truncated distributions. Thus, the median is commonly used with ordinal scale scores and interval or ratio data that are skewed or truncated. For example, housing prices or salaries are often reported using the median because although several highly priced homes or high-salaried employees can really affect the average score, they have little effect on the middlemost score.

## Mean

The **mean** is the arithmetic average of a set of scores. It is the exact balance point in a distribution of scores. To obtain the mean, simply add all of the scores in a distribution and divide by the number of scores:

$$M = \Sigma X/n, \tag{12.1}$$

where $M$ is the mean of the test scores, $\Sigma X$ means to sum all of the scores in the test distribution ($X$), and $n$ is the number of scores in the distribution. For example, to compute the mean of the IQ scores just provided, simply add the IQ test scores: $86 + 131 + 101 + 125 + 111 + 79 + 75 + 95 + 88 + 106 + 119 = 1,116$; then divide by the number of scores ($n = 11$). Thus, the mean is $1,116 \div 11 = 101.45$. Returning to the depression test example, $\Sigma X = 240$ and $n = 20$ scores. Thus, the mean for the depression score distribution is $240 \div 20 = 12.0$.

When computing the mean from a frequency distribution, the formula becomes

$$M = \Sigma f X/n, \tag{12.2}$$

where $f$ is the frequency of a given score on a test ($X$). Referring to Table 12.3, you will see that this can be simply accomplished by multiplying each depression score in the first column by the frequency ($f$) listed in the third column (e.g., for the score of 18, $fX$ is 2[18] or 36) and then adding these multiplied values down the column ($\Sigma fX = 240$) and dividing by the number of scores ($n = 20$). The result is the same: $M = 12.0$.

The mean is the most commonly used measure of central tendency with interval and ratio scale scores that are fairly normally distributed, and because the mean is directly applicable to advanced statistical procedures. The median and mode are not. Most developers of clinical, personality, and behavioral tests also use the mean, even though scores from these measures are most often ordinal. The mean has useful algebraic properties, and it is widely used in descriptive and inferential statistics. In general, as the number of scores in a distribution increases, so does the stability of the mean. Unfortunately, the mean is affected by extreme scores (i.e., outliers) and has limited usefulness with skewed distributions. Thus, one or several unusually high or low scores can substantially change or distort the mean and reduce its usefulness as a measure of central tendency. For example, if a 21st client received a score of 50 on the depression scale, and this score was averaged into the distribution, the resulting mean would equal 13.8 ($290 \div 21 = 13.8$). One high score caused the mean to rise from 12.0 to 13.8. In such a case, the median becomes a much better estimate of the distribution's center point.

### Standard Error of the Mean

The standard error of the mean ($SE_m$) is similar to the standard error of measurement in that it allows the researcher to establish a confidence interval around the mean within which likely percentages of randomly derived sample means are likely to fall. Thus, this confidence interval is an estimate of the likelihood that the obtained sample mean is representative of all possible sample means drawn from the population. The formula for computing the standard error of the mean is

$$SE_m = \sqrt{\frac{S^2}{n}},$$ (12.3)

where $S^2$ is the sample variance—a concept that will be defined in the sections that follow. The standard error of the mean is a default statistic provided in SPSS output, as is often presented in conjunction with the mean in empirical studies. For example, assuming for the moment that the variance for the depression sample mean is 19.26 with an $n = 20$, the resulting $SE_m$ is 0.98. To construct a confidence interval, professional counselors use

$$M \pm t \times SE_m,$$ (12.4)

where $t$ equals the desired level of confidence (LOC). Confidence intervals are generally reported as $\pm 1$ $SE_m$, which is the 68 percent LOC, but they are sometimes reported at the 95 or 99 percent LOC, depending on the degree of certainty required by the researcher. The 68 percent LOC means that if 100 means were sampled from the distribution of scores, the obtained mean would fall within the given range 68 times. In the case of the depression score mean, $12.0 \pm 0.98$ yields a 68 percent confidence interval of 11.02 – 12.98, meaning that the true population mean has a 68 percent probability of falling within the given range. The 95 percent LOC would be $12.0 + 2(0.98)$ or $10.04 - 13.96$, and the 99 percent LOC would be $12.0 \pm 2.58(0.98)$ or $9.47 - 14.53$.

## Comparison of Measures of Central Tendency in Various Types of Distributions

The mean, median, and mode each have their own characteristics and usefulness under various circumstances. Each has usefulness depending on the type of the measurement scale (i.e., nominal, ordinal, interval, and ratio) and the shape (symmetry) of the distribution (e.g., normal and skewed). Table 12.5 summarizes the measure of central tendency applicable to the various scales of measurement. Note that the mode is the only measure of central tendency for nominal data, and the mean does not (theoretically) apply to ordinal data.

**TABLE 12.5**  Measures of central tendency used with various scales of measurement.

| Measure of Central Tendency | Scales of Measurement |
| --- | --- |
| Mode | Nominal, Ordinal, Interval, Ratio |
| Median | Ordinal, Interval, Ratio |
| Mean | Interval, Ratio |

© Cengage Learning

**Figure 12.7**

Relationship of mean, median, and mode in normal and skewed distributions.

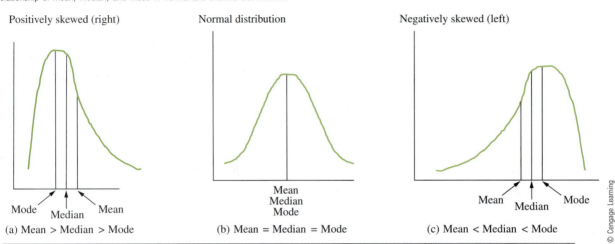

Positively skewed (right)    Normal distribution    Negatively skewed (left)

Mode  Median  Mean
(a) Mean > Median > Mode

Mean
Median
Mode
(b) Mean = Median = Mode

Mean  Median  Mode
(c) Mean < Median < Mode

© Cengage Learning

In a normal distribution of scores, the mean, median, and mode are at the same point: the highest rise of the curve. This makes sense when you think of the bell-shaped curve as being bilaterally symmetric, with an equal number of scores and variance on either side of the midpoint. As distributions become more skewed, the mean usually becomes a less accurate reflection of centrality, whereas the median usually becomes more meaningful. Figure 12.7 shows the relationship of the mean, median, and mode in normal and skewed distributions.

Note that when a distribution is skewed, the mode stays at the peak of the curve (by definition), whereas the median is pulled a bit toward the skew's tail, and the mean is pulled substantially toward the skew's tail. As just mentioned, this is because one or several extreme scores or outliers can have a substantial impact on the mean, a slight impact on the median, and virtually no impact on the mode.

# Measures of Variability (Dispersion)

While measures of central tendency explain where the center of a distribution of scores is, **measures of variability** tell what the distribution looks like as scores away from the middle are explored. Two distributions may have identical means or medians but very different shapes. One distribution may have all of the scores clustered close to the center point; the other spread out over a substantial range of scores in either direction. Measures of variance or dispersion describe how much variation is evident in a distribution of scores (i.e., how spread out the scores are). Look at Figure 12.8 and notice that even though the mean of each distribution is identical, the shape of the curve and range of scores vary greatly. These differences are a function of the scores' variability or how dispersed they are.

If you take a handful of birdseed, hold it at your side, and drop it on a sidewalk, the birdseed will likely fall to the surface and cluster around a center point near where you are standing, with little variation. Thus, the dispersion of seeds is small. If you take the same handful of birdseed and fling it down on the sidewalk, it will disperse over a wide range

**Figure 12.8**

Examples of kurtosis.

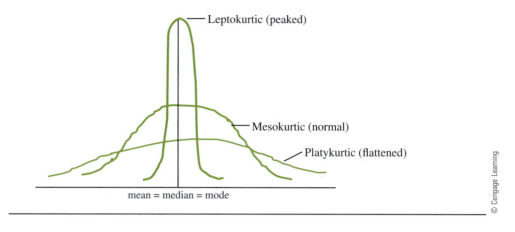

Leptokurtic (peaked)

Mesokurtic (normal)

Platykurtic (flattened)

mean = median = mode

© Cengage Learning

some distance from where you are standing, depending on how strong or practiced you are at hurling birdseed. In this latter case, the seed is dispersed over a much greater range; so it's the same handful of seeds and the same sidewalk but two different variabilities. In group counseling, a professional counselor may need to prepare for sessions quite differently if all clients are female (low variability) versus male and female (more variability). A professional school counselor will need to prepare a quite different developmental guidance lesson on conflict resolution if the audience is a group of elementary students aged 7–11 years, as opposed to a group of 11-year-olds. The concept of variability is essential to an understanding of data. It gives helpful indications of what scores mean and what to expect from differences between scores. When describing variability, statisticians, researchers, and test developers frequently report range, interquartile range, semi-interquartile range, average deviation, variance, and standard deviation. Each will be discussed in turn.

## Range

Simply put, the **range** is the distance between the highest and lowest scores in the distribution. Many texts indicate that the range can be computed using the formula, range = $X_H - X_L$, where $X_H$ is the highest score and $X_L$ is the lowest score. Thus, in the depression score distribution, $X_H$ is 20 and $X_L$ is 3. Thus, range = $X_H - X_L$ = 17. Easy, right?

Not so fast. Statisticians have a way of complicating even the simplest things. There is some disagreement in the field over the accuracy of this seemingly simple computation because if you start at 3 and count all the possible scores up to and including 20, you would get 18 because 3 and 20 are both scores found in the distribution. Thus, a more accurate formula is

$$\text{Range} = X_H - X_L + 1. \qquad (12.5)$$

In the depression scores example, the range using this corrected formula is range = 20 − 3 + 1 = 18. At any rate, arguing over the difference is hardly worth the effort because the range is not a particularly useful or widely reported measure of variability. This is because extreme scores always influence the range and limit its usefulness. Remember what happened to the mean when the 21st participant's depression score of 50 was entered. The same problem occurs with the range, which would then be range = $X_H - X_L + 1$ = 50 − 3 + 1 = 48. The range of 48 is hardly representative of the variability present in the other 20 scores! Thus, the range of scores is the simplest measure of variability to compute but the least helpful in understanding the variability of a distribution because it is susceptible to influence by extreme scores. An important caveat: the +1 in Equation 12.5 only applies when the scores are whole numbers; if the score values are reported as units of tenths, hundredths, etc., the equation should be modified accordingly. That is, if the scores range from .3 to 2.0, the range would be computed: range $= X_H - X_L + .1 = 2.0 - 0.3 + 0.1 = 1.8$.

## Interquartile and Semi-Interquartile Ranges

Because the range is affected by extreme scores, researchers may prefer to report the interquartile range (*IR*) or semi-interquartile range (*Q*). This is particularly appropriate when the median is reported as the measure of a distribution's central tendency. Although the *IR* is sometimes reported, *Q* is more relevant to our discussion. In practice, *Q* is simply one-half of *IR* (i.e., $Q = IR/2$).

*Semi* means "half," *inter* means "between," *quartiles* are the three points within a distribution that divide the distribution into four equal parts, and *range* refers to the difference between these demarcations. The two quartiles of interest are the first and the third demarcations. You are already familiar with the second quartile, which is more commonly known as the median. There are several methods for computing *Q*, and they vary in complexity. Simply put, *Q* is half the difference between the 1st ($Q_1$ or the 25th percentile) and 3rd ($Q_3$ or the 75th percentile) quartiles, or $Q = (Q_3 - Q_1) \div 2$.

The more challenging part is determining $Q_1$ and $Q_3$! The statistics involved in computing $Q_1$ and $Q_3$ can be quite complex. Simply put, $Q_1$ falls in the middle position of the bottom half of scores, while $Q_3$ falls in the middle of the top half of scores. The good news is that SPSS gives $Q_1$, $Q_2$, and $Q_3$ as part of its default parameters when using the frequencies analysis. In fact, nearly all of the measures of central tendency and variability covered in this section are available through common statistical packages, such as SPSS Excel, or R-stat. Use statistical programs whenever possible: it cuts down on errors and saves a *lot* of time.

In a normal distribution, $Q_1$ and $Q_3$ will be the same raw or standardized score distance from the median score. The lesser or greater the distance between the median and $Q_1$, as compared to the distance between the median and $Q_3$, the more skewed the distribution will be. In general, both *Q* and *IR* have the advantages of not being influenced by extreme scores and fitting nicely as an index of variability to accompany the median score—just as the mean and standard deviation are often wedded when describing a relatively normal distribution. Thus, the 21st client who receives a 50 for either the depression scale or substance use scale will have little effect on the median, interquartile range, or semi-interquartile range. Figure 12.9 provides an example of finding the semi-interquartile range for the depression scores.

**Figure 12.9**

Obtaining the semi-interquartile range for the depression scores.

| Rank: | 1 | 2 | 3 | 4 | 5 | 6 | 7 | 8 | 9 | 10 | 11 | 12 | 13 | 14 | 15 | 16 | 17 | 18 | 19 | 20 |
|-------|---|---|---|---|---|---|---|---|---|----|----|----|----|----|----|----|----|----|----|----|
| Score: | 3 | 6 | 7 | 8 | 8 | 9 | 10 | 10 | 12 | 12 | 13 | 13 | 14 | 14 | 14 | 15 | 16 | 18 | 18 | 20 |

      ↑        ↑        ↑

    25th %ile    50th %ile    75th %ile

    Place#5.25   Place#10.5   Place#15.75

    $Q_1 = 8.25$  Median ($Q_2$) = 12.5  $Q_3 = 14.75$

© Cengage Learning

## Average Deviation

The **average deviation**, sometimes called the mean deviation, is a very simple way of expressing the variation of scores in a distribution by adding the absolute differences between each score and the mean, and then dividing by the number of scores:

$$AD = \frac{\Sigma|x|}{n},$$

(12.6)

where $x = (X - M_X)$. The term *absolute* means that all values, whether negative or positive, become positive. This makes it possible for the variation in scores to be averaged. Table 12.6 presents the scores from the depression and substance use score distributions along with various other columns needed to compute the average deviation (and variance and standard deviation, which are discussed in the following section). Notice how the summation of $x$ (e.g., $\Sigma x$) at the bottom of the "Deviation Score of $x$" column is equal to zero (0). This is because half of the deviation falls above the mean and half below—so they cancel each other out. To counteract this, the average deviation sums the absolute values of $x$ (e.g., $|x|$) so that all of the negative values (values of $X$ below the mean) become positive values. When calculating $\Sigma|x|$ values for the depression scores, one gets 70.0. To obtain the average deviation, just divide this value by the number of scores in the distribution: $AD_X = \Sigma|x|/n = 70 \div 20 = 3.5$. Thus, the average deviation of the depression distribution is 3.5, meaning that the average distance that each score varies from the mean is 3.5 raw score points.

To obtain the average deviation for the substance use scores presented in Table 12.6, just divide the value 98.0 (see the bottom of the "Deviation Score of $Y$" column) by the number of scores in the distribution: $AD_Y = \Sigma|y|/n = 98 \div 20 = 4.9$. Thus, the average deviation of the substance use scale distribution is 4.9, meaning that the average distance that each score varies from the mean is 4.9 raw score points. You will see this statistic only occasionally because empirical researchers, action researchers, and measurement specialists ordinarily prefer to use the standard deviation. However, the calculation of the average deviation is important as a building block to understanding how the standard deviation is conceptualized and computed.

## Standard Deviation and Variance

Recall that the average deviation requires the absolute values of deviation scores. This was necessary to be able to add the variations around the mean; otherwise, the $x$ values would cancel each other out. Another way to ensure that variation around the mean is always expressed as positive values is to square the deviation scores (i.e., $x^2$, $y^2$). This is the basis of the concepts of variance and standard deviation. **Variance** (also called "mean square deviation") is mathematically related to standard deviation, and so if you know the variance of a distribution, you also know the standard deviation. The variance is simply the average of the scores' squared deviations (i.e., $\Sigma x^2/n$).

The standard deviation is the square root of the variance. **Standard deviation** has three primary advantages. First, it expresses the variation around the mean in score units comparable to the mean. This is why the mean and standard deviation are nearly always wedded in empirical research reports and test manuals. Second, the properties of the standard deviation imply that it should be applied to distributions that are basically "normal." This allows the use of the wedded terms *mean* and *standard deviation* to conjure up the wonderful statistical properties of the normal curve and standardized scores, which will be explained in Chapter 13. For now, suffice it to say that the closer the

**TABLE 12.6** Computing difference scores for depression and substance use.

| Student | Depression Score X | Depression Score Squared $X^2$ | Deviation Score of X $x = (X - M_X)$ | Deviation Squared of X $x^2$ | Substance Use Score Y | Substance Use Score Squared $Y^2$ | Deviation Score of Y $y = (Y - M_Y)$ | Deviation Squared of Y $y^2 \cdot y$ |
|---|---|---|---|---|---|---|---|---|
| 01 | 10 | 100 | -2.0 | 4.0 | 7 | 49 | -2.0 | 4.0 |
| 02 | 13 | 169 | 1.0 | 1.0 | 6 | 36 | -3.0 | 9.0 |
| 03 | 6 | 36 | -6.0 | 36.0 | 16 | 256 | 7.0 | 49.0 |
| 04 | 16 | 256 | 4.0 | 16.0 | 20 | 400 | 11.0 | 121.0 |
| 05 | 3 | 9 | -9.0 | 81.0 | 2 | 4 | -7.0 | 49.0 |
| 06 | 8 | 64 | -4.0 | 16.0 | 0 | 0 | -9.0 | 81.0 |
| 07 | 14 | 196 | 2.0 | 4.0 | 10 | 100 | 1.0 | 1.0 |
| 08 | 8 | 64 | -4.0 | 16.0 | 6 | 36 | -3.0 | 9.0 |
| 09 | 18 | 324 | 6.0 | 36.0 | 12 | 144 | 3.0 | 9.0 |
| 10 | 15 | 225 | 3.0 | 9.0 | 14 | 196 | 5.0 | 25.0 |
| 11 | 7 | 49 | -5.0 | 25.0 | 0 | 0 | -9.0 | 81.0 |
| 12 | 14 | 196 | 2.0 | 4.0 | 8 | 64 | -1.0 | 1.0 |
| 13 | 12 | 144 | 0.0 | 0.0 | 8 | 64 | -1.0 | 1.0 |
| 14 | 10 | 100 | -2.0 | 4.0 | 16 | 256 | 7.0 | 49.0 |
| 15 | 12 | 144 | 0.0 | 0.0 | 7 | 49 | -2.0 | 4.0 |
| 16 | 20 | 400 | 8.0 | 64.0 | 16 | 256 | 7.0 | 49.0 |
| 17 | 18 | 324 | 6.0 | 36.0 | 4 | 16 | -5.0 | 25.0 |
| 18 | 13 | 169 | 1.0 | 1.0 | 8 | 64 | -1.0 | 1.0 |
| 19 | 9 | 81 | -3.0 | 9.0 | 2 | 4 | -7.0 | 49.0 |
| 20 | 14 | 196 | 2.0 | 4.0 | 18 | 324 | 9.0 | 81.0 |
| $n = 20$ | $\Sigma X = 240$ | $\Sigma X^2 = 3,246$ | $\Sigma X = 0$ | $\Sigma X^2 = 366.0$ | $\Sigma Y = 180$ | $\Sigma Y^2 = 2,318$ | $\Sigma y = 0$ | $\Sigma y^2 = 698.0$ |
| | $M_x = 12.0$ | | $\Sigma|x| = 70.0$ | | $M_Y = 9.0$ | | $\Sigma|y| = 98.0$ | |

© Cengage Learning

distribution is to normal, the more accurate one can be about knowing the exact percentages of a population that fall between the mean and a given standard deviation.

This can be a big help when you have to interpret what an individual's score means. Finally, the standard deviation has marvelous algebraic/mathematical properties that make it a commonly used facet of statistical formulas and applications. Thus, it is important to understand how the standard deviation is calculated and the kinds of information it allows professional counselors to convey when interpreting scores. The importance of the standard deviation cannot be overemphasized, and every researcher and test user must become proficient in its use and applications.

Mathematically, the standard deviation is the square root of the variance and is a useful estimate of how far above and below the mean a typical score falls. There are two common ways for determining variance and standard deviation: the raw score method and the deviation score method. Of course, statistical programs such as SPSS (and some calculators) do all of this automatically, so use them whenever possible. The formula for variance ($S^2$) using the raw score method is

$$S^2 = (\Sigma X^2/n) - M_X^2. \tag{12.7}$$

The standard deviation (SD or S) is simply the square root of this result. Using the depression scores from Table 12.6, follow this simple seven-step procedure:

1. Calculate the mean (see Table 12.6, second column: $M = 12.0$).

2. Square each depression score (see the third column of Table 12.6: $X^2$, "Depression Score Squared").

3. Sum this column ($\Sigma X^2$). Notice that in this example $\Sigma X^2 = 3{,}246$.

4. Divide this sum by the number of scores. Notice that in this example $n = 20$. Therefore, $\Sigma X^2/n = 3{,}246 \div 20 = 162.3$.

5. Square the mean of the $X$ distribution (i.e., $M_X^2$). In this example, $M_X = 12$, so $M_X^2 = 144.0$.

6. From the sum in step 4 (i.e., 162.3), subtract $M_X^2$ obtained in step 5 (i.e., 144.0). In this example, $\Sigma X^2/n - M_X^2 = 162.3 - 144.0 = 18.3$. This is the variance ($S^2$).

7. Obtain the standard deviation (SD) by taking the square root of variance: $SD = \sqrt{S^2} = \sqrt{18.3}$ 4.3. Thus, the depression score distribution $M$ is 12.0 and the SD is 4.3.

The second method for determining the variance and standard deviation is the deviation score method. The formula for variance ($S^2$) using the deviation score method is

$$S^2 = \Sigma x^2/n. \tag{12.8}$$

Again, the standard deviation (SD or S) is simply the square root of this result. Using the depression scores from Table 12.6, follow this simple six-step procedure:

1. Calculate the mean ($M_X = 12.0$).

2. Subtract the mean ($M_X$) from each score ($X$) (see the fourth column of Table 12.6: $x$, "Deviation Score of $X$").

3. Square each deviation score of $X$ (see the fifth column of Table 12.6: $x^2$, "Deviation Squared of $X$").

4. Sum this column ($\Sigma x^2$). Notice that in this example $\Sigma x^2 = 366.0$.

5. Divide this sum by the number of scores. Notice that in this example $n = 20$. Therefore, $S^2 = \Sigma x^2/n = 366.0 \div 20 = 18.3$. Thus, the variance is 18.3.

6. Obtain the standard deviation (SD) by taking the square root of variance: $SD = \sqrt{S^2} = 4.3$. Thus, the depression score distribution $M$ is 12.0 and the SD is 4.3.

| TABLE 12.7 | *SPSS* output of descriptive statistics for the depression and substance use scores. | | |
|---|---|---|---|
| | | **Depression** | **Substance Use** |
| *N* | Valid | 20 | 20 |
| | Missing | 0 | 0 |
| Mean | | 12.0000 | 9.0000 |
| Std. Error of 7 Mean | | .98141 | 1.35530 |
| Median | | 12.5000 | 8.0000 |
| Mode | | 14.00 | 8.00* |
| Std. Deviation | | 4.38898 | 6.06109 |
| Variance | | 19.263 | 36.737 |
| Skewness | | −.125 | .236 |
| Std. Error of 7 Skewness | | .512 | .512 |
| Kurtosis | | −.389 | −.978 |
| Std. Error of Kurtosis | | .992 | .992 |
| Range | | 17.00 | 20.00 |
| Minimum | | 3.00 | .00 |
| Maximum | | 20.00 | 20.00 |
| Percentiles | 25 ($Q_1$) | 8.2500 | 4.5000 |
| | 50 ($Q_2$; *Mdn*) | 12.5000 | 8.0000 |
| | 75 ($Q_3$) | 14.7500 | 15.5000 |

*Multiple modes exist. The smallest value is shown.

© Cengage Learning

Using the same steps for the substance use score distribution, the result is $S^2 = \Sigma y^2/n = (698.0 \div 20) = 34.9$ (variance). The $SD = 5.9$. Note that regardless of whether one uses the raw score method or the deviation score method, the final result is the same.

On a final note, there is some discussion in the field about the appropriateness of use of the "unbiased estimate" or an **attenuated standard deviation**, which uses $(n - 1)$ in the denominator rather than $n$. Be aware of this when using SPSS because it generally defaults to the attenuated sample parameter $(n - 1)$ rather than a population parameter $(n)$, so you could end up with a slightly different result. More important, as the number of scores in a sample gets larger, this difference becomes quite small. Table 12.7 provides the SPSS output for the descriptive statistics derived from the depression and substance use score distributions. Note that with an $n$ of 20, the attenuated $(n - 1 = 19)$, and non-attenuated $(n = 20)$ standard deviations are yielding very similar score interpretations.

# Symmetry (Skewness)

Most of the time distributions are not perfectly normal (bell-shaped). Generally, this is because samples are drawn from the global population and sampling error occurs (e.g., too many scores higher or lower than normally expected). A **normal curve** is perfectly symmetrical (bell-shaped), meaning that for every score occurring above the mean, there is a mirror-image score occurring below the mean to balance it. Too many low scores can quickly change the shape of a distribution; the same is true for too many high scores. When this occurs, the curve is said to be asymmetrical, or skewed. **Positively skewed** (or skewed right) means a distribution of scores has a lot of low scores (e.g., low-end piling) so a preponderance of scores fall below the mean. In other words, few scores fall at the positive end of the distribution, so the distribution "tails-off" in the positive (high-score) direction. When graphing a positively skewed distribution of scores, the "hump" or mode shifts to the left, and the tail of the distribution trails off to the right. If one puts an arrow on the tail of the curve, it will point to the right. To correct for a positive skew, the test developer can make the scale more normal by adding easier items to the item pool.

**Negatively skewed** (or skewed left) means that a distribution of scores has a lot of high scores (e.g., high-end piling), and so a preponderance of scores fall above the mean. In other words, few scores fall at the negative end of the distribution, and so the distribution "tails-off" in the negative (low-score) direction. When graphing a negatively skewed distribution of scores, the "hump" or mode shifts to the right, and the tail of the distribution trails off to the left. If one puts an arrow on the tail of the curve, it will point to the left. To correct for a negative skew, the test developer can make the scale more normal by adding more difficult items to the item pool.

Figure 12.7 shows a comparison of a normal curve with both positively and negatively skewed distributions. Note that on the normal curve, the mean, median, and mode are all at the same score (e.g., mean = median = mode). This is because the center point of a normal curve is the highest peak, and the distribution is bilaterally symmetric (i.e., a mirror image). When a distribution is positively skewed, the mean and, to a lesser extent, the median are pulled toward the tail (e.g., mean > median > mode). Likewise, when a distribution is negatively skewed, the mean and, to a lesser extent, the median are also pulled toward the tail (e.g., mean < median < mode).

It is important to note that obtaining a skewed distribution is not always a bad thing. In fact, it may be something you want to plan for. For example, when attempting to identify students at risk for math deficiencies, a test developer is interested in identifying the students who are performing below the average level and is not at all interested in including difficult items that might help to identify the best math students in a class.

The formula for determining skewness is

$$\sqrt{b^1} = \frac{\Sigma(Y - M_Y)^3/N}{[\Sigma(Y - M_Y)^2/N]^{3/2}}. \tag{12.9}$$

Generally, it is easy to identify skewed data by looking at the graphed distribution. This is not very precise, however, and there are varying degrees of skewness. A quick way of determining whether a distribution of scores is skewed is to compare the difference between quartiles $(Q_3 - Q_2)$ and $(Q_2 - Q_1)$. If $(Q_3 - Q_2)$ approximately equals $(Q_2 - Q_1)$, the distribution is probably normal. If $(Q_3 - Q_2)$ is substantially greater than $(Q_2 - Q_1)$, the distribution is probably positively skewed. If $(Q_3 - Q_2)$ is substantially less than $(Q_2 - Q_1)$, the distribution is probably negatively skewed. Applying this model to the quartile determinations for depression scores derived from SPSS output, $(Q_3 - Q_2) = (14.75 - 12.50) = 2.25$ and $(Q_2 - Q_1) = (12.5 - 8.25) = 4.25$. Because $(Q_3 - Q_2)$ is somewhat less than $(Q_2 - Q_1)$, the midterm score distribution may be slightly negatively skewed. Using the quartile determinations for the substance use scores derived from *SPSS* output, $(Q_3 - Q_2) = (15.5 - 8.0) = 7.5$ and $(Q_2 - Q_1) = (8.0 - 3.0) = 5.0$. Because $(Q_3 - Q_2)$ is somewhat greater than $(Q_2 - Q_1)$, the depression score distribution may be slightly positively skewed. Note that this method has no hard and fast index to determine whether the skew is of significant concern and, as you will see in the following paragraph, is often inaccurate. For the most accurate determination of symmetry, one should rely on computerized statistical packages, or Equation 12.9.

Many computerized statistical packages, such as SPSS, provide indexes of symmetry or skewness. As a general rule-of-thumb, index scores that range from $+1.00$ to $-1.00$ are considered symmetrical. An index of greater than $+1.00$ is frequently interpreted as positively skewed, whereas an index of less than $-1.00$ is frequently interpreted as negatively skewed. The further above or below these values, the more substantial the skew. In practice, larger samples ($n > 35$ or so) are likely to provide more symmetrical distributions. Note that the depression score distribution from Table 12.2 has a skewness index of $-.125$, whereas the substance use score distribution has an index of $+.236$. Thus, both are considered symmetrical distributions because each falls within the ranges of $-1.00$ to $+1.00$.

## Kurtosis

A normal curve also has a characteristic bell shape of specified dimensions (i.e., height, breadth). Most distributions, however, are a bit flatter or more peaked than normal because of the variation of scores around the mean. **Kurtosis** describes the degree of flatness in a curve. When a distribution of scores is flatter than normal, it is referred to as **platykurtic**. When a distribution of scores is more peaked than normal, it is referred to as **leptokurtic**. A normal curve is referred to as **mesokurtic**. Figure 12.8 displays mesokurtic, platykurtic, and leptokurtic curves. The formula for determining kurtosis is

$$\sqrt{b_2} = \frac{\Sigma(Y - M_Y)^4/N}{[\Sigma(Y - M_Y)^2/N]^4}.$$ (12.10)

Many computerized statistical packages provide indexes of kurtosis. As a general rule of thumb, index scores that range from $+1.00$ to $-1.00$ are considered mesokurtic. An index of greater than $+1.00$ is frequently interpreted as leptokurtic, whereas an index of less than $-1.00$ is frequently interpreted as platykurtic. The further above or below these values, the more substantial the kurtosis. Again, larger samples are likely to provide more normal distributions. The depression score distribution from Table 12.2 has a kurtosis index of $-.389$, while the substance use score distribution has a kurtosis index of $-.978$. Thus, both are considered generally mesokurtic distributions, although the substance use distribution is right on the borderline of being labeled a platykurtic distribution.

## The Effects of Transformations on the Mean, Variance, and Standard Deviation

Sometimes researchers transform data by adding, subtracting, multiplying, or dividing the score by some constant. A common example is when entering CEEB (i.e., SAT) scores, which have a range of 200–800 and always end in a zero. The researcher could always drop the final 0 digit for each score, effectively dividing each score by 10. As a second example, a researcher may want to add five points to every participant's score because some of the scores were negative numbers; adding five would make them all positive. It is interesting to examine how transforming a variable in these ways will affect the distribution's mean, standard deviation, and variance, as these statistics are commonly used when making decisions and interpreting scores.

| **TABLE 12.8**    The effects of transforming scores by a constant of 5. | | | |
|---|---|---|---|
| | **M** | **SD** | **S²** |
| Original data set | 10.00 | 5.00 | 25.00 |
| Add 5 points to each score | 15.00 | 5.00 | 25.00 |
| Subtract 5 points from each score | 5.00 | 5.00 | 25.00 |
| Multiply each score by 5 | 50.00 | 25.00 | 625.00 |
| Divide each score by 5 | 2.00 | 1.00 | 1.00 |

© Cengage Learning

**Figure 12.10**

Graphs demonstrating the effects of transforming data on the distribution mean, standard deviation, and variance.

(a) Addition of a constant

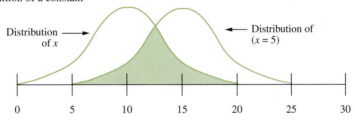

(b) Subtraction of a constant

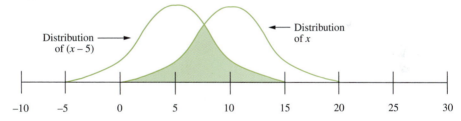

(c) Multiplication by a constant

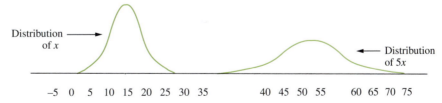

(d) Division by a constant

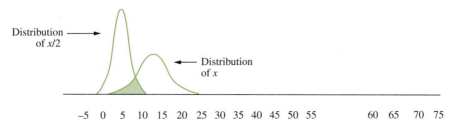

© Cengage Learning

Table 12.8 provides examples of the effects of adding, subtracting, multiplying, and dividing a constant to a distribution of scores. When adding or subtracting a constant, the mean always changes by the constant, but the variance and standard deviation remain unchanged. Also, the shape of the distribution is the same, whereas the position of the mean of the curve is shifted (see Figure 12.10). When scores are multiplied or divided by a constant, the mean, standard deviation, and variance all change. Also, the shape of the distribution is changed (i.e., flattens when a constant is multiplied, and peaks when a constant is divided), whereas the position of the mean of the curve is shifted (see Figure 12.10).

# Conclusion

Frequency distributions, histograms, frequency polygons, stem-and-leaf, and box-and-whisker plots are common ways of pictorially displaying distributions of scores, whereas the statistical analysis of scores yields a great deal of mathematical information helpful to test score interpretation. The mean (average), median (middlemost), and mode (most frequently occurring) are three common measures of central tendency, which mathematically describe the middle of a distribution. Standard deviation, range, and semi-interquartile range are commonly used methods of mathematically describing the variability of a distribution of scores away from the middle. Mesokurtic (normal), lepto-kurtic (peaked), and platykurtic (flattened) curves indicate kurtosis, or the general shape of a curve. Symmetry describes the skewness of curves that are not normally distributed.

*Now go to the Student Workbook found on cengagebrain.com that accompanies this text for additional application and review activities.*

# Deriving Standardized Scores

## CHAPTER **13**

T his chapter introduces the process by which raw scores are transformed into standardized scores, based on the mathematical properties of the normal curve, including *z*-scores, *T* scores, deviation IQs, and percentile ranks. Finally, we discuss transforming one type of standardized scores to another, as well as how to determine the area under the normal curve.

# Standard Deviation and the Normal Curve

At this point, you may be wondering what the preceding discussions of measures of central tendency, dispersion, and curve characteristics are leading to. These principles form the basis for understanding inferential statistics and the normal curve. The normal curve in turn serves as the basis for the interpretation of an individual's norm-referenced test scores, which will be discussed in the remainder of this chapter. Learning to compute, understand, and interpret standardized scores is important in research because score distributions are not always perfectly normal: some are skewed, have an unusual kurtosis, or are in some other way misshapen. After all, samples are drawn from a population, but the distribution of the sample may not look like the distribution of the population. However, those misshapen distributions can be smoothed or made to fit a normal curve.

Interpreting the standard deviation (*SD*) is something of a challenge, but it becomes more meaningful in the context of the normal curve. It is difficult to explain what *SD* is, but suffice it to say that it describes how the scores spread out from the middle of the distribution. Try to look at it this way: If the scores are nearly all the same and clustered around the mean, the *SD* will be very small, and the curve will probably appear leptokurtic. Then as many scores become farther from the mean, the variability increases, the *SD* becomes larger, and the curve may take on a more platykurtic shape. Unfortunately, differently shaped distributions may lead to confusing interpretations of test scores, particularly when the distribution becomes skewed. Statistically speaking, using the normal curve solves many of these interpretive dilemmas.

The **normal curve** is a bell-shaped, mathematically defined, smooth curve in which the mean, median, and mode lie in the exact center. The normal curve tapers as it proceeds away from the center of the distribution and, theoretically, approaches the horizontal axis without ever touching it (e.g., is *asymptotic*). It is the mathematical definition of the normal curve that helps examiners efficiently interpret norm-referenced scores. The area under the normal curve can be parsed into 100 units (blocks), and each unit can be viewed as equivalent to one person in a percentile rank range. These blocks can be stacked one on top of the other to indicate the number of individuals whose scores fall within a given range of scores. Figure 13.1 shows the classic normal curve with the actual, mathematically defined percentage of the population given in between the major *SD* units. The beauty of the normal curve is that the precise mathematical relationship allows comparisons to be made about different clients' scores on the same test, or about the same client's scores on different tests.

When you interpret scores using the normal curve, you always have the following information:

- 34.13 percent of all scores fall between the mean (0 *SD*) and one *SD* above (or below) the mean.

- 13.59 percent of all scores fall between one *SD* and two *SD*s (whether above or below the mean).

**Figure 13.1**

The normal curve, including standard deviation demarcations, percentage of population falling within standard deviations, and associated percentile ranks.

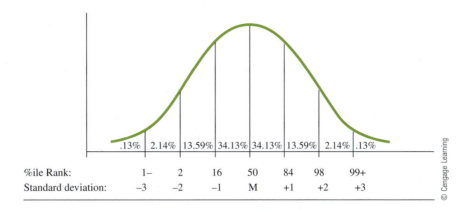

| | | | | | | |
|---|---|---|---|---|---|---|
| .13% | 2.14% | 13.59% | 34.13% | 34.13% | 13.59% | 2.14% | .13% |

| | | | | | | | |
|---|---|---|---|---|---|---|---|
| %ile Rank: | 1– | 2 | 16 | 50 | 84 | 98 | 99+ |
| Standard deviation: | –3 | –2 | –1 | M | +1 | +2 | +3 |

© Cengage Learning

- 2.14 percent of all scores fall between two *SD*s and three *SD*s (whether above or below the mean).
- Only 0.13 percent of all scores fall beyond three *SD*s (whether above or below the mean).

These mathematical constants define the normal curve and simplify interpretations of test scores across examinees and different tests. In combination, these demarcations also tell examiners the following:

- Half (50 percent) of the scores always fall below the mean, and half always fall above the mean.
- About 68 percent (68.26 percent) of all scores fall between one *SD* above the mean and one *SD* below the mean (±1 *SD*).
- About 95 percent (95.44 percent) of all scores fall between two *SD*s above the mean and two *SD*s below the mean (±2 *SD*).
- About 99 percent (99.74 percent) of all scores fall between three *SD*s above the mean and three *SD*s below the mean (±3 *SD*).

Although this discussion has focused on the "percentage of scores," or what is commonly referred to as percentile ranks, the normal curve has the wonderful property of equalizing all sorts of standard score scales (i.e., *T* scores, deviation IQs, and *z*-scores). That is, a deviation IQ of 130, *T* score of 70, and *z*-score of +2.00 will always mean that the score falls at the 98th percentile. Likewise, a deviation IQ of 85, *T* score of 40, and *z*-score of −1.00 will always mean the score falls at the 16th percentile. Such "interchangeability" is just one of the valuable characteristics of the normal curve. Applications of this information to test score interpretation will be expanded on in the next section. But for now, the reader should simply revel in the statistical beauty of the normal curve and appreciate the fact that it will make the professional counselor's life all the easier when faced with trying to help a client understand the meaning and implications of test scores! Standardized scores also sometimes simplify the analyses conducted by a researcher.

# Standardized Scores Based on the Normal Curve

Normally, data are entered into a database as raw scores and analyzed using various statistical procedures. Unfortunately, raw scores are meaningless without some context for interpretation. This is where the normal curve and score transformations come in handy.

As long as a distribution of scores does not violate an assumption of the normal curve (e.g., skewness), raw scores can be linearly transformed into standardized scores and interpreted with greater meaning. Linear transformation involves converting a (normal) raw score distribution with a given mean and *SD* into a standardized score distribution conforming to the normal curve characteristics with a standardized mean and *SD*. Making a raw data set "fit" the normal curve allows researchers and test interpreters to communicate a lot about a client's test score and performance. For example, if a researcher says the participants raw score was 50, that tells you very little. However, when the researcher says the participant's deviation IQ score was 100, or *z*-score was 0.00, it tells you that the participant performed at the mean of the score distribution, precisely at the 50th percentile rank. This is a great deal of helpful information! It places the score within some meaningful perspective relative to the distribution of scores with a commonly agreed upon, and usually easy to remember, mean and *SD*. Likewise, any standardized score received by a client on a given test, or even across various tests, can be understood within this context—a decided advantage when it comes to decision making about clients using test scores. Many types of standard score scales have been developed over the years, but a few are the most commonly used in research and counseling, and these will be reviewed now.

## *z*-Scores

A common type of standardized score used in research is the *z*-score. The *z*-score has a mean of zero, and an *SD* of one and is computed from the raw score distribution using the following formula:

$$z = \frac{X - M_x}{SD}, \tag{13.1}$$

where *X* is the participant's raw score, *M* is the sample mean, and *SD* is the sample *SD*. The formula basically allows the individual's raw score to be expressed as above the mean (a positive *z*-score) or below the mean (a negative *z*-score) in terms of the sample's *SD*. For example, assume that client A's raw score is 30 and client B's raw score is 45. By themselves, raw scores of 30 and 45 give little meaning. Perhaps one can only really conclude that the score of 45 is higher than a raw score of 30 by about 15 raw score scale points, but little else can be discerned without further information. To convert these raw scores to *z*-scores, you need to know the mean and *SD* of the raw score distribution. In this example, assume the sample of scores has a mean of 40 and an *SD* of 10. Using equation 13.1, the calculation is as follows:

$$\text{Raw score} = 30: \quad z = \frac{X - M_x}{SD} = \frac{30 - 40}{10} = -1.00$$

$$\text{Raw score} = 45: \quad z = \frac{X - M_x}{SD} = \frac{45 - 40}{10} = +0.50$$

By converting the raw scores into *z*-scores, we now know that a raw score of 30 is exactly one *SD* below the mean (−1.00 means "1.00 *SDs*"; the minus sign indicates "below the mean"), and a raw score of 45 is exactly one-half *SD* above the mean (+0.50 means ".50 *SDs*"; the plus sign indicates "above the mean").

## *T* Scores

*T* scores are frequently used in behavioral, personality, and clinical research and test development. A *T* score provides context for meaningful interpretation by declaring that the mean of a distribution of scores is 50 and the *SD* is 10. Thus, *T* scores greater than 50 are above the mean, and $T$ scores less than 50 are below the mean. In this way, the interpretation of scores is similar to $z$-scores, but the index of comparison has shifted (i.e., $z$-scores: $M = 0$, $SD = 1$; $T$ scores: $M = 50$, $SD = 10$). The formula for converting a raw score into a $T$ score is

$$T = (10)\frac{X - M_x}{SD} + 50. \tag{13.2}$$

Notice that embedded within this equation is the formula for computing a $z$-score. Thus, if one starts with a $z$-score rather than a raw score, the formula is

$$T = 10(z) + 50. \tag{13.3}$$

That is, the client's $z$-score is multiplied by the $SD$ of 10 and then added to the mean of 50. Obviously, this would result in a score below the mean (i.e., a negative $z$-score) being subtracted from 50 and a score above the mean (i.e., a positive $z$-score) being added to 50. Returning to the previous example of clients with raw scores of 30 and 45, $T$ scores are computed as follows:

Raw Score (X) = 30:

$$T = (10)\frac{X - M_x}{SD} + 50 = (10)\frac{30 - 40}{10} + 50 = 10(-1.00) + 50 = 40 = T$$

Raw Score (X) = 45:

$$T = (10)\frac{X - M_x}{SD} + 50 = (10)\frac{45 - 40}{10} + 50 = 10(+0.50) + 50 = 55 = T$$

Interpreting $T$ scores is similar to $z$-scores. In this example, a $T$ score of 40 is exactly one $SD$ below the mean, and a $T$ score of 55 is exactly one-half $SD$ above the mean.

## Deviation IQ and Standard Scores

Deviation IQs, which in the education and counseling fields are frequently referred to simply as **standard scores**, are commonly used to describe scores on intelligence, achievement, and perceptual skills tests. Notice that all linearly transformed scores have traditionally been called standard scores [(e.g., $z$-scores, $T$ scores) although I refer to these as "standardized scores" throughout this book], but in contemporary practice, deviation IQs are generically referred to as *standard* scores because it makes little sense to refer to a student's reading achievement score as a deviation IQ score.

A **deviation IQ** score provides context for meaningful interpretation by declaring that the mean of a distribution of scores is 100 and the $SD$ is 15. Notice that the $SD$ can be either 15 or 16, but at this point in history, nearly all tests use an $SD$ of 15. Thus, standard scores greater than 100 are above the mean, and standard scores of less than 100 are below the mean. Again, the interpretation of standard scores is similar to $z$-scores and $T$ scores. The formula for converting a raw score into an $SS$ (standard score) score is

$$SS = (15)\frac{X - M_x}{SD} + 100. \tag{13.4}$$

Again, note that embedded within this equation is the formula for computing a $z$-score. Thus, if one starts with a $z$-score rather than a raw score, the formula is

$$SS = 15(z) + 100. \tag{13.5}$$

That is, the client's $z$-score is multiplied by the $SD$ of 15, and then added to the mean of 100. This would result in a score below the mean (i.e., a negative $z$-score) being subtracted from 100 and a score above the mean (i.e., a positive *z*-score) being added to 100. Continuing with the previous example of clients with raw scores of 30 and 45, standard scores (i.e., deviation IQs) are computed as follows:

Raw Score (X) = 30:

$$SS = (15)\frac{X - M_x}{SD} + 100 = (15)\frac{30 - 40}{10} + 100 = 15(-1.00) + 100 = 85$$

Raw Score (X) = 45:

$$SS = (15)\frac{X - M_x}{SD} + 100 = (15)\frac{45 - 40}{10} + 100 = 15(+0.50) + 100 = 107.5$$

Interpreting standard scores is similar to *z*-scores and *T* scores. In this example, a standard score of 85 is exactly one *SD* below the mean, and a standard score of 107.5 is exactly one-half *SD* above the mean.

## Other Types of Standard Scores Used in Counseling, Research, and Education

As stated earlier, the number of potential standardized score scales is virtually unlimited. In addition to *z*-scores, *T* scores, and deviation IQ scores, the professional counselor should be aware of several additional standard score scales. **Normal curve equivalents (NCEs)** are standard scores with a mean of 50 and an *SD* of 21.06. Although this may appear strange at first glance, such a mathematical transformation allows for the normal curve to be divided into 100 equal units or intervals. Although not commonly used, NCEs are perhaps most applicable in achievement testing.

**Stanine** is short for "standard nine," a system that divides the normal curve into nine equidistant segments, using the formula $2z + 5$ and rounding to the nearest whole number. Stanines 2 through 8 represent a ½ *SD* range with the 5th stanine straddling the mean (i.e., ±¼ *SD* [*z*-scores of −0.25 to +0.24]). Thus, stanine 6 covers the *z*-score range of +0.25 to +0.74; stanine 7, +0.75 to +1.24; and so on. The stanine designations can be found in Table 13.1 along with many other scales based on the normal curve. Stanines are frequently used in large-scale achievement testing programs, but they should be interpreted with caution.

**Scaled scores** have a mean of 10 and an *SD* of 3 and are frequently used in intelligence, achievement, or perceptual skills measures to report on subtest or subscale scores. Then the scaled scores for these several subtests can be summed and converted into a standard score (*M* = 100; *SD* = 15). Perhaps the most popular example of scaled scores is the Wechsler Scales (e.g., Wechsler Adult Intelligence Scales, now in its fourth edition [WAIS-IV], and Wechsler Intelligence Scale for Children, now in its fourth edition [WISC-IV]).

Professional counselors should be aware of **CEEB (College Entrance Examination Board) scores**—yes, the unavoidable scale from the Scholastic Assessment Test (SAT)! CEEB scores have a mean of 500 and an *SD* of 100. What is somewhat different about CEEB scores is that the College Board only designates scores of 200–800, even though, theoretically speaking, the normal curve allows for scores to continue on in either direction to infinity.

## Percentile Ranks

**Percentile ranks,** or percentiles, indicate the percentage of observations that fall below a given score on a measure plus one-half of the observations falling at the given score. Percentiles are relatively easy to understand and to explain to those who have little or no

**TABLE 13.1**  Standardized score conversion table.

| IQ | %ile Rank | Scaled Score | Stanine | z-Score | T Score | NCE | Interpretive Range |
|-----|-----|-----|-----|-----|-----|-----|-----|
| 155 | 99.99 | 19 | 9 | +3.67 | 87 | 99 | Very superior |
| 154 | 99.98 | 19 | 9 | +3.60 | 86 | 99 | Very superior |
| 153 | 99.98 | 19 | 9 | +3.53 | 85 | 99 | Very superior |
| 152 | 99.97 | 19 | 9 | +3.47 | 85 | 99 | Very superior |
| 151 | 99.97 | 19 | 9 | +3.40 | 84 | 99 | Very superior |
| 150 | 99.96 | 19 | 9 | +3.33 | 83 | 99 | Very superior |
| 149 | 99.95 | 19 | 9 | +3.27 | 83 | 99 | Very superior |
| 148 | 99.93 | 19 | 9 | +3.20 | 82 | 99 | Very superior |
| 147 | 99.91 | 19 | 9 | +3.13 | 81 | 99 | Very superior |
| 146 | 99.89 | 19 | 9 | +3.07 | 81 | 99 | Very superior |
| 145 | 99.87 | 19 | 9 | +3.00 | 80 | 99 | Very superior |
| 144 | 99.83 | 19 | 9 | +2.93 | 79 | 99 | Very superior |
| 143 | 99.79 | 19 | 9 | +2.87 | 79 | 99 | Very superior |
| 142 | 99.74 | 18 | 9 | +2.80 | 78 | 99 | Very superior |
| 141 | 99.69 | 18 | 9 | +2.73 | 77 | 99 | Very superior |
| 140 | 99.62 | 18 | 9 | +2.67 | 77 | 99 | Very superior |
| 139 | 99.53 | 18 | 9 | +2.60 | 76 | 99 | Very superior |
| 138 | 99 | 17 | 9 | +2.53 | 75 | 99 | Very superior |
| 137 | 99 | 17 | 9 | +2.47 | 75 | 99 | Very superior |
| 136 | 99 | 17 | 9 | +2.40 | 74 | 99 | Very superior |
| 135 | 99 | 17 | 9 | +2.33 | 73 | 99 | Very superior |
| 134 | 99 | 17 | 9 | +2.27 | 73 | 99 | Very superior |
| 133 | 99 | 17 | 9 | +2.20 | 72 | 99 | Very superior |
| 132 | 98 | 16 | 9 | +2.13 | 71 | 93 | Very superior |
| 131 | 98 | 16 | 9 | +2.07 | 71 | 93 | Very superior |
| 130 | 98 | 16 | 9 | +2.00 | 70 | 93 | Very superior |
| 129 | 97 | 16 | 9 | +1.93 | 69 | 90 | Superior |
| 128 | 97 | 16 | 9 | +1.87 | 69 | 90 | Superior |
| 127 | 96 | 15 | 9 | +1.80 | 68 | 87 | Superior |
| 126 | 96 | 15 | 9 | +1.73 | 67 | 87 | Superior |
| 125 | 95 | 15 | 8 | +1.67 | 67 | 85 | Superior |
| 124 | 95 | 15 | 8 | +1.60 | 66 | 85 | Superior |
| 123 | 94 | 15 | 8 | +1.53 | 65 | 83 | Superior |
| 122 | 93 | 14 | 8 | +1.47 | 65 | 81 | Superior |
| 121 | 92 | 14 | 8 | +1.40 | 64 | 80 | Superior |
| 120 | 91 | 14 | 8 | +1.33 | 63 | 78 | Superior |
| 119 | 90 | 14 | 8 | +1.27 | 63 | 77 | High average |
| 118 | 88 | 14 | 8 | +1.20 | 62 | 75 | High average |
| 117 | 87 | 13 | 7 | +1.13 | 61 | 74 | High average |
| 116 | 86 | 13 | 7 | +1.07 | 61 | 73 | High average |
| 115 | 84 | 13 | 7 | +1.00 | 60 | 71 | High average |
| 114 | 82 | 13 | 7 | +0.93 | 59 | 59 | High average |
| 113 | 81 | 13 | 7 | +0.87 | 59 | 68 | High average |
| 112 | 79 | 12 | 7 | +0.80 | 58 | 67 | High average |

*(Continued)*

| TABLE 13.1 *continued* | | | | | | | |
|---|---|---|---|---|---|---|---|
| **IQ** | **%ile Rank** | **Scaled Score** | **Stanine** | **z-Score** | **T Score** | **NCE** | **Interpretive Range** |
| 111 | 77 | 12 | 7 | +0.73 | 57 | 66 | High average |
| 110 | 75 | 12 | 6 | +0.67 | 57 | 64 | High average |
| 109 | 73 | 12 | 6 | +0.60 | 56 | 63 | Average |
| 108 | 70 | 12 | 6 | +0.53 | 55 | 61 | Average |
| 107 | 68 | 11 | 6 | +0.47 | 55 | 60 | Average |
| 106 | 66 | 11 | 6 | +0.40 | 54 | 59 | Average |
| 105 | 63 | 11 | 6 | +0.33 | 53 | 57 | Average |
| 104 | 61 | 11 | 6 | +0.27 | 53 | 56 | Average |
| 103 | 58 | 11 | 5 | +0.20 | 52 | 54 | Average |
| 102 | 55 | 10 | 5 | +0.13 | 51 | 53 | Average |
| 101 | 53 | 10 | 5 | +0.07 | 51 | 52 | Average |
| 100 | 50 | 10 | 5 | 0.00 | 50 | 50 | Average |
| 99 | 47 | 10 | 5 | −0.07 | 49 | 48 | Average |
| 98 | 45 | 10 | 5 | −0.13 | 49 | 47 | Average |
| 97 | 42 | 9 | 5 | −0.20 | 48 | 46 | Average |
| 96 | 39 | 9 | 5 | −0.27 | 47 | 44 | Average |
| 95 | 37 | 9 | 4 | −0.33 | 47 | 43 | Average |
| 94 | 34 | 9 | 4 | −0.40 | 46 | 41 | Average |
| 93 | 32 | 9 | 4 | −0.47 | 45 | 40 | Average |
| 92 | 30 | 8 | 4 | −0.53 | 45 | 39 | Average |
| 91 | 27 | 8 | 4 | −0.60 | 44 | 37 | Average |
| 90 | 25 | 8 | 4 | −0.67 | 43 | 36 | Average |
| 89 | 23 | 8 | 4 | −0.73 | 43 | 34 | Low average |
| 88 | 21 | 8 | 3 | −0.80 | 42 | 33 | Low average |
| 87 | 19 | 7 | 3 | −0.87 | 41 | 32 | Low average |
| 86 | 18 | 7 | 3 | −0.93 | 41 | 31 | Low average |
| 85 | 16 | 7 | 3 | −1.00 | 40 | 29 | Low average |
| 84 | 14 | 7 | 3 | −1.07 | 39 | 27 | Low average |
| 83 | 13 | 7 | 3 | −1.13 | 39 | 26 | Low average |
| 82 | 12 | 6 | 3 | −1.20 | 38 | 25 | Low average |
| 81 | 10 | 6 | 2 | −1.27 | 37 | 23 | Low average |
| 80 | 9 | 6 | 2 | −1.33 | 37 | 22 | Low average |
| 79 | 8 | 6 | 2 | −1.40 | 36 | 20 | Deficient |
| 78 | 7 | 6 | 2 | −1.47 | 35 | 19 | Deficient |
| 77 | 6 | 5 | 2 | −1.53 | 35 | 17 | Deficient |
| 76 | 5 | 5 | 2 | −1.60 | 34 | 15 | Deficient |
| 75 | 5 | 5 | 2 | −1.67 | 33 | 15 | Deficient |
| 74 | 4 | 5 | 2 | −1.73 | 33 | 13 | Deficient |
| 73 | 4 | 5 | 2 | −1.80 | 32 | 13 | Deficient |
| 72 | 3 | 4 | 1 | −1.87 | 31 | 10 | Deficient |
| 71 | 3 | 4 | 1 | −1.93 | 31 | 10 | Deficient |
| 70 | 2 | 4 | 1 | −2.00 | 30 | 7 | Deficient |
| 69 | 2 | 4 | 1 | −2.07 | 29 | 7 | Very deficient |
| 68 | 2 | 4 | 1 | −2.13 | 29 | 7 | Very deficient |

*(Continued)*

**TABLE 13.1**  *continued*

| IQ | %ile Rank | Scaled Score | Stanine | z-Score | T Score | NCE | Interpretive Range |
|----|-----------|--------------|---------|---------|---------|-----|---------------------|
| 67 | 1 | 3 | 1 | −2.20 | 28 | 1 | Very deficient |
| 66 | 1 | 3 | 1 | −2.27 | 27 | 1 | Very deficient |
| 65 | 1 | 3 | 1 | −2.33 | 27 | 1 | Very deficient |
| 64 | 1 | 3 | 1 | −2.40 | 26 | 1 | Very deficient |
| 63 | 1 | 3 | 1 | −2.47 | 25 | 1 | Very deficient |
| 62 | 1 | 2 | 1 | −2.53 | 25 | 1 | Very deficient |
| 61 | .47 | 2 | 1 | −2.60 | 24 | 1 | Very deficient |
| 60 | .38 | 2 | 1 | −2.67 | 23 | 1 | Very deficient |
| 59 | .31 | 2 | 1 | −2.73 | 23 | 1 | Very deficient |
| 58 | .26 | 2 | 1 | −2.80 | 22 | 1 | Very deficient |
| 57 | .21 | 1 | 1 | −2.87 | 21 | 1 | Very deficient |
| 56 | .17 | 1 | 1 | −2.93 | 21 | 1 | Very deficient |
| 55 | .13 | 1 | 1 | −3.00 | 20 | 1 | Very deficient |
| 54 | .11 | 1 | 1 | −3.07 | 19 | 1 | Very deficient |
| 53 | .09 | 1 | 1 | −3.13 | 19 | 1 | Very deficient |
| 52 | .07 | 1 | 1 | −3.20 | 18 | 1 | Very deficient |
| 51 | .05 | 1 | 1 | −3.27 | 17 | 1 | Very deficient |
| 50 | .04 | 1 | 1 | −3.33 | 17 | 1 | Very deficient |
| 49 | .03 | 1 | 1 | −3.40 | 16 | 1 | Very deficient |
| 48 | .03 | 1 | 1 | −3.47 | 15 | 1 | Very deficient |
| 47 | .02 | 1 | 1 | −3.53 | 15 | 1 | Very deficient |
| 46 | .02 | 1 | 1 | −3.60 | 14 | 1 | Very deficient |
| 45 | .01 | 1 | 1 | −3.67 | 13 | 1 | Very deficient |

test sophistication, and they are commonly used with nearly all types of measures. Percentile ranks are easy to understand when one visualizes a line of 100 individuals with characteristics similar to the reference group under study (e.g., age, grade, and sex), with the first individual standing in line possessing the least amount of the construct under study and the 100th person standing in line possessing the greatest amount of the construct under study. If a participant scored at the 37th percentile rank (i.e., $P_{37}$), this means that his or her performance exceeded 37 percent of all those comprising the reference group. Table 13.1 contains percentile ranks and conversions to commonly used standardized scores. One can compute percentile ranks from a raw score distribution using the following formula:

$$PR = \left(\frac{100}{n}\right)\left(cf - \frac{f}{2}\right), \qquad (13.6)$$

where $PR$ is the percentile rank, $n$ is the sample size, $cf$ is the cumulative frequency, and $f$ is the frequency of occurrence of the value being determined. For example, using the frequency distribution data from the depression scale found in Table 12.6, you can determine the percentile rank of a raw score of 10 as follows:

$$PR = \left(\frac{100}{n}\right)\left(cf - \frac{f}{2}\right) = (100/20)(8 - [2/2]) = (5)(7) = 35.$$

Thus, a raw score of 10 in the depression data set has a percentile rank of 35 ($P_{35}$). Likewise, a raw score of 16 in that same distribution of scores has a percentile rank of 82.5 ($P_{82.5}$):

$$PR = \left(\frac{100}{N}\right)\left(cf - \frac{f}{2}\right) = (100/20)(17 - [1/2]) - (5)(16.5) = 82.5.$$

As you can see, the computation for percentile rank is more complex than for the standardized scores reviewed previously. Thus, most researchers and evaluators use conversion tables, such as Table 13.1, to convert a standardized score, that is, a z-score, standard score, or T score, into a percentile rank.

Percentile ranks should not be confused with percentage scores. A percentage is the percent correct out of the total. So if a client correctly responds to 17 out of 20 questions, and each question is equally weighted, the percentage score is 85 or (17/20)(100%) = 85%. Notice that percentiles indicate an individual's score as referenced to a comparison group of individuals with like characteristics—thus the term "norm-referenced." A percentage score indicates only the percentage of responses that met some criterion of correctness but not referenced or related to any group of individuals or scores—thus the term "criterion-referenced."

Also notice that unlike standardized scores, percentile ranks are not in equal intervals (i.e., an interval scale with equivalent distance between scale points). Thus, unlike standardized scores, percentile ranks cannot be subjected to mathematical operations such as addition, subtraction, or multiplication. To do so, percentile ranks must be converted to standard scores, subjected to mathematical operations, and then converted back into percentiles. Aside from this weakness, percentile ranks are very useful interpretive scores that statistically challenged individuals (e.g., clients, parents, teachers, and students) can understand. Related to percentile ranks, reporting a **quartile** is a common way of dividing a percentile rank distribution into four portions. $Q_1$ covers $P_0$–$P_{24}$; $Q_2$, $P_{25}$–$P_{49}$; $Q_3$, $P_{50}$–$P_{74}$; and $Q_4$, $P_{75}$–$P_{99}$. Finally, although neither a standardized score nor a percentile rank, an **interpretive range** can help convey performance information to those individuals who are unskilled in test score interpretation. Interpretive ranges are verbal performance descriptors such as Average, High Average, and Very Superior. When used with percentile ranks, interpretive ranges help describe client performance in very understandable terms.

## Converting One Standardized Score Into Another

Figure 13.2 and Table 13.1 serve as general conversion aids for the major types of standardized scores, percentile ranks, and interpretive ranges just discussed. Using the table, notice how easy it is to convert one type of score into another. In research and test score interpretation, it is extremely helpful to communicate in a single language, but this can be difficult if one scale uses a *T* score, another a percentile rank, and a third a deviation IQ. Conversion of these diverse types of scores to a single scale makes comparisons simple and meaningful. For example, consider a situation in which a professional counselor receives the following scores for a client: deviation IQ = 115; scaled score = 9; *T* score = 75; *z* = +0.20; stanine = 2; and percentile rank = 30. How could one make sense out of all of these scores? The answer is to put them on the same scale using a conversion table such as Table 13.1. Table 13.2 provides an example.

Notice how each of the scores can be transformed one on another, allowing an apples-to-apples comparison. Also notice that although percentile ranks are the easiest to understand, the mathematical limitation just discussed makes them the least desirable choice for further database computations. On the other hand, this is the primary reason that *z*-scores are so commonly used in research; one can easily manipulate *z*-scores mathematically and meaningfully.

**Figure 13.2**

The normal curve and myriad standardized score types.

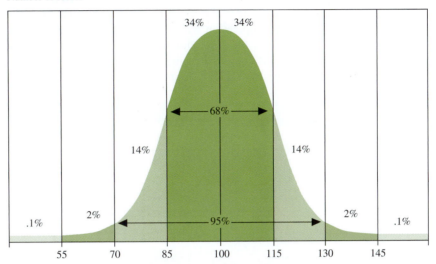

|  | Standard Deviations | | | | | | |
|---|---|---|---|---|---|---|---|
|  | −3 | −2 | −1 | 0 | +1 | +2 | +3 |
| **Standard Scores** | | | | | | | |
| $z$-scores | −3.00 | −2.00 | −1.00 | 0 | +1.00 | +2.00 | +3.00 |
| $T$ Scores | 20 | 30 | 40 | 50 | 60 | 70 | 80 |
| IQ ($SD = 15$) | 55 | 70 | 85 | 100 | 115 | 130 | 145 |
| Stanines |  | 1  2 | 3  4 | 5  6 | 7  8 | 9 |  |
| Percentiles | .13 | 2 | 16 | 50 | 84 | 98 | 99.87 |

© Cengage Learning

| **TABLE 13.2** | Conversion of various scores to common scales. | | | | | |
|---|---|---|---|---|---|---|
|  | **IQ = 115** | **Scale Score = 9** | **T Score = 75** | **z = +0.20** | **Stanine = 2** | **$P_{30}$** |
| Deviation IQ | 115 | 95 | 137 | 103 | 77 | 92 |
| Scale Score | 13 | 9 | 17 | 11 | 5 | 8 |
| $T$ Score | 60 | 47 | 75 | 52 | 35 | 45 |
| $z$-Score | +1.00 | −0.33 | +2.47 | +0.20 | −1.53 | −0.53 |
| Stanine | 7 | 4 | 9 | 5 | 2 | 4 |
| Percentile Rank | 84 | 37 | 99 | 58 | 6 | 30 |

© Cengage Learning

## Finding the Distance Between Given Scores

In research and measurement, it is sometimes of interest to determine the difference or distance between certain types of standardized scores, as well as the area between certain scores under the normal curve. For example, if a professional counselor wanted to know what percentage of the population fell between standard scores ($M = 100$; $SD = 15$) of 78.4 and 85.7, how could the counselor find out? Usually, standardized scores are converted into $z$-scores and compared using a table of values for areas under the normal curve. Table 13.3 is such a table; it contains the $z$-score designations for areas under a

**TABLE 13.3** Areas under the normal curve distribution.

| z | .00 | .01 | .02 | .03 | .04 | .05 | .06 | .07 | .08 | .09 |
|-----|-------|-------|-------|-------|-------|-------|-------|-------|-------|-------|
| 0.0 | .0000 | .0040 | .0080 | .0120 | .0160 | .0199 | .0239 | .0279 | .0319 | .0359 |
| 0.1 | .0398 | .0438 | .0478 | .0517 | .0557 | .0596 | .0636 | .0675 | .0714 | .0753 |
| 0.2 | .0793 | .0832 | .0871 | .0910 | .0948 | .0987 | .1026 | .1064 | .1103 | .1141 |
| 0.3 | .1179 | .1217 | .1255 | .1293 | .1331 | .1368 | .1406 | .1443 | .1480 | .1517 |
| 0.4 | .1554 | .1591 | .1628 | .1664 | .1700 | .1736 | .1772 | .1808 | .1844 | .1879 |
| 0.5 | .1915 | .1950 | .1985 | .2019 | .2054 | .2088 | .2123 | .2157 | .2190 | .2224 |
| 0.6 | .2257 | .2291 | .2324 | .2357 | .2389 | .2422 | .2454 | .2486 | .2517 | .2549 |
| 0.7 | .2580 | .2611 | .2642 | .2673 | .2703 | .2734 | .2764 | .2794 | .2823 | .2852 |
| 0.8 | .2881 | .2910 | .2939 | .2967 | .2995 | .3023 | .3051 | .3078 | .3106 | .3133 |
| 0.9 | .3159 | .3186 | .3212 | .3238 | .3264 | .3289 | .3315 | .3340 | .3365 | .3389 |
| 1.0 | .3413 | .3438 | .3461 | .3485 | .3508 | .3531 | .3554 | .3577 | .3599 | .3621 |
| 1.1 | .3643 | .3665 | .3686 | .3708 | .3729 | .3749 | .3770 | .3790 | .3810 | .3830 |
| 1.2 | .3849 | .3869 | .3888 | .3907 | .3925 | .3944 | .3962 | .3980 | .3997 | .4015 |
| 1.3 | .4032 | .4049 | .4066 | .4082 | .4099 | .4115 | .4131 | .4147 | .4162 | .4177 |
| 1.4 | .4192 | .4207 | .4222 | .4236 | .4251 | .4265 | .4279 | .4292 | .4306 | .4319 |
| 1.5 | .4332 | .4345 | .4357 | .4370 | .4382 | .4394 | .4406 | .4418 | .4429 | .4441 |
| 1.6 | .4452 | .4463 | .4474 | .4484 | .4495 | .4505 | .4515 | .4525 | .4535 | .4545 |
| 1.7 | .4554 | .4564 | .4573 | .4582 | .4591 | .4599 | .4608 | .4616 | .4625 | .4633 |
| 1.8 | .4641 | .4649 | .4656 | .4664 | .4671 | .4678 | .4686 | .4693 | .4699 | .4706 |
| 1.9 | .4713 | .4719 | .4726 | .4732 | .4738 | .4744 | .4750 | .4756 | .4761 | .4767 |
| 2.0 | .4772 | .4778 | .4783 | .4788 | .4793 | .4798 | .4803 | .4808 | .4812 | .4817 |
| 2.1 | .4821 | .4826 | .4830 | .4834 | .4838 | .4842 | .4846 | .4850 | .4854 | .4857 |
| 2.2 | .4861 | .4864 | .4868 | .4871 | .4875 | .4878 | .4881 | .4884 | .4887 | .4890 |
| 2.3 | .4893 | .4896 | .4898 | .4901 | .4904 | .4906 | .4909 | .4911 | .4913 | .4916 |
| 2.4 | .4918 | .4920 | .4922 | .4925 | .4927 | .4929 | .4931 | .4932 | .4934 | .4936 |
| 2.5 | .4938 | .4940 | .4941 | .4943 | .4945 | .4946 | .4948 | .4949 | .4951 | .4952 |
| 2.6 | .4953 | .4955 | .4956 | .4957 | .4959 | .4960 | .4961 | .4962 | .4963 | .4964 |
| 2.7 | .4965 | .4966 | .4967 | .4968 | .4969 | .4970 | .4971 | .4972 | .4973 | .4974 |
| 2.8 | .4974 | .4975 | .4976 | .4977 | .4977 | .4978 | .4979 | .4979 | .4980 | .4981 |
| 2.9 | .4981 | .4982 | .4982 | .4983 | .4984 | .4984 | .4985 | .4985 | .4986 | .4986 |
| 3.0 | .4987 | .4987 | .4987 | .4988 | .4988 | .4989 | .4989 | .4989 | .4990 | .4990 |

normal curve or distribution. To access the information within the table for this example, the professional counselor first needs to know the $z$-score equivalents for standard scores of 78.4 and 85.7. Recall that the formula for computing $SS$ from $z$ is $SS = 15(z) + 100$. Solving for $z$, this formula can be rearranged as follows: $z = (SS - 100)/15$. Thus, the desired $z$-scores are computed as follows:

Standard score of 78.4: $z = (SS - 100)/15 = (78.4 - 100)/15 = -1.44$

Standard score of 85.7: $z = (SS - 100)/15 = (85.7 - 100)/15 = -0.95$

Using Table 13.3, the area under the curve for a $z$-score of $-1.44$ can be located in the row labeled 1.4 and column labeled .04, which is .4251. Notice that because the $z$-score is negative (i.e., below the mean), to compute the exact percentile rank of $z = -1.44$, one would subtract this value from .5000, resulting in $P = 7.49$ (i.e., a $z$ of $-1.44$ is a percentile rank of 7.49). Similarly, the area under the curve for a $z$-score of $-0.95$ can be located in the row labeled 0.9 and column labeled .05, which is .3289. The exact percentile rank for this $z$-score is $.5000 - .3289$, or $P = 17.11$. Thus, the distance between the two original standard scores (78.4 [or $z$ of $-1.44$] and 85.7 [or $z$ of $-0.95$]) is .0962, or about 10 (9.62) percentile rank points.

Notice that if the $z$-score is positive, the value from Table 13.3 is added to .50 to indicate the area above the mean. For example, if a researcher wanted to know the area under the curve exceeded by an individual with $z = +2.29$, the correct value from Table 13.3 is .4890. Because the $z$-score is positive (i.e., above the mean), when the .4890 value is added to .5000, the result is .9890. This means that an individual with a $z$-score of $+2.29$ exceeded the performance of 98.90 percent of the comparison sample, or is in the top 1.10 percent of performers. Such information can be very helpful when exacting values are required.

## Conclusion

The chapter reviewed the major categories of standardized scores, including $z$-scores ($M = 0$, $SD = 1$), $T$ scores ($M = 50$, $SD = 10$), deviation IQs ($M = 100$, $SD = 15$), and lesser-used types like stanines, CEEB scores, and NCEs. Percentile ranks, quartiles, and interpretive ranges were also discussed. Now that you are familiar with the basics of descriptive statistics and curve characteristics, you can better grasp the concepts of correlation, regression, univariate and multivariate statistical analyses, and nonparametric statistics commonly used in research, all of which are discussed in the remaining chapters of this text.

*Now go to the Student Workbook found on cengagebrain.com that accompanies this text for additional application and review activities.*

# Statistical Hypothesis Testing

CHAPTER **14**

*by Richard S. Balkin and Bradley T. Erford*

Researchers frequently analyze theories or models, develop questions or hypotheses about how variables will behave as predicted by these theories or models, and design experiments to collect data that will answer the questions/hypotheses, thus confirming or rejecting the expected results. This process is known as **statistical hypothesis testing**, and it is based on logical, analytical questioning procedures. This chapter explains the process of hypothesis testing, including identification of null and alternative hypotheses, type I and type II errors, level of significance, and statistical power. A thorough understanding of hypothesis testing is critical to the appropriate use of inferential statistics, which will be addressed in the remainder of this book.

Assume that a counselor working with clients with anger management problems designs an anger management strategy to be used in group work. The counselor wishes to know whether the strategy is effective. So after the sample in this study was drawn from the population of interest and therefore assumed to represent the population, participants are randomly assigned to groups, with half of the participants receiving the new anger management strategy and the other half participating in a waitlist control group. Assuming that the methods used to gather the data will yield reliable and valid scores, this type of group comparison may fit under parametric univariate statistics (e.g., one normally distributed dependent variable measured on an interval or ratio scale). Hypothesis testing in univariate statistics is used to determine whether any change in the dependent variable is due to a change in the independent variable or simply due to chance.

The statistics used in a study are generally *inferential statistics* because a researcher makes a judgment on a population parameter based on sampling data. If a sample of participants has been randomly or in another way faithfully obtained, the assumption is that the results represent or extend to the population of interest. When conducting a study for empirical purposes, three steps are required: (1) translate the research question/hypothesis into a statistical (null) hypothesis; (2) design, conduct, and analyze the results (data) of the study using an inferential statistic; and (3) determine whether to reject or retain (never accept!) the null hypothesis. This chapter explores an expanded series of these logical steps that are employed in hypothesis testing and expanded on in Table 14.1.

## Identifying the Null and Alternative Hypotheses

Recall the discussion of research questions and hypotheses from Chapters 1 and 2. The first step in statistical hypothesis testing is to convert the research question or research hypothesis into a **statistical hypothesis**, more commonly known as the null hypothesis and alternative hypothesis. Because inferential statistics are about a population, the

**TABLE 14.1**    Steps in statistical hypothesis testing.

1. Identify the null and alternative hypotheses.
2. Establish a level of significance.
3. Select an appropriate statistic.
4. Calculate the test statistic and probability values.
5. Evaluate the outcome for statistical significance.
6. Evaluate practical significance.
7. Write the results.

© Cengage Learning

hypotheses are created using parameter statistics. The **null hypothesis** ($H_0$) is the hypothesis that is rejected or retained with inferential statistics and is often the opposite of what the researcher believes to be true (i.e., no difference exists). The **alternative hypothesis** ($H_1$) is generally the research hypothesis and is a statement of what occurs if the null hypothesis is rejected. Both the null and alternative hypotheses are written in statistical notation as population parameters:

$$H_0 : \mu_1 = \mu_2$$
$$H_1 : \mu_1 \neq \mu_2$$

(14.1)

where $H_0$ represents the null hypothesis and $H_1$ represents the alternative hypothesis. Notice that the terms $H_0$ and $H_1$ apply only to statistical hypothesis testing, not to the general terminology of research questions and hypotheses as discussed in Chapters 1 and 2.

In hypothesis testing, the null hypothesis is always tested. Consider the example in which the researcher wants to compare the mean score of a group of participants who are introduced to a new anger management strategy to the mean score of control group participants (i.e., a group of participants who do not receive the new strategy) on some dependent variable that measures anger. The null hypothesis ($H_0$) indicates that there is no difference between the groups. If the null hypothesis is retained, then no statistical group differences were found. If the null hypothesis is rejected, then the alternative hypothesis ($H_1$) can be considered (i.e., statistical differences do exist between the groups). Notice again that the researcher never "accepts" that the null hypothesis ($H_0$) is true. This is because the null hypothesis is a probability-based statement, and there are at least two additional reasons the experimenter must consider to explain the result: (1) a true difference may have existed, and the sample result did not faithfully express this true population result; and (2) there may have been bias in the experimental procedures that led to a conclusion of no difference when a difference did, in fact, exist.

Retaining or rejecting the null hypothesis is directly related to the amount of error the researcher chooses to allow in the study. Thus, the allowance of error is, in part, a subjective decision by the researcher. Whether $H_0$ is retained or rejected, researchers reach one of two decision outcomes: The researcher either makes a correct decision or an incorrect decision. Unfortunately, because statistical hypothesis testing is based on the probability of chance occurrence in a population based on observation of the current sample under study, one is never 100 percent sure that the decision outcome is correct. Figure 14.1 displays the logic behind the possible decision outcomes.

There are two types of error to consider in hypothesis testing: type I error and type II error. Other types of error exist as well, such as errors inherent in the experimental design of the research (as discussed in Chapter 7), but type I and type II error are most relevant to the current discussion and will be explained further here.

**Figure 14.1**

Possible decision outcomes in statistical hypothesis testing.

| | | In reality | |
| --- | --- | --- | --- |
| | | $H_0$ is true | $H_0$ is false |
| Decision about the sample outcome | $H_0$ is true (retain) | A correct decision $(1 - \alpha)$ We accurately retain a true null hypothesis. | An incorrect decision Type II error ($\beta$) We inaccurately retain a false null hypothesis. |
| | $H_0$ is false (reject) | An incorrect decision Type I error ($\alpha$) We inaccurately reject a true null hypothesis. | A correct decision $1 - \beta$ (called "power") We accurately reject a false null hypothesis. |

© Cengage Learning

# Type I Error

Type I error occurs when the null hypothesis is rejected but should have been retained. In other words, the researcher determined that statistically significant differences existed between the sample groups when the difference actually did not exist in the population. It is important to remember that, according to probability theory, there is always some possibility that sample differences will be due to chance rather than true sample differences. The amount of type I error is identified as $\alpha$ (alpha). The researcher has some control over $\alpha$, although sample size also influences $\alpha$. Still, the researcher always establishes the amount of type I error allowed at the outset of the study. The intricacies of establishing a level of statistical significance are discussed in the following section.

# Type II Error

Type II error occurs when the null hypothesis is retained but should have been rejected. In other words, the researcher determined that statistically significant differences did not exist between the groups of the sample when the difference actually did exist in the population. The amount of type II error is identified as $\beta$ (beta). Type II error is conversely related to statistical power $(1 - \beta)$: the likelihood of rejecting the null hypothesis given that the null hypothesis should be rejected. Put another way, statistical power is the likelihood of finding statistically significant differences, given that these differences actually exist (i.e., a correct decision). So if the likelihood of making a type II error is 20 percent, then statistical power is at 80 percent. There are mathematical formulae to compute statistical power and type II error, known as a power analysis. Computing a power analysis goes beyond the scope of this book (although an example is provided at the end of this chapter), but it is important to note that a given study should have at least .80 for statistical power (at least 80 percent power, or at most 20 percent type II error). Studies that lack sufficient power are more likely to make a type II error. The best way to avoid this problem is to have a sufficient sample size. Usually, a sample size of at least 15 participants for each group suffices nicely (Kirk, 1995).

Type I and type II errors may occur for several reasons. For example, the participants in the sample may not be representative of the population. If, for example, participants for the anger management groups were all patients in a psychiatric hospital, the results of the study may not be representative of the client population as a whole. Alternatively, the sampling procedure could be biased, such as if the researcher unintentionally placed adolescents with more severe anger issues in the control group. Although procedures exist to control for type I error, type II error is largely dependent on sample size.

So which is worse—a type I or type II error? Both have adverse consequences. Looking again at the anger management example, consider the following two scenarios.

## Scenario 1: Consequences of a Type I Error

The researcher determined that the group with the new anger management strategy had a statistically significant increase in their ability to manage their anger. But the researcher made a type I error, and the group with the new strategy actually did worse or experienced no change. Because the researcher was unaware of the error, the researcher publicized the findings and made a new policy of implementing the new strategy into all anger management groups. Thus, type I error can lead to ineffective treatments being implemented because researchers falsely believe the treatments to be effective.

## Scenario 2: Consequences of a Type II Error

The researcher determined that the group with the new anger management strategy showed no statistically significant difference in ability to manage anger. However, the researcher made a type II error, and the group with the new strategy actually did much better. Because the researcher was unaware of the error, the researcher discarded the new method, and future clients were never able to experience the benefit of the new method. Thus, type II errors can lead to effective treatments not being implemented because researchers falsely conclude effective treatments are ineffective.

# Establishing a Level of Significance

The level of significance in a study is directly related to the amount of type I error allowed in a study. The researcher identifies an **alpha level**, signified by $\alpha$, as the amount of type I error the researcher is willing to allow in the study. The alpha level, therefore, is the level of significance and is set at the beginning of the study. In social science research, typical alpha levels are around .05 to .01. Alpha levels can be larger or smaller. Alpha levels ranging from .10 down to .001 are not uncommon. The decision to allow for more or less type I error is somewhat subjective. Often, researchers review the literature and choose a level of significance based on previous research. If, for example, similar studies have a level of significance of .05, the researcher may decide to replicate the study using the same alpha level, or the researcher may choose a more conservative type I error. Higher alpha levels, such as .05 or .10, allow for a greater chance of type I error (5 percent or 10 percent, respectively) and are therefore considered more liberal tests of statistical significance ($\alpha = .10$ is frequently used to indicate a "trend" result). Lower alpha levels, such as .01 or .001, allow for a reduced chance of type I error (1 percent or .1 percent, respectively), and are therefore considered more conservative tests of statistical significance. However, such conservative measures have the undesirable affect of decreasing power. The relationship between alpha levels, statistical power (the likelihood of finding statistical significance if it actually exists), type I error, and type II error is shown in Table 14.2. The lower (more conservative) a researcher sets $\alpha$, the more likely the researcher is to make a type II error, meaning that it becomes more likely that an effective treatment will not be identified.

# Selecting, Calculating, and Evaluating the Test Statistic

The theory underlying statistical significance is that if a researcher draws 100 samples from the population, the means of those samples on the dependent variable will be normally distributed around a grand mean, which theoretically will be the mean of the population on that dependent variable. The researcher's experimental treatment is designed to change the sample mean, usually in the direction indicating improvement on the dependent variable. Therefore, the further the treatment sample mean is pushed from

| **TABLE 14.2** | Relationship between alpha levels, statistical power, type I error, and type II error. | | |
|---|---|---|---|
| **Level of Significance** | **Likelihood of Type I Error** | **Likelihood of Type II Error** | **Power** |
| Conservative (e.g., $\alpha = .01, .001$) | Decreased | Increased | Decreased |
| Liberal (e.g., $\alpha = .05, .10$) | Increased | Decreased | Increased |

**Figure 14.2**

Normal curve when $\alpha = .05$ (nondirectional).

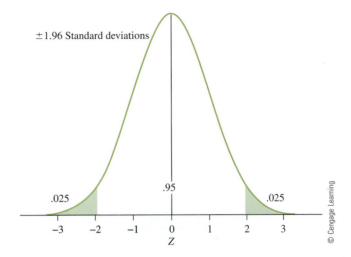

the population mean (usually represented by some control group sample mean), the more effective the treatment mean is proposed to be.

Once a level of significance is established, a critical value can be determined and a test statistic can be calculated. How to accomplish calculation of a test statistic depends on how the hypothesis is phrased and the dependent variable scaled (i.e., nominal, ordinal, interval, and ratio). (These computations will be covered in detail in Chapters 15–19.) Scores that are beyond the stated level of significance and critical value are considered to be statistically significant. The critical value will always match the level of significance, but the critical value changes based on the type of test statistic used, the number of groups being compared, and the number in the sample size. Figure 14.2 displays an alpha level of .05. On the normal curve, this amount of type I error can be divided into two halves known as a **nondirectional test** (i.e., the researcher predicts that the two groups will differ but does not predict which group will be higher; the treatment sample mean will be pushed away from the grand mean, but we are not able to predict in which direction the mean will move). Statistical significance can be found on either side of the normal curve. If $\alpha = .05$, then $\frac{\alpha}{2} = .025$ on either side of the normal curve. The shaded areas are referred to as the **region of unlikely values** because at the given level of probability it is unlikely that differences this great would occur by chance. Conversely, the unshaded area is referred to as the **region of likely values** because at the given level of probability it is likely that differences this great would occur by chance. In the Figure 14.2 example, scores that fall beyond z-scores of $-1.96$ or $+1.96$ would be statistically significant. For now, understand that scores that fall in the middle 95 percent of the normal curve are not statistically significant because the researcher set the alpha level at .05, indicating a 5 percent chance of type I error. Scores beyond that point, designated by $\alpha$ are statistically significant. Another way of thinking about it is if the researcher has established a 5 percent type I error rate, we can be 95 percent confident in the results. Chance sampling errors would only push the sample mean beyond the critical value 5 percent of the time—a very unlikely result, but one that is still possible. This is why a researcher never "accepts" the null hypothesis; it is always possible that chance error was at play.

Figure 14.3 displays an alpha level of .05 for a **directional test**. In a directional test, the researcher hypothesizes that a given score will be either higher or lower than the chosen level of significance. Consider the example of the researcher who decides to implement a new anger management strategy and is using a standardized instrument to measure progress. If the researcher hypothesized that the group who receives the new anger management intervention will demonstrate more progress (i.e., better outcome) than the

Normal curve when $\alpha = .05$ (directional).

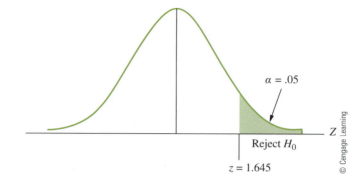

$\alpha = .05$

$Z$

Reject $H_0$

$z = 1.645$

© Cengage Learning

| TABLE 14.3 | Relationship between directional and nondirectional tests, statistical power, and the critical value. | |
| --- | --- | --- |
| **Type of Test** | **Critical Value** | **Power** |
| Directional | Lower | Decreased |
| Nondirectional | Higher | Increased |

© Cengage Learning

population upon whom the measure was standardized (i.e., the norm or average performance), a directional test would be used. The alternative hypothesis in this example may read, "Participants in the treatment group will perform better on the outcome measure than the mean of the standardization population." This means that the level of significance is placed to one side, rather than divided between both sides of the normal curve, as shown in Figure 14.3. Notice that the critical value is lower on a one-tailed $z$-test because 5 percent of the type I error rate is placed to one side of the normal curve, not divided by both sides. There is a relationship between directional versus nondirectional tests, statistical power, and the critical value, as shown in Table 14.3. In certain statistical tests, the researcher may need to determine whether the hypothesis is directional or nondirectional. For directional hypotheses, the null hypothesis is written the same, but the alternative hypothesis identifies the direction. Directional hypotheses have greater power because the lower critical value means the researcher is more likely to identify an effective treatment, if such a treatment exists. From the previous example, the researcher's alternative hypothesis indicated that the group who receives the new intervention would have a statistically significant higher score on a standardized instrument. So the null and alternative hypotheses would be written with the following statistical notation:

$$H_0 : \mu_1 = \mu_2$$
$$H_1 : \mu_1 > \mu_2$$

(14.2)

## Statistical Power

As mentioned earlier, **statistical power** is the likelihood of finding statistically significant differences given that statistically significant differences actually do exist. Put another way, power is the likelihood of rejecting the null hypothesis when it actually should be rejected. Power, therefore, is directly related to type II error. The more power in a study, the less chance there is to identify a nonsignificant difference when a significant difference exists. Statistically, power is expressed as $1 - \beta$ with type II error expressed as $\beta$.

The power of a study is dependent on several factors, including sample size, alpha level, effect size, error, and appropriate use of nondirectional and parametric tests.

As discussed earlier, a large sample size increases the likelihood of finding statistically significant differences. That is, a correct decision is more likely to occur when the sample size is 30 than when it is 15. Increasing sample size, however, will only substantially increase power when the original sample size is small. Adding more participants to a sample of 100 will only minimally increase power, whereas adding more participants to a sample of 10 will have a substantial effect on power.

The alpha level chosen at the outset of the study also has an impact. When the $\alpha$ is set at the .10 level of significance, as opposed to .05, the critical value is lowered and the likelihood of finding a statistically significant difference increases (e.g., $F_{obs}$ is more likely to be larger than $F_{crit}$). As the likelihood of making a type I error increases, the likelihood of making a type II error decreases, so there is an inverse relationship between $\alpha$ and $\beta$. Although procedures exist to decrease the chance of making a type I error, researchers run the risk of increasing the chance of making a type II error, especially when smaller sample sizes are involved.

Increasing effect size also increases power. The greater the magnitude of the difference between groups, the fewer participants needed to identify statistical significance. Effect size increases as the various levels of an independent variable work to create substantial differences in the dependent variable. Thus, the more effective a treatment is, the greater the resulting effect size. When planning for effective treatments, wise researchers ensure that the participants are exposed to sufficient intensities of the treatment and over a long enough period of time to maximize treatment effects.

Power is also influenced by error; the less error measured in a study, the more power. Researchers strive to minimize potential sources of systematic and random error by controlling extraneous variables, using dependent variables that produce reliable scores, and designing studies to account for threats to internal validity.

Finally, researchers must judiciously determine the appropriateness of test directionality and the statistical tests used to increase power. When all other things are equal, directional (one-tailed) tests are more powerful than nondirectional (two-tailed) tests. Likewise, parametric tests (e.g., $t$-test and ANOVA) are more powerful than nonparametric tests (chi-square and Mann-Whitney U tests).

Although issues such as the magnitude of the treatment effect or the error variance are minimally influenced by the researcher, the establishment of an alpha level and the sample size are easily controlled. Still, the most effective method of increasing power in a study is to increase sample size.

As an example, consider that the researcher of the anger management treatment study plans to implement a one-time, one-hour large-group guidance intervention with a class of 15 fourth graders, collect the dependent variable by administering an ordinal-scaled anger management instrument, and set $\alpha$ at .01 for a directional hypothesis (one-tailed), reasoning that the treatment should make the participants better managers of their anger. Although the preliminary literature review may actually back up each of these study design decisions, as mentioned previously, several adjustments could be made to increase the power of this study and increase the likelihood of determining that the treatment is effective, if indeed it truly is. First, sample size could be increased from 15 to 30 or even 50 participants. Second, the dependent variable should be changed from an ordinal-scaled measure (to which nonparametric statistical tests would be applied) to an interval-scaled measure (to which the more powerful parametric statistical tests would be applied). The researcher should also consider raising $\alpha$ to .05. Finally, the researcher should consider increasing the intensity of the intervention from 1 hour to 4–10 hours. This can be accomplished either by adding more sessions to the large-group format, or by altering the delivery so that it occurs in a small group delivery system. These modifications probably will substantially increase the power of the study and increase the likelihood that an effective treatment will be recognized as effective.

# Evaluating Practical Significance

Research methods may be wrought with emphasis on statistical significance. An unfortunate trend is to discount meaningful findings because no statistical difference or relationship exists. Perhaps not enough emphasis is placed on **practical significance**. Thompson (1999) identified the overemphasis on tests for statistical significance and emphasized the need to report practical significance along with statistical significance, because knowing where not to look for answers can be just as important as knowing where to look for answers. But moderate and large effect sizes may be found when statistically significant differences do not exist, usually because of a lack of statistical power. When sample size is increased, statistical significance will be evident. Thus, having sufficient power in a design can be very important to the manner in which results are reported and ultimately published.

For social sciences, power is usually deemed sufficient at .80; that is, an 80 percent chance of finding statistically significant differences when they actually do exist and a 20 percent chance of type II error. Popular statistical software programs (e.g., SPSS) may provide *post hoc* power analyses, which identify the amount of statistical power after hypothesis testing was conducted. Using the heuristic example of the anger management intervention between a treatment and control group, noting the amount of power in the test after data were collected is not very helpful. Rather, researchers should be informed of the necessary sample size needed *prior* to conducting a study. Hence, statistical power is analyzed *a priori*, that is, prior to collecting data.

*G\*Power* (available at http://www.psycho.uni-duesseldorf.de/abteilungen/aap /gpower3/) is a free statistical software program that conducts power analysis. Researchers can conduct an *a priori* power analysis to investigate the necessary sample size for a study, a sensitivity power analysis to identify the magnitude of the effect size (e.g., mean differences or strength of relationship in a correlation) necessary for statistical significance, or a *post hoc* power analysis, which provides statistical power estimates after hypothesis testing. *G\*Power* then provides information related to how many participants would be required in the treatment and control groups of the anger management study (*a priori*), to find statistical significance with a given alpha level and an estimated effect size, and usually estimates as small, medium, or large (Cohen, 1992). *G\*Power* could also be used to identify the necessary effect size, or the differences between the means, necessary to find statistical significance when the sample size and alpha level are known (sensitivity). Finally, *G\*Power* can be used to indicate statistical power after all analyses were conducted (*post hoc*). This alternative is probably the least useful. Balkin & Sheperis (2011) outlined steps for using *G\*Power* in counseling research and publication.

Without the use of statistical software, such as *G\*Power*, statistical power may be calculated through hand computations and use of power charts. To calculate power $(1 - \beta)$, the phi statistic $(\phi)$ must be calculated as follows:

$$\phi = \sqrt{\frac{\Sigma n_j (\overline{X}_j - \overline{X}.)^2}{j\sigma_e^2}}.$$

(14.3)

For an ANOVA, and using the self-efficacy study data from Chapter 16, this formula can be simplified:

$$\phi = \sqrt{\frac{\Sigma n_j(\overline{X_j} - \overline{X}.)^2}{j\sigma_e^2}} = \sqrt{\frac{SS_B}{j(MS_W)}} = \sqrt{\frac{114.6}{4(3.325)}} = 2.94.$$

Once $\phi$ is calculated, power can be determined using charts of power curves (see Pearson & Hartley, 1970). First, find the correct chart that depicts the appropriate degrees of freedom between groups—in this case, $4 - 1 = 3$. Next, use the family of curves that displays the appropriate alpha level. Each of the lines in the family of curves depicts degrees of freedom within: $n. - j$. Use $\phi$ at the bottom to match the appropriate line in the family of curves. Power $(1 - \beta)$ is on the corresponding vertical axis. Using the power curve chart that depicts $v_B = 3$, $\alpha = .05$, $\phi = 2.94$, and $v_W = 6$ (based on a sample size of 20 and $n. - j = 16$), $1 - \beta = .98$. There is a 98 percent probability of finding statistically significant differences given that statistically significant differences actually exist. Put another way, there is only a 2 percent chance of making a type II error. Statistical power analysis is frequently required by high-quality empirical journals and is essential to understanding the likely accuracy of decision outcomes in statistical hypothesis testing. The *G*Power* program immensely simplifies the power analysis determination.

# Conclusion

Researchers provide null $(H_0)$ and alternative $(H_1)$ hypotheses to explore relationships between or among variables. $H_0$ predicts no difference (or relationship) between or among groups, whereas $H_1$ ordinarily predicts a difference (or relationship). After the statistical analysis of the data is conducted, researchers either retain or reject the $H_0$. Correct decisions occur when the researcher accurately retains a true null hypothesis $(1 - \alpha)$ or when accurately rejecting a false null hypothesis (power, or $1 - \beta$). Incorrect decisions, however, occur when a researcher inaccurately rejects a true null hypothesis (type I error, or $\alpha$) or inaccurately retains a false null hypothesis (type II error, or $\beta$). Researchers have control over type I error by establishing $\alpha$ prior to conducting the study. Setting a liberal type I error probability (e.g., $\alpha = .05$ or $\alpha = .10$) helps to control for type II error $(\beta)$ and increases power. Other ways to increase power include increasing the sample size, increasing the treatment effect size, minimizing systematic and random error, conducting one-tailed (directional) tests, and using parametric statistical tests when appropriate. Calculation and evaluation of test statistics vary according to the nature of the hypothesis and the data collected (i.e., number and type of independent and dependent variables). The exploration of these important statistical analyses comprises the remainder of this book.

*Now go to the Student Workbook found on cengagebrain.com that accompanies this text for additional application and review activities.*

# Using SPSS for Introductory Statistical Analyses

## CHAPTER 15

The purpose of this chapter is to introduce you to the statistical computer program called SPSS. In this chapter, you will learn how to use SPSS to (a) enter data, (b) manage data, (c) report summary information both descriptively and graphically, and (d) analyze data using several common introductory inferential statistics. Throughout the chapter, we will use an example data set to illustrate various techniques and procedures in SPSS. Note that the basic statistical analyses can all be performed using other commercially available products such as SAS, Microsoft Excel, and R-stat (http://www.r-project.org/). Also note that Chapters 16–19 will demonstrate additional statistical applications.

Performing statistical tests requires many calculations. Not too long ago, researchers had to manually calculate these statistics, using complicated formulas and tedious procedures. More recently, mainframe computers provided the results to the calculations but at the expense of researchers' needing to learn rudimentary computer programming skills. Fortunately, technology has advanced to the point where virtually all researchers have access to statistical computer programs on desktop computers that usually just require choosing the correct menu options. The purpose of this chapter is to introduce you to one of the more common statistical computer packages: SPSS. Although managing data and performing statistical analyses have become much easier with the advent of programs such as SPSS, interpreting these results is still up to the researcher and consumer. Therefore, the statistical knowledge and skills you learn elsewhere will be necessary to make sense of the information provided to you by SPSS.

This chapter focuses on the most recent version of SPSS: version 21.0. Most of the features and functions of this version have been in place for several previous versions, so most of what is learned here will apply very nicely to earlier versions. (*Note*: The student version of SPSS may be different in places.)

One chapter cannot possibly present all the features available in SPSS. The primary goal of this chapter is to examine some of the more important functions and features necessary to perform several basic statistical tests. First, several functions and techniques that are useful in managing data for quantitative research are introduced. Next, some descriptive statistical procedures that will help describe data are presented. Finally, procedures for running a few of the more common introductory inferential statistical methods are demonstrated.

As you read through this chapter, you'll notice some shorthand methods used to talk about SPSS. Titles and headings of screens, dialog boxes, and sections of output will be shown in a monospaced font; for example, after opening SPSS, you are in the Data Editor window. Any named feature or function (e.g., a button, menu, option, procedure, or tab) will be identified with an *italicized font*. For example, at the bottom left of the main Data Editor screen there are two tabs, *Data View* and *Variable View* (Figure 15.1). Some procedures require multiple steps, which will be given here all at once but separated by vertical bars. For example, one way to produce basic descriptive statistics for a variable is to choose the *Analyze* menu, then the **Descriptive Statistics** submenu, and then finally

**Figure 15.1**

The Data Editor screen.

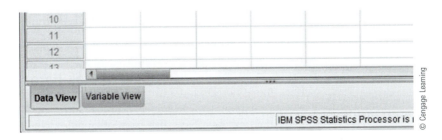

**Figure 15.2**

An example of multiple step procedures using *SPSS*.

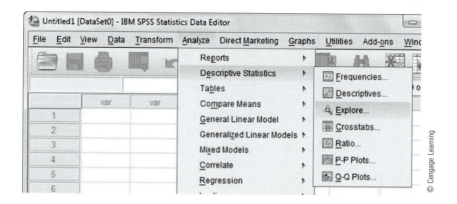

the *Explore* procedure option (Figure 15.2); this menu sequence will be shown as *Analyze|Descriptive Statistics|Explore*. Variables from our example data set will be printed in capital letters (e.g., GPA, GENDER).

As you play around with and learn the statistical program, you will discover that many of the approaches available in SPSS produce the same results. Certain approaches and procedures will be recommended here, but after working with the program for a while, you may find that you prefer slightly different approaches. Don't be afraid to experiment with SPSS; experimentation leads to comfort and confidence in future situations. As with so much else, learning to use a computer program like SPSS requires an investment of time and effort. SPSS includes several features to help individuals use the program. In particular, the *Help* menu provides access to a good *Tutorial* and to in-depth help on relevant *Topics*. The reader may find it helpful to implement the instructions in this chapter while actually using the SPSS program.

## Example Data

As the basic functions of SPSS are reviewed, data (included in Table 15.1) will be used for the following example. For many years, the Student Affairs division at a university has been providing alcohol awareness programs for students. Recently, however, national events have caused acute concern about binge drinking on college campuses. As a result, Student Affairs solicited help from substance abuse counseling professionals in the university's counseling center. The college counselors, in conjunction with Student Affairs staff, developed a workshop to focus on binge drinking and its negative impact on college students. To evaluate the new binge drinking workshop (hereinafter called "workshop"), they want to compare its impact on students' attitudes toward binge drinking with the impact of the existing alcohol decision making seminar (hereinafter called "control"). This two-level independent variable will be called Alcohol Awareness Program (AAP). Different students attended each intervention program, but we don't know how they were assigned to the treatments.

The workshop will be evaluated using students' attitudes toward binge drinking measured with a constructed instrument called the *Binge Drinking Assessment (BDA)*, which was administered about one week before and one week after each intervention program. The *BDA* contains five items scaled Strongly Disagree (1 point), Disagree (2 points), Neither Agree nor Disagree (3 points), Agree (4 points), and Strongly Agree (5 points). The *BDA* contains two negatively worded and three positively worded items. Data for several other variables have also been obtained, including the participants' biological sex

**TABLE 15.1** Example BDA data prior to data-screening.

| | ID | Gender | GPA | AWDU | Pre | AAP | BDA1 | BDA2 | BDA3 | BDA4 | BDA5 |
|---|---|---|---|---|---|---|---|---|---|---|---|
| 1 | A01 | 0 | 4.00 | 9.0 | 15 | 1 | 3 | 3 | 4 | 3 | 2 |
| 2 | A02 | 0 | 3.55 | 8.9 | 8 | 1 | 3 | 2 | 4 | 3 | 2 |
| 3 | A03 | 0 | 4.00 | 7.5 | 10 | 1 | 3 | 2 | 3 | 3 | 2 |
| 4 | A04 | 1 | 3.10 | 8.0 | 14 | 1 | 3 | 3 | 3 | 4 | 3 |
| 5 | A05 | 0 | 4.00 | 5.3 | 41 | 1 | 3 | 2 | 3 | 3 | 3 |
| 6 | A06 | 0 | 4.00 | 3.6 | 17 | 1 | 3 | 3 | 3 | 3 | 3 |
| 7 | A07 | 0 | 3.58 | 5.0 | 12 | 1 | 3 | 3 | 3 | 7 | 3 |
| 8 | A08 | 1 | 3.90 | 12.7 | 21 | 1 | 5 | 2 | 5 | 5 | 2 |
| 9 | A09 | 0 | 3.59 | 11.6 | 19 | 1 | 4 | 2 | 4 | 4 | 2 |
| 10 | A10 | 1 | 3.56 | 9.5 | 20 | 1 | 5 | 2 | 4 | 4 | 2 |
| 11 | A11 | 0 | 3.63 | 9.0 | 11 | 1 | 3 | 3 | 3 | 3 | 3 |
| 12 | A12 | 1 | 2.98 | 11.1 | 23 | 1 | 5 | -1 | 5 | 4 | 2 |
| 13 | A13 | 0 | 4.00 | 8.3 | 17 | 1 | 4 | 3 | 4 | 3 | 3 |
| 14 | A14 | 1 | 1.44 | 11.6 | 16 | 1 | 4 | 2 | 4 | 3 | 2 |
| 15 | A15 | 1 | 3.02 | 7.4 | 21 | 1 | 4 | 2 | 4 | 3 | 2 |
| 16 | A16 | 1 | 3.43 | 7.5 | 25 | 1 | 4 | 2 | 4 | 3 | 2 |
| 17 | A17 | 0 | 3.57 | 12.4 | 20 | 1 | 4 | 2 | 3 | 4 | 3 |
| 18 | A18 | 1 | 2.29 | -5.2 | 18 | 1 | 3 | 2 | 4 | 3 | 2 |
| 19 | A19 | 0 | 3.13 | 8.7 | 12 | 1 | 4 | 2 | 3 | 3 | 3 |
| 20 | A20 | 0 | 2.82 | 9.2 | 18 | 1 | 4 | 3 | 4 | 3 | 5 |
| 21 | A21 | 0 | 4.00 | 4.5 | 18 | 1 | 3 | 3 | 3 | 3 | 3 |
| 22 | A22 | 1 | 4.40 | 5.6 | 16 | 1 | 3 | 3 | 3 | 3 | 3 |
| 23 | A23 | 0 | 4.00 | 4.1 | 10 | 1 | 2 | 5 | 2 | 2 | 5 |
| 24 | A24 | 1 | 3.82 | 4.3 | 19 | 1 | 3 | 3 | 3 | 2 | 3 |
| 25 | A25 | 0 | 3.67 | 8.2 | 17 | 1 | 4 | 3 | 3 | 3 | 2 |
| 26 | B01 | 0 | 3.32 | 7.6 | 18 | 2 | 5 | . | 4 | 4 | 2 |
| 27 | B02 | 0 | 2.89 | 12.3 | 17 | 2 | 4 | 2 | 4 | 4 | 2 |
| 28 | B03 | 1 | 3.31 | 15.1 | 25 | 2 | 5 | . | 5 | 5 | 2 |
| 29 | B04 | . | 3.53 | 8.1 | 17 | 2 | 4 | 3 | 5 | 3 | 2 |
| 30 | B05 | 1 | 2.76 | 11.2 | 22 | 2 | 4 | 1 | 4 | 3 | 1 |
| 31 | B06 | 0 | 2.48 | 13.3 | 18 | 2 | 5 | 1 | 5 | 4 | 2 |
| 32 | B07 | 0 | 4.00 | 9.1 | 14 | 2 | 3 | 2 | 4 | 4 | 3 |
| 33 | B08 | 0 | 4.00 | 7.3 | 13 | 2 | 4 | 2 | 43 | 4 | 2 |
| 34 | B09 | 1 | 4.00 | 6.1 | 16 | 2 | 4 | 1 | 4 | 4 | 3 |
| 35 | B10 | 0 | 3.18 | 9.9 | 23 | 2 | 4 | 2 | 5 | 4 | 2 |
| 36 | B11 | 0 | 2.84 | 8.2 | 21 | 2 | 4 | 2 | 4 | 4 | 2 |
| 37 | B12 | 0 | 3.17 | 5.7 | 19 | 2 | 4 | 2 | 4 | 4 | 2 |
| 38 | B13 | 1 | 3.88 | 3.4 | 17 | 2 | 4 | 2 | 4 | 3 | 2 |
| 39 | B14 | 1 | 2.74 | 12.7 | 15 | 2 | 4 | 1 | 5 | 4 | 1 |
| 40 | B15 | 0 | 0.70 | 8.7 | 18 | 2 | 4 | 1 | 4 | 3 | 2 |
| 41 | B16 | 0 | 2.55 | 7.6 | 15 | 2 | . | 3 | 4 | 3 | 3 |
| 42 | B17 | 1 | 3.06 | 12.3 | 24 | 2 | 4 | 2 | 4 | 4 | 2 |
| 43 | B18 | 0 | 3.92 | 7.3 | 17 | 2 | 4 | 2 | 4 | 3 | 2 |
| 44 | B19 | 0 | 2.84 | 7.9 | 20 | 2 | 4 | 2 | 4 | 4 | 2 |
| 45 | B20 | 1 | 3.00 | 15.1 | 23 | 2 | 5 | 1 | 5 | 5 | 2 |

*(Continued)*

**TABLE 15.1**  *continued*

|    | ID  | Gender | GPA  | AWDU | Pre | AAP | BDA1 | BDA2 | BDA3 | BDA4 | BDA5 |
|----|-----|--------|------|------|-----|-----|------|------|------|------|------|
| 46 | B21 | 0      | 2.90 | 12.1 | 19  | 2   | 4    | 1    | 4    | 4    | 2    |
| 47 | B22 | 0      | 2.86 | 11.2 | 18  | 2   | 4    | 2    | 4    | 4    | 2    |
| 48 | B23 | 0      | 4.00 | 8.6  | 11  | 2   | 1    | 3    | 3    | 3    | 3    |
| 49 | B24 | 1      | 3.51 | 11.3 | 14  | 2   | 4    | 2    | 4    | 4    | 2    |
| 50 | B25 | 1      | 3.46 | 11.0 | 22  | 2   | 5    | 1    | 5    | 5    | 1    |

© Cengage Learning

**TABLE 15.2**  The *Binge Drinking Assessment (BDA)* data collection instrument.

Please provide the following information.

1.  Gender                    _____ Male                              _____ Female

2.  Current GPA               _____

3.  How many alcoholic beverages do you drink per week on average? _____

Circle the rating that most closely describes your feelings about these statements concerning the use of alcohol on the scale from Strongly Disagree (SD) to Strongly Agree (SA).

| | | | | | |
|---|---|---|---|---|---|
| 4.  Binge drinking is bad. | SD | D | N | A | SA |
| 5.  I frequently drink too much. | SD | D | N | A | SA |
| 6.  I usually drink responsibly. | SD | D | N | A | SA |
| 7.  I encourage friends not to binge drink. | SD | D | N | A | SA |
| 8.  I try to drink more than my friends. | SD | D | N | A | SA |

--------------------------------------------------------------------------------------------------

For Researcher Use:

Binge Drinking Assessment (pretest):   _____
Alcohol Awareness Program:             _____

© Cengage Learning

(GENDER), current grade point average (GPA), and the average number of alcoholic beverages consumed on a weekly basis (average weekly drink units, or AWDU). The BDA (data collection instrument) is presented in Table 15.2.

# Entering Data

By default, when one begins SPSS, an introductory dialog box will open with the heading "What would you like to do?" (Figure 15.3). From this dialog window, you can choose to type in new data or open an existing file. For now, just *Cancel* the dialog box, but in the future you may decide to open files from this dialog box or avoid this dialog box altogether by clicking the *Don't show this dialog in the future* option located at the bottom of the box. After leaving the introductory dialog box, you will be in the *Data View* tab of the SPSS Data Editor (Figure 15.4). Before you can perform any statistical analyses, you must create or open a database.

The Data Editor function in SPSS has several similarities to spreadsheet programs but also some key differences that will be described at appropriate places in this chapter. In SPSS, the spreadsheet rows represent the individual cases, and the columns represent

**Figure 15.3**

*SPSS* opening dialog box.

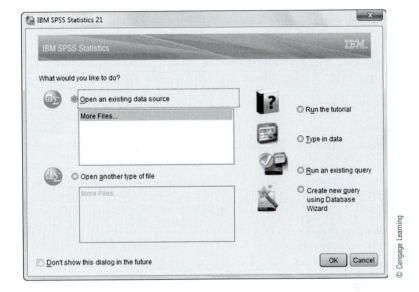

**Figure 15.4**

*SPSS* Data Editor box.

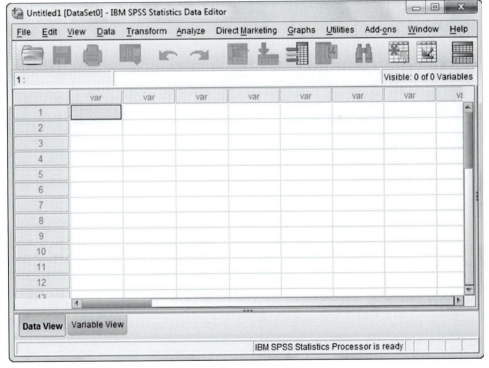

the variables. In Figure 15.4, notice that every column heading starts as *var* until the variable names are defined; the rows of the spreadsheet are labeled sequentially to represent the case numbers for the current data view. Because current case numbers change when you sort the data based on different variables, it is often helpful to provide every case a unique identification (ID) value. Sometimes you will have already done this by numbering surveys or experimental participants as you recorded their data; either way, it is handy to make the first variable in your database an ID variable.

**Figure 15.5**

*Variable View* of the binge-drinking study data.

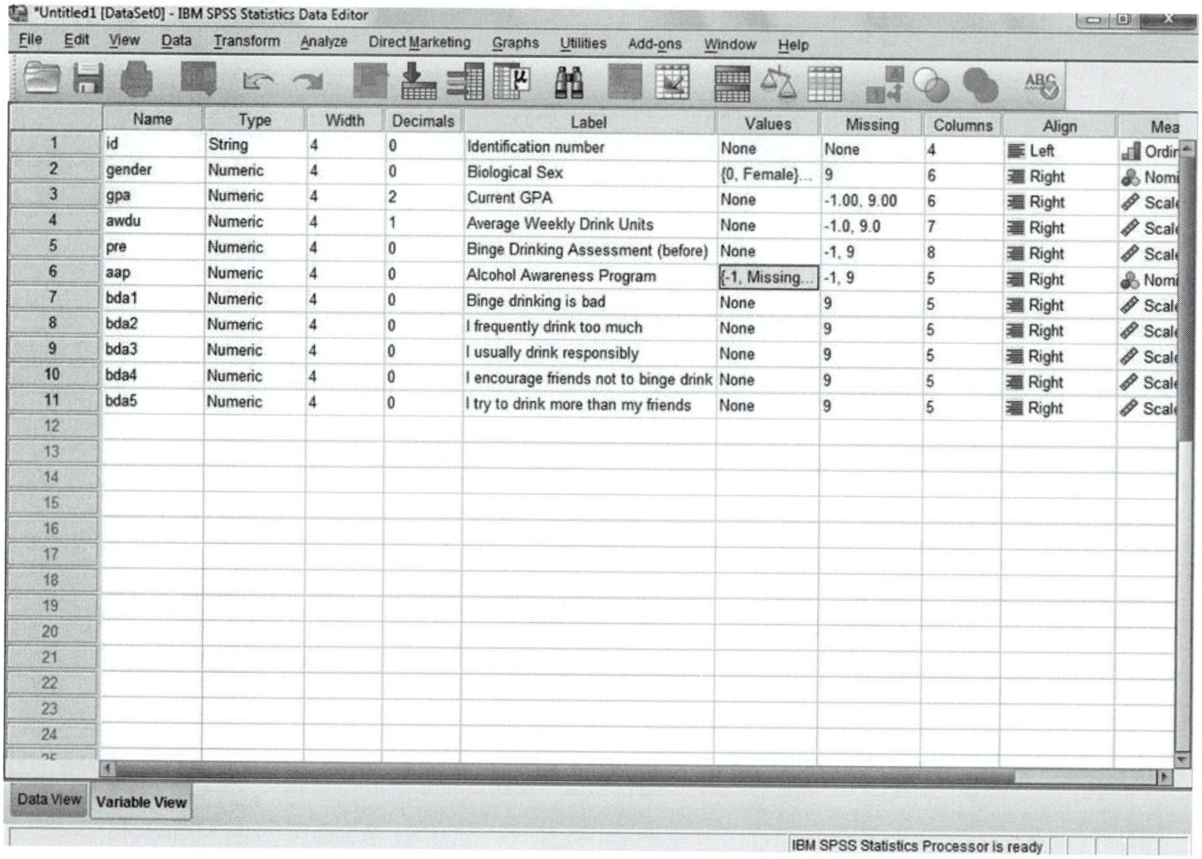

| | Name | Type | Width | Decimals | Label | Values | Missing | Columns | Align | Mea |
|---|---|---|---|---|---|---|---|---|---|---|
| 1 | id | String | 4 | 0 | Identification number | None | None | 4 | Left | Ordir |
| 2 | gender | Numeric | 4 | 0 | Biological Sex | {0, Female}... | 9 | 6 | Right | Nomi |
| 3 | gpa | Numeric | 4 | 2 | Current GPA | None | -1.00, 9.00 | 6 | Right | Scale |
| 4 | awdu | Numeric | 4 | 1 | Average Weekly Drink Units | None | -1.0, 9.0 | 7 | Right | Scale |
| 5 | pre | Numeric | 4 | 0 | Binge Drinking Assessment (before) | None | -1, 9 | 8 | Right | Scale |
| 6 | aap | Numeric | 4 | 0 | Alcohol Awareness Program | {-1, Missing... | -1, 9 | 5 | Right | Nomi |
| 7 | bda1 | Numeric | 4 | 0 | Binge drinking is bad | None | 9 | 5 | Right | Scale |
| 8 | bda2 | Numeric | 4 | 0 | I frequently drink too much | None | 9 | 5 | Right | Scale |
| 9 | bda3 | Numeric | 4 | 0 | I usually drink responsibly | None | 9 | 5 | Right | Scale |
| 10 | bda4 | Numeric | 4 | 0 | I encourage friends not to binge drink | None | 9 | 5 | Right | Scale |
| 11 | bda5 | Numeric | 4 | 0 | I try to drink more than my friends | None | 9 | 5 | Right | Scale |

© Cengage Learning

When defining a database, it is often useful to define the variables first. To begin defining variables, click *Variable View*. The *Variable View* tab allows one to define variables in a variety of ways. Figure 15.5 illustrates the definitions given to the variables in the database that will be used throughout this chapter. SPSS requires variable names to begin with a letter and not to contain spaces or other symbols (but numbers and underscores are allowed). One trick is to use the underscore character to separate parts of the variable name (e.g., pretest). Variable labels allow greater length and provide more flexibility than variable names because most characters and symbols are permitted. Be both clear and concise while providing short names and labels that completely describe the variable. Using shorter names and labels helps SPSS format output better; longer names and labels may cause output to be more difficult to read. One trick for working with survey data is to use the original item wording or abbreviated wording to help keep it short, like *variable labels*.

For categorical variables, one usually needs to provide numeric codes. SPSS will allow string data to be entered (characters, numbers, and symbols) but will not allow use of such data for analyses. Instead, code the categorical variables so that each number is given a label. To change the labels for the values of a categorical variable, click the appropriate cell in the *Variable View* tab, and then click the button with three dots in the Values column (e.g., the GENDER variable in Figure 15.5). Figure 15.6 shows the

**Figure 15.6**

The Value Labels dialog box for the GENDER variable.

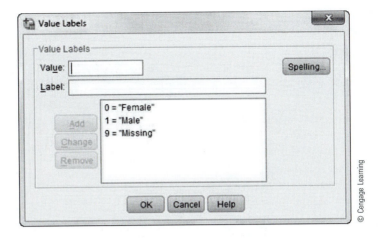

**Figure 15.7**

Variable descriptions using the *Working File* option.

## Variable Information

| Variable | Position | Label | Measurement Level | Role | Column Width | Alignment | Print Format | Write Format | Missing Values |
|---|---|---|---|---|---|---|---|---|---|
| id | 1 | Identification number | Ordinal | Input | 4 | Left | A4 | A4 | |
| Gender | 2 | Biological Sex | Nominal | Input | 6 | Right | F4 | F4 | 9 |
| GPA | 3 | Current GPA | Scale | Input | 6 | Right | F4.2 | F4.2 | −1.00, 9.00 |
| AWDU | 4 | Average Weekly Drink Units | Scale | Input | 7 | Right | F4.1 | F4.1 | −1.0, 9.0 |
| Pre | 5 | Binge Drinking Assessment (before) | Scale | Input | 8 | Right | F4 | F4 | −1, 9 |
| AAP | 6 | Alcohol Awareness Program | Nominal | Input | 5 | Right | F4 | F4 | −1, 9 |
| BDA1 | 7 | Binge drinking is bad | Scale | Input | 5 | Right | F4 | F4 | 9 |
| BDA2 | 8 | I frequently drink too much | Scale | Input | 5 | Right | F4 | F4 | 9 |
| BDA3 | 9 | I usually drink responsibly | Scale | Input | 5 | Right | F4 | F4 | 9 |
| BDA4 | 10 | I encourage friends not to binge drink | Scale | Input | 5 | Right | F4 | F4 | 9 |
| BDA5 | 11 | I try to drink more than my friends | Scale | Input | 5 | Right | F4 | F4 | 9 |

Variables in the working file

## Variable Values

| Value | | Label |
|---|---|---|
| Gender | 0 | Female |
| | 1 | Male |
| | 9[a] | Missing |
| AAP | −1[a] | Missing |
| | 1 | Control |
| | 2 | Treatment |
| | 9[a] | Missing |

a. Missing Value

*Value Labels* dialog box, from which one can make these changes. Notice that a value label can be applied to the codes defined as missing values but that one must still define them as missing codes in the *Missing Values* column in *Variable View* tab. The menu option *File|Display Data File Information|Working File* produces a table that describes the variables (Figure 15.7), such as the numeric values of 0 for female and 1 for male.

Clicking the *Data View* tab returns one to the main Data Editor window. Figure 15.8 shows some of the data used in examples in this chapter. View the value labels, or the

**Figure 15.8**

Partial data display.

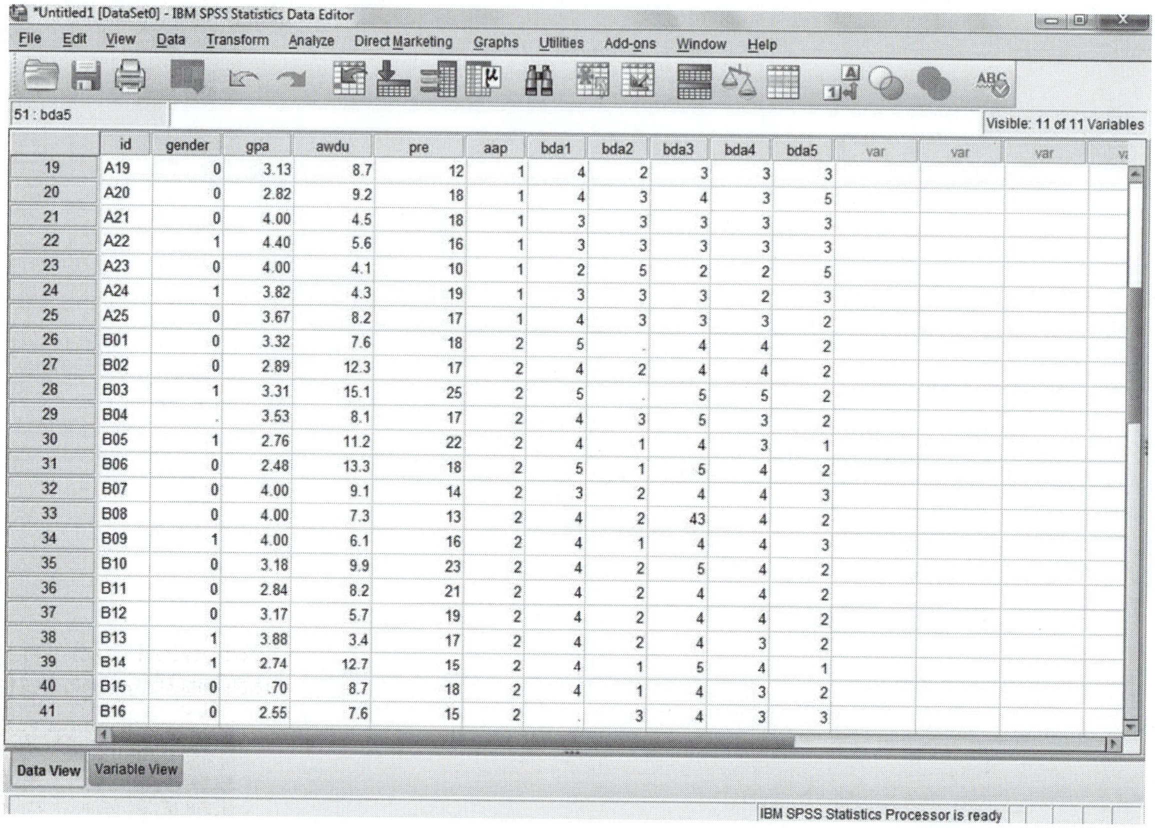


| | id | gender | gpa | awdu | pre | aap | bda1 | bda2 | bda3 | bda4 | bda5 | var | var | var |
|---|---|---|---|---|---|---|---|---|---|---|---|---|---|---|
| 19 | A19 | 0 | 3.13 | 8.7 | 12 | 1 | 4 | 2 | 3 | 3 | 3 | | | |
| 20 | A20 | 0 | 2.82 | 9.2 | 18 | 1 | 4 | 3 | 4 | 3 | 5 | | | |
| 21 | A21 | 0 | 4.00 | 4.5 | 18 | 1 | 3 | 3 | 3 | 3 | 3 | | | |
| 22 | A22 | 1 | 4.40 | 5.6 | 16 | 1 | 3 | 3 | 3 | 3 | 3 | | | |
| 23 | A23 | 0 | 4.00 | 4.1 | 10 | 1 | 2 | 5 | 2 | 2 | 5 | | | |
| 24 | A24 | 1 | 3.82 | 4.3 | 19 | 1 | 3 | 3 | 3 | 2 | 3 | | | |
| 25 | A25 | 0 | 3.67 | 8.2 | 17 | 1 | 4 | 3 | 3 | 3 | 2 | | | |
| 26 | B01 | 0 | 3.32 | 7.6 | 18 | 2 | 5 | . | 4 | 4 | 2 | | | |
| 27 | B02 | 0 | 2.89 | 12.3 | 17 | 2 | 4 | 2 | 4 | 4 | 2 | | | |
| 28 | B03 | 1 | 3.31 | 15.1 | 25 | 2 | 5 | . | 5 | 5 | 2 | | | |
| 29 | B04 | . | 3.53 | 8.1 | 17 | 2 | 4 | 3 | 5 | 3 | 2 | | | |
| 30 | B05 | 1 | 2.76 | 11.2 | 22 | 2 | 4 | 1 | 4 | 3 | 1 | | | |
| 31 | B06 | 0 | 2.48 | 13.3 | 18 | 2 | 5 | 1 | 5 | 4 | 2 | | | |
| 32 | B07 | 0 | 4.00 | 9.1 | 14 | 2 | 3 | 2 | 4 | 4 | 3 | | | |
| 33 | B08 | 0 | 4.00 | 7.3 | 13 | 2 | 4 | 2 | 43 | 4 | 2 | | | |
| 34 | B09 | 1 | 4.00 | 6.1 | 16 | 2 | 4 | 1 | 4 | 4 | 3 | | | |
| 35 | B10 | 0 | 3.18 | 9.9 | 23 | 2 | 4 | 2 | 5 | 4 | 2 | | | |
| 36 | B11 | 0 | 2.84 | 8.2 | 21 | 2 | 4 | 2 | 4 | 4 | 2 | | | |
| 37 | B12 | 0 | 3.17 | 5.7 | 19 | 2 | 4 | 2 | 4 | 4 | 2 | | | |
| 38 | B13 | 1 | 3.88 | 3.4 | 17 | 2 | 4 | 2 | 4 | 3 | 2 | | | |
| 39 | B14 | 1 | 2.74 | 12.7 | 15 | 2 | 4 | 1 | 5 | 4 | 1 | | | |
| 40 | B15 | 0 | .70 | 8.7 | 18 | 2 | 4 | 1 | 4 | 3 | 2 | | | |
| 41 | B16 | 0 | 2.55 | 7.6 | 15 | 2 | . | 3 | 4 | 3 | 3 | | | |



actual numeric data, by toggling the *View|Value Labels* menu option. Notice in Figure 15.8 that case 26 (with ID B01) and case 28 (with ID B03) have dots as values for variable BDA2. These dots represent missing values as designated by default by the SPSS system. It is often useful to designate a particular value (e.g., −1 or 9) for missing values so that it will be known later that the original data were actually looked at and identified as missing rather than being unsure whether they were just skipped when they were entered (which resulted in the dot). Note that if a missing value code in the data is used (e.g., −1 or 9, 99, or even 999, under the *Discrete Missing Values* option), be sure to set up the missing value code (Figure 15.9) in the *Variable View* tab (Figure 15.5); otherwise, the missing value will be analyzed as if it were legitimate and therefore included inappropriately in all calculations. You also may have noticed that case 33 (with ID B08 in Figure 15.8) has a much larger value than all the other cases. To try to identify such potential problems, screen the data for accuracy after finishing data entry but before doing any statistical analyses, and then change the data value to a missing code if it can't be corrected.

Entering data into SPSS is just a matter of typing the appropriate values and moving through the database using the mouse or keyboard navigation keys. One can practice by entering the example data from Table 15.1 into an SPSS data file, which can then allow one to perform analyses specified later in the chapter. Sometimes researchers have data from either SPSS or another source already saved. For example, some researchers prefer

**Figure 15.9**

Missing values dialog box.

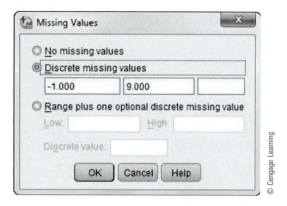

to enter their data into a text processor or a spreadsheet program and then import the data into SPSS. By choosing *File|Open|Data*, one can open saved SPSS data files or import several kinds of files; *File|Read Text Data* opens a wizard to import text files into the Data Editor. *File|Recently Used Data* provides quick access to the most current files.

# Interaction with SPSS

Most researchers interact with SPSS through the menu structure and dialog boxes, but there are other ways to communicate with SPSS. At its heart, SPSS is really a command processor; that is, all procedures are actually run based on a series of text commands that are generated by the menu options (or entered directly into the SPSS Syntax Editor through *File|New|Syntax* in the full version of the program). Using syntax ensures the ability to run the procedure exactly the same way in the future (because sometimes it is hard to remember which menu options were selected in a previous analysis) and provides access to some options that are not available through the menu structure. An example of the syntax is displayed in the top section of Figure 15.10. The section of text that begins with EXAMINE... and ends with .../NOTOTAL represents syntax that will run the *Explore* procedure. The full version of SPSS provides an option, *Edit| Options||Viewer|Display commands in the log*, that will automatically report the syntax input used to create the output shown in the SPSS Viewer, but all versions include the syntax in the Notes table that is usually hidden in the output by default.

In this chapter, the menus and the dialog boxes will be used exclusively for examples (most introductory procedures are implemented well with the menu options). There are some things to keep in mind when beginning to learn how to communicate with SPSS, most of which will be relevant to dialog boxes throughout SPSS. For example, notice in Figure 15.11, which is the main dialog box opened by *Analyze|Descriptive Statistics| Frequencies*, that all variables are listed in an unlabeled window on the left. By default, the variables are listed by their variable labels, with variable names in brackets after the label, in the order they are shown in the SPSS Data Editor; these are among the settings one can change in the *Edit|Options* dialog window. To analyze the data, you must move at least one variable into the Variable(s) window on the right. To run the same analysis on a set of variables, one can either enter one variable at a time and run the procedure multiple times, or make several variables active at the same time and run the analysis only once (and sometimes one must choose more than one variable for an analysis). Also notice the *Statistics*, *Charts*, and *Options* buttons across the bottom of the dialog

**Figure 15.10**

Example of *SPSS* syntax.

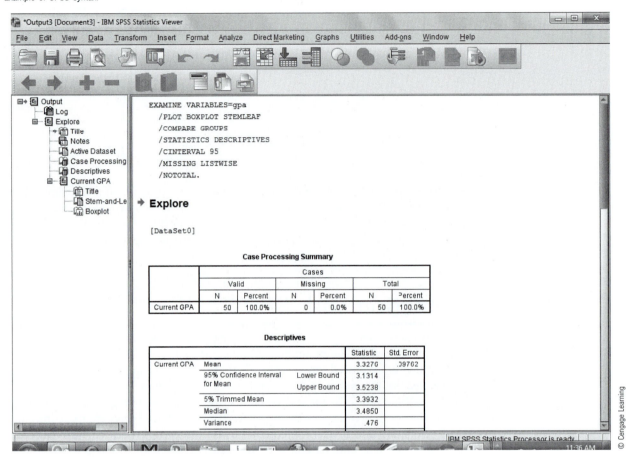

**Figure 15.11**

List of variables viewed in the *Frequencies* dialog box.

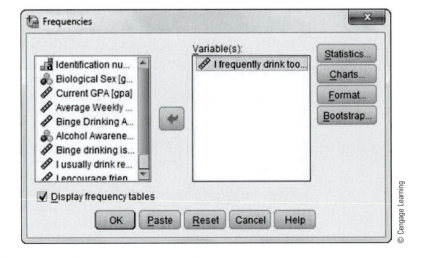

**Figure 15.12**

The *Statistics* dialog box.

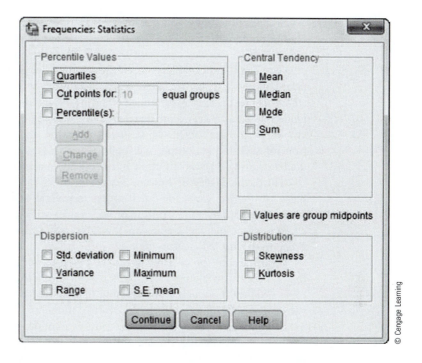

box. Most SPSS dialog boxes will have similar buttons that open additional dialog boxes. For example, after clicking the *Statistics* button, the dialog box in Figure 15.12 opens. Pay attention to these dialog boxes because one may not necessarily want to run the same default options every time a procedure is run.

## SPSS Output

The output in SPSS is opened in a new window that includes the words *SPSS Viewer* on the window title bar (Figure 15.10). There are a few other things to remember about the output window. First, SPSS repeats all menus from the SPSS Data Editor window so that one can perform most functions from either location; that is, you do not need to return to the Data Editor to run successive analyses. To return to the Data Editor (e.g., for the purpose of examining standardized scores that were saved in the database by the *Descriptives* procedure), either use the *Window* menu (Figure 15.13) or click on the appropriate Windows taskbar button.

**Figure 15.13**

The *Window* menu.

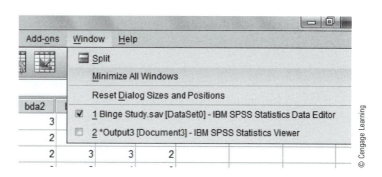

Second, the output can get quite long, especially if you run multiple procedures. The Output outline on the left of the SPSS Viewer window can help navigate through the output (Figure 15.10). You can print and save the entire output or select parts of the output to save or print. Output tables and graphs can be selected by single-clicking on them or edited by double-clicking on them; right-clicking while in edit mode provides access to the editing context menu. Also, notice Notes in the outline of Figure 15.10, which is currently hidden and has a gray icon that looks like a closed book, which means that it is neither visible nor printed (but it will be saved when the output is saved). Double-clicking on an icon for such hidden output will make it visible (thus, it will look like an open book), or double-clicking on visible output in the outline makes it become hidden.

Third, the *File|Print Preview* feature in SPSS can often help save paper (notice that there are toolbar icons for quick access to several of these more useful functions). One useful feature allows the printing of wide tables within the printed page margins: double-click on the table, right-click on the table while in edit mode, and then choose *Table Properties|Printing|Rescale wide table to fit page*.

Fourth, many procedures begin their output with a **Case Processing Summary** like the one shown in Figure 15.10. This part of the output is useful primarily to help determine whether more values are missing than should be. Of course, if no data are missing, you can usually ignore this table. Notice, though, that because of different methods of handling missing data, different procedures may process different numbers of cases.

Fifth, right-clicking on an output table enables a context menu that includes an option called *Results Coach*, which provides context-sensitive access to the *SPSS Tutorial* that may help the user interpret some results.

Sixth, to open saved output from the Data Editor, you must use the *File|Open|Output* menu commands. In the SPSS Viewer, the *Open Folder* icon on the task bar (the manila folder icon) will open output files; in the Data Editor, however, the same icon opens only data files.

Finally, output can be copied to another program, such as a word processor, by selecting the output and using the *Edit|Copy* command. With some output, however, the process works much more smoothly when you use the *Edit|Copy Objects* command. Be aware, though, that most of the output provided by SPSS does not meet the strict guidelines for *APA Style*.

# Screening and Cleaning Data

Dirty data lead to inaccurate results! This may sound very simple, but the most important thing to do after entering data is to make sure it was entered correctly; that is, be sure to analyze good, clean data. Problem data usually result from two sources: data that are entered incorrectly and participants who provide very strange information. Either way, screening the data leads to working with the best possible information. It may seem reasonable to look over all the data case by case and try to identify potential problem values, either by scrolling through the Data Editor window or by using the *Analyze| Reports|Case Summaries* menu option (which was used to create the example data in Table 15.1). Indeed, many potential problems may be identified that way, particularly with smaller databases. Unfortunately, even for smaller databases some problem values may be missed using such a process. Several SPSS procedures can help identify strange values quickly. Beware, though, that even these techniques will only help to identify extreme values not necessarily data entered incorrectly but within the reasonable range of values (e.g., no technique will easily identify a participant who had an actual score of 3 on a 5-point rating scale but for whom a 2 was incorrectly entered). The only way to

**Figure 15.14**

*Frequencies* output table for the variable, "I frequently drink too much."

## Statistics

I frequently drink too much

| N | Valid | 48 |
|---|---|---|
| | Missing | 2 |

I frequently drink too much

| | | Frequency | Percent | Valid Percent | Cumulative Percent |
|---|---|---|---|---|---|
| Valid | −1 | 1 | 2.0 | 2.1 | 2.1 |
| | 1 | 8 | 16.0 | 16.7 | 18.8 |
| | 2 | 24 | 48.0 | 50.0 | 68.8 |
| | 3 | 14 | 28.0 | 29.2 | 97.9 |
| | 5 | 1 | 2.0 | 2.1 | 100.0 |
| | Total | 48 | 96.0 | 100.0 | |
| Missing | System | 2 | 4.0 | | |
| Total | | 50 | 100.0 | | |

verify data completely is to review the information from a variety of approaches, including inspecting each case individually.

For categorical variables, and even ordinal or scale variables (what SPSS calls interval and ratio data) with only a few possible scores, the *Analyze|Descriptive Statistics|Frequencies* procedure can be used to examine the data. Figure 15.14 shows the frequency table output from the **Frequencies** procedure for one of the BDA scale items in our example data, BDA2. A few potential problems in these results can be noticed, including an invalid score and two system missing values. One can sort the data in the Data Editor by right-clicking on the column heading for BDA2 and then choosing **Sort Ascending** (Figure 15.15). We find that case 1 (with ID B01) and case 2 (with ID B03) both have the system missing values. To check these, review the original data source (e.g., survey and experimental notes) to determine whether these values were skipped while entering data or whether the values are really missing. After reviewing the original data source, either enter the correct value or change the system missing value to one of the missing value codes. Because both cases in the example should have a value of 2, edit the data appropriately (note that if it had been determined that the data values were indeed missing, the system missing value would be changed to a 9, which is the missing value

**Figure 15.15**

Example of sorting variable BDA2 values in ascending order.

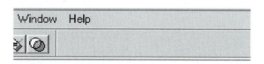

code for the BDA2 variable). Follow similar tactics to determine the accuracy of the −1 value observed in the frequency table. Sometimes such a value represents a missing value code used in the data but not reported to SPSS in the *Variable View* tab; in this case, however, it should have been a 1 and should be corrected in the Data Editor mode.

The SPSS *Explore* procedure, obtained through *Analyze|Descriptive Statistics|Explore* and primarily intended for scale variables, also provides several ways to help identify potential problem values (Figure 15.16). The **Statistics** button provides an opportunity to examine the most extreme values (i.e., outliers) for chosen variables (Figure 15.17). Figure 15.18 shows the Extreme Values output table, which actually just shows the highest and lowest scores (which may or may not be extreme values) for the GPA variable. Notice that two scores seem a bit odd: a highest score of 4.40 and a lowest score of 0.70. After checking the original data sources for our example, we discover that the 4.40 should have been a 4.00 and that the 0.70 should have been 2.70. There are helpful methods that can be used for discovering extreme values. Usually just noticing strange values descriptively is enough of a warning to check the accuracy of the data.

The boxplot shown in Figure 15.19 and the stem-and-leaf plot in Figure 15.20, both produced by default by *Explore*, show the extremely low 0.70 to be an outlier; the boxplot also identifies the current Data Editor case number (i.e., 40). Neither, however, shows the problematic 4.40 because it is a strange value because of the maximum 4.00

**Figure 15.16**

The *Explore* dialog box.

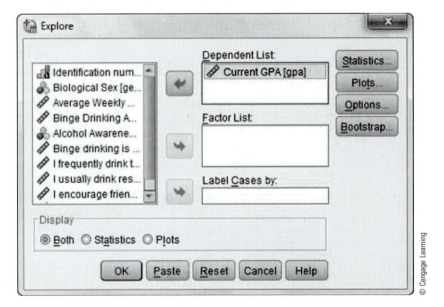

**Figure 15.17**

The *Statistics* dialog box used to identify outliers in a variable data set.

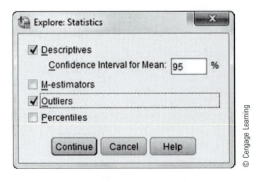

**Figure 15.18**

The `Ex Values` output table used to identify potential outliers.

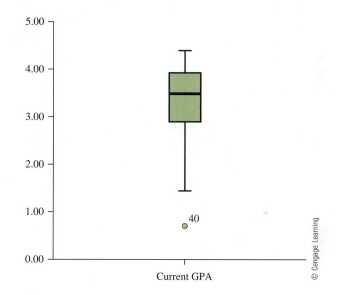

**Extreme Values**

| | | | Case Number | Value |
|---|---|---|---|---|
| Current GPA | Highest | 1 | 22 | 4.40 |
| | | 2 | 1 | 4.00 |
| | | 3 | 3 | 4.00 |
| | | 4 | 5 | 4.00 |
| | | 5 | 6 | 4.00[a] |
| | Lowest | 1 | 40 | .70 |
| | | 2 | 14 | 1.44 |
| | | 3 | 18 | 2.29 |
| | | 4 | 31 | 2.48 |
| | | 5 | 41 | 2.55 |

a. Only a partial list of cases with the value 4.00 are shown in the table of upper extremes.

**Figure 15.19**

Example boxplot of GPA data.

**Figure 15.20**

Example stem-and-leaf plot of GPA data.

Current GPA Stem-and-Leaf Plot

| Frequency | Stem & Leaf |
|---|---|
| 1.00 | Extremes    (=<.7) |
| 1.00 | 1 .    4 |
| .00 | 1 . |
| 2.00 | 2 .    24 |
| 10.00 | 2 .    5778888899 |
| 11.00 | 3 .    00011113344 |
| 13.00 | 3 .    5555555668899 |
| 12.00 | 4 .    000000000004 |

Stem width:       1.00
Each leaf:              1 case(s)

possible for the GPA variable's scale, not in relation to the distribution of the data. This exemplifies further the need to use multiple approaches to screen the data.

One final method most useful for scale variables is to create and examine standardized scores (i.e., *z*-scores). SPSS provides an easy way to calculate these standardized scores from *Analyze|Descriptive Statistics|Descriptives* (Figure 15.21). When the *Save*

**Figure 15.21**

The *Save standardized values as variables* option.

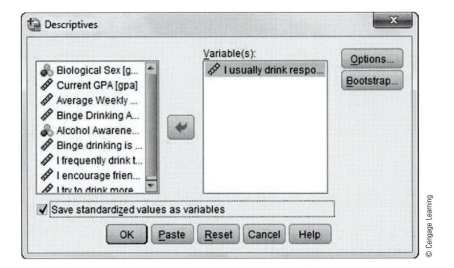

**Figure 15.22**

Display of the newly created ZDBA3 variable.

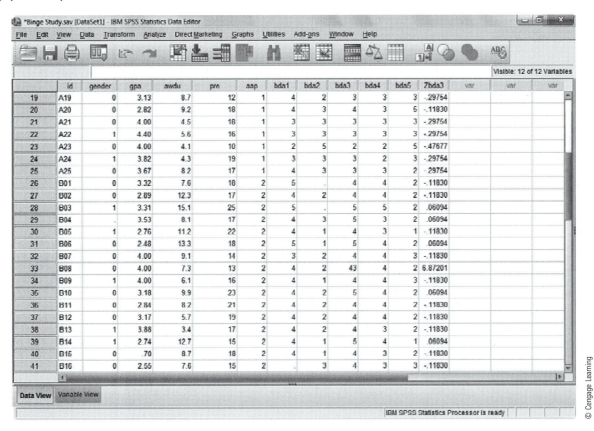

*standardized values as variables* option is checked, a new variable will be created in the database (Figure 15.22). Upon sorting the ZBDA3 variable (*z*-score for original variable BDA3) that was created when saving the standardized scores for the BDA3 variable, we discover that the case with an ID of B08 has a very large *z*-score of 6.872, which turns

**Figure 15.23**

Deleting an erroneous *z*-score
value.

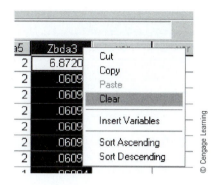

**Figure 15.23**

Deleting an erroneous *z*-score
value.

out to be associated with an impossible value of 43 on a 5-point scale (upon review, the
hypothetical score should have been 4 and was changed). ZBDA3 also could have been
analyzed using the *Explore* procedure to determine whether any of the values seem
unreasonable. Most scholars recommend that standardized scores (*z*) beyond 2.50 or
3.00 should be investigated further. Note that the ZBDA3 variable can be deleted
after it has been examined by right-clicking on the variable name in the Data Editor
(Figure 15.23) and choosing *Clear*.

All three of the basic descriptive statistics procedures (i.e., *Frequencies*, *Descriptives*,
and *Explore*) can provide a quick view of impossible values like the 43 on BDA3 by
reporting the minimum and maximum values of a variable, which can be compared to
the most extreme possible values. If the minimum or maximum is beyond the possible
scores, then further analyses can be performed to determine whether other such problem
values exist. For example, the *Analyze|Descriptive Statistics|Descriptives* results shown in
Figure 15.24 list 0.70 and 4.40 as the minimum and maximum GPA, respectively (note
that both output tables shown in Figure 15.24 are actually the same table; SPSS allows us
to edit and pivot the output tables to match our preferences).

After performing these data screening procedures, 11 potential problem values were
identified; each should be investigated and fixed, as appropriate. Fortunately, in this example
all the data values were able to be corrected by reviewing the original source of the data. In
real life, one may not have been as successful and perhaps would have been forced to code

**Figure 15.24**

A *Descriptive Statistics* output table for GPA, useful in identifying outliers.

**Descriptive Statistics**

|  | N | Minimum | Maximum | Mean | | Std. Deviation | Skewness | |
|---|---|---|---|---|---|---|---|---|
|  | Statistic | Statistic | Statistic | Statistic | Std. Error | Statistic | Statistic | Std. Error |
| Current GPA | 50 | 0.70 | 4.40 | 3.3276 | .09762 | .69028 | −1.474 | .337 |
| Valid N (listwise) | 50 | | | | | | | |

**Descriptive Statistics**

|  |  | Current GPA | Valid N (listwise) |
|---|---|---|---|
| *N* | Statistic | 50 | 50 |
| Minimum | Statistic | .70 | |
| Maximum | Statistic | 4.40 | |
| Mean | Statistic | 3.3276 | |
|  | Std. Error | .09762 | |
| Std. Deviation | Statistic | .69028 | |
| Skewness | Statistic | −1.474 | |
|  | Std. Error | .337 | |

© Cengage Learning

| | ID | Gender | GPA | AWDU | Pre | AAP | BDA1 | BDA2 | BDA3 | BDA4 | BDA5 |
|---|---|---|---|---|---|---|---|---|---|---|---|
| **TABLE 15.3** | | | | Cases from example data that were changed following screening and prior to recoding. | | | | | | | |
| 5 | A05 | | | | 14 | | | | | | |
| 7 | A07 | | | | | | | | | 4 | |
| 12 | A12 | | | | | | | 1 | | | |
| 18 | A18 | | | 5.2 | | | | | | | |
| 22 | A22 | | 4.00 | | | | | | | | |
| 26 | B01 | | | | | | | 2 | | | |
| 28 | B03 | | | | | | | 2 | | | |
| 29 | B04 | 1 | | | | | | | | | |
| 33 | B08 | | | | | | | | 4 | | |
| 40 | B15 | | 2.70 | | | | | | | | |
| 41 | B16 | | | | | | 4 | | | | |

© Cengage Learning

some of the values as missing values, which would have meant that some of those cases would be lost for many subsequent statistical analyses. All cases that needed to have data corrected are listed in Table 15.3. Although we identified several problems here, we may not have identified all data entry problems. Sometimes it is useful to run the same data screening procedures multiple times; it often happens that removing one extreme value causes another value to appear to be extreme, even though it appeared reasonable before. Notice that there is a difference between erroneous data and extreme data: One must fix or remove erroneous data, but handling extreme data is much more difficult to reconcile. Sometimes extreme data are erroneous, but sometimes they are legitimate—just extreme. As a researcher, you will need to decide whether to include or exclude these cases or adjust the analysis. See Chapter 18 for procedures used for dealing with potentially problematic outliers. Generally, you will include any cases for which you cannot justify removal.

# Manipulating Data

Now that the data have been screened and cleaned, you can begin to work with it. It is often the case that data must be transformed in some way before performing any statistical analyses. For instance, in our example, we must compute a total BDA score from the several BDA scale items in our database (i.e., BDA1, BDA2, BDA3, BDA4, and BDA5). Before we can compute a total, however, we must ensure that all the items are scaled in the same direction. That is, BDA2 and BDA5 are negatively worded items. The BDA scale was written such that higher total scores, which range from the lowest possible score of 5 to the highest possible score of 25, represent a healthier attitude toward binge drinking. When respondents agree with a positively worded item, they present a healthier attitude toward alcohol and they therefore receive more points for the item (i.e., either 4 or 5 points). When respondents agree with an item that presents an unhealthy stimulus, they are suggesting a more unhealthy attitude toward alcohol. Consequently, we must recode these negatively worded items (BDA2 and BDA5) so that disagreement correctly receives more points toward a higher total score, reflecting a more positive and healthy attitude.

A few small recommendations may be helpful before discussing transformations. First, it is always a good idea to save a data file prior to making any dramatic changes. Indeed, one may want to keep multiple versions of the file, just in case one needs to revert back to a pretransformation database for some reason. It is too easy to transform

**Figure 15.25**

The *Recode|Into Same Variables* dialog box.

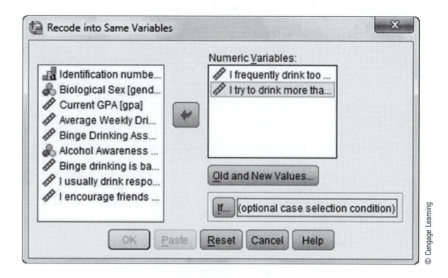

and recode variables incorrectly, without any possibility of undoing the damage. Second, record how variables were transformed or computed, perhaps in the variable label itself. Unfortunately, SPSS doesn't keep track of how variables are changed. The *Edit|Options| Viewer|Display commands in the log* option can help keep track of such changes, but even these reports are not complete. Third, the SPSS Data Editor is least like a spreadsheet in that it does not automatically calculate transformations for new or modified data. That is, if one adds or changes data, one will need to transform the data again using the same commands previously used, whereas a spreadsheet allows one to enter a formula that automatically computes scores for new or modified data.

In SPSS, the *Transform|Recode|Into Same Variables* procedure will allow recoding of these negatively worded items quickly. In Figure 15.25, BDA2 and BDA5 have been recoded at the same time because they will be changed in the same way. Once the two variables are entered into the Numeric Variables list, clicking the *Old and New Values* button opens the dialog box in Figure 15.26. To accomplish this, first enter each original value in the Old Value side of the dialog box. Then enter the New Value in the appropriate location, click *Add*, and then repeat for all values as shown in Figure 15.26. Although it may seem redundant to change the 3 into a 3, there are two reasons that this is a useful habit: (a) if one ever recodes *Into different variables*, you'll need to do this or you'll end up with missing values, and (b) if one ever uses the *All other values* option, all previous values need to be individually specified.

Now that the items are scaled in the same direction, the *Transform|Compute* menu option will allow us to calculate a total score variable. As shown in Figure 15.27, it is necessary to enter a name for the Target Variable to be computed and the Numeric Expression to be used. Notice that in addition to basic calculator functions, there are many predefined functions available. For example, instead of using the four plus signs in the example formula, you could have used the *SUM* function: Either *SUM(bda1, bda2, bda3, bda4, bda5)* or *SUM(bda1 to bda5)* would work, because the five BDA items are in contiguous columns in the Data Editor. It is important to know, however, that these two approaches (i.e., straightforward calculations versus SPSS functions) will produce different results when there are missing values for any of the variables used in the calculation. That is, using the plus signs will result in an underestimated total score if any of the items comprising the sum have missing values. Thus, the **SUM function** will total only those items for which we do have data (e.g., the total would be based on four

**Figure 15.26**

Converting reverse-scored items using the *Recode|Into Same Variables|Old and New Values* dialog box.

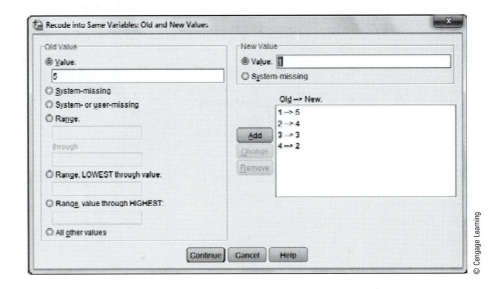

**Figure 15.27**

Using the *Transform| Compute* function to sum the five BDA variables.

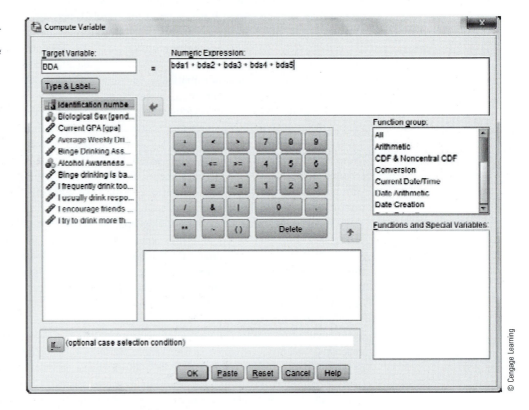

items instead of five). Figure 15.28 shows the results of the computation and sorting of BDA, along with the results of ranking the BDA variable (RBDA) and creating three roughly equally sized groups, or what SPSS calls *Ntiles*, from the BDA scores (NBDA), both created using *Transform|Rank Cases|Rank Types* (Figure 15.29). After computing BDA, Figure 15.30 shows how to compute a change score to represent the difference between BDA scores before treatment (PRE) and after treatment (BDA).

## Figure 15.28

Data file showing new variables BDA (total summed score), RBDA (ranking), and NBDA (effectively splitting the sample into three groups based upon the BDA score).

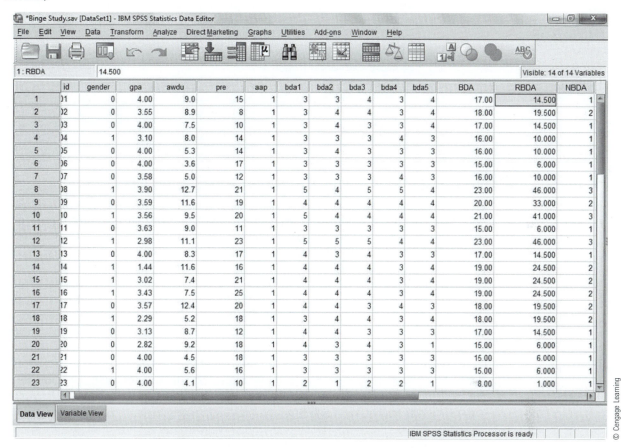

## Figure 15.29

The *Transform | Rank Cases | Rank Types* dialog box used to create NDBA.

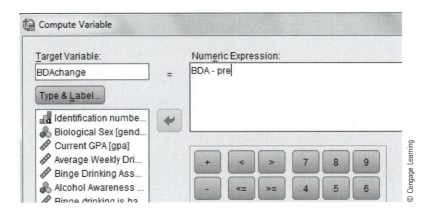

# Describing Data for Individual Variables

After the data are determined to be reasonably accurate and all necessary transformations have been made, we can begin to make sense of the data. The first step is to calculate appropriate summary (descriptive) statistics for the variables we will analyze. Many of the same procedures used in the data screening section will be used here, but with different purposes. It is important to decide what variables you need to summarize and describe, what information will be most useful for these summaries and descriptions, and how to report the summaries and descriptive statistics (e.g., report summary statistics in text, create tables, and create graphs or figures). These decisions will help determine the choice of which procedures and graphs to run when analyzing the data in SPSS.

Categorical variables should be summarized differently from scale variables. The SPSS *Frequencies* procedure is the most appropriate to use for categorical variables. In addition to features such as frequency tables (Figure 15.14), *Analyze|Descriptive Statistics|Frequencies|Charts* will produce bar charts and pie charts appropriate for categorical variables (Figure 15.31). Note that the *Frequencies* procedure does provide certain information about scale variables not easily obtained from other procedures; for example, this is the easiest place to create a histogram that includes a superimposed normal curve.

Any of the basic descriptive procedures (*Frequencies*, *Descriptives*, and *Explore*) can provide the most common summary statistics reported for scale variables (e.g., the *Explore*

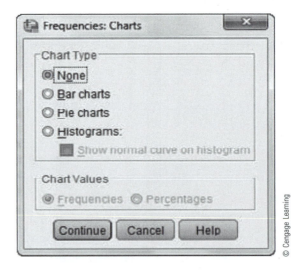

**Figure 15.32**

A sample *Descriptives* table derived from the *Explore* function.

**Descriptives**

| | | | Statistic | Std. Error |
|---|---|---|---|---|
| Current GPA | Mean | | 3.3596 | .08104 |
| | 95% Confidence Interval for Mean | Lower Bound | 3.1968 | |
| | | Upper Bound | 3.5224 | |
| | 5% Trimmed Mean | | 3.4002 | |
| | Median | | 3.4850 | |
| | Variance | | .328 | |
| | Std. Deviation | | .57301 | |
| | Minimum | | 1.44 | |
| | Maximum | | 4.00 | |
| | Range | | 2.56 | |
| | Interquartile Range | | 1.04 | |
| | Skewness | | −.835 | .337 |
| | Kurtosis | | .912 | .662 |

© Cengage Learning

output in Figure 15.32); each also provides slightly different output, useful for different purposes. For example, *Frequencies* will report the mode and allows specification of particular percentile values, whereas *Explore* provides only a predefined set of percentiles. There is really no advantage to running the *Descriptives* procedure, except for its ability to create standardized scores and perhaps for its condensed table output format.

The *Explore* procedure, however, provides many features well suited for descriptive analysis of scale variables. In addition to the features used in screening data (e.g., extreme values, stem-and-leaf displays, and descriptive statistics), *Explore* reports such unique information as the interquartile range and the lower and upper bounds of the confidence interval for the mean, which is calculated based on a critical *t*-value rather than a critical *z*-value. Histograms (Figure 15.33) and other graphs can be requested through *Analyze|Descriptive Statistics|Explore|Plots* (Figure 15.34). This same *Explore| Plots* dialog box allows users to obtain **Normality plots with tests** for help in checking the normality assumption required for so many common statistics. Figure 15.35 shows both the statistical tests provided by the *Explore* normality tests and the Normal Q-Q Plot, in which more normal data more closely match the diagonal line in the chart.

**Figure 15.33**

A sample histogram from the *Explore* function output.

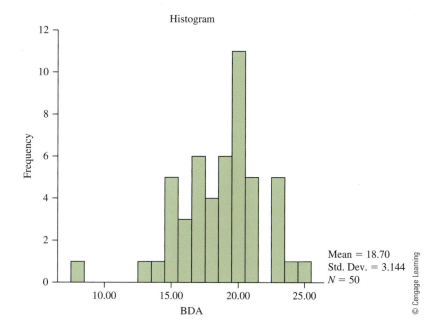

Mean = 18.70
Std. Dev. = 3.144
*N* = 50

© Cengage Learning

**Figure 15.34**

Selecting various graphs and plots using the *Explore|Plots* dialog box.

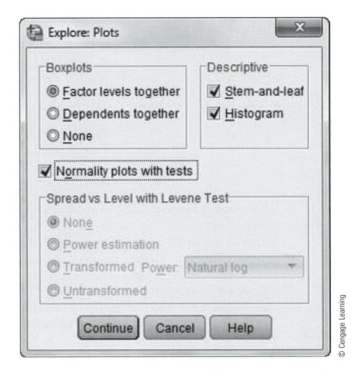

**Figure 15.35**

A sample *Normality plots with tests* output table and `Normal Q-Q Plot`.

**Tests of Normality**

| | Kolmogorov–Smirnov[a] | | | Shapiro–Wilk | | |
|---|---|---|---|---|---|---|
| | Statistic | *df* | Sig. | Statistic | *df* | Sig. |
| BDA | .120 | 50 | .068 | .955 | 50 | .057 |

a. Lilliefors Significance Correction

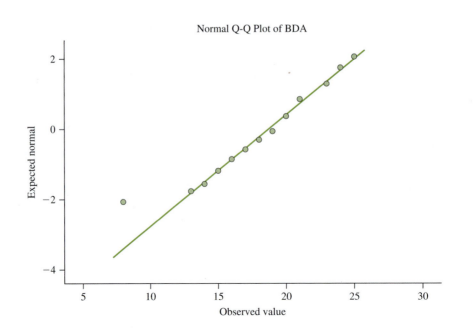

© Cengage Learning

**Figure 15.36**

The BDA boxplot available in the *Explore* function.

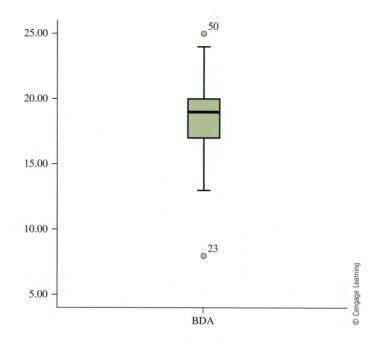

The *Explore* boxplot for BDA (Figure 15.36) shows a couple of interesting things. Most noticeably, the boxplot shows two data values that seem to be outliers: case 1 (with ID A23) and case 50 (with ID B25) based on the current Data Editor ordering of the cases (Figure 15.28). Notice that if data were sorted differently, the case numbers on the boxplot would differ, but they would still represent the same cases based on ID numbers. The circles designate the values as outliers, which are values more than 1.5 times the interquartile range below or above the box in the plot. The interquartile range (i.e., the difference between the 75th and 25th percentiles) can be visualized as the distance from the top of the box to the bottom of the box (the line across the box is the 50th percentile, the median). If any values were more than three times the interquartile range from the box, they would be designated as **extreme values** and marked with an asterisk. These outliers in Figure 15.36 may represent additional erroneous data values that were missed during the screening process, or they may be legitimate values very different from most of the cases in the data set. The researcher would need to decide how to handle these cases if they do turn out to be legitimate but extreme (e.g., one may decide to run analyses both with and without extreme cases and report any differences).

Sometimes one of the variables is a composite variable; that is, the variable is a function of other variables in the database. In such cases, generally the composite variable rather than the individual variables (e.g., scale items) will be analyzed. For example, the BDA variable in our example is calculated as the sum of the five individual items in the instrument. When using a summated scale such as the total BDA, it is usually important to evaluate the internal consistency reliability of the scores provided. The SPSS *Analyze| Scale|**Reliability Analysis*** procedure provides this information. In the present example, one must identify all items that are used to calculate the total BDA variable and choose the *Alpha* model (Figure 15.37). By clicking the *Statistics* button and requesting descriptive statistics for the items, we can analyze the scale to some extent (Figure 15.38). The output from the reliability procedure (Figure 15.39) not only gives us internal consistency **Reliability Statistics** as measured by Cronbach's Alpha but also **Item-Total Statistics** that can help us determine whether any items are not working well.

**Figure 15.37**

Conducting an internal consistency reliability analysis using the *Reliability Analysis* dialog box.

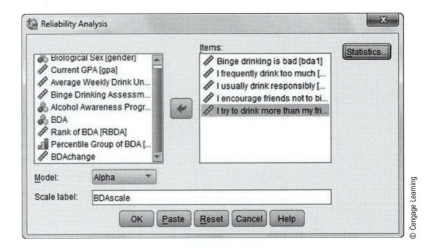

**Figure 15.38**

Selecting specific statistical analyses using the *Reliability Analysis/Statistics* dialog box.

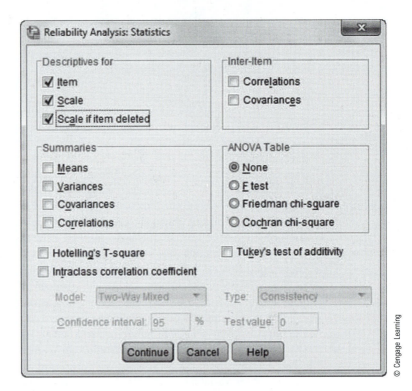

## Describing Data for Combinations of Variables

So far, the focus has been exclusively on examining individual variables, but often it is important to examine combinations of variables as well. Sometimes researchers want to summarize particular variables for each level of an independent variable separately. The *Explore* procedure provides an easy way to perform such analyses for the descriptive statistics and graphs it produces. For example, by identifying AAP as the grouping variable in the Factor List in the main *Explore* dialog box (Figure 15.40), you obtain output separated by the control and workshop groups. Figure 15.41 shows how the *Descriptives* table is divided according to the AAP group. In Figure 15.42, which provides both groups in the same boxplot, notice that within groups there are now potential problem cases.

### Figure 15.39

Output tables derived from the *Reliability Analysis* function.

**Reliability Statistics**

| Cronbach's Alpha | N of Items |
|---|---|
| .884 | 5 |

**Item Statistics**

| | Mean | Std. Deviation | N |
|---|---|---|---|
| Binge drinking is bad | 3.80 | .808 | 50 |
| I frequently drink too much | 3.84 | .792 | 50 |
| I usually drink responsibly | 3.88 | .718 | 50 |
| I encourage friends not to binge drink | 3.54 | .706 | 50 |
| I try to drink more than my friends | 3.64 | .776 | 50 |

**Item-Total Statistics**

| | Scale Mean if Item Deleted | Scale Variance if Item Deleted | Corrected Item-Total Correlation | Cronbach's Alpha if Item Deleted |
|---|---|---|---|---|
| Binge drinking is bad | 14.90 | 6.255 | .737 | .855 |
| I frequently drink too much | 14.86 | 6.245 | .762 | .849 |
| I usually drink responsibly | 14.82 | 6.477 | .792 | .843 |
| I encourage friends not to binge drink | 15.16 | 6.953 | .654 | .873 |
| I try to drink more than my friends | 15.06 | 6.629 | .665 | .872 |

**Scale Statistics**

| Mean | Variance | Std. Deviation | N of Items |
|---|---|---|---|
| 18.70 | 9.888 | 3.144 | 5 |

© Cengage Learning

### Figure 15.40

Analyzing/describing levels of independent variables using the *Explore* dialog box.

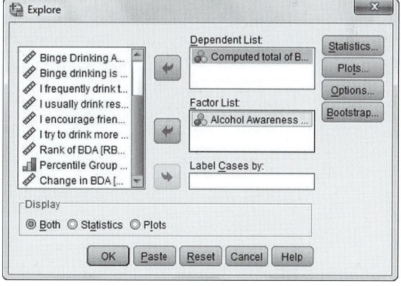

© Cengage Learning

Notice that case 2 in the current sort order (with ID B23), which is not shown as any sort of outlier in Figure 15.36, becomes an extreme value when compared only to those other cases in the workshop group. Once again, it would be appropriate to investigate the accuracy of this and the other outliers and then, if necessary, decide how to handle any strange but legitimate values. Because all other parts of the *Explore* output are also

**Figure 15.41**

Sample *Descriptives* table output divided by treatment condition.

**Descriptives**

| Alcohol Awareness Program | | | | Statistic | Std. Error |
|---|---|---|---|---|---|
| Computed total of BDA | Control | Mean | | 17.1200 | .61188 |
| | | 95% Confidence Interval for Mean | Lower Bound | 15.8571 | |
| | | | Upper Bound | 18.3829 | |
| | | 5% Trimmed Mean | | 17.2333 | |
| | | Median | | 17.0000 | |
| | | Variance | | 9.360 | |
| | | Std. Deviation | | 3.05941 | |
| | | Minimum | | 8.00 | |
| | | Maximum | | 23.00 | |
| | | Range | | 15.00 | |
| | | Interquartile Range | | 4.00 | |
| | | Skewness | | −.522 | .464 |
| | | Kurtosis | | 2.599 | .902 |
| | Treatment | Mean | | 20.2800 | .47441 |
| | | 95% Confidence Interval for Mean | Lower Bound | 19.3009 | |
| | | | Upper Bound | 21.2591 | |
| | | 5% Trimmed Mean | | 20.3889 | |
| | | Median | | 20.0000 | |
| | | Variance | | 5.627 | |
| | | Std. Deviation | | 2.37206 | |
| | | Minimum | | 13.00 | |
| | | Maximum | | 25.00 | |
| | | Range | | 12.00 | |
| | | Interquartile Range | | 1.50 | |
| | | Skewness | | −.750 | .464 |
| | | Kurtosis | | 3.031 | .902 |

© Cengage Learning

**Figure 15.42**

Separate boxplot graphs of the two levels of the independent variable for treatment.

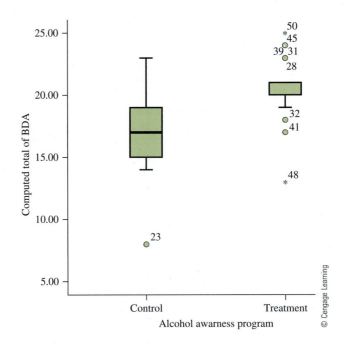

© Cengage Learning

separated by group in this way, this procedure can also be used to examine the assumption of normality within groups.

As nice as the *Explore* procedure is, it is limited to certain output. Although there are several ways to perform any analysis separately for each group (e.g., *Data|Select Cases*), the *Data|Split File* (Figure 15.43) function works well for many purposes. Once the database is split, choose the desired procedures; output will be separated appropriately in the SPSS Viewer. For example, when running *Descriptives* after splitting the data based on GENDER, the results for AWDU are displayed separately for each GENDER in Figure 15.44. You may notice that only 48 total cases are represented in Figure 15.44 (28 females instead of 30); this is because two cases with AWDU values of 9.0 (with ID A01 and A11) were excluded from analysis because of the missing value codes set up in Figure 15.7. Because the value of 8.0 is a reasonable AWDU value, that value may have been a poor choice to use as a missing value code, but these two cases will be treated as missing for the remainder of the chapter. Summary reports, statistical tests, and graphs can all be produced separately for each group using **Split File**. Perhaps the most important thing to remember about *Split File* is that you must unsplit the database when you

**Figure 15.43**

The *Data|Split File* dialog box.

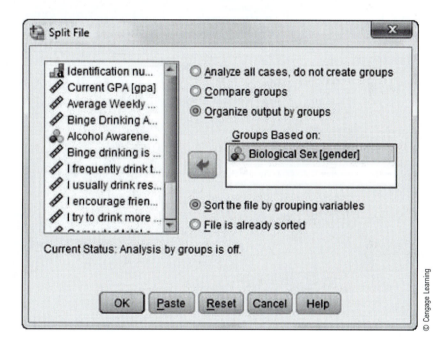

© Cengage Learning

**Figure 15.44**

Gender-specific descriptive statistics output derived through the *Data|Split File* function.

## Descriptives

### Biological Sex = Female

**Descriptive Statistics[a]**

|  | N | Minimum | Maximum | Mean | Std. Deviation |
|---|---|---|---|---|---|
| Average Weekly Drink Units | 28 | 3.6 | 13.3 | 8.361 | 2.5881 |
| Valid N (listwise) | 28 |  |  |  |  |

a. Biological Sex = Female

### Biological Sex = Male

**Descriptive Statistics[a]**

|  | N | Minimum | Maximum | Mean | Std. Deviation |
|---|---|---|---|---|---|
| Average Weekly Drink Units | 20 | 3.4 | 15.1 | 9.460 | 3.4678 |
| Valid N (listwise) | 20 |  |  |  |  |

a. Biological Sex = Female

© Cengage Learning

are finished running the grouped analyses (choose *Analyze all cases, do not create groups* in Figure 15.43).

Like *Explore*, most of the *Graphs* in SPSS provide methods by which to use or represent a grouping variable. For example, the **Error Bar** procedure (obtained through the *Graphs|Legacy Dialogs/Error Bar|Simple|Define*) allows identification of AAP as the Category Axis (Figure 15.45). Designating AAP as a grouping variable produces a separate error bar for each group (Figure 15.46). This sort of combined Error Bar graph is usually

**Figure 15.45**

Requesting error bars based on AAP using the *Graphs| Error Bar* dialog box.

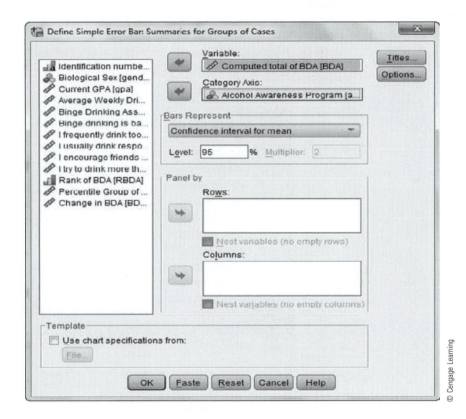

**Figure 15.46**

Sample error bar output graph.

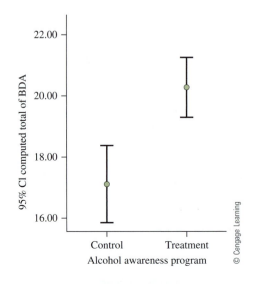

a better choice to display *t*-test results than a similarly grouped boxplot. There are several other ways to combine variables for both error bar graphs and other types of graphs. Also notice that most of the graphs can be created through either the *Graphs* menu options or the *Graphs|Interactive* procedure (there are some minor differences between the editing options available and the final graphs produced).

Other ways to describe combinations of variables include contingency tables and correlations. If you want to know how many men and women there are in each of the AAP treatment groups, for example, the *Analyze|Descriptive Statistics|**Crosstabs*** procedure (Figure 15.47) will provide those results. Although the results in Figure 15.48 provide only the default information (frequencies) in each cross-categorization, the *Statistics* and *Cells* buttons in the *Crosstabs* dialog (Figure 15.47) provide many additional options for appropriate descriptive and inferential statistics.

Similarly, the *Analyze|**Correlate**|Bivariate* procedure (Figure 15.49) provides descriptive bivariate correlations (e.g., Pearson, Spearman), as well as inferential statistical information. Correlation matrix output for Pearson correlations is shown in Figure 15.50 (notice again the 48 cases for all correlations with AWDU owing to the choice of missing values codes). The **bivariate** Pearson correlation is listed on the first line in each cell of the table and that the statistical significance of the correlation is on the second line, flagged with an asterisk by default if statistically significant. The scatterplot shown in Figure 15.51, obtained

**Figure 15.47**

The *Analyze|Descriptive Statistics|Crosstabs* dialog box.

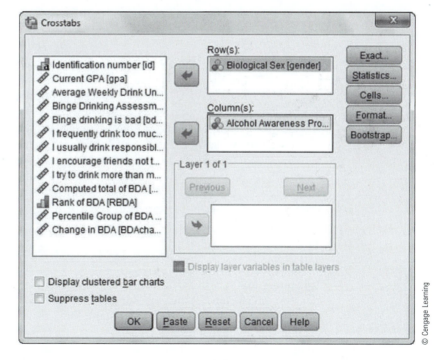

© Cengage Learning

**Figure 15.48**

Sample crosstabs output table.

**Biological Sex\* Alcohol Awareness Program Crosstabulation**

Count

|  |  | Alcohol Awareness Program | | Total |
|---|---|---|---|---|
|  |  | Control | Treatment |  |
| Biological | Female | 15 | 15 | 30 |
| Sex | Male | 10 | 10 | 20 |
| Total |  | 25 | 25 | 50 |

© Cengage Learning

**Figure 15.49**

The *Analyze|Correlate| Bivariate* dialog box.

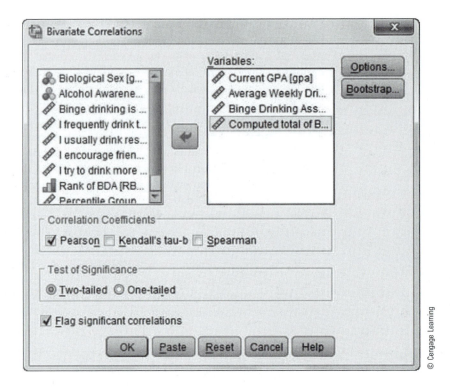

through the menu sequence *Graph|Legacy Dialogs/Scatter/Dot|Simple Scatter|Define* (Figure 15.52), provides a graphical representation of the relationship among two of these variables, GPA and AWDU. You may notice that one dot in Figure 15.52 seems rather far removed from the mass of dots. This case (with ID A14) may be a bivariate outlier, with a strange combination of values on the two variables (here, for case A14, a very low GPA combined with a relatively high AWDU). Notice that graphs created by SPSS can be edited in many ways by double-clicking on them to open the Chart Editor—for example, a regression line can be added to a scatterplot. The matrix of scatterplots in Figure 15.53 (*Graph|Legacy Dialog/Scatter/Dot|Matrix Scatter|Define*) provides miniature graphs for every pair of variables in the correlation matrix in Figure 15.50.

# Introductory Inferential Statistics

It is rather ironic, really. The reason we do research is to answer specific research questions. Although some of these questions will be answered descriptively using many of the procedures just described, most will require the use of inferential statistical tests in association with null hypothesis significance tests (see Chapters 14 and 16). The irony is that, compared to entering, screening, and describing our data, running the procedures necessary to decide about our statistical null hypotheses takes very little time. Interpreting the output and making sense of the results often requires some time and effort, but just running the procedures is a relatively quick and easy process. Several introductory statistical procedures will be presented in this section, including Single-Sample *t*-tests, Dependent *t* -tests, Independent *t*-tests, and bivariate regression. Interestingly, SPSS doesn't provide any means to easily perform statistical tests based on the normal distribution (i.e., *z*-statistics), which are typically the first statistical methods introduced in statistics textbooks; therefore, such tests must be performed manually.

**Figure 15.50**

A sample bivariate correlation output table.

➡ **Correlations**

**Correlations**

| | | Current GPA | Average Weekly Drink Units | Binge Drinking Assessment (before) | Computed total of BDA items |
|---|---|---|---|---|---|
| Current GPA | Pearson Correlation | 1 | −.434** | −.305* | −.389** |
| | Sig. (2-tailed) | | .002 | .031 | .005 |
| | N | 50 | 48 | 50 | 50 |
| Average Weekly Drink Units | Pearson Correlation | −.434** | 1 | .405** | .681** |
| | Sig. (2-tailed) | .002 | | .004 | .000 |
| | N | 48 | 48 | 48 | 48 |
| Binge Drinking Assessment (before) | Pearson Correlation | −.305* | .405** | 1 | .604** |
| | Sig. (2-tailed) | .031 | .004 | | .000 |
| | N | 50 | 48 | 50 | 50 |
| Computed total of BDA items | Pearson Correlation | −.389** | .681** | .604** | 1 |
| | Sig. (2-tailed) | .005 | .000 | .000 | |
| | N | 50 | 48 | 50 | 50 |

**. Correlation is significant at the 0.01 level (2-tailed).

*. Correlation is significant at the 0.05 level (2-tailed).

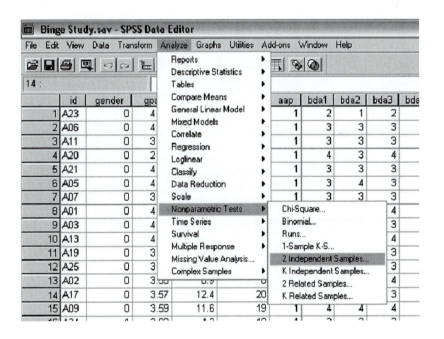

© Cengage Learning

## One-Sample *t*-test

When you want to know whether the mean for the target population differs from some hypothesized value, a Single-Sample *t*-test is run, which SPSS calls a *One-Sample* **t-test**. For example, assume that a researcher wants to compare the average weekly alcohol consumption (AWDU) for the student population to a national average of eight drinks per week (i.e., the statistical null hypothesis would be that the mean equals 8). We would use the *Analyze|Compare Means|One-Sample* t-test procedure to calculate the *t*-statistic necessary for the inferential analysis (Figure 15.54); it is important to change the Test Value in the dialog box to match the hypothesized value (here it was changed to 8).

**Figure 15.51**

Scatterplot of a sample bivariate correlation.

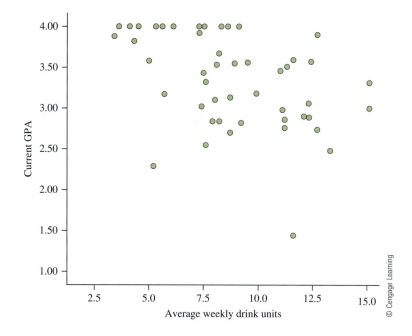

**Figure 15.52**

Scatterplot dialog box from the *Graph* function.

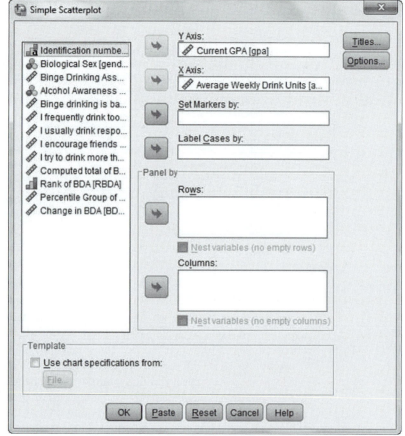

**Figure 15.53**

Scatterplot matrix available
from the *Graph* function.

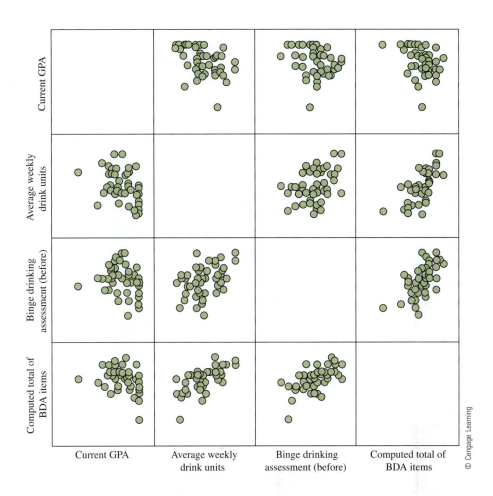

**Figure 15.54**

The *One-Sample t Test* dialog
box with the test value
set to 8.

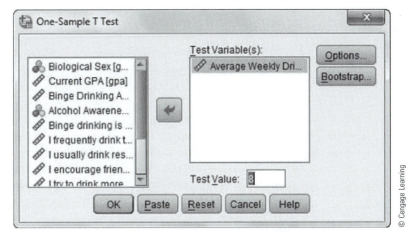

The results of the *One-Sample t-test* procedure are shown in Figure 15.55. By default, the One-Sample Statistics table lists relevant descriptive statistics for the analysis. The One-Sample Test table reports the statistical significance testing information. Many of the SPSS statistical significance tables report information in much the same way as shown in Figure 15.55. In particular, the *t*-statistic is reported in one column (but not

## T-Test

**One-Sample Statistics**

|  | N | Mean | Std. Deviation | Std. Error Mean |
|---|---|---|---|---|
| Average Weekly Drink Units | 48 | 8.819 | 3.0015 | .4332 |

**One-Sample Test**

| | Test Value = 8 | | | | | |
|---|---|---|---|---|---|---|
| | | | | | 95% Confidence Interval of the Difference | |
| | *t* | *df* | Sig. (2-tailed) | Mean Difference | Lower | Upper |
| Average Weekly Drink Units | 1.890 | 47 | .065 | .8188 | −.053 | 1.690 |

© Cengage Learning

always the first), with the degrees of freedom (df) usually displayed in a contiguous column: here, $t(47) = 1.890$. The actual significance, which would typically be reported as $p = 0.065$ in a research report, is called Sig. by SPSS; the parenthetical (two-tailed) indicates that the significance is reported for a nondirectional null hypothesis (for a One-Tailed Test, divide the Sig. in half). Finally, the mean difference ($8.8188 − 8.0000 = 0.8188$) being tested by the *t*-statistic is reported in one column, often followed by the confidence interval for that mean difference (the 95 percent confidence interval can be changed to another criterion from the *Options* button in the dialog box shown in Figure 15.54).

After reviewing the results, you must interpret them in terms of the original research question and statistical null hypothesis. In this example, using a two-tailed level of significance of 0.05, we fail to reject the null hypothesis that our student population's mean AWDU is equal to 8; therefore, we conclude that the population mean for the university students is not statistically significantly different from eight drinks per week. (More on the use of univariate inferential statistics will be presented in Chapter 16.)

## Paired-Samples *t*-test

You may also want to know whether binge-drinking attitudes changed for students who were involved in the new workshop. The appropriate test to answer this question would be a Dependent *t*-test, which SPSS calls a *Paired-Samples* t-*test* (accessible through the *Analyze|Compare Means|Paired-Samples* t-*test* menu sequence). Notice that we need to split the database based on the AAP variable or select only the workshop group (*Data| Select Cases|If condition is satisfied|If|AAP=2*) so only those in the workshop group will be included in the analysis. Also notice that to run the Paired *t*-test, when we collect and record the data, we must have a coding system or process that allows us to match the pretests with the posttests, while ideally maintaining the anonymity of the participants.

To move the variables PRE and BDA into the Paired Variables box on the dialog box shown in Figure 15.56, we must click both variables before clicking the small black triangle between the variable list boxes (notice that the order of the variables in the Paired Variables box depends on the column ordering of the variables in the Data Editor). By clicking the *Options* button (Figure 15.57), you can change the size of the confidence interval and how missing data will be handled. If you choose *Exclude cases analysis by analysis* (called pairwise in some procedures), cases will be included in analyses of all variables for which they have valid data; if you choose *Exclude cases listwise*, cases will be excluded if they are missing data for any variable listed in the Paired Variables box.

**Figure 15.56**

The *Paired-Samples* t-*test* dialog box.

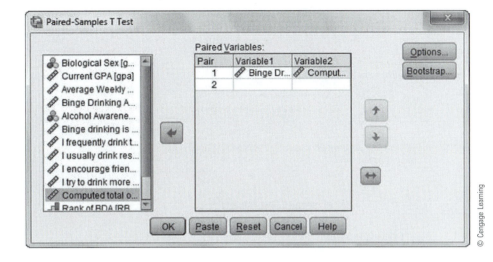

**Figure 15.57**

The *Options* dialog box under the *Paired-Samples* t-*test* function with the *Exclude cases analysis by analysis* option selected.

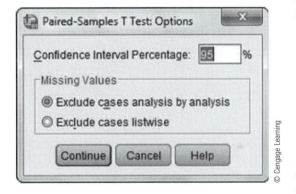

This choice becomes most important when more than one variable, or variable pair, is chosen for analysis (i.e., when doing multiple Paired-Samples *t*-tests concurrently).

Like all *t*-tests, the *Paired-Samples* t-*test* output (Figure 15.58) begins with relevant descriptive statistics in the **Paired Samples Statistics** table (right below the heading to indicate that we split the file based on AAP). If we had requested multiple Dependent *t*-tests, there would be more pairs displayed, but as we only requested a single analysis, the table shows only Pair 1. The Paired Samples Correlations table reports the bivariate correlation between these two variables (i.e., PRE and BDA) that were presumed to be dependent, or correlated. In other words, this is not the important statistical test for our statistical null hypothesis that the mean PRE equals the mean BDA; rather, this is just the test to confirm that the two variables are correlated. The statistical test necessary to decide about the null hypothesis of equal means is in the Paired Samples Test table. The first five columns in this table all pertain to the Paired Differences, as indicated by the heading. For example, the Mean reported is the mean paired difference as calculated by (PRE – BDA). In this example, there is a statistically significant difference between the variable means, where $t(24) = -3.635$, $p = 0.001$. Therefore, we conclude that the BDA after the new workshop ($M = 20.28$, $SD = 2.372$) is higher than before ($M = 18.24$, $SD = 3.609$), indicating that attitudes toward binge drinking were healthier after the workshop. Notice that we cannot conclude that the workshop caused the improvement in students' binge-drinking attitudes without knowing more about the research design.

**Figure 15.58**

Output table for the *Paired-Samples* t-*test* function.

## T-Test

**Alcohol Awareness Program = Treatment**

**Paired Samples Statistics**

|  |  | Mean | N | Std. Deviation | Std. Error Mean |
|---|---|---|---|---|---|
| Pair 1 | Binge Drinking Assessment (before) | 18.24 | 25 | 3.609 | .722 |
|  | Computed total of BDA | 20.2800 | 25 | 2.37206 | .47441 |

**Paired Samples Correlations**

|  |  | N | Correlation | Sig. |
|---|---|---|---|---|
| Pair 1 | Binge Drinking Assessment (before) and Computed total of BDA | 25 | .629 | .001 |

**Paired Samples Test**

|  |  | Paired Differences | | | | | | | |
|---|---|---|---|---|---|---|---|---|---|
|  |  |  |  |  | 95% Confidence Interval of the Difference | | | | |
|  |  | Mean | Std. Deviation | Std. Error Mean | Lower | Upper | t | df | Sig. (2-tailed) |
| Pair 1 | Binge Drinking Assessment (before) – Computed total of BDA | −2.04 | 2.80595 | .56119 | −3.19824 | −.88176 | −3.635 | 24 | .001 |

© Cengage Learning

## Independent-Samples *t*-test

The primary goal of the example study was to determine whether the new workshop improved students' binge-drinking attitudes more than the control (i.e., the existing program). To compare the attitude improvement, we needed to calculate a change score (Figure 15.30). The statistical null hypothesis is that the mean change in binge-drinking attitudes is equal for both the control and workshop groups. For this analysis, we decided to remove case A02, not because it had a relatively low PRE score but rather based on comments written on that student's BDA that strongly suggested the student did not take the assessment seriously (to remove the case, right-click on the correct row number and then choose *Clear*). Following this decision, we can run an independent *t*-test through *Analyze|Compare Means|Independent-Samples* t-*test* (Figure 15.59). The key element in running this *t*-test is to define the groups. We put the independent variable, AAP, in the Grouping Variable box and then click the *Define Groups* button (Figure 15.60). The *Cut Point* option is useful to categorize a scale variable into two groups.

The *Independent-Samples* t-*test* output is displayed as Figure 15.61. Relevant descriptive statistics are provided by group in the Group Statistics table. The Independent Samples Test table provides the important information for testing our statistical null hypothesis. There are two primary sections in the table: the Levene's Test for **Equality of Variances** section and the *t*-test for *Equality of Means* section. Levene's test provides a way for us to evaluate whether the assumption of homogeneous variances across groups is reasonable. Standard practice is to use the row of the table labeled *Equal variances assumed* if Levene's test is not statistically significant (hence, the assumption of equal variance is not violated); otherwise, if Levene's test is statistically significant, we

**Figure 15.59**

The *Independent-Samples t-test* dialog box available under the *Analyze|Compare Means* function.

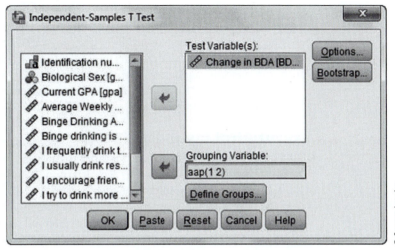

**Figure 15.60**

The *Define Groups* dialog box.

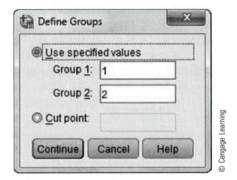

---

**Figure 15.61**

*Independent-Samples* t-*test* output table.

### → T-Test

**Group Statistics**

|  | Alcohol Awareness Program | N | Mean | Std. Deviation | Std. Error Mean |
|---|---|---|---|---|---|
| BDAchange | Control | 24 | .2917 | 3.14130 | .64121 |
|  | Workshop | 25 | 2.0400 | 2.80595 | .56119 |

**Independent Samples Test**

|  |  | Levene's Test for Equality of Variances | | t-test for Equality of Means | | | | | | |
|---|---|---|---|---|---|---|---|---|---|---|
|  |  |  |  |  |  |  |  |  | 95% Confidence Interval of the Difference | |
|  |  | F | Sig. | t | df | Sig. (2-tailed) | Mean Difference | Std. Error Difference | Lower | Upper |
| BDAchange | Equal variances assumed | .881 | .353 | −2.057 | 47 | .045 | −1.74833 | .85011 | −3.45854 | −.03812 |
|  | Equal variances not assumed |  |  | −2.052 | 45.913 | .046 | −1.74833 | .85211 | −3.46363 | −.03304 |

© Cengage Learning

use the row labeled *Equal variances not assumed*. In this example, the assumption of equal variances is tenable, so we reject the null hypothesis of equal group means based on the *Equal variances assumed* line: $t(47) = -2.057$, $p = 0.045$. Referring to the Group Statistics table, we are able to determine that the workshop group ($M = 2.04$, $SD = 2.81$) had a statistically significantly larger positive change in binge-drinking attitude than did the control group ($M = 0.29$, $SD = 3.14$). Again, remember that without more information about the research design, you cannot conclude anything about cause.

## Bivariate Linear Regression

SPSS uses the same procedure for linear regression whether there is one predictor or many: *Analyze|Regression|Linear*. To determine whether average alcohol consumption (AWDU) is able to predict GPA, we enter GPA into the box labeled *Dependent* and AWDU into the Independent(s) box in Figure 15.62. For simple, or bivariate, linear regression (i.e., one predictor), the *Enter* Method is appropriate. The *Statistics*, *Plots*, *Save*, and *Options* buttons each produce additional output that can be helpful in making sense of the regression results but are mostly beyond the scope of this chapter (as you become more comfortable with running regression analyses, you'll want to investigate these options; see Chapters 17 and 19 for more information on simple regression and multiple regression, respectively). For example, residuals, outliers, and influential cases can be examined by saving diagnostic data to the database through the *Save* button; several methods by which regression assumptions can be tested are available from the *Plots* button. Perhaps the most important of these plots, obtained through *Analyze|Regression|Linear|Plots* (Figure 15.63), allows testing of the assumptions of linearity and homoscedasticity. This plot of the standardized predicted values with the standardized residuals (Figure 15.64) indicates no apparent problems for either linearity or homoscedasticity (i.e., equality of variances across the independent variable values).

The linear regression results are presented in Figure 15.65. In a bivariate regression, the *Variables Entered/Removed* table shows which variable was used as the independent

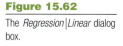

**Figure 15.62**

The *Regression|Linear* dialog box.

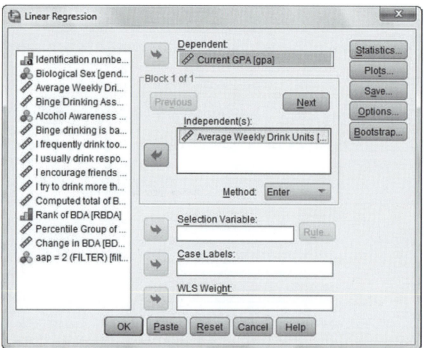

**Figure 15.63**

Obtaining a graph/plot through the *Analyze | Regression | Linear | Plots* dialog box.

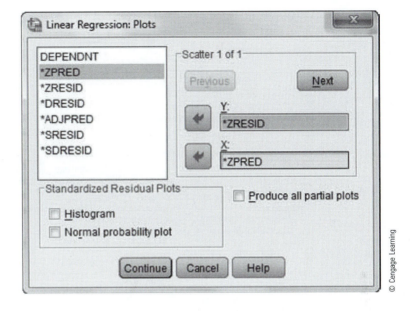

**Figure 15.64**

A sample scatterplot using the *Analyze | Regression | Linear | Plots* function.

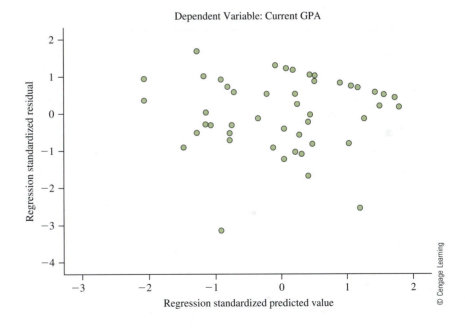

variable. Notice that the regression output does not include descriptive statistics by default like the *t*-test procedures did (descriptive statistics, which include both a table of means and standard deviations and a correlation matrix, are available as an option in the dialog box accessed from the *Statistics* button in Figure 15.62). The *Model Summary* table includes information about the predictive relationship between AWDU and GPA. The amount of shared variance between the two variables, or the coefficient of determination, is reported as *R* Square ($R^2 = 0.189$). The **Std. Error of the Estimate** provides a measure of how well the prediction model fits the data (technically, it is the standard deviation of the residuals, $Y - Predicted\ Y$). The ANOVA table provides the statistical significance for the null hypothesis of no correlation among the variables as defined in

# Regression

**Variables Entered/Removed**[a]

| Model | Variables Entered | Variables Removed | Method |
|---|---|---|---|
| 1 | Average weekly drink units[b] | | Enter |

[a] Dependent Variable: Current GPA
[b] All requested variables entered.

**Model Summary**[b]

| Model | R | R Square | Adjusted R Square | Std. Error of the Estimate |
|---|---|---|---|---|
| 1 | .435[a] | .189 | .171 | .52914 |

[a] Predictors: (Constant), Average Weekly Drink Units
[b] Dependent Variable: Current GPA

**ANOVA**[a]

| Model | | Sum of Squares | df | Mean Square | F | Sig. |
|---|---|---|---|---|---|---|
| 1 | Regression | 2.944 | 1 | 2.944 | 10.514 | .002[b] |
| | Residual | 12.599 | 45 | .280 | | |
| | Total | 15.543 | 46 | | | |

[a] Dependent Variable: Current GPA
[b] Predictors: (Constant), Average Weekly Drink Units

**Coefficients**[a]

| Model | | Unstandardized Coefficients | | Standardized Coefficients | t | Sig. |
|---|---|---|---|---|---|---|
| | | B | Std. Error | Beta | | |
| 1 | (Constant) | 4.071 | .240 | | 16.999 | .000 |
| | Average Weekly Drink Units | −.083 | .026 | −.435 | −3.243 | .002 |

[a] Dependent Variable: Current GPA

**Residuals Statistics**[a]

| | Minimum | Maximum | Mean | Std. Deviation | N |
|---|---|---|---|---|---|
| Predicted Value | 2.8123 | 3.7878 | 3.3362 | .25298 | 47 |
| Residual | −1.66412 | .88760 | .00000 | .52336 | 47 |
| Std. Predicted Value | −2.071 | 1.785 | .000 | 1.000 | 47 |
| Std. Residual | −3.145 | 1.677 | .000 | .989 | 47 |

[a] Dependent Variable: Current GPA

the *Model Summary*. In this case, we reject the null hypothesis that there is no correlation between AWDU and GPA, with $F(1,46) = 10.51$, $p = 0.002$. Therefore, we can conclude that the regression model with AWDU as the predictor does explain a statistically significant portion of the variance (about 19 percent [$R^2$]) in the dependent variable GPA.

The *Coefficients* table in Figure 15.65 provides the information necessary to test the statistical null hypothesis that the regression coefficient is equal to zero and to define the prediction model: *Predicted Y = a + bX*. The **Unstandardized Coefficient** on the (Constant) line represents the Y-intercept value in our prediction model ($a = 4.071$); the Unstandardized Coefficient associated with AWDU is the slope in our regression model ($b = -0.083$). The **Standardized Coefficient** (Beta) represents the regression coefficient when standardized scores are used in the regression and, therefore, in this case is simply the bivariate correlation between the variables AWDU and GPA ($r = -0.435$). With just one predictor, the statistical test for the regression coefficient provided in the *Coefficients* table is equivalent to the statistical test for the overall model provided in the ANOVA table: $t(46) = -3.24$, $p = 0.002$; therefore, the null hypothesis is rejected, and it is concluded that AWDU is a statistically significant predictor of GPA (i.e., the regression coefficient for AWDU is statistically different from zero). Predicted values for each case based on the regression model can be saved to the database using the *Save* button in Figure 15.62.

# Conclusion

There are many ways SPSS can help make sense out of a data set. In this chapter, the basics of SPSS were considered so that some introductory statistics might be used to examine data. The initial portion of the chapter explored how to create a database of scores and then how to try to verify the accuracy of those scores. Later, after ensuring that the data were accurate, variables were analyzed in the example data set in a variety of ways, including calculating descriptive statistics, creating tables and graphs, and performing inferential null hypothesis tests.

Many more procedures are available in SPSS than discussed here. For example, studies with more than two groups usually require an Analysis of Variance (ANOVA) procedure performed using either *Analyze|Compare Means|Oneway ANOVA* or *Analyze| General Linear Model|Univariate*. Sometimes a dependent variable that is categorical or ordinal rather than interval or ratio must be analyzed; in such cases one may choose to run one of the **Nonparametric Tests** available in SPSS. Also, for example, SPSS provides more sophisticated ways to select and filter cases for analysis and to transform data. The most important thing is to start using SPSS to become familiar with its capabilities and gain confidence in your abilities to use the program to help answer research questions.

*Now go to the Student Workbook found on cengagebrain.com that accompanies this text for additional application and review activities.*

# Univariate Inferential Statistics

*by Richard S. Balkin and Bradley T. Erford*

When you have questions about the effect of a treatment or intervention, or if you want to compare groups, you would use hypothesis testing. Parametric statistics are used in hypothesis testing when the groups that are being studied are normally distributed on a measure that uses interval or ratio data. In contrast, nonparametric statistics, covered later in the text, are not based on a normal distribution and may often have less-stringent criteria but may also reduce statistical power (e.g., produce results that are less likely to be statistically significant and inflate the chance of a type II error). The types of parametric statistics discussed in this chapter are univariate; that is, they are all focused on the measurement of one dependent variable.

## Selecting, Calculating, and Evaluating for Statistical Significance

The discussion of univariate statistical tests in this chapter is focused on the four most popular univariate tests (i.e., one dependent variable) in counseling literature: (a) $z$-test, (b) $t$-test, (c) analysis of variance (ANOVA), and (d) analysis of covariance (ANCOVA). Table 16.1 provides a brief purpose of each test and the hypothetical question each addresses.

The statistical tests discussed in this chapter share common properties. Each test statistic is computed from a fraction (see Equation 16.1). The numerator represents a computation for mean differences, such as by comparing two groups and subtracting one group mean from another. The denominator is an error term, computed by taking into account the standard deviation ($SD$) or variance, and sample size. The numerator is an expression of differences between groups, often referred to as between-groups differences, the denominator looks at error, or differences that exist within each group, often referred to as within-group differences.

$$\text{Test statistic} = \frac{mean\ differences}{error} \text{ or } \frac{\mu_1 - \mu_2}{s_{\text{error}}} \text{ or } \frac{between\text{-}group\ differences}{within\text{-}group\ differences} \tag{16.1}$$

So why does this computation work? Simply put, the numerator value expresses differences between groups, whereas the denominator expresses the error value; the greater the differences between groups compared to lower level of errors, the more confident the researcher can be that any difference is not because of chance errors (i.e., low error values lead to low chance of differences because of errors; high group mean difference values lead

| TABLE 16.1 | Synopsis of univariate parametric tests. | |
|---|---|---|
| **Type of Test** | **Purpose** | **Answers the Question** |
| $z$-test | Tests hypotheses between a sample mean and a population mean. | (i.e., Is there a difference between the sample and the population mean?) |
| $t$-test | Tests hypotheses between two sample means only. | (i.e., Is there a difference between two means?) |
| ANOVA | Tests hypotheses between two or more sample means. | (i.e., Is there a difference among the means?) |
| ANCOVA | Tests hypotheses between two or more sample means while controlling for another variable that affects the outcome of the dependent variable. | (i.e., Is there a difference among the means, when controlling for [a mediating variable]?) |

to high chances that groups do truly differ). Take as an example the hypothesis that the experimental group had a higher performance than the population group. Thus, the mean score from the population was subtracted from the mean score of the experimental group. The mean score in either group, however, is simply a representative score for many participants in each group. Each participant in either group may have scored above the mean or below the mean. Consider the following scores: 20, 18, 21, 18, 23, and 20. The mean (*M*) for this distribution is 20. Some participants scored at the mean, and some participants scored above or below the mean. The error term—in this case, the *SD*—is approximately 1.90 representing the average amount of error within the group. While the mean is a score that represents group outcome, the *SD* is an estimate of error that signifies that some participants did not score at the mean. Thus, a test statistic is computed by taking into account a score that represents the average divided by a score that represents error. Keep this example in mind as we proceed through this chapter exploring univariate statistical analysis. First, we will explore the uses of a *t*-test, which is used to compare only two means, and its permutations. Which *t*-test you use depends on how the means were obtained.

# *z*-Test: Comparing a Sample Mean to a Population Mean

The **z-test** is used to compare a sample mean to a previously known population mean. In this comparison test, the population mean serves as the "control group" or group of comparison. The *z*-test identifies whether there is a statistically significant difference between means of the sample and the population. A graduate counseling program, for example, may wish to compare their students' scores to those of the national average on the National Counselor Examination (NCE). The counseling program can determine whether a statistically significant difference exists between their students' scores and the students who take the exam nationwide. Recall from the discussion of directional and nondirectional hypotheses from Chapter 14 that as the faculty members do not know whether their students will be above or below the mean, they opt to use a nondirectional *z*-test and set alpha at .05 ($\alpha = .05$).

## Calculating the *z*-Test

In the *z*-test, the population mean is subtracted from the sample mean and then divided by the *standard error of the mean*, where $\overline{X}(M)$ is the sample mean, $\mu$ is the population mean, and $\sigma_{\overline{X}}$ is the standard error of the mean.

$$z = \frac{\overline{X} - \mu}{\sigma_{\overline{X}}} \tag{16.2}$$

The standard error of the mean represents the *SD* of the sampling distribution of the mean. In a typical scenario, data would be gathered from a representative sample, and a mean and *SD* would be computed. From these data, a researcher may try to make inferences about the population. But what if many samples were taken from the same population? Then a distribution of sample means and a distribution of sample *SD*s would exist. Furthermore, a normal curve could be contrived to represent the distribution of means and *SD*s. It is often impractical to examine several samples to make inferences about the population. After all, a researcher often does not wish to collect data repeatedly (although replication studies can be valuable!). Generally, inferences are made from one sample only. As the sample mean is compared to the population mean in the numerator, the error estimates would be more accurate if it accounted for an estimate of the *SD* of probable sample means. To calculate the standard error of the mean, the *SD* is divided by the square root of the sample size:

$$\sigma_{\overline{X}} = \frac{\sigma}{\sqrt{n.}}, \tag{16.3}$$

where $\sigma$ is the *SD* of the population mean and *n.* is the number of participants in the sample. Notice that a larger sample size contributes to a smaller standard error of the mean. Thus, larger sample sizes lead to smaller amounts of sampling error.

So assume that 25 graduate students from a counseling program take the *NCE*, and the graduate program faculty wants to know how their students performed compared to the national norms. The sample of 25 students constitute (*n.*). The mean score for the sample of 25 students was 117 ($\overline{X} = 117$). The mean score ($\mu$) for the national sample was 110 with an *SD* of 15 ($\mu = 110; \sigma = 15$). The faculty members of the counseling program know that their students scored higher than the population. But is this difference statistically significant? Can it be stated with a 95 percent level of confidence ($\alpha = .05$) that the difference in these scores is outside the realm of chance? A *z*-test is conducted to answer this question using the means from the sample and population and *SD* from the population.

First, compute the standard error of the mean:

$$\sigma_{\overline{X}} = \frac{\sigma}{\sqrt{n.}} = \frac{15}{\sqrt{25}} = 3$$

Next, conduct the *z*-test:

$$z = \frac{\overline{X} - \mu}{\sigma_{\overline{X}}} = \frac{117 - 110}{3} = 2.33$$

Interpretation of this *z*-test score of 2.33 will be discussed in the next section.

As a second example, assume a counseling researcher is interested in knowing whether the sample of children with attention-deficit/hyperactivity disorder (AD/HD) she has selected is significantly more hyperactive than the normal population (a directional hypothesis). She selected the Hyperactivity subscale from the *Conners-3* (Conners, 2007) as the dependent variable and will use *T* scores as the metric of comparison. Recall from Chapter 13 that *T* scores have a (population) $\mu = 50$ and $\sigma = 10$. The researcher's sample $M = 64$ and the sample consisted of 20 participants. The question is, is this difference between the sample mean of 64 and population mean of 50, statistically significant? Can it be stated with a 95 percent level of probability ($\alpha = .05$) that the difference in these scores is outside the realm of chance? Once again, the *z*-test is conducted to answer this question using the means from the sample and population and *SD* from the population.

First, compute the standard error of the mean:

$$\sigma_{\overline{X}} = \frac{\sigma}{\sqrt{n.}} = \frac{10}{\sqrt{20}} = 2.24$$

Next, conduct the *z*-test:

$$z = \frac{\overline{X} - \mu}{\sigma_{\overline{X}}} = \frac{64 - 50}{2.24} = 6.25$$

Interpretation of this *z*-test score of 6.25 will be discussed in the next section.

## Evaluating the *z*-Test for Statistical Significance

To determine whether the observed value, $z_{obs} = 2.33$ for the preceding NCE example, is statistically significant at the $\alpha = .05$ level of significance, the observed score must be greater than the critical value, $z_{crit}$. The critical value is based on the probability of making a type I error. When a test statistic is computed, it is compared to a critical value either by comparing the selected alpha level to the actual probability of making a type I error, known as a *p*-value, or by comparing the observed score to the critical value. Remember, statistical significance exists when the null hypothesis is rejected, which is evidenced by $z_{obs} > z_{crit}$ or by $p < \alpha$. For a visual representation, Table 16.2 shows a decision grid for retaining or rejecting the null hypothesis. The top row represents the actual status of the null hypothesis. The vertical column represents the decision the researcher made based on observed data. As discussed earlier, there can be error in the researcher's methods of analysis that can interfere with making a correct decision.

Assume for the sake of this example that even though the faculty members knew that their students' mean score was above the national mean, the *z*-test was nondirectional; thus 2.5 percent of the distribution is left over each side of the normal curve: a total of 5 percent, the designated alpha ($\alpha$) level (i.e., .05). To determine the critical value for the *z*-test, use Table 16.3. As the test is nondirectional, the critical value $\frac{\alpha}{2} = .\frac{05}{2} = .025$. In a normal curve, 50 percent (.50) of the data lies on both sides of the mean, median, and mode, so .50 − .025 = .475. In Table 16.3, the leftmost column represents the first two values of *z*, and the top numbers represent the second decimal place number in *z* (i.e., left column of 1.9 and top row of .06 means that a *z*-score of 1.96 has a critical value of .4750). Thus, using the values in the center portion of the table, the critical value consistent with the .4750 amount is 1.96. The observed value, $z_{obs} = 2.33$, is greater than (i.e., lies in the extreme shaded area of the normal curve) the critical value, $z_{crit} = 1.96$. Therefore, the null hypothesis is rejected, and the faculty conclude that the students' mean score from the university program is (statistically) significantly different from the mean score of the population.

What if the *z*-test was directional instead of nondirectional? For example, what if the researcher hypothesized that the sample group would be statistically significantly higher than the population? In this case, the observed value, $z_{obs} = 2.33$, would be the same, but the critical value would change to $z_{crit} = 1.645$ (Table 16.3) because the *z*-score of 1.645 is associated with the critical value ($z_{crit}$) of .450 ($\alpha$ .05 or .5 − $\alpha$ = .450). Thus, the critical value changes based on the level of significance established for the study (alpha level) and the type of test: directional or nondirectional. Table 16.4 contains the most common

**TABLE 16.2**   Decision grid for the null hypothesis.

| Researcher's Decision | Actual Status of the Null Hypothesis | |
|---|---|---|
| | **True** | **False** |
| Reject the null hypothesis | Type I error $\alpha$ | Correct (1 − $\alpha$) obs > crit $p < \alpha$ |
| Retain the null hypothesis | Correct (1 − $\beta$) obs < crit $p > \alpha$ | Type II error $\beta$ |

© Cengage Learning

**TABLE 16.3**  *Using z to find areas under the normal curve.*

| z | Second Decimal Place of z | | | | | | | | | |
|---|------|------|------|------|------|------|------|------|------|------|
|   | 0.00 | 0.01 | 0.02 | 0.03 | 0.04 | 0.05 | 0.06 | 0.07 | 0.08 | 0.09 |
| 0.0 | 0.000 | 0.004 | 0.008 | 0.012 | 0.016 | 0.020 | 0.024 | 0.028 | 0.032 | 0.036 |
| 0.1 | 0.040 | 0.044 | 0.048 | 0.052 | 0.056 | 0.060 | 0.064 | 0.678 | 0.071 | 0.075 |
| 0.2 | 0.079 | 0.083 | 0.087 | 0.090 | 0.095 | 0.099 | 0.103 | 0.106 | 0.110 | 0.114 |
| 0.3 | 0.118 | 0.122 | 0.126 | 0.129 | 0.133 | 0.137 | 0.141 | 0.144 | 0.148 | 0.152 |
| 0.4 | 0.155 | 0.159 | 0.163 | 0.166 | 0.170 | 0.174 | 0.177 | 0.181 | 0.184 | 0.188 |
| 0.5 | 0.192 | 0.195 | 0.199 | 0.202 | 0.205 | 0.209 | 0.212 | 0.216 | 0.219 | 0.222 |
| 0.6 | 0.226 | 0.229 | 0.232 | 0.236 | 0.239 | 0.242 | 0.245 | 0.249 | 0.252 | 0.255 |
| 0.7 | 0.258 | 0.261 | 0.264 | 0.267 | 0.270 | 0.273 | 0.276 | 0.279 | 0.282 | 0.285 |
| 0.8 | 0.288 | 0.291 | 0.294 | 0.297 | 0.300 | 0.302 | 0.305 | 0.308 | 0.311 | 0.313 |
| 0.9 | 0.316 | 0.319 | 0.321 | 0.324 | 0.326 | 0.329 | 0.332 | 0.334 | 0.337 | 0.339 |
| 1.0 | 0.341 | 0.344 | 0.346 | 0.349 | 0.351 | 0.353 | 0.355 | 0.358 | 0.360 | 0.362 |
| 1.1 | 0.364 | 0.367 | 0.369 | 0.371 | 0.373 | 0.375 | 0.377 | 0.379 | 0.381 | 0.383 |
| 1.2 | 0.385 | 0.387 | 0.389 | 0.391 | 0.393 | 0.394 | 0.396 | 0.398 | **0.400** | 0.402 |
| 1.3 | 0.403 | 0.405 | 0.407 | 0.408 | 0.410 | 0.412 | 0.413 | 0.415 | 0.416 | 0.418 |
| 1.4 | 0.419 | 0.421 | 0.422 | 0.424 | 0.425 | 0.427 | 0.428 | 0.429 | 0.431 | 0.432 |
| 1.5 | 0.433 | 0.435 | 0.436 | 0.437 | 0.438 | 0.439 | 0.441 | 0.442 | 0.443 | 0.444 |
| 1.6 | 0.445 | 0.446 | 0.447 | 0.448 | **0.450** | 0.451 | 0.452 | 0.453 | 0.454 | 0.455 |
| 1.7 | 0.455 | 0.456 | 0.457 | 0.458 | 0.459 | 0.460 | 0.461 | 0.462 | 0.463 | 0.463 |
| 1.8 | 0.464 | 0.465 | 0.466 | 0.466 | 0.467 | 0.468 | 0.469 | 0.469 | 0.470 | 0.471 |
| 1.9 | 0.471 | 0.472 | 0.473 | 0.473 | 0.474 | 0.474 | **0.475** | 0.476 | 0.476 | 0.477 |
| 2.0 | 0.477 | 0.478 | 0.478 | 0.479 | 0.479 | 0.480 | 0.480 | 0.481 | 0.481 | 0.482 |
| 2.1 | 0.482 | 0.483 | 0.483 | 0.483 | 0.484 | 0.484 | 0.485 | 0.485 | 0.485 | 0.486 |
| 2.2 | 0.486 | 0.486 | 0.487 | 0.487 | 0.488 | 0.488 | 0.488 | 0.488 | 0.489 | 0.489 |
| 2.3 | 0.489 | 0.490 | **0.490** | 0.490 | 0.490 | 0.491 | 0.491 | 0.491 | 0.491 | 0.492 |
| 2.4 | 0.492 | 0.492 | 0.492 | 0.493 | 0.493 | 0.493 | 0.493 | 0.493 | 0.493 | 0.494 |
| 2.5 | 0.494 | 0.494 | 0.494 | 0.494 | 0.495 | 0.495 | 0.495 | **0.495** | 0.495 | 0.495 |
| 2.6 | 0.495 | 0.496 | 0.496 | 0.496 | 0.496 | 0.496 | 0.496 | 0.496 | 0.496 | 0.496 |
| 2.7 | 0.497 | 0.497 | 0.497 | 0.497 | 0.497 | 0.497 | 0.497 | 0.497 | 0.497 | 0.497 |
| 2.8 | 0.497 | 0.498 | 0.498 | 0.498 | 0.497 | 0.498 | 0.498 | 0.498 | 0.498 | 0.498 |
| 2.9 | 0.498 | 0.498 | 0.498 | 0.498 | 0.498 | 0.498 | 0.499 | 0.499 | 0.499 | 0.499 |
| 3.0 | 0.499 | 0.499 | 0.499 | 0.499 | 0.499 | 0.499 | 0.499 | 0.499 | 0.499 | 0.499 |

*Note:* An entry in the table is the proportion under the entire curve that is between $z = 0$ and a positive value of $z$. Because the normal curve is bilaterally symmetric, areas for negative values of $z$ are obtained by symmetry. Bolded entries indicate values associated with commonly used alphas for hypothesis testing.
© Cengage Learning

critical values ($z_{crit}$) used in research studies, and these critical values are highlighted in Table 16.3 for easy reference.

The second example used the Connors AD/HD scale $z_{crit} = 1.64$ for the directional hypothesis, so the obtained $z$-score ($z_{obt}$) of 6.25 exceeds the $z_{crit}$. Thus, the $H_0$ is rejected,

| TABLE 16.4 | z-Critical values for rejection of null hypothesis. | | |
|---|---|---|---|
| **Type of Test** | **α = 0.10** | **α = 0.05** | **α = 0.01** |
| Nondirectional | 1.64 | 1.96 | 2.58 |
| Directional | 1.28 | 1.64 | 2.33 |

© Cengage Learning

and the researcher concludes that the sample of children with AD/HD is significantly more hyperactive than the normal population. Notice that directional tests have smaller critical values because all of the type I error is loaded onto one side of the normal curve, moving the critical value line closer to the mean, and making it more likely to find statistical significance if statistical significance actually exists. This is known as *statistical power*—the likelihood of rejecting the null hypothesis given that the null hypothesis should be rejected. As discussed in Chapter 14, power is directly related to the alpha (α) level, the direction of the test, the magnitude of differences between the means, and the sample size.

# Comparing Two or More Sample Means: Student's *t*-Test and the *F*-Test

Often in social science research, information regarding populations is not readily available for comparisons. After all, the number of variables to consider when investigating various phenomena is vast and arbitrary. Unlike the *z*-test, which compares the sample mean to the population mean, Student's *t*-test compares two sample means, and the **F-test** (also known as ANOVA) compares two or more sample means.

The term **Student's *t*-test** has an interesting origin. William Sealey Gosset was employed by Guinness Breweries of Dublin, Ireland. The chemists at the brewery were given the task of identifying the various aspects of developing a quality brew at the cheapest price. Various factors were considered, such as various types of barley and hops and fermentation. The problem was that statistical tests prior to this point focused on large populations, not small samples. "Gosset determined that the distribution curves of small sample means were somewhat different from the normal curve. Small sample distributions were observed to be lower at the means and higher at the tails, or ends, of the distributions" (Best & Kahn, 2006, p. 400; see Figure 16.1). Gosset published his research under the name Student—hence the name "Student's *t*-test," because Guinness brewery did not want to advertise the fact that they were employing statisticians to gain an advantage in the beer market!

**Figure 16.1**

Examples of observed variations in sample and population means.

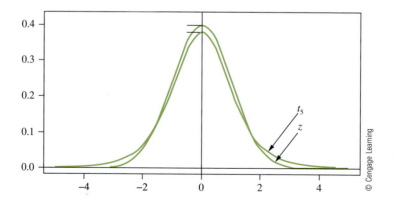

© Cengage Learning

## Model Assumptions

When using a *t*-test or ANOVA, certain assumptions must be in place. In other words, a statistical test cannot be arbitrarily used, but a specific set of conditions must be met for the statistical test to be deemed appropriate and meaningful. These conditions are known as model assumptions. The model assumptions for *t*-test or ANOVA include independence, normality, and homogeneity of variances.

Independence refers to randomness in selection and assignment. In other words, the selection of a participant should not be dependent on the selection of another participant. In a study in which treatment conditions are used (e.g., treatment and control groups), individuals in a population should have an equal chance of being selected and assigned to a group at random. Social science research, however, often deals with examining differences in characteristics, such as gender, in which random assignment is not possible. Independence also specifies that each participant should be observed (measured) only once. For example, assume a researcher wants to compare two classes with respect to performance on a test. If one student was in both classes, that student should not be measured twice (once for each class). Rather, it would be best to eliminate such a participant. The most important issue of independence is that "observations within or between groups are not paired, dependent, correlated, or associated in any way" (Glass & Hopkins, 2008, p. 295). There are specific tests for paired observations, known as repeated measures, which can be used with paired observations. The essential point here is that when independence is compromised, probability estimates of type I and type II errors are not accurate.

Normality is concerned with the distributions of the groups being compared in a study. Parametric tests assume that each group is normally distributed. The mathematical properties of the formulae used to compare groups are based on the mean, median, and mode being approximately equal and the distribution resembling a bell-shaped curve. In a normal sample distribution from a population, means and variances over repeated samples will be uncorrelated and, thus, statistically independent. Although measures exist to test for normality prior to running a *t*-test or ANOVA (e.g., Shapiro-Wilk statistic ($W$), *z*-test for skewness, and *z*-test for kurtosis), in reality, the consequences of violating the normality assumption are rather minimal, especially when conducting a study with a balanced design (i.e., conducting research with sample sizes being equal in all groups) (Glass & Hopkins, 2008).

Homogeneity of variances is concerned with the estimation of within-group differences. When conducting an ANOVA or *t*-test, the researcher is focused on establishing whether statistically significant differences exist between the groups. Thus, a mean for each group is calculated. However, most participants (if any) do not score at the exact mean, which is only an estimation of the group's average performance. Thus, when participants do not score at the mean, this results in error, and the average amount of error in the group is known as the *SD*. The variance (i.e., the *SD* squared) is the estimated amount of error under the normal curve. Put another way, the *SD* is the average amount of error in scores, whereas the variance is the amount of error in the area under the normal curve. In univariate parametric statistics, the variances (also the amount of error under the normal curve or the estimated within group differences) should be approximately equal to each other. When parametric tests are used, a single term representing the pooled variance (i.e., the combined variances of the group) is used. Consider an example where one group has a distribution in which all participants scored close to the mean, but the other group had a lot more variability and deviated from the mean quite extensively. The result is that the researcher is comparing apples to oranges. The two groups have very different distributions and cannot be compared without using additional statistical procedures (e.g., the Welch *t*-test or Brown–Forsy the *F*-test) or nonparametric tests.

Like normality, when sample sizes are equal among groups, *t*-test and ANOVA are robust to heterogeneous variances; that is, equal sample sizes reduce the problem of unequal variances. When sample sizes are unequal and heterogeneous variances occur, however, the results of the *t*-test or ANOVA are compromised with respect to the likelihood of making a type I error. In a given data set, when groups with larger sample sizes also have larger variances and groups with smaller sample sizes have smaller variances, the likelihood of making a type I error (alpha) is actually lower; this is referred to as a conservative statistical test. When groups with larger sample sizes have smaller variances and groups with smaller sample sizes have larger variances, the likelihood of making a type I error (alpha) is higher; this is referred to as a liberal statistical test (Glass & Hopkins, 2008).

Although statistical tests to address problems with homogeneity of variances exist, some tests are seldom used (e.g., Hartley's $F_{max}$ test or Cochran test) because they require a balanced design (i.e., equal sample sizes) and are inaccurate when distributions are not normal. Balanced designs seldom occur in social science research, and as stated before, *t*-test and ANOVA are robust to heterogeneous designs when sample sizes are equal. Two additional tests that are commonly used in statistical software are the Levene test and Brown–Forsythe test. In some statistical software, such as *SPSS*, the Levene test is the only test that is used for homogeneity of variance. The Levene test uses the absolute value of the deviation scores (i.e., the group mean is subtracted from the raw score), and an *F*-test is conducted using the absolute value of the deviation scores (using the median score). Unfortunately, the Levene test falls under the same criticisms as the other tests for homogeneity of variance: To yield accurate results, the group samples should be equal and the distributions normal (Glass & Hopkins, 2008). The Brown–Forsythe test can be used when sample sizes are unequal and is robust to nonnormality. It is similar to the Levene test, but it uses an *F*-test on the absolute value of the deviation scores using the median, as opposed to the mean. Thus, the Brown-Forsythe test is less influenced by groups with greater ranges of scores. Overall, when conducting or reviewing research, awareness of the degree to which model assumptions were met can influence the generalizability of the results and the replicability of the research.

## Degrees of Freedom (*df*)

When comparing samples, the researcher must account for sample size and the number of groups being compared. Sample size and group comparisons can differ from study to study, and so can the distributions (Figure 16.2). Thus, probability values under the

**Figure 16.2**

Distribution variations owing to sample sizes.

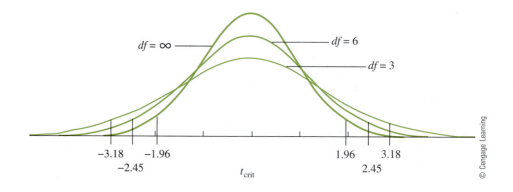

$df = \infty$        $df = 6$

$df = 3$

$-3.18$    $-1.96$         $1.96$    $3.18$

$-2.45$        $t_{crit}$        $2.45$

© Cengage Learning

normal curve can change. As a result, **degrees of freedom** are calculated to provide an estimate of the normal curve given the number of groups and the sample size of each group. There are various formulae for computing the degrees of freedom, each dependent on the number of comparison groups, sample size, and type of statistical test. Each method for computing the degrees of freedom (*df*) will be addressed in the respective calculations that follow.

# Calculating the Independent *t*-Test

In the independent *t*-test (sometimes called a *t*-test for independent samples), a statistical test is run to determine whether a statistically significant difference exists between two independent sample means. *Independent* in this context means that the two means are not connected to the same sample of participants. The sample mean of one group is subtracted from the sample mean of the second group and then divided by the pooled standard error, where $\overline{X}_1$ is the sample mean for the first group, $\overline{X}_2$ is the sample mean for the second group, and $s_{\overline{x}_1} - s_{\overline{x}_2}$ is the pooled standard error.

$$t = \frac{\overline{X}_1 - \overline{X}_2}{s_{\overline{x}_1} - s_{\overline{x}_2}} \tag{16.4}$$

The pooled standard error represents the combined variance terms from each of the two groups. By combining these terms, sampling error is reduced and an approximation of the population variance is achieved. To calculate the standard error, the variance and samples of each group need to be known. The subscripts by each term represent the variance or sample size of each group (group 1 or group 2). The degrees of freedom are calculated by subtracting 1 from the sample size of the group. Thus, $s^2_1$ represents the variance for group 1; $s^2_2$ represents the variance for group 2; $n_1 - 1$ represents the degrees of freedom for group 1 ($df_1$); and $n_2 - 1$ represents the degrees of freedom for group 2 ($df_2$).

$$s_{\overline{x}_1} - s_{\overline{x}_2} = \sqrt{\left(s_1^2(n_1 - 1) + s_2^2(n_2 - 1)\right)\left(\frac{1}{n_1} + \frac{1}{n_2}\right)} \tag{16.5}$$

So assume that 25 graduates from a counseling program in University A and 30 graduates from a counseling program in University B take the NCE, and the graduate program that is doing a better job of preparing students for the NCE is to be determined. The mean score for the 25 students from University A was 120 with an *SD* of 10. The mean score for the 30 students from University B was 125 with an *SD* of 15. So is there a statistically significant difference between the two groups? Can it be stated with 95 percent confidence ($\alpha = .05$) that the difference in these scores is outside the realm of chance? An independent *t*-test is conducted to answer this question using the means, *SD*s, and sample sizes from the two independent groups. Although this computation procedure can be conducted using SPSS in a matter of minutes, the conceptual process can be summarized in the following six steps.

*Step 1: Decide if the test is directional or nondirectional and set the alpha level.*

Similar to the *z*-test, the *t*-test can be directional or nondirectional. So in this case, if group 1 scored lower than group 2, there would be no method to test if group 1 was statistically significantly lower because the test was designed to detect statistical significance only if group 1 was higher. For this example, we will conduct a nondirectional test.

*Step 2: Compute the variance from the standard deviation.*

$$s_1 = 10, \text{ so } s_1^2 = 100$$

$$s_2 = 15, \text{ so } s_2^2 = 225$$

*Step 3: Compute the degrees of freedom.*

$$df_1 = n_1 - 1 = 25 - 1 = 24$$

$$df_2 = n_2 - 1 = 30 - 1 = 29$$

$$df = df_1 + df_2 = 53$$

*Step 4: Compute the pooled error variance.*

$$s_{\bar{x}_1} - s_{\bar{x}_2} = \sqrt{\frac{s_1^2(n_1 - 1) + s_2^2(n_2 - 1)}{(n_1 - 1) + (n_2 - 1)}\left(\frac{1}{n_1} + \frac{1}{n_2}\right)}$$

$$= \sqrt{\frac{100(24) + 225(29)}{53}\left(\frac{1}{25} + \frac{1}{30}\right)}$$

$$= \sqrt{2400 + 6525(.04 + .03)}$$

$$= \sqrt{(168.40)(.07)} = \sqrt{11.79} = 3.43$$

*Step 5: Conduct the t-test.*

$$t = \frac{\overline{X}_1 - \overline{X}_2}{s_{\bar{x}_1} - s_{\bar{x}_2}} = \frac{120 - 125}{3.43} = -1.46$$

*Step 6: Determine the critical value.*

Table 16.5 includes the degrees of freedom in the left column and the alpha level on top. Directional *t*-tests are interpreted using the $\alpha_1$ values, and nondirectional *t*-tests use the $\alpha_2$ values. Critical values are located underneath the alpha levels, using the respective degrees of freedom. In the event the degrees of freedom are not represented in the table—*t*(115), for example—use the lower degrees of freedom between the two values for a more conservative estimate. Using Table 16.5, when $\alpha = .05$ (nondirectional), $t(53) = 2.01$. Of course, statistical packages such as SPSS calculate *t*-tests without the tedious hand calculations.

As a second demonstration of the use of the independent *t*-tests, consider an example of the children with AD/HD in which the researcher has a sample mean $(M_a)$ T score of 70 $(SD = 8; N_a = 20)$, and a control group mean $(M_b)$ T score of 55 $(SD = 11; N_b = 20)$. Assuming a directional hypothesis (A > B) at the $\alpha$ .05 level of significance, using the preceding six-step process, the resulting $t(38) = +4.81$—that is,

$$t(38) = \frac{70 - 55}{\sqrt{\frac{64(19) + 121(19)}{19 + 19}\left[\frac{1}{19} + \frac{1}{19}\right]}} = \frac{15}{3.12} = +4.81.$$

## Evaluating the Independent *t*-Test for Statistical Significance

Like the *z*-test, if you want to determine whether the observed score for the NCE example, $t_{obs} = -1.46$, is statistically significant at the .05 level of significance, the observed score must be greater than the critical value, $t_{crit}$. In this example, the $t_{crit}$ can be located in

**TABLE 16.5**  Critical values for Student's *t*-test.

| df | Nondirectional | | Directional | |
| --- | --- | --- | --- | --- |
| | 0.05 | 0.01 | 0.05 | 0.01 |
| 1 | 12.71 | 63.56 | 6.31 | 31.82 |
| 2 | 4.30 | 9.92 | 2.92 | 6.96 |
| 3 | 3.18 | 5.84 | 2.35 | 4.54 |
| 4 | 2.78 | 4.60 | 2.13 | 3.75 |
| 5 | 2.57 | 4.03 | 2.02 | 3.36 |
| 6 | 2.45 | 3.71 | 1.94 | 3.14 |
| 7 | 2.36 | 3.50 | 1.90 | 3.00 |
| 8 | 2.31 | 3.36 | 1.86 | 2.90 |
| 9 | 2.26 | 3.25 | 1.83 | 2.82 |
| 10 | 2.23 | 3.17 | 1.81 | 2.76 |
| 11 | 2.20 | 3.11 | 1.80 | 2.72 |
| 12 | 2.18 | 3.06 | 1.78 | 2.68 |
| 13 | 2.16 | 3.01 | 1.77 | 2.65 |
| 14 | 2.14 | 2.98 | 1.76 | 2.62 |
| 15 | 2.13 | 2.95 | 1.75 | 2.60 |
| 16 | 2.12 | 2.92 | 1.75 | 2.58 |
| 17 | 2.11 | 2.90 | 1.74 | 2.57 |
| 18 | 2.10 | 2.88 | 1.73 | 2.55 |
| 19 | 2.09 | 2.86 | 1.73 | 2.54 |
| 20 | 2.09 | 2.84 | 1.72 | 2.53 |
| 21 | 2.08 | 2.83 | 1.72 | 2.52 |
| 22 | 2.07 | 2.82 | 1.72 | 2.51 |
| 23 | 2.07 | 2.81 | 1.71 | 2.50 |
| 24 | 2.06 | 2.80 | 1.71 | 2.49 |
| 25 | 2.06 | 2.79 | 1.71 | 2.48 |
| 26 | 2.06 | 2.78 | 1.71 | 2.48 |
| 27 | 2.05 | 2.77 | 1.70 | 2.47 |
| 28 | 2.05 | 2.76 | 1.70 | 2.47 |
| 29 | 2.04 | 2.76 | 1.70 | 2.46 |
| 30 | 2.04 | 2.75 | 1.70 | 2.46 |
| 40 | 2.02 | 2.70 | 1.68 | 2.42 |
| 60 | 2.00 | 2.66 | 1.67 | 2.39 |
| 120 | 1.98 | 2.62 | 1.66 | 2.36 |
| ∞ | 1.96 | 2.58 | 1.64 | 2.33 |

© Cengage Learning

Table 16.5 under the nondirectional $\alpha = .05$ column. Notice that because $df = 53$ for this example, the researcher must interpolate the *t* value; that is, if a *df* of 40 yields a $t_{crit}$ of 2.021 and a *df* of 60 yields a $t_{crit}$ value of 2.000, then a *df* of 53 will be 13/20 of the distance between 2.021 and 2.000, or about 2.008. Therefore, $| -1.46 | < | -2.008 |$, so there is no statistically significant difference between the two groups of university students on the NCE.

Using the AD/HD example results, the $t_{obs}$ (38) = +4.81 and the $t_{crit}$ = 1.68 for the directional hypothesis at $\alpha.$ = 05. Applying the comparison $\mid t_{obs} \mid > \mid t_{crit} \mid$, the result of $\mid 4.81 \mid > \mid 1.68 \mid$ means that Group A is statistically significantly higher than Group B.

## Calculating the Dependent *t*-Test

A dependent *t*-test (sometimes called a *t*-test for correlated means) also compares two means, but in this case the means are compared from the same sample of participants across time, such as with a pretest and posttest administered to the same group. Although in an independent *t*-test two sets of independent means are compared between two randomized groups, in a dependent *t*-test two sets of correlated means are compared for a set of participants. The two sets of means in a dependent *t*-test may result from a study in which individuals initially take a pretest, then experience a treatment/intervention, and finally take a posttest. For example, assume that a researcher would like to know the effect of self-talk strategies in decreasing depression. Participants could be administered the Beck Depression Inventory—II (BDI-II) (Beck, Steer, & Brown, 1996), learn and practice self-talk strategies, and then retake the BDI-II. To determine whether the self-talk intervention was successful, mean scores from each administration of the BDI-II could be compared using a dependent *t*-test.

A second common scenario involves a comparison between pairs of individuals who have been matched because of commonality in one or more characteristics. Using the preceding BDI-II example, another way to do the study would be to administer the BDI-II to two groups. Participants are then matched according to similar BDI-II scores. One of the participants in each of the pairs is randomly assigned to the experimental group and learns and practices self-talk strategies; the other participant in the pair functions as a member of the control group. A dependent *t*-test is conducted to determine significant differences between participants who received the intervention (i.e., treatment) versus participants who did not receive the intervention (i.e., control). The advantage of this design is the presence of a control group. In the first design, the researcher cannot be certain that the intervention was the reason for improvement if significant differences do exist. Potential differences in the no control group study could be the result of a testing effect (i.e., the fact that the participants thought they should be doing better by the time the second BDI-II was administered) or statistical regression (i.e., depressed participant scores regress toward the mean or re-administration of the same test). The latter design provides a control for this problem.

To conduct a dependent *t*-test, the correlation coefficient (*r*) must be calculated between the pretest and posttest scores or the scores of the matched pairs.

$$t = \frac{\overline{X}_1 - \overline{X}_2}{s_{\overline{x}_1 - \overline{x}_2}} = \frac{\overline{X}_1 - \overline{X}_2}{\sqrt{\dfrac{s_1^2}{n_1} + \dfrac{s_2^2}{n_2} - 2r\left(\dfrac{s_1}{\sqrt{n_1}}\right)\left(\dfrac{s_2}{\sqrt{n_2}}\right)}} \tag{16.6}$$

Remember, tests of statistical significance follow a similar pattern for their formulae: The mean differences are divided by the standard error. For the dependent *t*-test, the sample size (*n*), standard deviation (*s*), the variance for each group (*s*²), and the correlation coefficient (*r*) between the two groups are needed.

So, assume that 25 clients from a counseling center at a university are administered the BDI-II upon initial screening and then again three months later. The counseling center wishes to know whether the clients with depression are doing better after three months of counseling. The mean score for the 25 clients at the initial screening is 35 with a standard deviation of 12. The mean score for the 25 clients after three months is 26 with a standard deviation of 10. The correlation between the two administrations is

$r = .93$. So is there a statistically significant difference between the two scores over time? Can it be stated with 95 percent confidence ($\alpha = .05$) that the difference in these scores is outside the realm of chance? A dependent *t*-test is conducted to answer this question. Again, the researcher should use the following six steps.

*Step 1: Decide if the test is directional or nondirectional and set the alpha level.*

In testing the null hypothesis, we will assume that there is no statistically significant difference in the two administrations. So the null and alternative hypotheses may be written as follows:

$$H_0: \mu_1 = \mu_2.$$

$$H_1: \mu_1 \neq \mu_2.$$

So, in this case, if the latter assessment is not statistically significantly different (either higher or lower) than the initial assessment, then the null hypothesis is accepted. If a statistically significant difference does exist, then the null hypothesis is rejected.

*Step 2: Compute the variance from the standard deviation.*

$$s_1 = 12, \text{ so } s_1^2 = 144$$

$$s_2 = 10, \text{ so } s_2^2 = 100$$

*Step 3: Compute the degrees of freedom.*

The total number of pairs is subtracted by 1: $df = n - 1$ or, in this case, $25 - 1 = 24$.

*Step 4: Compute the pooled error variance.*

$$s_{\bar{x}_1 - \bar{x}_2} = \sqrt{\frac{s_1^2}{n_1} + \frac{s_2^2}{n_2} - 2r\left(\frac{s_1}{\sqrt{n_1}}\right)\left(\frac{s_2}{\sqrt{n_2}}\right)}$$

$$= \sqrt{\frac{144}{25} + \frac{100}{25} - 2(.93)\left(\frac{12}{\sqrt{25}}\right)\left(\frac{10}{\sqrt{25}}\right)}$$

$$= \sqrt{5.76 + 4 - 2(.93)(2.4)(2)}$$

$$= \sqrt{.832} = .91$$

*Step 5: Conduct the t-test.*

$$t = \frac{\overline{X}_1 - \overline{X}_2}{s_{\bar{x}_1 - \bar{x}_2}} = \frac{35 - 26}{.91} = 9.89$$

*Step 6: Calculate the critical value using Table 16.5.*

When $\alpha = .05$ (nondirectional), $t(24) = 2.064$.

In a second example (using an SPSS application), consider a study of anxiety treatment in which 20 matched participants were randomly assigned to treatment and control conditions, with the treatment group exposed to progressive muscle relaxation training (PMRT) meant to reduce the level of anxiety experienced by that group. The data for this study are presented in Table 16.6. Computation of a *t*-test for correlated samples using SPSS output is found in Table 16.7.

## Evaluating the Dependent *t*-Test for Statistical Significance

To determine whether the observed score, $t_{obs} = 9.89$, is statistically significant at the $\alpha = .05$ level of significance, the observed score must be greater than the critical value

| TABLE 16.6 | Data for a study of anxiety treatment using PMRT. |
| --- | --- |

© Cengage Learning

$t_{crit}$. In this example, $9.89 > 2.064$, so there is a statistically significant difference between the two groups.

In the second study using the PMRT anxiety-reduction technique, one can see from the output in Table 16.7 that the difference in matched pair means was significant ($p < .05$, two-tailed). Participants in the PMRT treatment group displayed significantly less perceived anxiety after treatment implementation. In this case, the resulting $t_{obs}$ was $t(9) = 2.924$.

# The *F*-Test: One-Way Analysis of Variance (ANOVA)

A one-way ANOVA answers the question "Is there a difference among group means?" and is used in designs with a single independent variable (with two or more groups or levels) and a single dependent variable (using an interval or ratio scale). An ANOVA is conducted when two or more group means (*J*) are being compared. When $J = 2$, either a *t*-test or an *F*-test may be computed because they are comparable. The relationship between a *t*-test and an *F*-test when $J = 2$ is $F = t^2$ (or $t = \sqrt{F}$). When $J > 2$ (i.e., there are three or more means being compared), however, statistical significance can be ascertained by conducting

**TABLE 16.7**    SPSS output for a study of anxiety treatment using PMRT.

**Paired Samples Statistics**

| | | Mean | N | Std. Deviation | Std. Error Mean |
|---|---|---|---|---|---|
| Pair 1 | AnxietyControl & | 21.0000 | 10 | 5.29150 | 1.67332 |
| | AnxietyPMRT | 16.9000 | 10 | 3.87155 | 1.22429 |

**Paired Samples Correlations**

| | | N | Correlation | Sig. |
|---|---|---|---|---|
| Pair 1 | AnxietyControl & AnxietyPMRT | 10 | .569 | .086 |

**Paired Samples Test**

| | | Paired Differences | | | | | | | |
|---|---|---|---|---|---|---|---|---|---|
| | | Mean | Std. Deviation | Std. Error Mean | 95 Percent Confidence Interval of the Difference | | t | df | Sig. (2-tailed) |
| | | | | | Lower | Upper | | | |
| Pair 1 | AnxietyControl & AnxietyPMRT | 4.1 | 4.43346 | 1.40198 | 0.92849 | 7.27151 | 2.924 | 9 | 0.017 |

© Cengage Learning

one statistical test, ANOVA, or alternatively but decidedly less desirably, by repeated *t*-tests. You may ask, "Why can't you conduct several *t*-tests?" Well, each statistical test is conducted with a specified chance of making a type I error (the alpha level [$\alpha$]). For example, consider the case of a researcher who wished to use a self-efficacy screening measure on students in a math class. Research has shown that higher levels of self-efficacy are related to better math performance. So students are randomly placed in four groups. Group 1 receives a lecture on enhancing self-efficacy. Group 2 receives a lecture and experiential exercise on self-efficacy. Group 3 receives an experiential self-efficacy exercise only. Finally, Group 4 is a control group, and so it receives no treatment whatsoever. After the treatment, a self-efficacy measure is administered to the four different math classes. If *t*-tests were used to conduct the analysis and a level of significance was set at $\alpha = .05$, then six separate *t*-tests would need to be conducted: (a) group 1 to group 2, (b) group 1 to group 3, (c) group 1 to group 4, (d) group 2 to group 3, (e) group 2 to group 4, and (f) group 3 to group 4. Then the number of comparisons is always $\dfrac{J(J-1)}{2}$. Thus, if $J = 4$, then $\dfrac{4(3)}{2} = 6$. The problem with conducting multiple *t*-tests is that type I error is multiplied by the number of tests being conducted. So if a researcher conducts six *t*-tests with an $\alpha = .05$ on the same data, the chance of having a type I error among the six tests is 30 percent, a rather large likelihood of identifying statistically significant differences when none actually exist! The implication here is profound. When considering whether such research results can help in identifying what models may be helpful to clients, one would need to be extremely cautious in implementing a "best practice" when there is a 30 percent chance of being wrong. Rather than conducting several *t*-tests, an ANOVA could be conducted to identify statistically significant differences among all the groups at the $\alpha = .05$ level of significance—resulting in only a 5 percent chance of type I error! To compute the *F*-test on the self-efficacy example, the data set presented in Table 16.8 will be used.

**TABLE 16.8** Data for the self-efficacy experiment.

| Group 1 | Group 2 | Group 3 | Group 4 | |
|---------|---------|---------|---------|---|
| 4 | 9 | 8 | 1 | |
| 6 | 11 | 6 | 2 | |
| 8 | 8 | 9 | 3 | |
| 3 | 9 | 5 | 5 | |
| 9 | 8 | 7 | 1 | |
| $\overline{X}_1 = 6.0$ | $\overline{X}_2 = 9.0$ | $\overline{X}_3 = 7.0$ | $\overline{X}_4 = 2.4$ | $\overline{X}. = 6.1$ |
| $s_1^2 = 6.5$ | $s_2^2 = 1.5$ | $s_3^2 = 2.5$ | $s_4^2 = 2.8$ | |

© Cengage Learning

## Calculating the *F*-Test

Nearly all statisticians use computerized statistical packages, such as SPSS, SAS, or R-stat to compute the *F*-test statistic. But seeing the actual logical formula steps may be instructive. To calculate the *F*-test statistic, use the following seven-step method.

*Step 1: State the null hypothesis and alpha level.*

Unlike the *t*-test, the *F*-test is calculated using squared deviations. Remember that in the *t*-test, the numerator was calculated by subtracting one group mean from another; so an observed value for a *t*-test could be positive or negative and fall on either side of the normal curve. The numerator of the *F*-test uses squared values, so the observed value in an *F*-test is always positive. Therefore, the curve is somewhat different (Figure 16.3).

Thus, the null hypothesis in an *F*-test is never directional. Using the preceding data set (Table 16.8), the null and alternative hypotheses would be expressed as follows:

$$H_0 : \mu_1 = \mu_2 = \mu_3 = \mu_4$$
$$H_1 : \mu_1 \neq \mu_2 \neq \mu_3 \neq \mu_4$$

So in this case, if any of the groups are not statistically significantly different (either higher or lower) from one another, then the null hypothesis is retained. If a statistically significant difference does exist between or among *any* groups, then the null hypothesis is rejected.

As the computation of the ANOVA is explained, keep in mind the common properties statistical tests share. Essentially, ANOVA is calculated by dividing the mean

**Figure 16.3**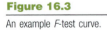

An example *F*-test curve.

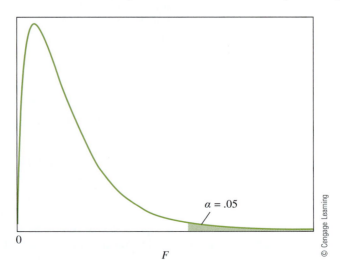

differences squared by the error variance. Thus, the numerator will comprise mean differences, and the denominator will comprise error variance.

*Step 2: Compute the grand mean.*

To evaluate whether statistically significant differences among groups are evident, *group means* $[(\overline{X}_j)]$ (i.e., the mean of each group) are compared with a **grand mean** $(\overline{X}.)$ (i.e., the mean of the entire sample). The grand mean can be computed with the following formula:

$$\overline{X}. = \frac{\sum n_j \overline{X}_j}{\sum n_j}, \tag{16.7}$$

where the numerator is the sum of the sample size for each group (in this case, $n_j = 5$, and the total sample $n. = 20$) multiplied by the mean of each group $(\overline{X}_j)$, and the denominator is the sum of the sample size from each group $(n.)$. If we were to break down this formula for this particular data set, it would look like the following:

$$\overline{X}. = \frac{\sum n_j \overline{X}_j}{\sum n_j} = \frac{n_1(\overline{X}_1) + n_2(\overline{X}_2) + n_3(\overline{X}_3) + n_4(\overline{X}_4)}{n_1 + n_2 + n_3 + n_4} \tag{16.8}$$

So

$$\overline{X}. = \frac{5(6) + 5(9) + 5(7) + 5(2.4)}{5 + 5 + 5 + 5} = \frac{30 + 45 + 35 + 12}{20} = 6.1$$

*Step 3: Calculate the Sum of Squares Between ($SS_B$).*

As just stated, rather than comparing one group mean with another, as was done in a *t*-test, the *F*-test requires that group means be compared against the grand mean. The Sum of Squares Between ($SS_B$) is the squared sum of the differences between each group mean and the grand mean. By comparing each group mean to the mean of the entire sample, the amount of variation *between* the groups can be assessed. Calculate $SS_B$ as follows:

$$SS_B = \sum n_j(\overline{X}_j - \overline{X}.)^2, \tag{16.9}$$

where the sum of $n_j$, the number of participants in a group, is multiplied by $(\overline{X}_j - \overline{X}.)^2$, the square of the group mean minus the grand mean. Because $(\overline{X}_j - \overline{X}.)$ is the magnitude of the difference between a group mean and grand mean, it is sometimes referred to as a **treatment effect**. Equation 16.9 is written in expanded form for the current example:

$$SS_B = \sum n_j(\overline{X}_j - \overline{X}.)^2 = n_1(\overline{X}_1 - \overline{X}.)^2 + n_2(\overline{X}_2 - \overline{X}.)^2 + n_3(\overline{X}_3 - \overline{X}.)^2 + n_4(\overline{X}_4 - \overline{X}.)^2$$

$$= 5(6 - 6.1)^2 + 5(9 - 6.1)^2 + 5(7 - 6.1)^2 + 5(2.4 - 6.1)^2$$

$$= .05 + 42.05 + 4.05 + 68.45$$

$$= 114.6$$

*Step 4: Calculate the Sum of Squares Within ($SS_W$).*

The Sum of Squares Within ($SS_W$) is the sum of the squared differences between each observation (i.e., raw score) and the group mean. In other words, a deviation score is computed and squared for each group. For group 1, each observation is subtracted by 6 and then squared. For group 2, each observation is subtracted by 9 and then squared. This process is repeated for all of the groups. Then the sum of the squared deviations is added together to compute $SS_W$. By comparing each observation to the group mean, the amount of variation *within* each group can be assessed.

This process can be quite tedious when doing hand computation with a larger data set, which is why statistical software, such as *SPSS* or R-stat, is almost always used. Here is a simpler formula:

$$SS_W = \sum s_j^2 (n_j - 1), \tag{16.10}$$

where the variance for each group ($s_j^2$) is multiplied by the sample size of each group minus 1 ($n_j - 1$) and then summed. To calculate $SS_W$ for the current example, do the following:

$$SS_W = \sum s_j^2 (n_j - 1) = s_1^2 (n_1 - 1) + s_2^2 (n_2 - 1) + s_3^2 (n_3 - 1) + s_4^2 (n_4 - 1)$$
$$= 6.5(4) + 1.5(4) + 2.5(4) + 2.8(4)$$
$$= 53.2.$$

Both $SS_B$ and $SS_W$ account for group size when computed. Remember, however, that when variance was computed, the total sample size was accounted for in the formula. The same must be done when computing an ANOVA. Degrees of freedom must be computed for $SS_B$ and $SS_W$ to establish the ratio of the *F*-test. This ratio is referred to as *mean squares*. Simply put, the *F*-test is the mean square between ($MS_B$) divided by the mean square within ($MS_W$).

*Step 5: Compute mean square between ($MS_B$).*

To compute $MS_B$, the degrees of freedom between ($df_b$ or $[j - 1]$) must be computed—that is, the number of groups minus 1 or ($j - 1$). In this example, $j - 1 = 4 - 1 = 3$. Thus,

$$MS_B = \frac{SS_B}{j - 1} = \frac{114.6}{4 - 1} = \frac{114.6}{3} = 38.2.$$

*Step 6: Compute mean square within ($MS_W$).*

To compute $MS_W$, the degrees of freedom within ($df_w$ or $[n. - j]$) must be computed; that is, the total sample size minus the number of groups or ($n. - j$). In this example, $n. - j = 20 - 4 = 16$. Thus, $MS_W = \dfrac{SS_W}{n. - j} = \dfrac{53.2}{20 - 4} = \dfrac{53.2}{16} = 3.325.$

*Step 7: Compute the* F-*ratio.*

We have now obtained all of the components necessary for computing the *F*-test. The *F*-test formula is

$$F = \frac{MS_B}{MS_W} = \frac{SS_B / j - 1}{SS_W / n. - j} \tag{16.11}$$

So in this example,

$$F = \frac{38.2}{3.325} = 11.49$$

These computations are quickly and easily performed using *SPSS* (Table 16.9).

### Evaluating the F-Test for Statistical Significance

To determine whether or not the observed score, $F(3, 16) = 11.49$, is statistically significant at the $\alpha = .05$ level of significance (the level decided on prior to the study), the observed score must be greater than the critical value, $F_{crit}$. The critical values for $F$ are located in Table 16.10. The *df* values on top of Table 16.10 represent the degrees of freedom between (i.e., $j - 1$). The values in the left column are the degrees of freedom within (i.e., $n. - j$). Check the critical value with respect to the appropriate alpha level identified

| **TABLE 16.9** | SPSS output for the data set provided in Table 16.8. |
|---|---|

**ANOVA**

**Self-Efficacy**

|  | **Sum of Squares** | **df** | **Mean Square** | **F** | **Sig.** |
|---|---|---|---|---|---|
| Between Groups | 114.600 | 3 | 38.200 | 11.489 | .000 |
| Within Groups | 53.200 | 16 | 3.325 |  |  |
| Total | 167.800 | 19 |  |  |  |

© Cengage Learning

in the study. In this example, 11.49 > 3.239, so a statistically significant score exists among the four groups. Of course, at this point we only know that a difference exists, not specifically which groups display differences. To determine this, we must conduct *post hoc* analyses, which are discussed next. Table 16.10 provides $F_{crit}$ values for $\alpha = .05$; Table 16.11 provides $F_{crit}$ values for $\alpha = .01$.

## *Post Hoc* Analysis

When statistically significant differences are found in an ANOVA, what is really known is that statistically significant differences exist among the groups. There may be significant differences between two groups only, or significant differences may exist between more or even all of the groups. In the current example, the results of the *F*-test are indicative of statistically significant results among the groups. Exactly what groups are different or where the statistically significant differences lie is not explained in ANOVA results. Further analysis is necessary. **Post hoc analyses** are the statistical tests conducted to indicate exactly where statistically significant differences exist. *Post hoc* analyses are *only* conducted when ANOVA results indicate statistical significance. There are several commonly used *post hoc* procedures (e.g., Tukey, Newman-Kevls, and Scheffé), with each varying primarily in how conservative the resulting decisions may be.

The most common method for *post hoc* analysis is the Tukey method of multiple comparisons (TMC). *Post hoc* comparisons are common in statistical packages, such as SPSS, R-stat, and SAS. The TMC tests all possible pairwise comparisons:

$$C = \frac{j(j-1)}{2}, \tag{16.12}$$

where $C$ is the number of pairwise comparisons, and $j$ is the number of groups. Thus, the number of pairwise comparisons for the ANOVA in this example is $C = \dfrac{4(4-1)}{2} = 6$.

Demonstrating this formula more concretely, six pairwise comparisons are possible among the four group means:

**1.** group 1 to group 2 $\overline{X}1 \rightarrow \overline{X}2$

**2.** group 1 to group 3 $\overline{X}1 \rightarrow \overline{X}3$

**3.** group 1 to group 4 $\overline{X}1 \rightarrow \overline{X}4$

**4.** group 2 to group 3 $\overline{X}2 \rightarrow \overline{X}3$

**5.** group 2 to group 4 $\overline{X}2 \rightarrow \overline{X}4$

**6.** group 3 to group 4 $\overline{X}3 \rightarrow \overline{X}4$

**TABLE 16.10**  *F*-distribution ($\alpha = 0.05$ in the right tail) for numerator *df* of 1–9.

**Numerator Degrees of Freedom**

| $df_2 \backslash df_1$ | 1 | 2 | 3 | 4 | 5 | 6 | 7 | 8 | 9 | 10 | 12 | 15 | 20 | 24 | ∞ |
|---|---|---|---|---|---|---|---|---|---|---|---|---|---|---|---|
| 1 | 161.45 | 199.50 | 215.71 | 224.58 | 230.16 | 233.99 | 236.77 | 238.88 | 240.54 | 241.88 | 243.91 | 245.95 | 248.01 | 249.05 | 254.31 |
| 2 | 18.513 | 19.000 | 19.164 | 19.247 | 19.296 | 19.330 | 19.353 | 19.371 | 19.385 | 19.396 | 19.413 | 19.429 | 19.446 | 19.454 | 19.496 |
| 3 | 10.128 | 9.552 | 9.277 | 9.117 | 9.014 | 8.941 | 8.887 | 8.845 | 8.812 | 8.786 | 8.745 | 8.703 | 8.660 | 8.639 | 8.526 |
| 4 | 7.709 | 6.944 | 6.591 | 6.388 | 6.256 | 6.163 | 6.094 | 6.041 | 5.999 | 5.964 | 5.912 | 5.858 | 5.803 | 5.775 | 5.628 |
| 5 | 6.608 | 5.786 | 5.410 | 5.192 | 5.050 | 4.950 | 4.876 | 4.818 | 4.773 | 4.735 | 4.678 | 4.619 | 4.558 | 4.527 | 4.365 |
| 6 | 5.987 | 5.143 | 4.757 | 4.534 | 4.387 | 4.284 | 4.207 | 4.147 | 4.099 | 4.060 | 4.000 | 3.938 | 3.874 | 3.842 | 3.669 |
| 7 | 5.591 | 4.737 | 4.347 | 4.120 | 3.972 | 3.866 | 3.787 | 3.726 | 3.677 | 3.637 | 3.575 | 3.511 | 3.445 | 3.411 | 3.230 |
| 8 | 5.318 | 4.459 | 4.066 | 3.838 | 3.688 | 3.581 | 3.501 | 3.438 | 3.388 | 3.347 | 3.284 | 3.218 | 3.150 | 3.115 | 2.928 |
| 9 | 5.117 | 4.257 | 3.863 | 3.633 | 3.482 | 3.374 | 3.293 | 3.230 | 3.179 | 3.137 | 3.073 | 3.006 | 2.937 | 2.901 | 2.707 |
| 10 | 4.965 | 4.103 | 3.708 | 3.478 | 3.326 | 3.217 | 3.136 | 3.072 | 3.020 | 2.978 | 2.913 | 2.845 | 2.774 | 2.737 | 2.538 |
| 11 | 4.844 | 3.982 | 3.587 | 3.357 | 3.204 | 3.095 | 3.012 | 2.948 | 2.896 | 2.854 | 2.788 | 2.719 | 2.646 | 2.609 | 2.405 |
| 12 | 4.747 | 3.885 | 3.490 | 3.259 | 3.106 | 2.996 | 2.913 | 2.849 | 2.796 | 2.753 | 2.687 | 2.617 | 2.544 | 2.506 | 2.296 |
| 13 | 4.667 | 3.806 | 3.411 | 3.179 | 3.025 | 2.915 | 2.832 | 2.767 | 2.714 | 2.671 | 2.604 | 2.533 | 2.459 | 2.420 | 2.206 |
| 14 | 4.600 | 3.739 | 3.344 | 3.112 | 2.958 | 2.848 | 2.764 | 2.699 | 2.646 | 2.602 | 2.534 | 2.463 | 2.388 | 2.349 | 2.131 |
| 15 | 4.543 | 3.682 | 3.287 | 3.056 | 2.901 | 2.791 | 2.707 | 2.641 | 2.588 | 2.544 | 2.475 | 2.403 | 2.328 | 2.288 | 2.066 |
| 16 | 4.494 | 3.634 | 3.239 | 3.007 | 2.852 | 2.741 | 2.657 | 2.591 | 2.538 | 2.494 | 2.425 | 2.352 | 2.276 | 2.235 | 2.010 |
| 17 | 4.451 | 3.592 | 3.197 | 2.965 | 2.810 | 2.699 | 2.614 | 2.548 | 2.494 | 2.450 | 2.381 | 2.308 | 2.230 | 2.190 | 1.960 |
| 18 | 4.414 | 3.555 | 3.160 | 2.928 | 2.773 | 2.661 | 2.577 | 2.510 | 2.456 | 2.412 | 2.342 | 2.269 | 2.191 | 2.150 | 1.917 |
| 19 | 4.381 | 3.522 | 3.127 | 2.895 | 2.740 | 2.628 | 2.544 | 2.477 | 2.423 | 2.378 | 2.308 | 2.234 | 2.156 | 2.114 | 1.878 |
| 20 | 4.351 | 3.493 | 3.098 | 2.866 | 2.711 | 2.599 | 2.514 | 2.447 | 2.393 | 2.348 | 2.278 | 2.203 | 2.124 | 2.083 | 1.843 |
| 21 | 4.325 | 3.467 | 3.073 | 2.840 | 2.685 | 2.573 | 2.488 | 2.421 | 2.366 | 2.321 | 2.250 | 2.176 | 2.096 | 2.054 | 1.812 |
| 22 | 4.301 | 3.443 | 3.049 | 2.817 | 2.661 | 2.549 | 2.464 | 2.397 | 2.342 | 2.297 | 2.226 | 2.151 | 2.071 | 2.028 | 1.783 |
| 23 | 4.279 | 3.422 | 3.028 | 2.796 | 2.640 | 2.528 | 2.442 | 2.375 | 2.320 | 2.275 | 2.204 | 2.128 | 2.048 | 2.005 | 1.757 |
| 24 | 4.260 | 3.403 | 3.009 | 2.776 | 2.621 | 2.508 | 2.423 | 2.355 | 2.300 | 2.255 | 2.183 | 2.108 | 2.027 | 1.984 | 1.733 |
| 25 | 4.242 | 3.385 | 2.991 | 2.759 | 2.603 | 2.490 | 2.405 | 2.337 | 2.282 | 2.237 | 2.165 | 2.089 | 2.008 | 1.964 | 1.711 |
| 26 | 4.225 | 3.369 | 2.975 | 2.743 | 2.587 | 2.474 | 2.388 | 2.321 | 2.266 | 2.220 | 2.148 | 2.072 | 1.990 | 1.946 | 1.691 |
| 27 | 4.210 | 3.354 | 2.960 | 2.728 | 2.572 | 2.459 | 2.373 | 2.305 | 2.250 | 2.204 | 2.132 | 2.056 | 1.974 | 1.930 | 1.672 |
| 28 | 4.196 | 3.340 | 2.947 | 2.714 | 2.558 | 2.445 | 2.359 | 2.291 | 2.236 | 2.190 | 2.118 | 2.041 | 1.959 | 1.915 | 1.654 |
| 29 | 4.183 | 3.328 | 2.934 | 2.701 | 2.545 | 2.432 | 2.346 | 2.278 | 2.223 | 2.177 | 2.105 | 2.028 | 1.945 | 1.901 | 1.638 |
| 30 | 4.171 | 3.316 | 2.922 | 2.690 | 2.534 | 2.421 | 2.334 | 2.266 | 2.211 | 2.165 | 2.092 | 2.015 | 1.932 | 1.887 | 1.622 |
| 40 | 4.085 | 3.232 | 2.839 | 2.606 | 2.450 | 2.336 | 2.249 | 2.180 | 2.124 | 2.077 | 2.004 | 1.925 | 1.839 | 1.793 | 1.509 |
| 60 | 4.001 | 3.150 | 2.758 | 2.525 | 2.368 | 2.254 | 2.167 | 2.097 | 2.040 | 1.993 | 1.917 | 1.836 | 1.748 | 1.700 | 1.389 |
| 120 | 3.920 | 3.072 | 2.680 | 2.447 | 2.290 | 2.175 | 2.087 | 2.016 | 1.959 | 1.911 | 1.834 | 1.751 | 1.659 | 1.608 | 1.254 |
| ∞ | 3.842 | 2.996 | 2.605 | 2.372 | 2.214 | 2.099 | 2.010 | 1.938 | 1.880 | 1.831 | 1.752 | 1.666 | 1.571 | 1.517 | 1.000 |

**Denominator Degrees of Freedom**

**TABLE 16.11**  *F*-distribution ($\alpha = 0.01$ in the right tail) for numerator $df$ of 1–9.

Numerator Degrees of Freedom

| $df_2$ \ $df_1$ | 1 | 2 | 3 | 4 | 5 | 6 | 7 | 8 | 9 | 10 | 12 | 15 | 20 | 24 | ∞ |
|---|---|---|---|---|---|---|---|---|---|---|---|---|---|---|---|
| 1 | 4052.2 | 4999.5 | 5403.4 | 5624.6 | 5763.6 | 5859.0 | 5928.4 | 5981.1 | 6022.5 | 6055.8 | 6106.3 | 6157.3 | 6208.7 | 6234.6 | 6365.9 |
| 2 | 98.503 | 99.000 | 99.166 | 99.249 | 99.299 | 99.333 | 99.356 | 99.374 | 99.388 | 99.399 | 99.416 | 99.433 | 99.449 | 99.458 | 99.499 |
| 3 | 34.116 | 30.817 | 29.457 | 28.710 | 28.237 | 27.911 | 27.672 | 27.489 | 27.345 | 27.229 | 27.052 | 26.872 | 26.690 | 26.598 | 26.125 |
| 4 | 21.198 | 18.000 | 16.694 | 15.977 | 15.522 | 15.207 | 14.976 | 14.799 | 14.659 | 14.546 | 14.374 | 14.198 | 14.020 | 13.929 | 13.463 |
| 5 | 16.258 | 13.274 | 12.060 | 11.392 | 10.967 | 10.672 | 10.456 | 10.289 | 10.158 | 10.051 | 9.888 | 9.722 | 9.553 | 9.467 | 9.020 |
| 6 | 13.745 | 10.925 | 9.780 | 9.148 | 8.746 | 8.466 | 8.260 | 8.102 | 7.976 | 7.874 | 7.718 | 7.559 | 7.396 | 7.313 | 6.880 |
| 7 | 12.246 | 9.547 | 8.451 | 7.847 | 7.460 | 7.191 | 6.993 | 6.840 | 6.719 | 6.620 | 6.469 | 6.314 | 6.155 | 6.074 | 5.650 |
| 8 | 11.259 | 8.649 | 7.591 | 7.006 | 6.632 | 6.371 | 6.178 | 6.029 | 5.911 | 5.814 | 5.667 | 5.515 | 5.359 | 5.279 | 4.859 |
| 9 | 10.561 | 8.022 | 6.992 | 6.422 | 6.057 | 5.802 | 5.613 | 5.467 | 5.351 | 5.257 | 5.111 | 4.962 | 4.808 | 4.729 | 4.311 |
| 10 | 10.044 | 7.559 | 6.552 | 5.994 | 5.636 | 5.386 | 5.200 | 5.057 | 4.942 | 4.849 | 4.706 | 4.558 | 4.405 | 4.327 | 3.909 |
| 11 | 9.646 | 7.206 | 6.217 | 5.668 | 5.316 | 5.069 | 4.886 | 4.745 | 4.632 | 4.539 | 4.397 | 4.251 | 4.099 | 4.021 | 3.602 |
| 12 | 9.330 | 6.927 | 5.953 | 5.412 | 5.064 | 4.821 | 4.640 | 4.499 | 4.388 | 4.296 | 4.155 | 4.010 | 3.858 | 3.781 | 3.361 |
| 13 | 9.074 | 6.701 | 5.739 | 5.205 | 4.862 | 4.620 | 4.441 | 4.302 | 4.191 | 4.100 | 3.960 | 3.815 | 3.665 | 3.587 | 3.165 |
| 14 | 8.862 | 6.515 | 5.564 | 5.035 | 4.695 | 4.456 | 4.278 | 4.140 | 4.030 | 3.939 | 3.800 | 3.656 | 3.505 | 3.427 | 3.004 |
| 15 | 8.683 | 6.359 | 5.417 | 4.893 | 4.556 | 4.318 | 4.142 | 4.005 | 3.895 | 3.805 | 3.666 | 3.522 | 3.372 | 3.294 | 2.868 |
| 16 | 8.531 | 6.226 | 5.292 | 4.773 | 4.437 | 4.202 | 4.026 | 3.890 | 3.780 | 3.691 | 3.553 | 3.409 | 3.259 | 3.181 | 2.753 |
| 17 | 8.400 | 6.112 | 5.185 | 4.669 | 4.336 | 4.102 | 3.927 | 3.791 | 3.682 | 3.593 | 3.455 | 3.312 | 3.162 | 3.084 | 2.653 |
| 18 | 8.286 | 6.013 | 5.092 | 4.579 | 4.248 | 4.015 | 3.841 | 3.705 | 3.597 | 3.508 | 3.371 | 3.227 | 3.077 | 2.999 | 2.566 |
| 19 | 8.185 | 5.926 | 5.010 | 4.500 | 4.171 | 3.939 | 3.765 | 3.631 | 3.523 | 3.434 | 3.297 | 3.153 | 3.003 | 2.925 | 2.489 |
| 20 | 8.096 | 5.849 | 4.938 | 4.431 | 4.103 | 3.871 | 3.699 | 3.564 | 3.457 | 3.368 | 3.231 | 3.088 | 2.938 | 2.859 | 2.421 |
| 21 | 8.017 | 5.780 | 4.874 | 4.369 | 4.042 | 3.812 | 3.640 | 3.506 | 3.398 | 3.310 | 3.173 | 3.030 | 2.880 | 2.801 | 2.360 |
| 22 | 7.945 | 5.719 | 4.817 | 4.313 | 3.988 | 3.758 | 3.587 | 3.453 | 3.346 | 3.258 | 3.121 | 2.978 | 2.827 | 2.749 | 2.306 |
| 23 | 7.881 | 5.664 | 4.765 | 4.264 | 3.939 | 3.710 | 3.539 | 3.406 | 3.299 | 3.211 | 3.074 | 2.931 | 2.781 | 2.702 | 2.256 |
| 24 | 7.823 | 5.614 | 4.718 | 4.218 | 3.895 | 3.667 | 3.496 | 3.363 | 3.256 | 3.168 | 3.032 | 2.889 | 2.738 | 2.659 | 2.211 |
| 25 | 7.770 | 5.568 | 4.676 | 4.177 | 3.855 | 3.627 | 3.457 | 3.324 | 3.217 | 3.129 | 2.993 | 2.850 | 2.699 | 2.620 | 2.169 |
| 26 | 7.721 | 5.526 | 4.637 | 4.140 | 3.818 | 3.591 | 3.421 | 3.288 | 3.182 | 3.094 | 2.958 | 2.815 | 2.664 | 2.585 | 2.132 |
| 27 | 7.677 | 5.488 | 4.601 | 4.106 | 3.785 | 3.558 | 3.388 | 3.256 | 3.149 | 3.062 | 2.926 | 2.783 | 2.632 | 2.552 | 2.097 |
| 28 | 7.636 | 5.453 | 4.568 | 4.074 | 3.754 | 3.528 | 3.358 | 3.226 | 3.120 | 3.032 | 2.896 | 2.753 | 2.602 | 2.522 | 2.064 |
| 29 | 7.598 | 5.420 | 4.538 | 4.045 | 3.725 | 3.500 | 3.330 | 3.198 | 3.092 | 3.005 | 2.869 | 2.726 | 2.574 | 2.495 | 2.034 |
| 30 | 7.563 | 5.390 | 4.510 | 4.018 | 3.699 | 3.474 | 3.305 | 3.173 | 3.067 | 2.979 | 2.843 | 2.700 | 2.549 | 2.469 | 2.006 |
| 40 | 7.314 | 5.179 | 4.313 | 3.828 | 3.514 | 3.291 | 3.124 | 2.993 | 2.888 | 2.801 | 2.665 | 2.522 | 2.369 | 2.288 | 1.805 |
| 60 | 7.077 | 4.977 | 4.126 | 3.649 | 3.339 | 3.119 | 2.953 | 2.823 | 2.719 | 2.632 | 2.496 | 2.352 | 2.198 | 2.115 | 1.601 |
| 120 | 6.851 | 4.787 | 3.949 | 3.480 | 3.174 | 2.956 | 2.792 | 2.663 | 2.559 | 2.472 | 2.336 | 2.192 | 2.035 | 1.950 | 1.381 |
| ∞ | 6.635 | 4.605 | 3.782 | 3.319 | 3.017 | 2.802 | 2.639 | 2.511 | 2.407 | 2.321 | 2.185 | 2.039 | 1.878 | 1.791 | 1.000 |

Denominator Degrees of Freedom

To determine whether statistically significant differences are evident in each pairwise comparison, the absolute value of the mean differences is divided by the standard error term:

$$q = \frac{|\overline{X}_j - \overline{X}_K|}{\sqrt{\dfrac{MS_W}{2}\left(\dfrac{1}{n_j} + \dfrac{1}{n_K}\right)}} \tag{16.13}$$

where $\overline{X}_j$ and $\overline{X}_K$ are the group means being compared, $MS_W$ is the mean square within, and $n_j$ and $n_k$ are the sample sizes in each comparison group. When conducting a TMC using hand calculations, it is best to start with the two groups that have the largest mean differences. When the comparison between group means for the largest group mean difference is not statistically significant, there is no need to test further pairwise comparisons with smaller mean differences. As stated before, there are six possible pairwise comparisons to test in the present example. When conducting pairwise comparisons, the same problem that existed for repeated *t*-tests also is evident in pairwise comparisons: inflated type I error! If $\alpha = .05$, and six pairwise comparisons are evaluated, then type I error is inflated to 30 percent (i.e., $6 \times .05 = .30$, or 30 percent). This can be addressed by conducting a *Bonferroni adjustment*. In a Bonferroni adjustment, the $q$ statistic is evaluated at $\dfrac{\alpha}{c}$, where $c$ is the number of pairwise comparisons. In this example, $\dfrac{\alpha}{c} = \dfrac{.05}{6} = .008$. Therefore, when evaluating output from a statistical package (e.g., *SPSS*, SAS, and R-stat), the *p*-value should be less than .008 ($p < .008$) for statistical significance. For hand computations, the appropriate critical value should be obtained by using Table 16.12.

$$q_1 = \frac{\overline{X}_2 - \overline{X}_4}{s_{\overline{X}}} = \frac{9.0 - 2.4}{.82} = 8.05$$

When using Table 16.12, the values on top represent the number of groups in the data set ($j$). The values to the left side are the degrees of freedom within ($n. - j$). For convenience, in Table 16.12, the critical $q$ values are provided at both $\alpha = .05$ (top value) and $\alpha = .01$ (bottom value). Check the critical value with respect to the appropriate alpha level identified in the study. In this example, $q_{\text{crit}}$ (4, 16) = 6.80, $p = .001$ (conservative estimate of .008; this value is not provided in Table 16.12), and $8.05 > 6.80$. So a statistically significant difference exists between the two groups.

As $q_1$ is statistically significant, we will compare the next pair of groups with the next greatest difference until we have either compared all of the pairs of groups or until one pair of groups is not statistically significant. $q_{\text{crit}}$ will remain the critical value for each of the comparisons.

$$q_2 = \frac{\overline{X}_3 - \overline{X}_4}{s_{\overline{X}}} = \frac{7.0 - 2.4}{.82} = 5.61$$

$$5.61 < 6.80$$

As $q_2$ is not statistically significant, there is no need to conduct the other comparisons, because the mean difference is less than $q_{\text{crit}}$. That is, further group mean comparisons become unnecessary because the mean difference values that are lower than the one just tested will also be nonsignificant.

Although the hand computations may appear to be a little complex, the important factors to remember when evaluating research from a statistical package or when reading research is to (a) address the inflated type I error through the Bonferroni adjustment and (b) evaluate statistical significance at the appropriate alpha level. When *post hoc* analyses are conducted and no adjustment is made for type I error, the results are not reliable. SPSS output for the *post hoc* analyses of the self-efficacy data from Table 16.8 is presented in Table 16.13.

## TABLE 16.12 The critical values for $q$ corresponding to alpha = .05 and alpha = .01.

| *df* for Error Term | k = Number of Treatments | | | | | | | | |
|---|---|---|---|---|---|---|---|---|---|
| | 2 | 3 | 4 | 5 | 6 | 7 | 8 | 9 | 10 |
| The critical values for $q$ corresponding to $\alpha = .05$ | | | | | | | | | |
| 5 | 3.64 | 4.60 | 5.22 | 5.67 | 6.03 | 6.33 | 6.58 | 6.80 | 6.99 |
| 6 | 3.46 | 4.34 | 4.90 | 5.30 | 5.63 | 5.90 | 6.12 | 6.32 | 6.49 |
| 7 | 3.34 | 4.16 | 4.68 | 5.06 | 5.36 | 5.61 | 5.82 | 6.00 | 6.16 |
| 8 | 3.26 | 4.04 | 4.53 | 4.89 | 5.17 | 5.40 | 5.60 | 5.77 | 5.92 |
| 9 | 3.20 | 3.95 | 4.41 | 4.76 | 5.02 | 5.24 | 5.43 | 5.59 | 5.74 |
| 10 | 3.15 | 3.88 | 4.33 | 4.65 | 4.91 | 5.12 | 5.30 | 5.46 | 5.60 |
| 11 | 3.11 | 3.82 | 4.26 | 4.57 | 4.82 | 5.03 | 5.20 | 5.35 | 5.49 |
| 12 | 3.08 | 3.77 | 4.20 | 4.51 | 4.75 | 4.95 | 5.12 | 5.27 | 5.39 |
| 13 | 3.06 | 3.73 | 4.15 | 4.45 | 4.69 | 4.88 | 5.05 | 5.19 | 5.32 |
| 14 | 3.03 | 3.70 | 4.11 | 4.41 | 4.64 | 4.83 | 4.99 | 5.13 | 5.25 |
| 15 | 3.01 | 3.67 | 4.08 | 4.37 | 4.59 | 4.78 | 4.94 | 5.08 | 5.20 |
| 16 | 3.00 | 3.65 | 4.05 | 4.33 | 4.56 | 4.74 | 4.90 | 5.03 | 5.15 |
| 17 | 2.98 | 3.63 | 4.02 | 4.30 | 4.52 | 4.70 | 4.86 | 4.99 | 5.11 |
| 18 | 2.97 | 3.61 | 4.00 | 4.28 | 4.49 | 4.67 | 4.82 | 4.96 | 5.07 |
| 19 | 2.96 | 3.59 | 3.98 | 4.25 | 4.47 | 4.65 | 4.79 | 4.92 | 5.04 |
| 20 | 2.95 | 3.58 | 3.96 | 4.23 | 4.45 | 4.62 | 4.77 | 4.90 | 5.01 |
| 24 | 2.92 | 3.53 | 3.90 | 4.17 | 4.37 | 4.54 | 4.68 | 4.81 | 4.92 |
| 30 | 2.89 | 3.49 | 3.85 | 4.10 | 4.30 | 4.46 | 4.60 | 4.72 | 4.82 |
| 40 | 2.86 | 3.44 | 3.79 | 4.04 | 4.23 | 4.39 | 4.52 | 4.63 | 4.73 |
| 60 | 2.83 | 3.40 | 3.74 | 3.98 | 4.16 | 4.31 | 4.44 | 4.55 | 4.65 |
| 120 | 2.80 | 3.36 | 3.68 | 3.92 | 4.10 | 4.24 | 4.36 | 4.47 | 4.56 |
| ∞ | 2.77 | 3.31 | 3.63 | 3.86 | 4.03 | 4.17 | 4.29 | 4.39 | 4.47 |
| The critical values for $q$ corresponding to $\alpha = .01$ | | | | | | | | | |
| 5 | 5.70 | 6.98 | 7.80 | 8.42 | 8.91 | 9.32 | 9.67 | 9.97 | 10.24 |
| 6 | 5.24 | 6.33 | 7.03 | 7.56 | 7.97 | 8.32 | 8.61 | 8.87 | 9.10 |
| 7 | 4.95 | 5.92 | 6.54 | 7.01 | 7.37 | 7.68 | 7.94 | 8.17 | 8.37 |
| 8 | 4.75 | 5.64 | 6.20 | 6.62 | 6.96 | 7.24 | 7.47 | 7.68 | 7.86 |
| 9 | 4.60 | 5.43 | 5.96 | 6.35 | 6.66 | 6.91 | 7.13 | 7.33 | 7.49 |
| 10 | 4.48 | 5.27 | 5.77 | 6.14 | 6.43 | 6.67 | 6.87 | 7.05 | 7.21 |
| 11 | 4.39 | 5.15 | 5.62 | 5.97 | 6.25 | 6.48 | 6.67 | 6.84 | 6.99 |
| 12 | 4.32 | 5.05 | 5.50 | 5.84 | 6.10 | 6.32 | 6.51 | 6.67 | 6.81 |
| 13 | 4.26 | 4.96 | 5.40 | 5.73 | 5.98 | 6.19 | 6.37 | 6.53 | 6.67 |
| 14 | 4.21 | 4.89 | 5.32 | 5.63 | 5.88 | 6.08 | 6.26 | 6.41 | 6.54 |
| 15 | 4.17 | 4.84 | 5.25 | 5.56 | 5.80 | 5.99 | 6.16 | 6.31 | 6.44 |
| 16 | 4.13 | 4.79 | 5.19 | 5.49 | 5.72 | 5.92 | 6.08 | 6.22 | 6.35 |
| 17 | 4.10 | 4.74 | 5.14 | 5.43 | 5.66 | 5.85 | 6.01 | 6.15 | 6.27 |
| 18 | 4.07 | 4.70 | 5.09 | 5.38 | 5.60 | 5.79 | 5.94 | 6.08 | 6.20 |
| 19 | 4.05 | 4.67 | 5.05 | 5.33 | 5.55 | 5.73 | 5.89 | 6.02 | 6.14 |
| 20 | 4.02 | 4.64 | 5.02 | 5.29 | 5.51 | 5.69 | 5.84 | 5.97 | 6.09 |
| 24 | 3.96 | 4.55 | 4.91 | 5.17 | 5.37 | 5.54 | 5.69 | 5.81 | 5.92 |
| 30 | 3.89 | 4.45 | 4.80 | 5.05 | 5.24 | 5.40 | 5.54 | 5.65 | 5.76 |
| 40 | 3.82 | 4.37 | 4.70 | 4.93 | 5.11 | 5.26 | 5.39 | 5.50 | 5.60 |
| 60 | 3.76 | 4.28 | 4.59 | 4.82 | 4.99 | 5.13 | 5.25 | 5.36 | 5.45 |
| 120 | 3.70 | 4.20 | 4.50 | 4.71 | 4.87 | 5.01 | 5.12 | 5.21 | 5.30 |
| ∞ | 3.64 | 4.12 | 4.40 | 4.60 | 4.76 | 4.88 | 4.99 | 5.08 | 5.16 |

**TABLE 16.13**   SPSS output for *post hoc* analyses.

**Multiple Comparisons**

Dependent Variable: Self-Efficacy
Tukey HSD

| (I) Group | (J) Group | Mean Difference (I–J) | Std. Error | Sig. | 95 Percent Confidence Interval | |
|-----------|-----------|----------------------|-----------|------|-------------|-------------|
| | | | | | Lower Bound | Upper Bound |
| 1.00 | 2.00 | –3.00000 | 1.15326 | .082 | –6.2995 | .2995 |
| | 3.00 | –1.00000 | 1.15326 | .822 | –4.2995 | 2.2995 |
| | 4.00 | 3.60000(*) | 1.15326 | .030 | .3005 | 6.8995 |
| 2.00 | 1.00 | 3.00000 | 1.15326 | .082 | –2995 | 6.2995 |
| | 3.00 | 2.00000 | 1.15326 | .339 | –1.2995 | 5.2995 |
| | 4.00 | 6.60000(*) | 1.15326 | .000 | 3.3005 | 9.8995 |
| 3.00 | 1.00 | 1.00000 | 1.15326 | .822 | –2.2995 | 4.2995 |
| | 2.00 | –2.00000 | 1.15326 | .339 | –5.2995 | 1.2995 |
| | 4.00 | 4.60000(*) | 1.15326 | .005 | 1.3005 | 7.8995 |
| 4.00 | 1.00 | –3.60000(*) | 1.15326 | .030 | –6.8995 | –3005 |
| | 2.00 | –6.60000(*) | 1.15326 | .000 | –9.8995 | –3.3005 |
| | 3.00 | –4.60000(*) | 1.15326 | .005 | –7.8995 | –1.3005 |

*The mean difference is significant at the .05 level.

**Self-Efficacy**

Tukey HSD

| Group | N | Subset for Alpha = .05 | |
|-------|---|------|------|
| | | 1 | 2 |
| 4.00 | 5 | 2.4000 | |
| 1.00 | 5 | | 6.0000 |
| 3.00 | 5 | | 7.0000 |
| 2.00 | 5 | | 9.0000 |
| Sig. | | 1.000 | .082 |

Means for groups in homogeneous subsets are displayed
using a harmonic mean sample size = 5.000.

© Cengage Learning

# Evaluating Practical Significance

Statistical significance refers to the probability that the rejection of the null hypothesis occurred outside the realm of chance (alpha [$\alpha$] level). *Practical significance* refers to the meaningfulness of the differences by specifying the magnitude of the differences between the means or the strength of the association between the independent variable(s) and the dependent variable. Larger sample sizes increase the likelihood of finding statistical significance but do not always lead to practical relevance. For example, consider the $z$-test discussed earlier in the chapter as used in a new study by a professional school counselor who wants to compare a set of scores on the SAT to the national norm. What follows is a simplification of reality, but assume the population (norm of SAT) has a mean ($\mu$) of 500 and a standard deviation ($\sigma$) of 100. If the counselor has 25 students in the sample with a mean $(\overline{X})$ of 520, then the *z*-test would be conducted as follows:

$$z = \frac{\overline{X} - \mu}{\sigma_{\overline{X}}} = \frac{\overline{X} - \mu}{\dfrac{\sigma}{\sqrt{n}}} = \frac{520 - 500}{\dfrac{100}{\sqrt{25}}} = \frac{20}{20} = 1.00.$$

With an alpha level of .05 (nondirectional) and $z_{crit} = 1.96$, there is no statistically significant difference between the sample group and the population ($z = 1.00$, $p > .05$). Now, take the same scores, but increase the sample size to 100:

$$z = \frac{\overline{X} - \mu}{\sigma_{\overline{X}}} = \frac{\overline{X} - \mu}{\dfrac{\sigma}{\sqrt{n}}} = \frac{520 - 500}{\dfrac{100}{\sqrt{100}}} = \frac{20}{10} = 2.00.$$

With an alpha level of .05 (nondirectional) and $z_{crit} = 1.96$, there is a statistically significant difference between the sample group and the population ($z = 2.00$, $p < .05$) because the observed value is greater than the critical value ($2.00 > 1.96$).

Although the *magnitude* of the mean differences did not change, the interpretation of the results changed, strictly based on the increase in sample size. When sample size increased, the error decreased. Thus, statistically significant differences are more likely to occur when large samples are used. In fact (and this is an important but little-known reality of quantitative research), nearly any null hypothesis can be rejected when a large enough sample is attained. Practical significance is important because it addresses the magnitude of a treatment effect without the complication of sample size, thereby providing more meaningful information practitioners and researchers can use,

The following procedures are used to provide measures of effect size to determine practical significance. Currently, statistical packages do not compute Cohen's *d* or Cohen's *f*, which measure effect size in standard deviation units, although several programs are available for free access through the Internet. They are, however, relatively simple computations to do by calculator from the statistical output. The reporting of practical significance is very important when reporting results and mandatory in many social science journals.

### Cohen's d

Cohen's *d* is used to determine the effect size for the differences between two groups, such as in a *t*-test or pairwise comparisons (e.g., Tukey *post hoc*), and it is expressed in standard deviation units. Cohen (1988) created the following categories to interpret *d*: Small effect, $d = .2$; Medium effect, $d = .5$; Large effect, $d = .8$. The following formula is used to calculate Cohen's *d*:

$$\frac{|\overline{X}_1 - \overline{X}_2|}{s_{pooled}}, \tag{16.14}$$

where

$$s_{pooled} = \sqrt{\frac{s_1^2(n_1 - 1) + s_2^2(n_1 - 1)}{(n_1 - 1) + (n_2 - 1)}}. \tag{16.15}$$

To demonstrate the usefulness of Cohen's *d*, consider the previous NCE example from the independent *t*-test in which a mean score for the 25 students from University A was 120 with a standard deviation of 10 and the mean score for the 30 students from

University B was 125 with a standard deviation of 15. Using Equations 16.14 and 16.15, we have the following:

$$\frac{|120 - 125|}{\sqrt{\dfrac{100(25 - 1) + 225(30 - 1)}{(25 - 1) + (30 - 1)}}} = \frac{5}{\sqrt{\dfrac{2400 + 6525}{53}}} = \frac{5}{12.98} = .385.$$

So a small effect size ($d > .2$ [small effect], but $d < .5$ [medium effect]) was found between the two groups, with the difference between the two means to be approximately .385 standard deviations. To interpret the result of $d$, we say, "The average students from University B scored .385 standard deviations higher than the average student from University A," or, more commonly, "The average student from University B scored better than 65 percent of students from University A." We know this because $d$ is actually a $z$-score, and a $z$-score of $+0.385$ is equivalent to a percentile rank of 65 (Table 13.1).

### Cohen's f, Eta-Squared ($\eta^2$), and Omega Squared ($\omega^2$)

Cohen's $f$ also expresses effect size in standard deviation units, but it does so for two or more groups. Thus, when conducting an ANOVA, Cohen's $f$ can be computed to determine the practical significance in the differences among the groups. Like the ANOVA, Cohen's $f$ will identify the magnitude of the differences among the groups, but it will not explain differences between specific groups. To identify differences between specific groups, a Tukey *post hoc* analysis followed by Cohen's $d$ for each pairwise comparison would be necessary.

Cohen (1988) created the following categories to interpret $f$: Small effect, $f = .10$; Medium effect, $f = .25$; Large effect, $f = .40$. These categories were based on using Cohen's $d$ as a standard metric:

$$f = \tfrac{1}{2}d \tag{16.16}$$

Hence, a medium effect size for Cohen's $d$ is .5. For Cohen's $f$ it is $\tfrac{1}{2}(.5) = .25$, as stated above.

Practical significance is not always measured in standard deviation units and may be expressed in variance units. There are mathematical relationships between effect sizes expressed in standard deviation units and strengths of association expressed in variance units. When conducting parametric statistics in which the focus of the study is on group differences, however, it is best to express effect size in standard deviation units as it better compliments the descriptive data, such as means and standard deviations. As a rule of thumb, Cohen's $d$ and Cohen's $f$ may be more informative for ANOVA. Many statistical packages, however, provide measures of strength of association, especially $\eta^2$ (eta-squared), and so this measure is widely used. Cohen (1988) created the following categories to interpret strength of association across the three statistics covered in this section ($\eta^2$, $\omega^2$): Small effect = .01; Medium effect = .059; and Large effect = .138. These decimals are normally converted to percentages (e.g., $.14 = 14$ percent) and interpreted as the percent of variance accounted for by the scores under study.

Eta-squared is easily computed and from this computation, Cohen's $f$ may be easily derived. Keep in mind that all these metrics are equivalent measures. Eta-squared may be calculated directly from the computations used in the $F$-test.

$$\eta^2 = \frac{SS_B}{SS_{\text{TOT}}} = \frac{114.6}{167.8} = .68, \tag{16.17}$$

where $SS_B$ as previously noted is the sum of squares between groups (see Equation 16.9) and $SS_{\text{TOT}}$ (total sum or squares) is $SS_B + SS_W$ (i.e., sum of squares within). From this statistic, we can conclude that the four groups of students account for 68 percent of the variance in self-efficacy scores—a very large effect!

The formula to calculate Cohen's $f$ is derived from eta-squared:

$$f = \sqrt{\frac{\eta^2}{1 - \eta^2}} = \sqrt{\frac{.68}{1 - .68}} = 1.46 \qquad (16.18)$$

So a very large effect size ($f > .40$) was found among the four groups, with an effect size of approximately 1.46 standard deviations.

When strength of association is used in ANOVA, *Omega squared* ($\omega^2$) is also a common measure (Kirk, 1995). The computation of $\omega^2$ uses terms from the ANOVA computation:

$$\omega^2 = \frac{SS_B - (j - 1)(MS_W)}{SS_{TOT} + MS_W} \qquad (16.19)$$

where $SS_{TOT}$ is the sum of $SS_B + SS_W$, and $j$ is the number of groups. Applied to the data from the self-efficacy ANOVA study from this chapter:

$$\omega^2 = \frac{114.6 - (4 - 1)(3.325)}{167.8 + 3.325} = \frac{104.625}{171.125} = .61.$$

From this statistic, we can conclude that the four groups of students account for 61 percent of the variance in self-efficacy scores. The rationale for using omega-squared, as opposed to eta-squared, is that eta-squared is criticized for overestimating practical significance in ANOVA. However, in counseling research, eta-squared is much more common.

# Interpreting and Writing Results

Statistical analyses may lend credibility and evidence to a particular process or procedure. However, a strong experimental design that is not investigated completely or communicated effectively loses credibility. The various procedures discussed in this chapter should be mentioned in a results section, but all of these components are rarely addressed.

Consumers of research may be tempted to skip the results section when investigating effective procedures and programs. However, the results section should provide adequate information related to statistical and practical significance. A well-written results section should include the following: (a) the type of analysis conducted and the level of significance; (b) a statement related to meeting model assumptions; (c) a report on the statistical test; (d) follow-up procedures, if appropriate; and (e) a statement related to practical significance.

When reporting the results of a statistical test, the reader will encounter a general format: *statistical test (e.g., t, F) (degrees of freedom)* = observed value, *probability of type I error (p)* = probability value. For example, $F(3, 16) = 11.49$, $p < .001$, signifies that an ANOVA with four groups ($4 - 1 = 3$ degrees of freedom) and a sample size of 20 ($20 - 4 = 16$ degrees of freedom) has an observed value of 11.49, and there is less than a one-thousandth of 1 percent probability of making a type I error. In other words, it is highly unlikely that this result occurred simply based on chance. An example of a more comprehensive results section is presented in Table 16.14.

A common practice when providing results is to refer readers to a table that reports means and standard deviations of each group. Often, ANOVA results may be reported in

| **TABLE 16.14**   Sample results findings for the self-efficacy study presented in this chapter. |
|---|

A one-way ANOVA was conducted on self-efficacy scores in math across students in four groups. Group 1 received a lecture on enhancing self-efficacy. Group 2 received a lecture and experiential exercise on self-efficacy. Group 3 received an experiential exercise only. Group 4 was a control group. An alpha level of .05 was used. All four groups were normally distributed: $W(5) = .94$, $p = .69$ for group 1; $W(5) = .83$, $p = .15$ for group 2; $W(5) = .99$, $p = .97$ for group 3; and $W(5) = .88$, $p = .31$ for group 4. Variances for all four groups were homogeneous, $F_{Levene}(3, 16) = 1.37$, $p = .289$. There was a statistically significant difference among the four groups, $F(3, 16) = 11.49$, $p < .001$. A large effect size was noted among the four groups, $f = 1.31$, indicating a strong degree of practical significance. Power was adequate for this study, $1 - \beta = .98$.

Given the statistically significant differences among the groups, a Tukey *post hoc* analysis was conducted to identify significant differences between each group. A Bonferroni adjustment was conducted to provide a more conservative estimate of statistical significance. An alpha level of .0125 was used. Statistically significant differences were evident between group 2 and group 4, $q = 8.10$, $p < .001$, and group 3 and group 4, $q = 5.64$, $p < .01$.

© Cengage Learning

a table format as well. Although the reporting of model assumptions, as demonstrated in the top portion of the results section, is not necessarily common practice, it is good practice to report model assumptions to identify that the statistical test was appropriate to the data.

# Factorial ANOVA

An ANOVA does not need to be limited to one independent variable. A factorial ANOVA is conducted when two or more independent variables are examined across a single dependent variable. These analyses are bit more complex than a one-way ANOVA. When an ANOVA is conducted across two independent variables, the *F*-tests are calculated. There is an *F*-test for each independent variable, called a **main effect**, and an *F*-test for an **interaction effect**; that is, the two independent variables may interact, leading to sometimes complex conclusions. When the data are graphed and similar patterns are noted across each independent variable, then there is no statistically significant interaction. For example, if a factorial ANOVA was to be computed for differences in a self-efficacy test score across gender and socioeconomic status (SES), then a nonsignificant interaction may be displayed, as seen in Figure 16.4.

SES, one of the independent variables, is on the horizontal axis, and the self-efficacy score, the dependent variable, is on the vertical axis. Gender (males and females) is graphed on separate lines. Note that the same pattern exists for males across SES as for females; in this case, females scored higher than males in each SES category. When the data are graphed and different patterns are noted across each independent variable, then there is a statistically significant interaction. Such an interaction effect is noted in Figure 16.5. Notice that there is a different pattern for males across SES than for females.

When there is no statistically significant interaction, then the main effects of each independent variable can be interpreted in a manner similar to a one-way ANOVA. When a statistically significant interaction does exist, however, the researcher needs to graph the interaction and examine each level of an independent variable across the other independent variable. For example, in the results displayed in Figure 16.5, two one-way ANOVAs would need to be conducted: one using only males with the independent variable as SES and one using only females with the independent variable as SES. This process is known as simple effects, and it can be used to determine the significant differences that occur for males and females across SES. In Figure 16.5, it appears that self-efficacy for math increases for females as socioeconomic levels increase, whereas

**Figure 16.4**

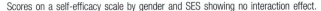

Scores on a self-efficacy scale by gender and SES showing no interaction effect.

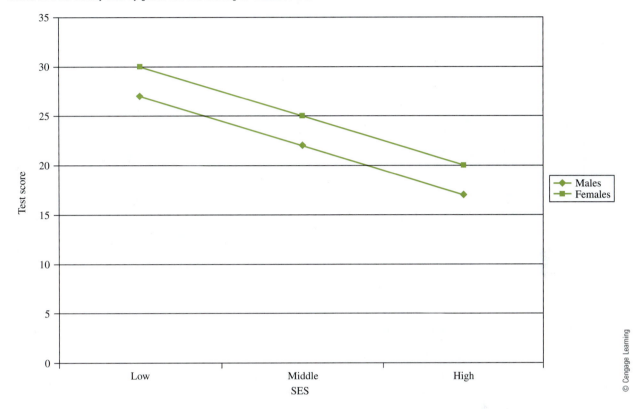

© Cengage Learning

the opposite is observed for males; that is, for males, self-efficacy appears to decrease as socioeconomic levels increase.

## Other Forms of ANOVA Designs

Although you should be familiar with several other, more complex forms of ANOVA designs, space limitations prevent a lengthy discussion of them here. **Randomized block factorial ANOVA** is used when "blocking variables" have been introduced into a design. A blocking variable is one that is suspected of being extraneous or confounding and is therefore incorporated into the ANOVA design. Thus, the designated blocking variable allows an additional control for variance in the resulting main effects and interaction effects that would otherwise be unaccounted for but is now accounted for through the introduction of a new independent (albeit extraneous) variable. For example, if sex is suspected of being a confounding variable, the sample could be stratified to include males and females—thus blocking on sex.

A **repeated measures ANOVA** is used in studies using a within-subjects design, in which participants are sequentially exposed to different levels of the independent variable (treatment). For example, participants may be observed prior to treatment (a control group measure), then after exposure to treatment #1, then again after exposure to treatment #2. Changes among the scores for the repeated administrations of the single dependent variable for each level become the foci of the analysis.

**Figure 16.5**

Scores on a self-efficacy scale by gender and SES showing an interaction effect.

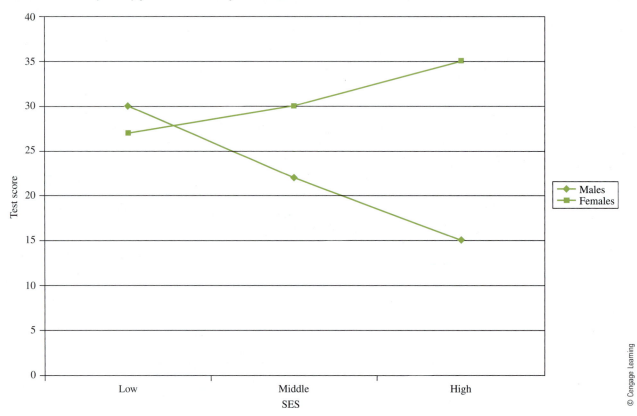

A **mixed (split-plot) ANOVA** is appropriate for studies that use a mixed design—that is, a design using one or more independent variables in a between-groups design and one or more independent variables in a within-subjects design. For example, sex and socioeconomic status may be used as independent variables for the between-groups comparisons, and each participant may be sequentially exposed to control, treatment #1, and treatment #2 conditions. The statistical analyses for these designs can become quite complex to interpret.

## Analysis of Covariance (ANCOVA)

ANCOVA is a statistical analysis that combines ANOVA and regression. It is often used to nullify the effects of a confounding variable (Best & Kahn, 2006) by statistically removing the variability in the dependent variable caused by the confounding variable, such as if a sample of participants differ on a pretest or to rule out the effects of socioeconomic status when looking at academic achievement. The computations for ANCOVA are complex. But most statistical packages can compute ANCOVA.

Generally, an ANCOVA is used if the results of the ANOVA appear to be biased. Consider the example in which a researcher wishes to examine the effect of three different methods in treating adolescents with substance abuse diagnoses. Because there are substantial variations in substance abuse, such as the type of drug abused and the extent of abuse versus dependency, the researcher uses participant pretest scores on the

Substance Abuse Subtle Screening Inventory—Adolescent Version (SASSI-A) as a covariate to equalize the groups. When an ANCOVA is used, the risk of comparing groups that have greater degrees of substance abuse to groups with lesser degrees of substance abuse is nullified, and the effectiveness of the three interventions can be better determined.

Consumers of research must be aware that studies using ANCOVA do not necessarily remove all of the bias. The best method of reducing bias is randomization, such as in a true experimental design. Quasi-experimental designs may include bias from other variables or methods. Thus, ANCOVA may not be appropriate or helpful in quasi-experimental studies. Also, it is essential to understand that ANCOVA should not be used merely because randomization was not used in a study (Glass & Hopkins, 2008).

# Conclusion

Inferential univariate statistics can be very useful in the social sciences. Using such tests should be preceded by meeting certain assumptions relevant to the data collected. Many statistical packages can be used to run statistical analyses, but the true usefulness of a study stems from an appropriate design, an appropriate statistical test, and a clearly written results section. Statistical packages have limitations, as well, particularly in the area of reporting practical significance and power. Consumers of research should be aware of both statistical and practical significance when considering the true merit of a study. The degree to which model assumptions have been met and the statistical power should be identified in a study. Readers should be cautious when multiple tests are run on the same data set. Conservative estimates of type I error should be used. Finally, when evaluating a research article, readers are encouraged to evaluate the discussion based on the results to ascertain whether the results truly reflect the merit of the research.

*Now go to the Student Workbook found on cengagebrain.com that accompanies this text for additional application and review activities.*

# Correlation and Regression

This chapter deals with the concepts of correlation and regression based on a linear relationship between two variables. The focus is on the logic behind these two concepts, their interpretation, and *SPSS*-aided applications (although Excel, SAS, or R-stat works just as well) in the context of counseling. Also discussed are several methodological issues, including factors affecting the Pearson product-moment correlation and the interplay of correlation, prediction, and causation. That is, correlation is NOT causation!

Often, you will want to know whether two variables are related and, if so, the type and strength of the relationship. For example, is verbal ability related to academic performance (grade point average [GPA])? Is anxiety related to test performance? Is college stress related to psychological adjustment? Is motivation related to task involvement? Is social support related to psychological adjustment following a relationship breakup? Is social functioning related to mental health? To answer these questions, a measure of relationship, called a **correlation**, between two variables is needed.

This chapter also briefly addresses application of partial and semipartial correlations, procedures that allow more accurate predictions of the relationship between two variables by removing the variance contributed by a third variable influencing that relationship.

# Correlation Between Two Variables

Most people have an intuitive understanding of a correlation between two variables. For example, when asked about the correlation between IQ and GPA, people usually say something like "The higher the IQ, the higher the GPA of the students"—thus demonstrating an understanding that the correlation has to do with the degree to which the students maintain the same relative position (or ranks) on both their IQ score and GPA. Or when asked about the correlation between test anxiety and GPA, many people might say "the higher the test anxiety, the lower the GPA of the students," so they understand that there is a negative correlation between test anxiety and GPA. To upgrade your general comprehension of correlation, this section provides explanations, examples, definitions, graphical representations, and quantitative descriptions of the direction (positive, negative) and the strength (magnitude) of a linear relationship between two variables.

The relationship between two variables (**bivariate correlation**), literacy and average life expectancy, with data from the World95 survey (a sample SPSS database) for 107 countries, is graphically represented as a scatterplot in Figure 17.1. The literacy measure (i.e., percent of people who can read at a defined level of proficiency) is on the horizontal axis ($X$), and the average life expectancy (in years) is on the vertical axis ($Y$). The **scatterplot** (i.e., a diagram with the predictor variable on the horizontal axis and criterion variable on the vertical axis) reveals that there is a linear relationship between the measures on $X$ and $Y$, where high literacy tends to be associated (paired) with high life expectancy and low literacy tends to be associated with low life expectancy. Each dot on the scatterplot represents one person's score on the $X$ and $Y$ variables. The dots group along a straight line with a **positive slope** (i.e., the direction of the dots is from the lower left to the upper right, or "uphill"). In statistical parlance, there is a positive linear relationship (**positive correlation**) between the two variables $X$ and $Y$ (literacy and average life expectancy, respectively) for the data provided with this survey. In previous associational research studies, positive correlations have been found, for example, between (a) motivation and academic success, (b) interpersonal dependency and lack of social self-confidence, (c) parental involvement and locus of control of high school students, (d) depression and state-trait anger (i.e., the intensity of angry feelings at a particular time), and (e) social functioning and mental health.

**Figure 17.1**

Positive linear relationship (positive correlation) between literacy and average life expectancy using survey data from 107 countries.

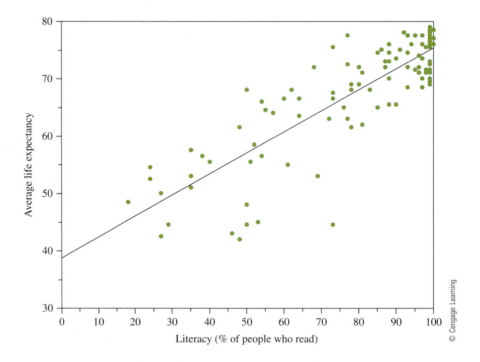

The scatterplot in Figure 17.2 shows a linear relationship between measures of depression and vitality for a sample of persons ($N = 395$), where high scores on $X$ (depression) tend to associate with low scores on $Y$ (vitality), and low scores on $X$ tend to associate with high scores on $Y$. The dots group along a straight line with a **negative slope** (i.e., the direction of the dots is from the upper left to the lower right, or "downhill"). In statistical parlance, this is referred to as a negative linear relationship (**negative correlation**) between the two variables $X$ and $Y$ (depression and vitality, respectively). Negative correlations have been found in previous research, for example,

**Figure 17.2**

Negative linear relationship (negative correlation) between depression and vitality ($N = 395$).

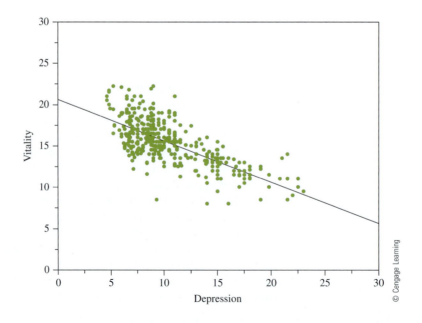

**Figure 17.3**

No linear relationship (no correlation) between literacy and AIDS cases (survey data from 107 countries).

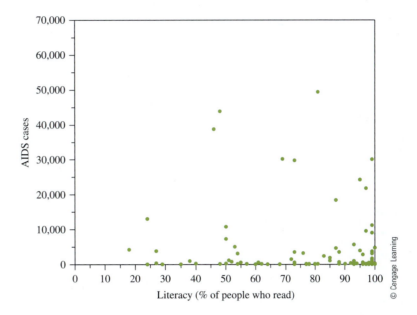

between (a) test anxiety and test performance, (b) avoidance and emotional empathy, (c) college stress and academic success, (d) anger control and depression, and (e) interpersonal dependency and assertiveness.

There is no correlation between two variables when neither a positive nor a negative linear relationship is in place. Figure 17.3 illustrates a lack of linear relationship (i.e., no correlation) between literacy and AIDS (acquired immunodeficiency syndrome) cases, using the data from the World95 survey. Figure 17.4 shows the wide variety of relationships a researcher is likely to encounter in the counseling research literature.

# The Pearson Product-Moment Correlation Coefficient

## Nature and Interpretation of the Pearson *r*

Although a scatterplot of the relationship between two variables, *X* and *Y*, is very useful, more accuracy is needed to determine the presence (or absence) of a linear relationship between *X* and *Y*, its direction (positive, negative), and strength. For variables that are interval or ratio scaled in nature, such information is provided by the Pearson product-moment correlation coefficient (Pearson *r*), which was developed by the English statistician Karl Pearson to summarize the relationship between two variables as a single number. The Pearson *r* can take on values from −1.00 and + 1.00, with positive *r* indicating a positive linear relationship (i.e., directly related; as scores on *X* get higher, so do scores on *Y*), and negative *r* indicating a negative linear relationship between *X* and *Y* (i.e., inversely related; as scores on *X* get higher, scores on *Y* decrease). The decimal indicates the magnitude or strength of the relationship. The closer the absolute value of *r* to 1.0, the stronger the correlation. On a scatterplot this means that the closer the dots are to the straight line, called a line of regression, the stronger is the relationship. When *r* = 0, there is no linear relationship between *X* and *Y*; that is, the scatterplot usually looks circular or without a linear pattern. The extreme positive value *r* = 1.0 indicates that there

**Figure 17.4**

Scatterplots showing various strengths and directions of correlation coefficients.

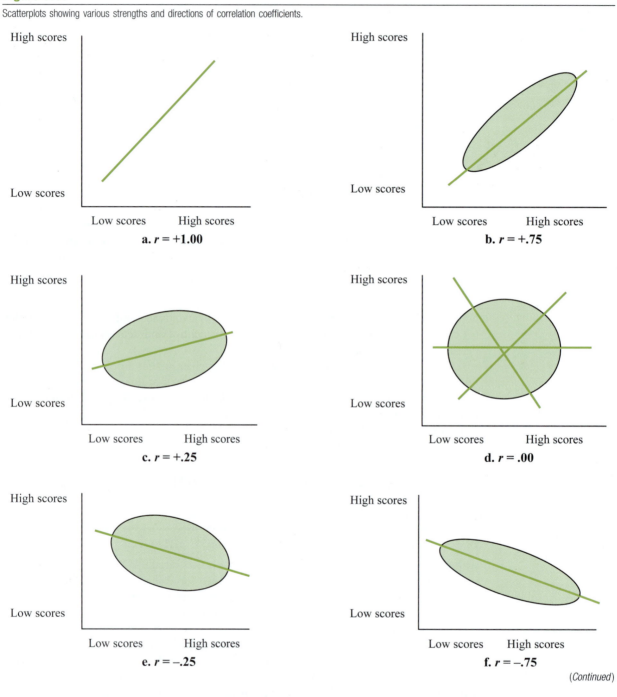

a. *r* = +1.00

b. *r* = +.75

c. *r* = +.25

d. *r* = .00

e. *r* = −.25

f. *r* = −.75

*(Continued)*

is a perfect positive correlation between *X* and *Y*, and all dots in the scatterplot fall exactly on a straight line with a positive slope. The extreme negative value $r = -1.0$ indicates that there is a perfect negative correlation between *X* and *Y*, and all dots in the scatterplot fall on a straight line with a negative slope.

With the data in Figure 17.1, $r = .84$, indicates the presence of a strong positive linear relationship (high positive correlation) between literacy and average life expectancy.

**Figure 17.4**

(*continued*)

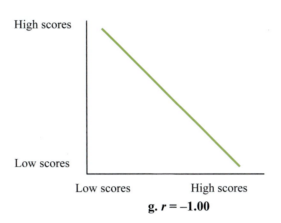

**g. $r = -1.00$**

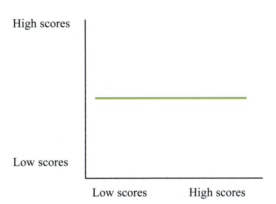

**h. Truncated score: $r = .00$**

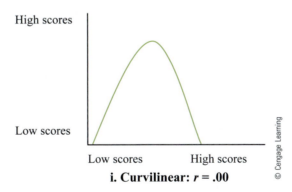

**i. Curvilinear: $r = .00$**

With the data in Figure 17.2, $r = -.71$, indicates that there is a strong negative linear relationship (high negative correlation) between depression and vitality. With the data in Figure 17.3, $r$ is very close to zero ($r = .06$), which indicates that there is a very weak (if any) linear relationship between literacy and AIDS cases. Notice that a rule of thumb for interpreting the size of the Pearson $r$ is based on its absolute value (sign ignored) as follows: (a) .90 to 1.00 = very high correlation; (b) .70 to .90 = high correlation; (c) .50 to .70 = moderate correlation; (d) .30 to .50 = low correlation; and

(e) .00 to .30 = very low (if any) correlation. For example, $r_{XY} = -.92$ indicates a very high negative correlation between $X$ and $Y$, and $r_{XZ} = .65$ indicates a moderate positive correlation between $X$ and $Z$. Thus, the negative relationship between $X$ and $Y$ is stronger than the positive relationship between $X$ and $Z$.

## Calculation of the Pearson *r*

One conceptually useful way of calculating the Pearson $r$ is to use the concept of covariance (i.e., variance between $X$ and $Y$) in representing the relationship between two variables, $X$ and $Y$. Specifically, given the $X$ and $Y$ scores for any sample of size $n$, the covariance of $X$ and $Y$ (denoted $s_{XY}$) is the average cross-product of the deviation scores—that is,

$$s_{XY} = \frac{\Sigma(X - \overline{X})(Y - \overline{Y})}{n - 1}. \tag{17.1}$$

The denominator in Equation 17.1 is the degrees of freedom ($n - 1$), with $n$ being the sample size. $\overline{X}$ and $\overline{Y}$ indicate the mean of the $X$ and $Y$ distributions, respectively.

The covariance of two variables ($\overline{X}$ and $\overline{Y}$) expresses the relationship between them. Specifically, if there is a positive linear relationship between $X$ and $Y$, $s_{XY}$ is positive. This is because persons with $X$ scores above the mean ($\overline{X}$) tend to have $Y$ scores above the mean ($\overline{Y}$), and those with $X$ scores below $\overline{X}$ tend to have $Y$ scores below $\overline{Y}$, which results in positive cross-products [$(X - \overline{X})(Y - \overline{Y})$]. In the case of a negative linear relationship between $X$ and $Y$, $s_{XY}$ is negative because persons with $X$ scores above $\overline{X}$ tend to have $Y$ scores below $\overline{Y}$ and vice versa, which results in negative cross-products [i.e., $(X - \overline{X})(Y - \overline{Y})$]. Unlike Pearson $r$, however, the size of $s_{XY}$ is not bounded by $-1.0$ and $1.0$, as it depends on the units of measurement for $X$ and $Y$. In fact, one way of obtaining the Pearson $r$ is by dividing the covariance by the product of the standard deviations of $X$ and $Y$:

$$r_{XY} = \frac{s_{XY}}{s_X s_Y}. \tag{17.2}$$

After replacing $s_{XY}$ in Equation 17.2 with its expression in Equation 17.1, we have the familiar formula for Pearson $r$:

$$r_{XY} = \frac{\Sigma(X - \overline{X})(Y - \overline{Y})}{(n - 1)s_X s_Y}. \tag{17.3}$$

A second version of the Pearson $r$ formula using $z$-score conversions (see Chapter 13) presumes that $z_X = (X - \overline{X})/s_X$ and $z_Y = (Y - \overline{Y})/s_Y$. Therefore, Equation 17.2 can also be written as

$$r_{XY} = \frac{\Sigma z_X z_Y}{n - 1}. \tag{17.4}$$

Thus, the Pearson $r$ is, in fact, the sum of cross-products of the standard scores for $X$ and $Y$ ($z_X$ and $z_Y$) divided by the degrees of freedom ($n - 1$). There are some other formulas that are more suitable for manual calculations of the Pearson $r$, given the sample values of $X$ and $Y$, but they are not provided here, as the calculations in this chapter are facilitated through the use of computer programs such as SPSS, SAS, or R-stat, rather than using manual calculations. Still, notice that whether one uses the cross-products method or the $z$-score method of computing Pearson $r$, the result is the same. A step-by-step guide on graphing scatterplots and calculating the Pearson $r$ using *SPSS* was provided in Chapter 15 (see Figures 15.50–15.53).

## Testing the Pearson *r* for Statistical Significance

Although the Pearson *r* provides information about the direction and strength of a linear relationship between two variables, *X* and *Y*, for a sample of measures on *X* and *Y*, it is important to use the Pearson *r* as an inferential statistic to determine whether a linear relationship between *X* and *Y* exists in the entire population to which the sample belongs. With $\rho_{XY}$ denoting the correlation between *X* and *Y* in the population, the task is then to test the null hypothesis $H_0$: $\rho_{XY} = 0$ versus the alternative $H_a$: $\rho_{XY} \neq 0$. When $\rho_{XY} = 0$ (and only then), the sampling distribution of the correlation coefficient *r*, calculated for a sample of size *n*, is symmetrical and follows the *t* distribution with $n - 2$ degrees of freedom. The test statistic for testing $H_0$: $\rho_{XY} = 0$ is

$$t = r\sqrt{\frac{n - 2}{1 - r^2}}. \tag{17.5}$$

For example, if $r = .27$ is calculated with *X* and *Y* measures for 30 persons ($n = 30$), the test statistic, obtained with Equation 17.5, is $t = 1.484$ ($t = .27 \sqrt{28/(1 - .0729)} = 1.484$). The **t critical value**, found in the statistical table (see Table 16.5) at the level of significance .05 ($\alpha = .05$), is 2.048. Because the absolute value of the test statistic (1.484) does not exceed the critical value (2.048), there is no sufficient evidence to reject $H_0$: $\rho_{XY} = 0$. The correlation coefficient $r = .27$ is not statistically significant (at $\alpha = .05$), so there is no evidence of a linear relationship between *X* and *Y* in the population. Interestingly, statistical significance is frequently a function of sample size because, all other things being equal, larger sample sizes tend to be more representative of the population. So would this inference hold if $r = .27$ is found with $n = 120$? To determine this, compute $t = .27 \sqrt{118/(1 - .0729)} = 2.975$. The critical value for *t* when $n = 120$ is 1.98. Thus, in this sample of 120 participants, $r = .27$ *is* statistically significant, and the null hypothesis can be rejected.

With $H_0$: $\rho_{XY} = 0$ being the null hypothesis that the correlation coefficient is zero for the population, *SPSS* provides the actual probability of type I error (to falsely reject $H_0$), referred to as the *p* value. If $\alpha$ is the desired level of significance (e.g., $\alpha = .05$) and $p < \alpha$, then there is sufficient evidence to reject $H_0$ and thus to conclude that there is a linear relationship between the two variables in the population.

## Using SPSS to Compute the Pearson *r*

Figure 17.5 provides the SPSS data entry for 20 persons on three variables, $X_1 =$ motivation, $X_2 =$ self-reliance, and $X_3 =$ task involvement, from a study of workplace conditions ($n = 20$). The correlation coefficients (for each pair of variables) are summarized in a correlation matrix obtained through the use of SPSS (Excel, SAS, R-stat, etc.).

The correlation matrix with the SPSS printout provides the correlation coefficients, their *p* values, and the sample size. The correlation coefficient for motivation ($X_1$) and self-reliance ($X_2$) is $r_{12} = .350$, which is not statistically significant because its *p* value (.131) is greater than the desired level of significance ($\alpha = .05$). It is safer then to conclude that there is no linear relationship between motivation and self-reliance in the study population. This may seem odd, given the value of the sample-based correlation coefficient (.350), but one must take into account that the sample size is small ($n = 20$). Further, the correlation coefficient for self-reliance ($X_2$) and task involvement ($X_3$) is $r_{23} = .475$, which is statistically significant at the .05 level because the associated *p* value (.034) is smaller than the desired level of significance ($\alpha = .05$). Therefore, there is a (low to moderate) positive linear relationship between self-reliance and task involvement in the study population. Finally, the correlation coefficient for motivation ($X_1$) and

## Figure 17.5

*SPSS* data table and correlation matrix for a study of workplace conditions.

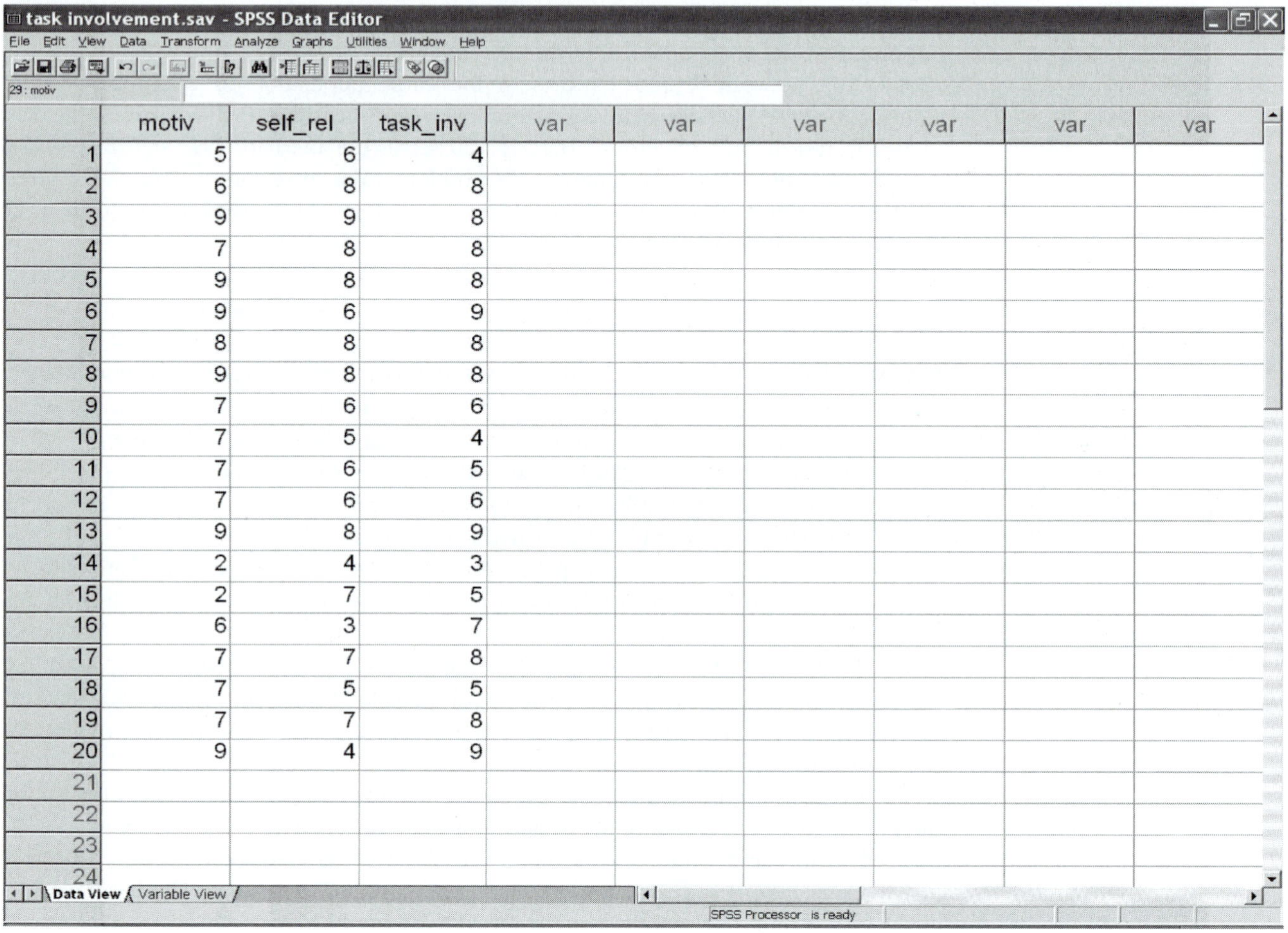

| | motiv | self_rel | task_inv | var | var | var | var | var | var |
|---|---|---|---|---|---|---|---|---|---|
| 1 | 5 | 6 | 4 | | | | | | |
| 2 | 6 | 8 | 8 | | | | | | |
| 3 | 9 | 9 | 8 | | | | | | |
| 4 | 7 | 8 | 8 | | | | | | |
| 5 | 9 | 8 | 8 | | | | | | |
| 6 | 9 | 6 | 9 | | | | | | |
| 7 | 8 | 8 | 8 | | | | | | |
| 8 | 9 | 8 | 8 | | | | | | |
| 9 | 7 | 6 | 6 | | | | | | |
| 10 | 7 | 5 | 4 | | | | | | |
| 11 | 7 | 6 | 5 | | | | | | |
| 12 | 7 | 6 | 6 | | | | | | |
| 13 | 9 | 8 | 9 | | | | | | |
| 14 | 2 | 4 | 3 | | | | | | |
| 15 | 2 | 7 | 5 | | | | | | |
| 16 | 6 | 3 | 7 | | | | | | |
| 17 | 7 | 7 | 8 | | | | | | |
| 18 | 7 | 5 | 5 | | | | | | |
| 19 | 7 | 7 | 8 | | | | | | |
| 20 | 9 | 4 | 9 | | | | | | |
| 21 | | | | | | | | | |
| 22 | | | | | | | | | |
| 23 | | | | | | | | | |
| 24 | | | | | | | | | |

**task involvement.sav - SPSS Data Editor**

File  Edit  View  Data  Transform  Analyze  Graphs  Utilities  Window  Help

29 : motiv

Data View / Variable View /

SPSS Processor  is ready

**Correlations**

| | | Motivation | Self-reliance | Task Involvement |
|---|---|---|---|---|
| Motivation | Pearson Correlation | 1 | .350 | .729** |
| | Sig. (2-tailed) | . | .131 | .000 |
| | N | 20 | 20 | 20 |
| Self-reliance | Pearson Correlation | .350 | 1 | .475* |
| | Sig. (2-tailed) | .131 | . | .034 |
| | N | 20 | 20 | 20 |
| Task Involvement | Pearson Correlation | .729** | .475* | 1 |
| | Sig. (2-tailed) | .000 | .034 | . |
| | N | 20 | 20 | 20 |

*Correlation is significant at the 0.05 level (2-tailed).

**Correlation is significant at the 0.01 level (2-tailed).

task involvement ($X_3$) is $r_{13} = .729$, which is statistically significant because its $p$ value (.000) is smaller than the desired level of significance ($\alpha = .05$). Thus, there is a strong evidence of a high positive linear relationship (high correlation) between motivation and task involvement in the study population.

## Factors Affecting the Pearson *r*

To better understand what factors affect the Pearson $r$ (and why), it is important to keep in mind that the Pearson $r$ is an index of the linear relationship between two variables. Therefore, $r = .00$ indicates that there is no linear relationship between the two variables, but there still might be some kind of (nonlinear) relationship between them. In Figure 17.6a, for example, $r = .00$ because there is a **curvilinear relationship** between two variables (e.g., age and physical strength). Figure 17.6b illustrates a scenario in which $r = .00$ when calculated over a **restricted range** of variable values, although there is a linear relationship between the two variables over a larger range of their measures. In another scenario, there may not be a linear relationship between two variables for a sample of persons ($r = .00$), but there might be a linear relationship between the variables for some

**Figure 17.6**

Scatterplots illustrating (a) curvilinear relationship, (b) restricted range, and (c) correlations by subgroups (e.g., females and males).

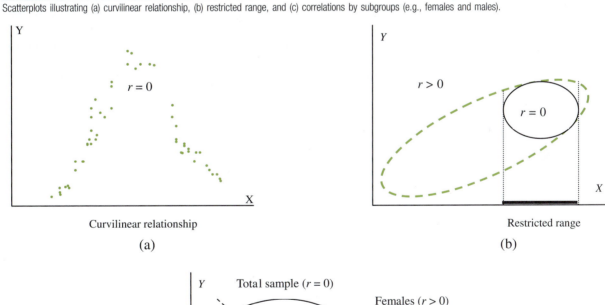

Curvilinear relationship

(a)

Restricted range

(b)

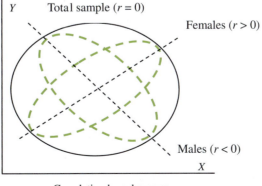

Correlation by subgroups

(c)

subgroups of persons from the total sample. This is illustrated in Figure 17.6c, with a positive linear relationship between $X$ and $Y$ for one subgroup (e.g., females) and, conversely, a negative linear relationship between $X$ and $Y$ for another subgroup (e.g., males), even though there is no linear relationship ($r = 0.00$) for the total sample. In this case, correlation coefficients by separate subgroups are more useful than $r = 0.00$ for the entire sample.

## Linear Transformations and the Pearson *r*

Linear transformations on variables $X$ and/or $Y$ do not affect the size of the Pearson $r$. In measurement, linear transformations commonly occur when a client's raw score on a norm-referenced psychological or educational test is transformed into a standard score, such as a deviation IQ score ($M = 100$; $SD = 15$), $T$ score ($M = 50$; $SD = 10$), or z-score ($M = 0$; $SD = 1$). Suppose that $X^* = bX + a$ is a linear transformation on $X$ and $Y^* = cX + d$ is a linear transformation on $Y$. Such transformations are often used to represent $X$ and $Y$ on a common scale for comparison or report purposes (e.g., to convert the raw $X$ and $Y$ scores into their scores, $z_X$ and $z_Y$, respectively). If the slopes in these two linear transformations ($b$ and $c$) have the same sign (both positive or both negative), the transformation does not affect the correlation coefficient—that is, $r_{X^*Y^*} = r_{XY}$. If, however, $b$ and $c$ have opposite signs (e.g., $b$ is positive and $c$ is negative), the size of the correlation remains the same, but its sign changes—that is, $r_{X^*Y^*} = r_{XY}$. For example, if $r_{XY} = -.57$ and the linear transformations are $X^* = 2X + 5$ and $Y^* = 0.5X - 10$, the correlation coefficient does not change ($r_{X^*Y^*} = -.57$), as the slopes (2 and 0.5) are both positive. When only $X$ is transformed, $r_{X^*Y} = r_{XY}$ if $b > 0$, and $r_{X^*Y} = -r_{XY}$, if $b < 0$. A useful practical implication is then that the correlation coefficient does not change when the values of $X$ and $Y$ are transformed into standard (z-) scores ($\mu = 0$; $\sigma = 1$) or other scales such as the $T$ score ($\mu = 50$; $\sigma = 10$) and norm curve equivalent ($NCE$) scale ($\mu = 50$; $\sigma = 21$).

## Reliability and the Pearson *r*

The reliability of the observed measures for $X$ and $Y$ influences the size of their correlation coefficient, $r$. Remember that the reliability of measures indicates the degree to which these measures are free of error (e.g., due to imperfection of the measurement instrument, fatigue during taking a test, or other sources of measurement error). If it is assumed that the observed score for a person ($X$) is a sum of the person's true score ($T$) and a random error of measurement ($E$)—that is, $X = T + E$, the reliability of $X$, denoted by $\rho_{XX}$, can be viewed as the proportion of the variance in $X$ scores that is *not* error variance. In other words, $\rho_{XX}$ is a coefficient from 0.0 to 1.0, which indicates what proportion of the observed variance is true score variance: $\rho_{XX} = \sigma_T^2 / \sigma_X^2$. Thus, a reliability coefficient of .85 indicates that 15 percent of the variance in the observed scores is due to measurement error or, equivalently, 85 percent of the observed score variance is true score variance.

The correlation between $X$ and $Y$ is attenuated (underestimated) in the presence of error in the observed values on $X$ and $Y$. That is, the lower the reliability for $X$ and/or $Y$, the lower the Pearson $r$ gets compared to its "true" size. An estimate of the Pearson $r$ that would be found if $X$ and $Y$ were perfectly reliable (i.e., no measurement error) is provided with the so-called correction for attenuation formula:

$$r_{T_X T_Y} = \frac{r_{XY}}{\sqrt{\rho_{XY}\rho_{YY}}} \tag{17.6}$$

where $r_{T_X T_Y}$ is the correlation between the true score for $X$ and the true score for $Y$ (i.e., the "true" Pearson $r$), $r_{XY}$ is the Pearson $r$ calculated with the observed values of $X$ and $Y$, $\rho_{XX}$ is the reliability for $X$, and $\rho_{YY}$ is the reliability for $Y$.

It is important to note that the reliability of test (or questionnaire) data is usually estimated with the Cronbach's alpha coefficient for internal consistency reliability (to obtain Cronbach's alpha in *SPSS*, see Chapter 15, Figure 15.37). It should be kept in mind, however, that Cronbach's alpha is an accurate measure of reliability only when the components of the instrument (e.g., items) are tau equivalent (i.e., they measure the same trait and their true scores have equal variances in the population of respondents). Otherwise, the Cronbach's alpha coefficient will underestimate the reliability (i.e., $\alpha < \rho_{XX}$). The correlation between measures collected with two administrations of the same instrument (say, two weeks apart) is used as an estimate of the so-called test–retest reliability (or stability) of the test data, using the standard Pearson product moment correlation coefficient.

As there is always some measurement error in the observed data, the corrected for attenuation correlation is a theoretical "ceiling" toward which the observed correlation coefficient can move with improved reliability of the measures for the two variables. It is important that accurate estimates of the reliabilities be used in Equation 17.6 because, as the examination of this formula shows, the corrected for attenuation correlation will be overestimated when the reliability of $X$ and/or $Y$ is underestimated. It is also important that the error of measurement that affects the observed correlation coefficient ($r_{XY}$) be the same error of measurement that affects the estimates of the reliabilities, $\rho_{XX}$ and $\rho_{YY}$. Thus, when $r_{XY}$ is obtained with measures of $X$ and $Y$ during one testing session, the Cronbach's alpha estimates of $\rho_{XX}$ and $\rho_{YY}$ should be obtained with the $X$ and $Y$ data from that session.

### Computing the Pearson r Using the Correction for Attenuation Formula

A study on *Differentiation of Self* in counseling research reported, among other things, a correlation of .45 between two subscales of a *Differentiation of Self-Inventory*: Emotional Reactivity (ER) and Fusion with Others (FO). The Cronbach's alpha coefficient of reliability for the study data with these two subscales was reported to be .85 and .71, respectively. Let us estimate the "true" correlation between ER and FO. With the notations $X = $ ER and $Y = $ FO, the reported results translate into $r_{XY} = .45$, $\rho_{XX} = .85$, and $\rho_{YY} = .71$. Then, using the correction for attenuation formula (Equation 17.6), the "true" correlation between $ER(X)$ and $FO(Y)$ is $.45/\sqrt{(.85)(.71)} = .58$. Thus, the correlation coefficient reported with the observed data (.45) may increase but will not exceed .58, with improving the reliability of the two subscales, $ER(X)$ and $FO(Y)$.

## Coefficient of Determination, $r^2$

The Pearson $r$ is a measure of the linear relationship between two variables, but it is also used to determine the degree to which the individual differences in one variable can be associated with the individual differences in another variable. Specifically, the square of the correlation coefficient, referred to as **coefficient of determination** ($r^2$), indicates what proportion of the variance in one of the variables is associated with the variance in the other variable. For instance, by squaring the correlation of .45 between "emotional reactivity" and "fusion with others" from the preceding example, we obtain $r^2 \approx .20$. This tells us that about 20 percent of people's differences in fusion with others are associated with their differences in emotional reactivity (or vice versa). Similarly, given the correlation of .729 between motivation and task involvement in an earlier example, $r^2 = (.729)^2 \approx .53$—thus indicating that about 53 percent of the people's differences in task involvement are associated with their differences in motivation. Importantly, the remaining 47 percent ($100\% - 53\% = 47\%$) of differences were *not* explained by the relationship (i.e., unexplained variance).

Graphical illustration of the coefficient of determination ($r^2$) is provided with the Venn diagrams in Figure 17.7, where each circle represents the variance of a variable.

**Figure 17.7**

Graphical illustration of the coefficient of determination, $r^2$, with the overlapping area representing the shared (common) variance in $X$ and $Y$.

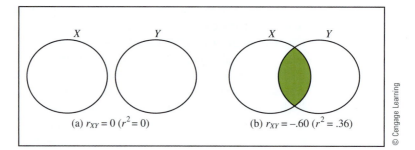

(a) $r_{XY} = 0$ $(r^2 = 0)$          (b) $r_{XY} = -.60$ $(r^2 = .36)$

© Cengage Learning

Let the focus in interpreting $r^2$ be on the degree to which the variance in $Y$ is associated with the variance in $X$ (i.e., $Y$ is a dependent criterion variable and $X$ an independent predictor variable). The larger the overlap between two circles, the higher the proportion of the variance in $Y$ associated with the variance in $X$. The lack of overlap in Figure 17.7a shows that there is no correlation between $X$ and $Y$ (i.e., $X$ and $Y$ are not linearly related), or, equivalently, none of the variance in $Y$ is explained by the variance in $X$. The overlap in Figure 17.7b, however, illustrates that 36 percent of the variance in $Y$ is explained by the variance in $X$, and 64 percent is unexplained variance.

## Other Types of Correlation Coefficients

As just mentioned, the Pearson $r$ is used to determine the relationship between two variables derived from interval or ratio scales. Many other coefficients, however, have been developed to analyze the relationships between variables from various combinations of scaling methods (e.g., nominal, ordinal, interval, and ratio). A number of the more commonly used coefficients along with their associated scaling variables are presented in Table 17.1.

The **Spearman rho** ($\rho$) is used when data on both variables is rank-ordered (ordinal scale). It is frequently used in behavioral and animal research when researchers want to minimize the effects of outliers (extreme scores) on the variance of a distribution. The Spearman rho formula is

$$\rho = 1 - \frac{6\Sigma D^2}{N(N^2 - 1)}, \qquad (17.7)$$

where $D = $ the difference between the ranks for a given individual's scores.

The test scores in Table 17.2 have been converted to rank-ordered data. Notice that in some instances several "ties" occurred. When two of the same test scores occur, add

| TABLE 17.1 | Types of correlation coefficients used with scales. | |
|---|---|---|
| **Type of Coefficient** | **Variable $X$** | **Variable $Y$** |
| Pearson Product-Moment ($r$) | Interval or ratio | Interval or ratio |
| Eta ($\eta$) (used to assess nonlinear relationships) | Interval or ratio | Interval or ratio |
| Spearman Rank Order ($\rho$) | Rank-ordered | Rank-ordered |
| Contingency ($C$) | Nominal | Nominal |
| Point Biserial ($r_{pbi}$) | True dichotomy | Interval or ratio |
| Biserial ($r_{bi}$) | Artificial dichotomy | Interval or ratio |
| Phi ($\Phi$) | True dichotomy | True dichotomy |
| Tetrachoric ($r_t$) | Artificial dichotomy | Artificial dichotomy |

Examples: True dichotomy (male, female); artificial dichotomy (favorable, unfavorable); nominal (DSM diagnosis); interval (IQ); ratio (height); rank-order (places in a contest).

© Cengage Learning

**TABLE 17.2**  Rank-ordered student scores on the midterm and final exam of an assessment course.

| Midterm Score X | Midterm Rank Xr | Final Score Y | Final Rank Yr | Rank Difference D | Rank Difference D² |
|---|---|---|---|---|---|
| 90 | 13.5 | 87 | 12.5 | +1.0 | 1.00 |
| 93 | 9.5 | 86 | 14.5 | −5.0 | 25.00 |
| 86 | 19 | 96 | 4 | +15.0 | 225.00 |
| 96 | 4 | 100 | 1 | +3.0 | 9.00 |
| 83 | 20 | 82 | 16.5 | +3.5 | 12.25 |
| 88 | 16.5 | 70 | 20 | −3.5 | 12.25 |
| 94 | 7 | 90 | 8 | −1.0 | 1.00 |
| 88 | 16.5 | 86 | 14.5 | +2.0 | 4.00 |
| 98 | 2.5 | 92 | 7 | −4.5 | 20.25 |
| 95 | 5 | 94 | 6 | −1.0 | 1.00 |
| 87 | 18 | 76 | 19 | −1.0 | 1.00 |
| 94 | 7 | 88 | 10 | −3.0 | 9.00 |
| 92 | 11.5 | 88 | 10 | +1.5 | 2.25 |
| 90 | 13.5 | 96 | 4 | +9.5 | 90.25 |
| 92 | 11.5 | 87 | 12.5 | −1.0 | 1.00 |
| 100 | 1 | 96 | 4 | −3.0 | 9.00 |
| 98 | 2.5 | 78 | 18 | −15.5 | 240.25 |
| 93 | 9.5 | 88 | 10 | −0.5 | 0.25 |
| 89 | 15 | 82 | 16.5 | −1.5 | 2.25 |
| 94 | 7 | 98 | 2 | +5.0 | 25.00 |
| N = 20 | | | | | $\sum D^2 = 691.0$ |

the two ranks together and divide by 2. For example, on the midterm exam, the score 98 occurred twice, so instead of ranking one 2 and the other 3, one simply splits the difference and assigns an average rank of 2.5 to each value. Likewise, the score 88 occurred three times on the final exam, so instead of assigning ranks 9, 10, and 11, the averaged rank of 10 is assigned to all three scores.

When assigning ranks, always make sure both sets of scores are ranked in the same direction (i.e., high to low, or low to high). If one set of scores is ranked in a different direction, the direction (e.g., positive, negative) of the correlation will be altered. For example, the midterm and final exam scores in Table 17.2 were both assigned ranks from highest to lowest, so the highest score received a rank of 1 and so forth. Because the two sets of scores were positively related, the resulting correlation showed a positive direction. If the midterm scores were ranked high to low and the final exam scores low to high, however, the resulting correlation would have a negative direction because high scores (ranks) on the midterm would be associated with low scores (ranks) on the final.

Applying the formula for the Spearman rho, one can obtain the correlation coefficient for the new rank-ordered midterm and final exam scores:

$$\rho = 1 - \frac{(6)(691)}{20(400 - 1)} = 1 - \frac{4,146}{7,980} = 1 - .52 = .48$$

Thus, the correlation coefficient for the rank-ordered scores is $\rho = .48$, and the coefficient of determination ($\rho^2$) is .23. Table 17.3 provides the SPSS output for both the

| **TABLE 17.3** | Pearson *r* and Spearman rho SPSS output computations for the data in Table 17.2. |
|---|---|

**Correlations**

| | | Midterm Score | Final Score |
|---|---|---|---|
| **Midterm Score** | Pearson Correlation | 1 | .411 |
| | Sig. (two-tailed) | . | .071 |
| | N | 20 | 20 |
| **Final Score** | Pearson Correlation | .411 | 1 |
| | Sig. (two-tailed) | .071 | . |
| | N | 20 | 20 |

| | | | Midterm Rank | Final Rank |
|---|---|---|---|---|
| **Spearman's Rho** | Midterm Rank | Correlation Coefficient | 1.000 | .477(*) |
| | | Sig. (two-tailed) | . | .034 |
| | | N | 20 | 20 |
| | Final Rank | Correlation Coefficient | .477(*) | 1.000 |
| | | Sig. (two-tailed) | .034 | . |
| | | N | 20 | 20 |

*Correlation is significant at the 0.05 level (2-tailed).

© Cengage Learning

Pearson *r* on the raw score data and the Spearman rho on the ranked data. Notice how using the Spearman rho resulted in a different (in this case a slightly higher) correlation coefficient. This is probably because a number of the scores on the midterm and final exams could be considered outliers (extremely low or high scores) given the overall closeness of the remainder of the scores. These scores contributed a huge amount of variance to the Pearson *r* correlation computations, whereas their rank ($\rho$)-ordered equivalents contributed less variance. Finally, you will notice that in comparison to the Pearson *r*, the computation of $\rho$ is rather simple.

In addition to $\rho$, there are a number of coefficients called "Pearson family coefficients" because they are computationally equivalent to *r*. The **phi** ($\Phi$) **coefficient** is used when one variable is a true dichotomy (e.g., male–female, correct–incorrect) and the other variable is either a true dichotomy or an artificial dichotomy (e.g., favorable–unfavorable, successful–unsuccessful). The simplest formula for computing phi is $\Phi = \chi^2/N$. The **point-biserial correlation coefficient** ($r_{pb}$) is used when one variable is a true dichotomy and the other is continuous. The point-biserial correlation is frequently used when achievement, ability, or intelligence test items (e.g., scored correct–incorrect) are correlated with subtest or total scores to determine how highly related various items are to the interpreted scales. The Pearson *r* formulae presented in the preceding section can be used to compute $r_{pb}$.

Several other coefficients that are not part of the Pearson family are the biserial, tetrachoric, and eta coefficients. These coefficients are rarely seen in test manuals. The **biserial correlation coefficient** ($r_{bi}$) expresses the relationship between two variables when one variable is an artificial dichotomy and the other a continuous variable. When attempting to relate success (e.g., successful/unsuccessful) at some given task to achievement on some continuous scale (e.g., Woodcock–Johnson: Tests of Achievement, third edition, Math Calculation subtest), $r_{bi}$ may be useful. The **tetrachoric coefficient** ($r_t$) is used to compute relationships when both variables are scaled on an artificial dichotomy (i.e., successful/unsuccessful achievement vs. favorable/unfavorable opinion). Finally, the **eta coefficient** ($\eta$) is used to assess nonlinear relationships (e.g., curvilinear distributions). Inspection of scatterplots may be helpful in determining whether the eta is needed.

## Correlation and Causation

It is important to emphasize that the coefficient of determination ($r^2$) indicates what proportion of the variance in $Y$ is associated with the variance in $X$, but this does not necessarily mean that individual differences in $Y$ are caused by individual differences in $X$; that is, correlation does not mean causation. Correlation only indicates the degree of association—not what causes the association! For example, with the World95 survey data (Figure 17.1), the correlation between literacy and average life expectancy was found to be $r = .84$. Then $r^2 = (.84)^2 = .705$, indicating that 70.5 percent of the differences in average life expectancy is associated with differences in literacy for the countries participating in the World95 survey. There is no logical basis, however, to believe that differences in literacy (percent of people who read) have caused differences in average life expectancy among these countries. Most likely, literacy and average life expectancy are correlated because they are both causally affected by a third variable (say, standard of living) or even by several other variables.

Hereafter, the terms "associated with," "accounted for by," and "explained by" are used synonymously in interpreting $r^2$ as a proportion of the variance in $Y$ associated with (accounted for by, explained by) the variance in $X$. But they do not imply causality.

# Simple Linear Regression

## Correlation, Prediction, and Causation

When there is a correlation between two variables, the linear relationship between them can be used to predict values on one of the variables ($Y$) from values on the other variable ($X$). If the goal is to predict scores on $Y$ from scores on $X$, then $Y$ is referred to as the *criterion variable* and $X$ is referred to as the *predictor variable*. Which of two variables is $Y$ (criterion) and which one is $X$ (predictor) depends on the research question and the methodological soundness of the prediction model. For example, given the high correlation between motivation and task involvement in a study on workplace conditions, the purpose is to predict task involvement from motivation. With this, the criterion variable is $Y =$ task involvement, and the predictor variable is $X =$ motivation.

It is important to reiterate that correlation does not necessarily mean causation. Correlational analyses indicate the degree of association, not the cause of the association! High (positive or negative) correlation between $X$ and $Y$ indicates that scores on $Y$ can be accurately predicted from scores on $X$, but this does not imply that changes in $X$ *cause* changes in $Y$. For example, using data from the World95 survey (Figure 17.1), one can predict average life expectancy from literacy, although there is probably no causal relationship between these two variables. In a more extreme example, one can predict mental ability from shoe size for children of age, say, 5–16 years, although the correlation between these two variables is spurious (i.e., does not make theoretical sense and vanishes after partialing out their common cause [age]). Thus, it is important to keep in mind that the emphasis in predictive research is on practical applications, not on causal explanation and conceptual understanding of relationships between variables. Of course, results in predictive research can be very useful in generating theoretical cause-and-effect hypotheses. Conversely, the chances of good prediction increase when the selection of predictor variables is based on their theoretical relationship with the criterion variable.

## The Regression Line

Suppose that a sample of scores on $X$ and $Y$ is available and the goal is to predict $Y$ scores from $X$ scores with future samples in which only $X$ scores are available. The regression line (i.e., line of best fit) for such a prediction is illustrated for the data in Figure 17.8, in which the scatterplot of dots (●) reveals a high positive linear relationship between the $X$ and $Y$ scores ($r = .729$). The straight line fitting the scatterplot is used to predict scores on $Y$ (task involvement) from scores on $X$ (motivation). Specifically, for any value of $X$, the predicted $Y$ value (denoted $\hat{Y}$) is located on the straight line (○). The difference between the actual $Y$ score and the predicted score ($\hat{Y}$) is called prediction *error*: $e = Y - \hat{Y}$. Evidently, the $Y$ values for dots (●) above the prediction line are associated with positive errors ($e > 0$), whereas those below the prediction line are associated with negative errors ($e < 0$). Note that if the correlation between $X$ and $Y$ is $+1.00$ or $-1.00$, all data points would fall on the regression line because there would be no error.

The total error is defined with the sum of squared errors: $SS_E = \Sigma e^2 = \Sigma(Y - \hat{Y})^2$. Among all possible prediction lines, the one that produces the smallest total error (sum of squared errors) is the line of the best fit, or **regression line**. With this approach, known as the least squares method, the sum of squared distances from the data points (●) to the prediction line is minimal. The prediction with a regression line is referred to as **simple linear regression** because only one predictor ($X$) is used to predict $Y$ (or, to "regress $Y$ on $X$").

The general analytic form of the regression line is provided with the equation

$$\hat{Y} = bX + a, \tag{17.8}$$

where $b$ is the **slope** and $a$ is the **intercept** of the line. The slope ($b$) governs the steepness of the regression line. The intercept ($a$) is the predicted value ($\hat{Y}$) for $X = 0$; that is, $(0, a)$

**Figure 17.8**

Regression line for predicting
task involvement from
motivation.

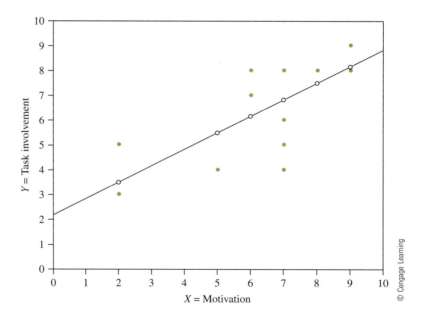

$X =$ Motivation

is the intersection point of the prediction line and the vertical axis ($Y$). With the least squares method, the slope and the intercept for the line of the best fit are calculated as

$$b = r_{XY} \frac{s_Y}{s_X},\tag{17.9}$$

$$a = \overline{Y} - b\overline{X},\tag{17.10}$$

where $r_{XY}$ = correlation between $X$ and $Y$; $s_X$ = standard deviation of the $X$ scores; $s_Y$ = standard deviation of the $Y$ scores; $\overline{X}$ = mean of the $X$ scores; and $\overline{Y}$ = mean of the $Y$ score.

In Equation 17.9, the standard deviations are positive ($s_X > 0$ and $s_Y > 0$), and, therefore, the slope ($b$) and the correlation coefficient ($r_{XY}$) are of the same sign (both positive or both negative). Given this, positive $b$ indicates positive direction, and negative $b$ indicates negative direction of the regression line. As can also be seen from Equation 17.9, the regression slope equals the correlation coefficient ($b = r$) when $X$ and $Y$ have equal variances and, thus, equal standard deviations ($s_X = s_Y$). Notice that the point with coordinates ($\overline{X}, \overline{Y}$) always belongs to the regression line. This can be seen by replacing $X$ with $\overline{X}$ in Equation 17.8, $\hat{Y} = b\overline{X} + a$, and then comparing this expression for $\hat{Y}$ with that for $\overline{Y}$, obtained from Equation 17.10: $\overline{Y} = b\overline{X} + a$. Thus, $\hat{Y} = \overline{Y}$, which shows that $\overline{Y}$ is in fact the predicted $Y$ score for $X = \overline{X}$.

### Simple Linear Regression

With the data for prediction of task involvement from motivation (Figure 17.5), $r_{XY}$ = .729, $\overline{X}$ = 6.95, $\overline{Y}$ = 6.80, $s_X$ = 2.06, and $s_Y$ = 1.88. Using Equations 17.9 and 17.10, we obtain $b = (.729)(1.88)/2.06 = 0.665$, and $a = 6.80 - (0.665)(6.95) = 2.18$. Thus, the equation of the regression line in Figure 17.7 is

$$\hat{Y} = 0.665X + 2.18.$$

For example, with $X = 10$ in this equation, we obtain $\hat{Y} = 0.665(10) + 2.18 = 8.83$. In other words, if the motivation score for a person is 10, the predicted score on task involvement for this person is $\hat{Y} = 8.83$.

You may recall that the use of SPSS for linear regression analysis was discussed in Chapter 15. In the Linear Regression dialog box (e.g., Figure 15.62), $Y$ is referred to as a *dependent* variable and $X$ the *independent* variable. Keep in mind, however, that the terminology used in this chapter is (a) $Y$ = *criterion* variable and $X$ = *predictor* variable, when $Y$ is predicted from $X$, and (b) $Y$ = *dependent* variable and $X$ = *independent* variable, when $Y$ is causally explained by $X$. Thus, the SPSS programming language assumes causality even though that may not be the case.

## Interpretation of the Slope

The prediction of $Y$ from $X$ with the regression equation $\hat{Y} = 1.5X + 2$ is graphically represented in Figure 17.9. The positive sign of the slope ($b = 1.5$) indicates that when the $X$ scores increase, the predicted scores associated with them also increase. Thus, a positive change in $X$ pairs with a positive change in $\hat{Y}$. Let us use $\Delta X$ for a change in $X$ (delta, $\Delta$, means "change") and $\Delta \hat{Y}$ for the associated change in the predicted score ($\hat{Y}$.). For the regression line in Figure 17.9, one can see that (a) if $X$ increases from 2 to 3 ($\Delta X = 1$), then $\Delta \hat{Y} = 1.5$, and (b) if $X$ increases from 4 to 8 ($\Delta X = 4$), then $\Delta \hat{Y} = 6$. In both cases, the ratio "change in $\hat{Y}$ to change in $X$" equals the slope of the regression line: $\Delta \hat{Y}/\Delta X = 1.5/1 = 6/4 = 1.5$. In fact, this holds for any (positive or negative) change in $X$ and its associated change in $\hat{Y}$ with any regression equation. Notice that when the slope is negative, an increase in $X$ ($\Delta X > 0$) is associated with a decrease in the predicted $Y$ score ($\Delta \hat{Y} < 0$).

**Figure 17.9**

The regression *slope* as a change-rate ($\Delta \hat{Y}/\Delta X$).

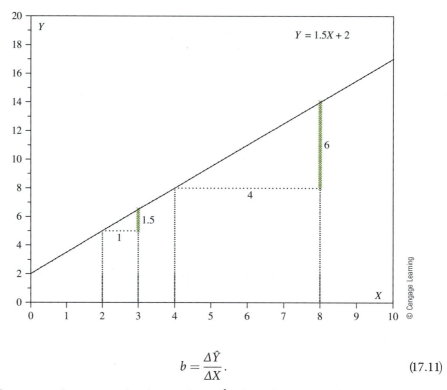

$$b = \frac{\Delta \hat{Y}}{\Delta X}. \qquad (17.11)$$

Of course, with $\Delta X = 1$, the slope is $b = \Delta \hat{Y}$. Thus, the slope in the regression equation indicates the change in the predicted $Y$ score associated with a unit change in the predictor variable, $X$. Note that at any point in the future when one is collecting data about a client using the predictor ($X$) variable, to find the predicted score ($\hat{Y}$) given $X$, one need simply recall the regression equation and replace $X$ with its given value. To find the change in the predicted score, given the change in $X$, it suffices to know the slope of the regression equation and use $\Delta \hat{Y} = b\Delta X$. As practice, for the regression equation in Figure 17.9, (a) find the predicted $Y$ score for $X = 6$, and (b) find the change in the predicted score if $X$ increases by six units. Did you determine $\Delta \hat{Y}$ to be 11 and 20, respectively?

## SPSS Output for Simple Linear Regression

The steps in using SPSS (SAS, R-stat, etc.) for linear regression analysis are described in Chapter 15 (Figures 15.62–15.65). This section illustrates the interpretation of results provided with the SPSS output for the linear regression prediction of task involvement from motivation. The SPSS output in Figure 17.10 includes only tables related to simple linear regression (the output for linear regression with two or more predictors, referred to as **multiple regression**, is discussed in Chapter 19). Also, the scatterplot with the regression line is not included in Figure 17.10, as it is provided with Figure 17.8.

The Model Summary table in Figure 17.10 provides (a) the coefficient of correlation between motivation ($X$) and task involvement ($Y$), $r_{XY} = .729$; (b) the squared correlation coefficient $= .532$, which indicates that 53.2 percent of the individual differences on task involvement are accounted for by differences in motivation; (c) the squared correlation coefficient, adjusted for the population, $r^2_{adj.} = .506$; and (d) the standard error of estimate, $s_{Y.X} = 1.322$.

The Coefficients table (Figure 17.10) provides information to test the regression coefficient for statistical significance and to obtain the regression equation $\hat{Y} = bX + a$.

**Figure 17.10**

*SPSS* output for linear regression of task involvement on motivation.

**Variables Entered/Removed[a]**

| Model | Variables Entered | Variables Removed | Method |
|---|---|---|---|
| 1 | Motivation[b] | | Enter |

b. All requested variables entered.
a. Dependent variable: task involvement

**Model Summary**

| Model | R | R Square | Adjusted R Square | Std. Error of the Estimate |
|---|---|---|---|---|
| 1 | .729[a] | .532 | .506 | 1.322 |

a. Predictors: (Constant), motivation

**Coefficients[a]**

| Model | | Unstandardized Coefficients | | Standardized Coefficients | | | 95% Confidence Interval for B | |
|---|---|---|---|---|---|---|---|---|
| | | B | Std. Error | Beta | $t$ | Sig. | Lower Bound | Upper Bound |
| 1 | (Constant) | 2.181 | 1.063 | | 2.052 | .055 | −.052 | 4.414 |
| | motivation | .665 | .147 | .729 | 4.524 | .000 | .356 | .973 |

a. Dependent Variable: task involvement

© Cengage Learning

Specifically, the regression coefficient ($b = 0.665$) is statistically significant because the $p$ value (.000) that is associated with its statistic ($t = 4.524$) is less than the .05 level of significance ($p < \alpha$). In other words, there is a sufficient evidence to reject the null hypothesis that the regression coefficient is equal to zero for the study population. Given the standard error for the regression coefficient, $SE(b) = 0.147$, the 95 percent confidence interval for $b$ is from 0.356 to 0.973; [the 95 percent confidence interval is $\pm 2$ standard errors; therefore, $0.665 \pm 2(0.147) = 0.356$ to 0.973]. The regression equation for the prediction of task involvement ($Y$) from motivation ($X$) in this example is $\hat{Y} = 0.665X + 2.181$ (see column B in Unstandardized Coefficients). Notice that this is the same simple linear regression equation used in the example of task involvement and motivation. Finally, notice that the higher the correlation between $X$ and $Y$, the more accurate the predictions resulting from linear regression equations. If the correlation between $X$ and $Y$ is 1.00 (or −1.00), perfect prediction has been achieved.

Of course more than one predictor variable ($X_1$, $X_2$, $X_3$, …) can be used to estimate the criterion score ($Y$). This is called multiple regression and will be addressed in Chapter 19.

# Partial Correlation

Two variables ($X$ and $Y$) may correlate because they are both affected by a third variable ($Z$). For example, math achievement and reading achievement are related but without causal inference. A third factor, perhaps intelligence, may be hypothesized to "cause" both math and reading achievement to vary. Such a "common cause hypothesis" is graphically represented in Figure 17.11a. In another scenario, the correlation between $X$ and $Y$ may be mediated by $Z$ (Figure 17.11b). A mediating variable is one that is related to a first variable and subsequently influences the second variable. In any case, when the effect of $Z$ is removed (partialled out) from $X$ and $Y$, the resulting correlation is referred to as **partial correlation** between $X$ and $Y$, controlling for $Z$, and denoted $r_{XYZ}$.

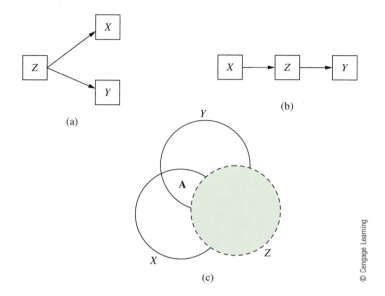

(a)

(b)

(c)

In Figure 17.11c, $r_{XY.Z}$ is presented with part A: the overlap between the residualized $X$ and $Y$, after $Z$ has been removed from both of them.

When the correlation between $X$ and $Y$ exists solely because it is affected by a common cause, $Z$, it is referred to as a **spurious** correlation. Clearly, if the correlation between $X$ and $Y$ is spurious, their partial correlation is zero or very close to it. In this case, expanding on the graphical representation in Figure 17.11c, the circles representing $X$ and $Y$ would not overlap at all, making $A = 0$. For example, it is known in behavioral research that there is a very high positive correlation between shoe size and mental ability for children aged, say, from 3 to 16 years. This, however, is a spurious correlation because it vanishes when controlling for age. This can be tested by calculating (a) the correlation for children of the same age or (b) the partial correlation between shoe size and mental ability controlling for age.

Another situation for potential use of partial correlations is when the correlation between two variables is **mediated** by other variables. For example, if it is hypothesized that parental support (PS) affects GPA of the students only through the mediation of the students' motivation (MOT), one can use the model in Figure 17.11b, with $X$ = PS, $Y$ = GPA, and $Z$ = MOT (i.e., PS→MOT→GPA). The hypothesis will be supported if the partial correlation between PS and GPA, while controlling for MOT, is zero (or close to zero). Notice that the correlation between two variables, $X$ and $Y$, when a third variable, $Z$, is removed (partialled out) from both $X$ and $Y$ is referred to as "partial correlation between $X$ and $Y$, controlling for $Z$" (notation: $r_{XY.Z}$). Partial correlations are used to more accurately predict the relationship (correlation) between two variables when a third variable is hypothesized to influence one or both of the first two variables.

## Semipartial Correlation

There are situations in which the interest is on the correlation between two variables, while removing the effect of other variables from only one of the two variables. In the context of an example involving three variables ($X_1$ = motivation, $X_2$ = self-reliance, and $X_3$ = task involvement), for instance, assume the correlation between motivation ($X_1$) and task involvement ($X_3$) is $r_{13} = .729$. Thus, computing the coefficient of

**Figure 17.12**

Semipartial (part) correlation between $X_1$ and $X_3$, partialing out $X_2$ from $X_1$ only.

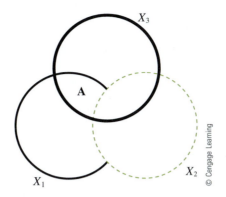

determination $(r^2) = (.729)^2 = .5314$ shows that 53.14 percent of the variance in task involvement is accounted for by the variance in motivation. But because $(X_1)$ is also correlated with self-reliance $(X_2)$ $(r_{12} = .35)$, it might be interesting to know what proportion of the variance in task involvement $(X_3)$ is accounted for by motivation $(X_1)$, over and above the proportion of variance accounted for by self-reliance $(X_2)$. This directly translates into a question about the correlation between motivation and task involvement $(r_{13})$, with self-reliance removed from motivation but not from task involvement, thus keeping the variance of task involvement intact. With the $X_1$, $X_2$, and $X_3$ notations, such correlation is referred to as **semipartial** (*part*) **correlation** between $X_3$ and $X_1$, partialing out $X_2$ from $X_1$ but not partialing out $X_2$ from $X_3$. The notations for this semipartial correlation is $r_{3(1.2)}$. With the data from this example, *SPSS* provided $r_{3(1.2)} = .601$. The squared semipartial correlation, $(.601)^2 = .3612$, shows that 36.12 percent of the variance in task involvement is uniquely accounted for by motivation, over and above the variance accounted for by self-reliance. In Figure 17.12, this semipartial (part) correlation $r_{3(1.2)}$ is depicted by part A: the overlap between the residualized $X_1$ and the intact $X_3$, after removing $X_2$ from $X_1$ but not from $X_3$. Thus, the squared semipartial correlation (.3612) indicates what proportion is part A from the total (intact) circle $X_3$.

If, on the other hand, we want to know what proportion of the individual differences in task involvement $(X_3)$ is uniquely associated with self-reliance $(X_2)$ over and above the proportion accounted for by motivation, then we need to square $r_{3(2.1)}$: the semipartial correlation between $X_3$ and $X_2$, partialing out $X_2$ from $X_1$ but not from $X_3$. (Look at Figure 17.12, and imagine what the graphical representation of $r_{3(2.1)}$ will look like.)

In general, which type of correlation (i.e., partial or semipartial) to use depends on the specific research question being asked. Notice that the correlation between two variables, $X$ and $Y$, (e.g., parental support [PS] and grade point average [GPA] from the first example in this chapter) when a third variable, $Z$ (student motivation [MOT]), is removed (partial out) from $X$ but not from $Y$, is referred to as semipartial (part) correlation between $X$ and $Y$, partialing out $Z$ from $X$ [notation: $r_{Y(X.Z)}$].

## Conclusion

This chapter introduced the concepts of linear relationship (correlation) between two variables and simple linear regression. These analyses are often misused in the counseling literature to indicate causative inferences that are not justified: correlation is NOT causation! In general, the correlation between two variables reveals the nature and the strength of their relationship (e.g., linear or curvilinear) if such a relationship exists.

The discussion of correlation in this chapter is restricted to a linear relationship between two variables. The Pearson product-moment correlation coefficient (briefly, Pearson $r$) indicates the direction (positive or negative) and the strength of a linear relationship between two variables ($X$ and $Y$) measured on interval or ratio scales. Specifically, Pearson $r$ takes on values from $-1.0$ to $1.0$ and indicates (a) a positive correlation, when $r > 0$; (b) a negative correlation, when $r < 0$; and (c) no correlation, when $r = 0$. As the Pearson $r$ is sample dependent, it is important to determine whether a linear relationship between two variables ($X$ and $Y$) exists in the population from which the sample has been (randomly) selected.

The size of the Pearson $r$ is affected by factors such as the sample size, range of $X$ and $Y$ values in the sample, and the nature of the relationship between $X$ and $Y$. It is important to keep in mind that when the Pearson $r$ is equal (or close) to zero—thus indicating the lack of linear relationship between $X$ and $Y$ for the sample at hand—this might be because of (a) the presence of a curvilinear relationship between $X$ and $Y$, (b) restricted range of $X$ and $Y$ values, or (c) the presence of, say, two groups in the sample for one of which the Pearson $r$ is positive and for the other, negative (see Figure 17.6). Linear transformations on the values of one (or both) of the variables $X$ and $Y$ do not affect the size of the Pearson $r$. The square of the correlation coefficient ($r^2$), referred to as coefficient of determination, indicates what proportion of the variance in one of the variables is associated with the variance in the other variable. Simple linear regression is in place when the linear relationship between two variables $X$ and $Y$ is used to predict values of one variable ($Y$ = criterion) from the other variable ($X$ = predictor). In the equation of the regression line, $\hat{Y} = bX + a$, the slope ($b$) indicates the direction (i.e., steepness of the regression line), whereas the intercept ($a$) indicates its location (i.e., where the regression line intersects the vertical [$Y$] axis). For interpretation purposes, it is important to note that the slope ($b$) shows the change in the predicted score ($\hat{Y}$) associated with a one-unit change in the predictor variable ($X$). Also, the sign of the slope (positive or negative) is always the same as the sign of the Pearson correlation between $X$ and $Y$.

This chapter also reviewed the application of partial and semipartial correlations, procedures that allow more accurate predictions of the relationship between two variables by removing the variance contributed by a third variable that influences that relationship. Partial correlations remove the effects of a mediating (third) variable from the relationship between the two primary variables of interest. Semipartial (or part) correlations remove the effects of a mediating (third) variable from only one of the two primary variables of interest. These statistical procedures help researchers understand more specific relationships between experimental variables.

*Now go to the Student Workbook found on cengagebrain.com that accompanies this text for additional application and review activities.*

# Nonparametric Tests of Statistical Inference

This chapter introduces the chi-square statistic and explores its usefulness in testing differences between expected frequencies of occurrence for categorical data or proportions. In addition, several nonparametric tests useful in analyzing ordinal and skewed data sets, such as Kolmogorov–Smirnov, Wilcoxen Rank Sum, Mann–Whitney *U*, and Kruskal–Wallis tests, are briefly explained. Nonparametric statistics are used to analyze nominal or ordinal data or when the assumptions required for parametric analysis have been violated, such as when one cannot assume that a distribution conforms to the properties of a normal curve or that the variances of two distributions are not equivalent (e.g., the distributions of one or both variables are skewed and one or both variable distributions are affected by extreme outliers).

When skewed distributions are evident, nonparametric tests can be helpful. Parametric tests, however, are ordinarily more powerful than nonparametric tests, and simple data transformations can be used to transform skewed distributions into more normal distributions so that these more powerful parametric tests can be used.

## CHAPTER 18

# Analysis of Proportions and Count Data—Chi-Square Applications

Proportion and count variables (e.g., nominal and categorical) tend to violate several assumptions of analyses and produce highly skewed distributions. A **chi-square** statistic ($\chi^2$) is used to determine whether a count or proportion variable distribution is equivalent to the distribution of expected frequencies. Expected frequencies are ordinarily predicted by the null hypothesis of no expected difference. So if a treatment group frequency of occurrence is compared with a control group frequency of occurrence, there should be no difference. Likewise, if two categories are studied (e.g., two candidates running for a political office), a 50-50 occurrence is expected, and if three categories are used (e.g., three candidates running for political office), a 33-33-33 occurrence is expected. Importantly, the chi-square statistic requires the provision of frequency data from independent categories (e.g., one cannot vote for more than one choice).

A very simple example using the chi-square analysis for count data involves the flipping of a coin 100 times. It is easy to understand that the expected frequency of heads and tails with 100 flips would be 50-50. The null hypothesis being tested is that the results obtained by flipping the coin 100 times will not differ significantly from the expected 50-50 frequency. SPSS output for a sample coin flip experiment is provided in Table 18.1.

Notice that when flipping the coin 100 times, heads came up 39 times (coded 0) and tails came up 61 times (coded 1), rather than the expected 50-50 frequency. Upon applying the chi-square statistic, the analysis resulted in $\chi^2 = 4.840$ [$p = 0.028$, $df = 1$, $N = 100$], thus indicating that the obtained and expected frequencies are significantly different. Thus, the null hypothesis is rejected.

Table 18.2 shows the proportion and count data from a second example along with suggested transformations (presented later in this chapter). In the example data set, whether the patient previously attempted suicide is coded as Suicide = 0 (has not attempted suicide) and Suicide = 1 (has attempted suicide). Therefore, the group means for this dichotomous variable will be the group proportions of patients who previously attempted suicide. Typically, these data are analyzed using contingency table

**TABLE 18.1**    Chi-square analysis of a coin flip example.

| | Coin Flip | | |
|---|---|---|---|
| | Observed N | Expected N | Residual |
| .00 | 39 | 50.0 | −11.0 |
| 1.00 | 61 | 50.0 | 11.0 |
| Total | 100 | | |

**Test Statistics**

| | Coin Flip |
|---|---|
| Chi-Square(a) | 4.840 |
| df | 1 |
| Asymp. Sig. | .028 |

(a) 0 cells (.0%) have expected frequencies less than 5. The minimum expected cell frequency is 50.0.

© Cengage Learning

**TABLE 18.2**    Data on the count and proportion data along with square root and arcsine transformations.

| | ID | Group | BDI | Num SI | TotState | Prop SI | Improve | Suicide | Num Suic | Arc Prop SI | Num SI sqrt | Num Suic Sqrt |
|---|---|---|---|---|---|---|---|---|---|---|---|---|
| 1 | A | 0 | 62 | 8 | 10 | .800 | 0 | 1 | 2 | 1.1071 | 2.8284 | 1.4142 |
| 2 | B | 0 | 48 | 4 | 8 | .500 | 0 | 0 | 0 | .7854 | 2.0000 | .0000 |
| 3 | C | 0 | 47 | 3 | 8 | .375 | 1 | 1 | 2 | .6591 | 1.7321 | 1.4142 |
| 4 | D | 0 | 46 | 3 | 10 | .300 | 2 | 0 | 0 | .5796 | 1.7321 | .0000 |
| 5 | E | 0 | 43 | 2 | 8 | .250 | 0 | 0 | 0 | .5236 | 1.4142 | .0000 |
| 6 | F | 0 | 42 | 1 | 9 | .111 | 2 | 1 | 1 | .3398 | 1.0000 | 1.0000 |
| 7 | G | 0 | 41 | 6 | 8 | .750 | 1 | 0 | 0 | 1.0472 | 2.4495 | .0000 |
| 8 | H | 1 | 44 | 4 | 8 | .500 | 0 | 0 | 0 | .7854 | 2.0000 | .0000 |
| 9 | I | 1 | 39 | 5 | 8 | .625 | 1 | 0 | 0 | .9117 | 2.2361 | .0000 |
| 10 | J | 1 | 38 | 3 | 10 | .300 | 2 | 1 | 3 | .5796 | 1.7321 | 1.7321 |
| 11 | K | 1 | 37 | 3 | 8 | .375 | 2 | 1 | 1 | .6591 | 1.7321 | 1.0000 |
| 12 | L | 1 | 34 | 2 | 9 | .222 | 2 | 0 | 0 | .4909 | 1.4142 | .0000 |
| 13 | M | 1 | 31 | 1 | 8 | .125 | 2 | 0 | 0 | .3614 | 1.0000 | .0000 |
| 14 | N | 1 | 29 | 1 | 9 | .111 | 1 | 0 | 0 | .3398 | 1.0000 | .0000 |

ID = identification code; Group: 0 = Control, 1 = Treatment; BDI = Beck Depression Inventory, 2nd edition; NumSi = number of suicidal ideations; TotState = number of total statements; PropSI = proportion of suicidal ideations; Improve = improvement rating: 0 = worsen, 1 = unchanged, 2 = slight improvement, 3 = definite improvement; Suicide: 0 = never attempted suicide, 1 = has attempted suicide; NumSuic = number of attempted suicides; ArcPropSI = arcsine of the square root of the proportion of suicidal ideations; NumSIsqrt = square root of the number of suicidal ideations; NumSuicsqrt = square root of the number of suicide attempts.

© Cengage Learning

analysis. Statistical significance is evaluated with a chi-square statistic, which tests the following null hypothesis: $H_0$: $(\mu_1 = \mu_2)$ or equivalently $(\mu_1 - \mu_2) = \mu_D = 0$, where $\mu$ is a population proportion. Notice that this is similar to the null hypothesis for means. In fact, its structure is identical. The only difference is that population means ($\mu$) are the parameters of interest when the dependent variable is continuous, whereas population proportions ($\theta$) are the parameters of interest when the dependent variable is categorical.

Using the *SPSS* Crosstabs module on the data in Table 18.2, the resultant contingency table analysis (Table 18.3) reveals that 42.9 percent (3/7) of the control group had previously attempted suicide, whereas only 28.6 percent (2/7) of the treatment group had previously attempted suicide. This difference in proportions was not statistically significant [$\chi^2 = 0.311$, $p = 0.577$, $df = 1$, $N = 14$, phi$^2 = 0.0222$]. Therefore, there does not appear to be any preexisting difference in the groups concerning attempting suicide. Another categorical variable in this data set is the Improvement Rating. The resultant contingency table analysis (Table 18.3) reveals that none of the patients showed definite improvement (Improve $= 3$). Also, 42.9 percent (3/7) of the control group worsened (Improve $= 0$), as compared to only 14.3 percent (1/7) of the treatment group; 28.6 percent (2/7) of the control and treatment groups were unchanged (Improve $= 1$); and 57.1% (4/7) of the treatment group showed slight improvement (Improve $= 2$), as compared to only 28.6 percent (2/7) of the control group. These differences in proportions were not statistically significant [$\chi^2 = 1.667$, $p = 0.435$, $df = 2$, $N = 14$, $\Phi^2 = 0.119$]. There appears, however, to be a small, but potentially interesting, treatment effect (i.e., $\Phi^2 = 0.119$) in terms of the improvement rating. Applying a power analysis, if the sample size were increased to $N = (n + m) = 52$, then results would be statistically significant at $\alpha = 0.05$. To elaborate, the critical value for chi-square statistics with $df = 2$ is 5.991. From the note in Table 18.2, $N(\varphi^2) = \chi^2$; thus, solving for $N$ results in $N = \chi^2/(\Phi^2) = 5.991/.119 = 50.34$. Rounding up and keeping sample sizes equal results in $N = 52$. Proportion and count data are becoming increasingly common in education and social science research and must be dealt with appropriately.

# The ANOVA Model

**Nonparametric statistics** are used to analyze nominal or ordinal data, or when the assumptions required for parametric analysis have been violated (e.g., skewed data and outliers). Data transformations can be helpful in converting skewed or nonnormal data sets into more normalized distributions that can then be analyzed using parametric statistics. It is important to briefly review the conceptual basics of parametric statistics before discussing transformations, robust alternatives, and nonparametric statistics. Although there are a variety of experimental designs, regression models, and correlational analyses that can be discussed, for the sake of simplicity, we will concentrate on one of the most widely used designs in behavioral research: the analysis of variance (ANOVA) model. The ANOVA model involves obtaining data on samples from two or more ($J \geq 2$) populations that differ with respect to some characteristic. This ANOVA model is typically used to test whether means (i.e., location parameters) differ across the $J$ populations. It is important to note, however, that most statistical analyses used in the behavioral sciences can be subsumed under the general linear model (GLM), which has the following parameter model:

$$Y_i = \beta_0 + \beta_1 X1_i + \beta_2 X2_i + \ldots \beta_k Xk_i + \varepsilon_i, \tag{18.1}$$

where $Y_i$ is an individual participant's score on the dependent (i.e., outcome response) variable modeled as a linear function of a set of independent (i.e., predictor) variables ($X$). Thus, ANOVA models, which use a set of coding variables to represent group membership, are simply a subset of this more general approach.

**TABLE 18.3** Previous suicide attempts and improvement rating crosstabulated with group (0 = control; 1 = treatment).

**A. Suicide * Group Crosstabulation**

| | | | Group 0 | Group 1 | Total |
|---|---|---|---|---|---|
| Suicide | 0 | Count | 4 | 5 | 9 |
| | | Expected Count | 4.5 | 4.5 | 9.0 |
| | | % within Group | 57.1% | 74.1% | 64.3% |
| | 1 | Count | 3 | 2 | 5 |
| | | Expected Count | 2.5 | 2.5 | 5.0 |
| | | % within Group | 42.9% | 28.6% | 35.7% |
| Total | | Count | 7 | 7 | 14 |
| | | Expected Count | 7.0 | 7.0 | 14.0 |
| | | % within Group | 100% | 100% | 100% |

Suicide: 0 = never attempted suicide, 1 = has attempted suicide.
Pearson $\chi^2 = 0.311$, $p = 0.577$, $df = 1$, $N = 14$, phi = $-0.149$, phi$^2$ = 0.0222.
*Note:* $N(\text{phi}^2) = \chi^2$, which is important for asymptotic properties of nonparametric statistics.

**B. Improve * Group Crosstabulation**

| | | | Group 0 | Group 1 | Total |
|---|---|---|---|---|---|
| Improve | 0 | Count | 3 | 1 | 4 |
| | | Expected Count | 2.0 | 2.0 | 4.0 |
| | | % within Improve | 42.9% | 14.3% | 28.6% |
| | 1 | Count | 2 | 2 | 4 |
| | | Expected Count | 2.0 | 2.0 | 4.0 |
| | | % within Improve | 28.6% | 28.6% | 28.6% |
| | 2 | Count | 2 | 4 | 6 |
| | | Expected Count | 3.0 | 3.0 | 6.0 |
| | | % within Improve | 28.6% | 57.1% | 42.9% |
| Total | | Count | 7 | 7 | 14 |
| | | Expected Count | 7.0 | 7.0 | 14.0 |
| | | % within Improve | 100% | 100% | 100% |

Improve = improvement rating: 0 = worsen, 1 = unchanged, 2 = slight improvement, 3 = definite improvement;
Pearson $\chi^2 = 1.667$, $p = 0.435$, $df = 2$, $N = 14$, phi = 0.345, phi$^2$ = 0.119.
*Note*: $N(\text{phi}^2) = \chi^2$, which is important for asymptotic properties of nonparametric statistics.
© Cengage Learning

A primary GLM assumption $[\varepsilon_i \sim NID(0, \sigma^2)]$ states that the individual population *errors* $(\varepsilon_i)$ are assumed to be (1) Normally and (2) Independently Distributed with (3) a mean of zero, and (4) a constant variance of $\sigma^2$. Of course, the assumption of independence can be violated when related individuals are in the same sample. For example, sampling students from the same classroom (or clients in the same group therapy session) may create a dependency in the data. That is, a student's response may be more similar to that of a classmate than to a student sampled from another school, or the same teacher may be rating several students from the same class. The most common methods to address dependency in the data involve generalized least squares (GLS). A discussion of GLS is beyond the scope of this chapter, but the reader is referred to Dobson (2002) or McCulloch and Searle (2001) for additional information on the use of GLS.

The assumption of constant variance is often called **homogeneity of variance** in ANOVA (i.e., group mean comparison) applications and **homoscedasticity** in linear regression applications. This assumption states that at each level of $X$, the residuals will have the same (i.e., common or constant) variance. In an ANOVA application, this implies that all groups will have the same within-group variance. That is, all groups should have the same (or at least very similar) variance and standard deviation (*SD*). Fortunately, when the constant variance assumption is violated in ANOVA models, parametric test statistics are fairly robust (i.e., valid type I error rates) as long as the groups have equal sample sizes. In this situation, however, there is a serious reduction in power (Scheffé, 1959).

To elaborate, consider two normally distributed populations with means of 50 and *SD*s of 5. In this situation assume the parametric null hypothesis $H_0$: $(\mu_1 = \mu_2)$ or equivalently $(\mu_1 - \mu_2) = \mu_D = 0$ is true and the model assumptions are met. Suppose a researcher randomly sampled 20 cases from each population, repeated this study 100 times, and computed a *t*-test (or *F*-ratio) for each resampling. If the significance level was set at $\alpha = 0.05$, then 5 of the 100 studies should have "statistically significant" results by chance (random variation). Now, consider one normally distributed population with a mean of 50 and an *SD* of 5 ($\sigma^2 = 25$) and a second normally distributed population with a mean of 50 and an *SD* of 10 ($\sigma^2 = 100$). In this situation, the parametric null hypothesis is true, but the model assumption of homoscedasticity does not hold. In fact, the second population has four times the variance as the first (i.e., $100/25 = 4$). Again, suppose a researcher sampled 20 cases from each population, repeated this study 100 times, and computed a *t*-test (or *F*-ratio) for each resampling; for a significance level set at $\alpha = 0.05$, the type I error rate will still be approximately 5 percent.

When the sample sizes are unequal, however, the type I error rate of the standard parametric statistics will be inflated (i.e., too many rejections under the null hypothesis) when the larger groups have the smaller variances (i.e., negative or liberal pairing). By contrast, the type I error rates may be considerably lower than the nominal alpha (i.e., too few rejections under the null hypothesis) when the larger groups have the larger variances (i.e., positive or conservative pairing), which also leads to a substantial loss in statistical power. This is because the test statistic ($t$ or $F$) uses a pooled error term, and so the variance of the larger sized group is overrepresented. Thus, when the larger group has the larger variance, the pooled error term is larger and the test statistic is smaller, which will lead to fewer than the expected number of rejections (i.e., too conservative). Similarly, when the larger group has the smaller variance, the pooled error term is smaller and the test statistic is larger, which will lead to more than the expected number of rejections (i.e., too liberal). Problems with heteroscedasticity in regression models cannot be as easily summarized. Test statistics to correct for heterogeneity of variance in ANOVA models (Welch, 1947) are based on weighted least squares (WLS). There are also WLS and GLS approaches for regression models. Again, these approaches are beyond the scope of this chapter but are reviewed in detail by Draper and Smith (1998).

Assuming that the population errors are normally distributed guarantees that parametric ordinary least squares (OLS) test statistics (e.g., $t$ or $F$) lead to valid statistical inference. That is, these tests will have valid type I error rates. What is often not emphasized is that by assuming normality of error distributions, the population distributions do not differ in shape (i.e., skew or kurtosis). Also, by assuming constant variance, the population distributions do not differ in spread (i.e., variance). Therefore, by making these assumptions, a statistically significant result by definition must be because of differences in location (i.e., mean). Also, with the normality assumption, a significant result must be because of differences in means because all measures of central tendency (i.e., mean, median, and mode) are the same. Thus, assuming away differences in distributional shape and spread allows the test to focus on a single **parameter** that defines the differences between population distributions (i.e., the mean defines the location of the center of a normal distribution)—hence the name **parametric test**. This is another reason why nonconstant variance is such a problem; it does not allow the researcher to focus on a single parameter (i.e., the mean only). It should be noted that there are several tests of differences in variance and that heterogeneity of variance can be a meaningful result (Thompson, 1994). For example, an educational program may show some progress when it reduces the variability in test scores rather than changing the average level of the scores. That is, even though the average student's score does not increase, the more consistent (similar) scores obtained by students could point to a program's success.

The principle that drives parametric statistics and allows for the computation of exact test statistics (e.g., $t$ or $F$) is as follows. The parameters of interest (i.e., means, regression coefficients, and correlation coefficients), which are estimated from the data, are linear transformations of $Y$ (i.e., linear combination; a client's score comprises the components specified in Equation 18.1). It follows that if $Y$ (or multiple $Y$'s, as in correlational studies) is normally distributed, then the distribution of parameter estimates will be normally distributed under the null hypothesis (Muller & Fetterman, 2002). For example, suppose $Y$ is a normally distributed random variable. The mean of $Y$ is a linear composite of the values of $Y$ $[\overline{Y} = (1/N)\Sigma Y)]$. If one repeatedly resampled from the distribution of $Y$ and computed means each time, these means (i.e., sampling distribution of the mean) will also be normally distributed. Likewise, a regression coefficient, which is a linear composite based on $Y$, computed on a normally distributed $Y$ variable should be normally distributed. Furthermore, the Central Limit Theorem (CLT) states that the sampling distribution of statistics based on linear composites (e.g., means, correlations, regression coefficients, and mean differences) will approximate a normal distribution, regardless of the shape of the original variables ($Y$), as the sample size becomes "sufficiently large." This implies that parametric statistics are robust to violations to the normality assumption when sample sizes are "sufficiently large." Of course, what constitutes "sufficiently large" is debatable and a focus of much research in nonparametric statistics. Furthermore, and of critical importance, when the data are nonnormal, parametric statistics may be less powerful than nonparametric alternatives.

# Evaluating Parametric Assumptions

There is often confusion about assessing parametric assumptions. Assumptions concern populations, not samples. Unfortunately, the sample is all the professional counselor has to work with, and diagnostics must be performed on sample data. It is quite possible for a sample, especially a small one, to look as though it does not represent a normal curve even though it was sampled from a normal distribution. Of course, it is also quite possible for a nonnormal distribution to produce small samples that look "normal." Some variables by their own nature are nonnormal. For example, if a researcher used the diameter ($d$) of a bone as a dependent variable and it is normally distributed, then the area of the bone (i.e., area $\approx \pi[d/2]^2$) would approximate a chi-square distribution.

A common situation in which a researcher might doubt the assumption of normality is when the measure has a ceiling or floor effect (e.g., skewed distributions). Another reason for nonnormality is the presence of outliers, scores that are extreme relative to the rest of the sample. If outliers are extremely large (or small) in value and thus create a positively (or negatively) skewed distribution, parameter estimates such as means can be biased. Also, because standard OLS methods use squared deviations from the mean, outliers can seriously inflate estimates of variance. In turn, this will reduce the power of test statistics, such as *t* or *F*. Thus, outliers are a major problem because they can bias parameter estimates, inflate variances, and contribute to misleading results. There is great debate in the literature on whether outliers should be removed or not. Judd and McClelland (1989) argued that outlier removal is desirable, honest, and important. However, not all researchers feel that way (Orr, Sackett, & DuBois, 1991).

Correlational studies do not explicitly define a dependent variable of primary interest; thus, if inferential tests are performed, all variables are assumed to be normal. If no inferential test will be performed, then normality is not an issue. Therefore, in correlational research where no inferences are made (e.g., exploratory factor analysis), the normality is of less concern. One should still examine the distributions of the variables for normality (symmetry). Also, highly skewed variables may drastically affect the magnitude of a correlation coefficient. It is also wise to construct bivariate plots for each pair of variables to examine potential problems with nonlinearity, heteroscedasticity, and outliers, which could bias the estimate of the correlation coefficient.

The fact that the variables themselves are examined when evaluating parametric assumptions in correlational studies has led to confusion over assessing the validity of linear model assumptions. When the null hypothesis is true (e.g., when two groups have identical population means), the dependent variable (*Y*) and the population residuals (*ε*) are identical. One never knows, however, whether the null is true, but only whether enough evidence exists to reject it. Thus, linear model assumptions are evaluated by performing diagnostics on the sample residuals (*e*), not on *Y*. Mathematical properties of the OLS computation used in standard linear models guarantees that the sample residuals will have a mean of zero. *Recall from basic statistics that the deviations from the mean will sum to zero, and thus the average of these mean deviations (the residuals) will be zero.* It is important to note that most linear models used in educational and behavioral research (e.g., ANOVA) investigate fixed effects as the predictor (*X*) variables. More important, linear models make no assumption about the distribution of fixed effects; thus, normality of the *X* (independent or predictor) variables is not required.

There are many tests to assess the normality assumption. There are also problems and fundamental issues to consider. When sample sizes are small, there may not be enough statistical power to reject the null hypothesis of normality and thus the reasonableness of the normality assumption is unknown. When sample sizes are large, tests tend to reject because they are powered to detect minor departures from normality. In this situation, however, the CLT will help out in that the sampling distribution of the test statistic (e.g., *t*-test) is more likely to be normal with a larger sample size. The key issue is that the statistical power one has to reject the null hypothesis of interest assumes that the normality assumptions are tenable (Thompson, 1994). Furthermore, testing of assumptions compounds the overall multiple testing issue. Thus, many researchers simply "eyeball" the assumption diagnostics in context with the sample size and make a judgment on whether alternative methods should be used (Orr et al., 1991). Researchers and reviewers, however, often are more comfortable with a more objective assessment of normality, which can range from simple examination of skew and kurtosis to examination of quantile-quantile (Q-Q) plots and inferential tests of normality (e.g., Kolmogorov-Smirnov and Shapiro-Wilks test). Professional counselors wanting more information on tests of normality should consult Goodman (1954), Lilliefors (1967), Rosenthal (1968), and Wilcox (1997).

There are multiple options for dealing with nonnormal data and outliers. First, the researcher must make certain that the nonnormality (or outliers) is because of a valid reason (e.g., real observed data points). Invalid reasons for nonnormality and outliers include things such as mistakes in data entry and missing data values not declared missing. Not all nonnormality, however, is because of data entry error or nondeclared missing values. If a researcher chooses not to remove outliers, or removes outliers and still finds substantial nonnormality, data transformation, robust alternatives, or nonparametric methods are viable options for dealing with violations of the normality assumption.

# Motivating Example

A professional counselor has identified 14 inpatient participants in a psychiatric ward with clinical depression and who are at risk of suicide. He randomly assigned $n = 7$ to a control condition (TAU; treatment-as-usual) in which they receive their usual medication regimen. The other $n = 7$ are assigned to a treatment condition in which they also continue to receive their usual medication but also receive a new experimental counseling strategy. As background information, the researcher reviewed previous records to find out whether the patients had previously attempted suicide and the number of previous suicide attempts. After three weeks, the patients are administered the *Beck Depression Inventory, 2nd edition* (BDI-II; Beck, Steer, & Brown, 1996), which ranges from raw scores of 0–63. The clinic staff conducts a standardized one-hour interview of each patient. Video and audio records are reviewed by the investigator, and the number of suicidal ideations expressed in the interview is counted. This number is also converted to the proportion of statements that express suicidal ideation to the total number of statements. The investigator also gives a global judgment on whether the patients have worsened (0), remained unchanged (1), improved slightly (2), or definitely improved (3). Table 18.4 displays these data.

Using the independent *t*-test module of *SPSS*, the results for *BDI-II* show that the control group had a mean of 47 with an *SD* of 7.12, and the treatment group had a mean of 36 with an *SD* of 5.10. Although the control group had nearly twice as much

**TABLE 18.4** Data for the motivating example.

|  | ID | Group | BDI | NumSI | NonSI | TotState | PropSI | Improve | Suicide | NumSuic |
|---|---|---|---|---|---|---|---|---|---|---|
| 1 | A | 0 | 62 | 8 | 2 | 10 | .800 | 0 | 1 | 2 |
| 2 | B | 0 | 48 | 4 | 4 | 8 | .500 | 0 | 0 | 0 |
| 3 | C | 0 | 47 | 3 | 5 | 8 | .375 | 1 | 1 | 2 |
| 4 | D | 0 | 46 | 3 | 7 | 10 | .300 | 2 | 0 | 0 |
| 5 | E | 0 | 43 | 2 | 6 | 8 | .250 | 0 | 0 | 0 |
| 6 | F | 0 | 42 | 1 | 8 | 9 | .111 | 2 | 1 | 1 |
| 7 | G | 0 | 41 | 6 | 2 | 8 | .750 | 1 | 0 | 0 |
| 8 | H | 1 | 44 | 4 | 4 | 8 | .500 | 0 | 0 | 0 |
| 9 | I | 1 | 39 | 5 | 3 | 8 | .625 | 1 | 0 | 0 |
| 10 | J | 1 | 38 | 3 | 7 | 10 | .300 | 2 | 1 | 3 |
| 11 | K | 1 | 37 | 3 | 5 | 8 | .375 | 2 | 1 | 1 |
| 12 | L | 1 | 34 | 2 | 7 | 9 | .222 | 2 | 0 | 0 |
| 13 | M | 1 | 31 | 1 | 7 | 8 | .125 | 2 | 0 | 0 |
| 14 | N | 1 | 29 | 1 | 8 | 9 | .111 | 1 | 0 | 0 |

ID = identification code; group: 0 = control, 1 = treatment; BDI = Beck Depression Inventory, 2nd edition; NumSi = number of suicidal ideations; TotState = number of total statements; PropSI = proportion of suicidal ideations; Improve = improvement rating: 0 = worsen, 1 = unchanged, 2 = slight improvement, 3 = definite improvement; Suicide: 0 = never attempted suicide, 1 = has attempted suicide; NumSuic = number of attempted suicides.

Histogram of the unstandardized residuals with a normal
curve superimposed.

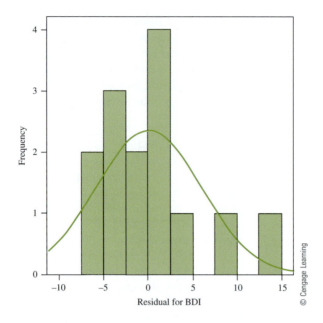

variance as the treatment group ($\sigma_C^2/\sigma_T^2 = 50.67/26.00 = 1.95$), the Levene test for heterogeneity of variance was not statistically significant [$F(1,12) = 0.07$, $p = 0.799$]. Furthermore, with equal sample sizes, heterogeneity of variance is less problematic. Therefore,
a *t*-test (assuming equal variances) was computed [$t(12) = 3.32$, $p = 0.006$], which
showed a statistically significant result. The 95 percent confidence interval for the mean
difference of 11 ranged from 3.31 to 18.21. It is worth noting that the treatment group
scores seem fairly symmetric (skew = 0.13; kurtosis = −0.41), whereas the control group
scores were positively skewed (skew = 1.92; kurtosis = 4.20). Next, the residuals were
examined. In this case, the residuals are the scores minus the predicted values (i.e.,
group means). Figure 18.1 shows a histogram of the residuals combined, which shows
substantial asymmetry (skew = 1.49; kurtosis = 2.56). Figure 18.2 shows a boxplot of
the residuals separated by group. Both plots suggest that outliers may be present.

**Figure 18.2**

Boxplot of the unstandardized
residual for each group.

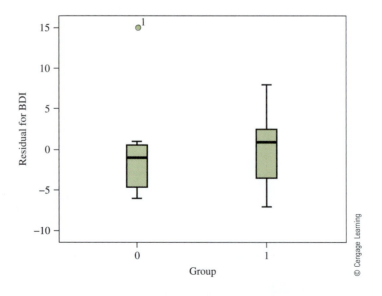

# Data Transformations

Data transformations are mathematical modifications to the values of a variable. There is a great variety of possible data transformations, including linear (e.g., adding constants and/or multiplying) and nonlinear transformations (e.g., squaring or raising to a power, taking the square root of the values, inverting and reflecting, converting to logarithmic scales, and applying trigonometric transformations such as sine wave transformations). Recall from basic statistics that linear transformations will change scaled statistics (e.g., mean, variance, and regression coefficients). Adding a constant to a variable changes only the mean, not the standard deviation, variance, skew, or kurtosis. Multiplying by a constant changes the mean, standard deviation, and variance but not the skew or kurtosis. The size of the constant, however, and the place on the number line that the constant moves the distribution to can influence the effect of any subsequent data transformations. Linear transformations will not affect scale-free statistics such as correlation coefficients, $R^2$, $t$-tests, and $F$-ratios. Therefore, in terms of conforming to model assumptions, linear transformations will not help normalize a distribution of scores (or residuals).

On the other hand, nonlinear transformations will affect the value (and hopefully reduce bias) of test statistics as well as scaled statistics. If a nonlinear transformation changes the value of a regression coefficient, researchers must change their interpretation accordingly. If a nonlinear transformation changes the value of a test statistic (e.g., $t$-test), then it may also affect whether the results are statistically significant. This is a much deeper problem that highlights one of the fundamental issues of data transformation. If a data transformation drastically changes the interpretation of the results, it begs the question of which results (the original or transformed) are more valid or believable. Data transformation often makes journal reviewers and consumers skeptical because it conveys the suspicion that the data were manipulated to gain the desired results. This is why the justification for a data transformation is so important. Often researchers are asked to discuss the difference between the results with and without the transformation. Because transformations primarily should be used to get the data to conform to model assumptions, the goal of this discussion is to focus on the use of data transformation for normalization of variables (or residuals).

Parametric statistical procedures assume that the variables (or residuals) are normally distributed. A significant violation of the assumption of normality can seriously increase the chances of the researcher committing either type I or II errors (depending on the nature of the analysis and the nonnormality). Micceri (1989), however, points out that approximate normality is exceedingly rare in education and psychology. Thus, one reason (although not the only reason) why researchers use data transformations is to improve the normality of variables (or residuals). Additionally, authors such as Zimmerman (1995, 1998) have pointed out that nonparametric tests (where no explicit assumption of normality is made) can suffer as much as parametric tests when normality assumptions are violated in combination with heteroscedasticity. Several common procedures for transforming data and compensating for outliers will be discussed in the following sections, including trimming, Winsorizing, and ladder of power transformations.

## Trimming and Winsorization

Trimming and Winsorization are used to make parameter estimates (e.g., mean, $SD$) more robust (i.e., less sensitive to outliers) sometimes at the expense of reduced statistical efficiency. Symmetrically **trimming** a data set involves removing the $k$ cases with the $k/2$ largest values and the $k/2$ smallest values. The trimmed mean is the mean value for the data ignoring the $k$ extreme values. The even positive integer $k$ determines the amount of trimming. When $k$ is one fewer than the size of the data sample, the trimming is maximum, and the trimmed mean is just the median. Thus, when one has a sample of 20 scores and uses a 10 percent symmetrical trim, the highest and lowest scores are eliminated. Trimming can be an effective way to deal with outliers and obtain a robust estimate of location (Huber, 2004); this procedure, however, involves removing potential outliers, which may be controversial. Furthermore, trimming is not recommended for computing variances. Rather, bootstrapping is often used to calculate variances and standard errors.

Winsorizing is also used to down-weight the influence of outliers. **Winsorization** is a procedure similar to trimming, but instead of throwing away the $k$ extreme values, the $k$ extreme values are replaced by the remaining extreme values. This moves the extreme values toward the center of the distribution. This technique is sensitive to the number of outliers but not to their actual values. To Winsorize the data, tail values are often set equal to some specified percentile of the data. For example, for 10 percent symmetric Winsorization, the bottom 5 percent of the values are set to the value corresponding to the 5th percentile while the upper 5 percent of the values are set to the value corresponding to the 95th percentile. Thus, when one has a sample of 20 scores and uses a 10 percent symmetrical Winsorization, the highest score is changed to become the same as the second highest score, and the lowest score is changed to become the same as the second lowest score.

Keselman, Wilcox, Kowalchuk, and Olejnik (2002) suggested conducting a preliminary examination of symmetry to determine whether symmetric or asymmetric trimming/Winsorization should be performed. Determining the appropriate percentage of data to trim or Winsorize is also an issue. For the current BDI-II example, the residuals appear to be positively skewed, and thus, asymmetric trimming/Winsorization on the positive end of the distribution would be suggested; symmetric trimming/Winsorization, however, will also be demonstrated for completeness.

The most common percentages for trimming and Winsorization are 10 percent symmetric (5 percent of each tail), 20 percent symmetric (10 percent of each tail), 10 percent asymmetric (10 percent of the skewed tail), and 20 percent asymmetric (20 percent of the skewed tail). For demonstration purposes using the BDI-II data, however, 15 percent trimming/Winsorization will be used, which means that two cases (15 percent of 14) will be trimmed or Winsorized. (This was done because using a data set of 14 scores means that 10 percent of scores is 1.4, 15 percent of scores is 2.1, and 20 percent of scores is 2.8; thus, using 15 percent simplifies things for the purpose of this example.) Table 18.5 shows the data sorted by BDI-II score along with 15 percent asymmetrically (BDITrim15A) and symmetrically trimmed BDI-II scores (BDITrim15S) along with asymmetrically (BDIWin15A) and symmetrically Winsorized BDI-II scores (BDIWin15S).

In Table 18.5, notice that for asymmetric trimming/Winsorization, the two highest cases (A and B) get changed and for symmetric trimming/Winsorization, the two end cases (A and N) get changed. Table 18.6 summarizes the descriptive statistics for the four transformed variables, which shows that trimming and Winsorization did help reduce the skewness of the residuals in the control group. In general, the mean differences are smaller than the mean difference of 11 in the original data presented earlier in this chapter; all transformed variables, however, still yield statistically significant results (Table 18.6). What is also apparent is that the variance of the treatment group remained relatively unchanged, whereas the variance of the control group was substantially reduced. Thus, by transforming these data, a concern about heterogeneity of variance was created! In fact, now the treatment group has substantially more variance. The Welch (1947) correction for unequal variances was applied where deemed necessary.

| TABLE 18.5 | | Data for demonstrating trimming and Winsorization. | | | | | |
|---|---|---|---|---|---|---|---|
| | ID | Group | BDI | BDITrim15A | BDITrim15S | BDIWin15A | BDIWin15A |
| 1 | A | 0 | 62 | . | . | 47 | 48 |
| 2 | B | 0 | 48 | . | 48 | 47 | 48 |
| 3 | C | 0 | 47 | 47 | 47 | 47 | 47 |
| 4 | D | 0 | 46 | 46 | 46 | 46 | 46 |
| 5 | H | 1 | 44 | 44 | 44 | 44 | 44 |
| 6 | E | 0 | 43 | 43 | 43 | 43 | 43 |
| 7 | F | 0 | 42 | 42 | 42 | 42 | 42 |
| 8 | G | 0 | 41 | 41 | 41 | 41 | 41 |
| 9 | I | 1 | 39 | 39 | 39 | 39 | 39 |
| 10 | J | 1 | 38 | 38 | 38 | 38 | 38 |
| 11 | K | 1 | 37 | 37 | 37 | 37 | 37 |
| 12 | L | 1 | 34 | 34 | 34 | 34 | 34 |
| 13 | M | 1 | 31 | 31 | 31 | 31 | 31 |
| 14 | N | 1 | 29 | 29 | . | 29 | 31 |

ID = identification code; group: 0 = control, 1 = treatment; BDI = Beck Depression Inventory, 2nd edition; BDITrim15A = BDI 15% asymmetrically trimmed; BDITrim15S = BDI 15% symmetrically trimmed; BDIWin15A = BDI 15% asymmetrically Winsorized; BDIWin15S = BDI 15% symmetrically Winsorized.

© Cengage Learning

Thus, trimming and Winsorization can be helpful in resolving some data issues but must be used cautiously because each can lead to other potentially problematic issues.

## Ladder of Power Transformations

The "ladder of power transformations" for data have been suggested when linear model assumptions are violated (e.g., scores are skewed). The dependent variable $Y$ is transformed to $Y^*$:

$$Y^* = \begin{cases} Y^d & d \neq 0 \\ \ln(Y) & d = 0 \end{cases}, \qquad (18.2)$$

where $d$ is a constant for the power transformation. Moving up (higher values of $d$) the ladder thickens the left tail and thins the right. Conversely, moving down (lower values of $d$) the ladder thins the left tail and thickens the right. Thus, with positive skewness in the residuals of the BDI-II example, thickening the right tail would be desirable, and thus, lower values for $d$ ($d \leq 0$) would be more likely to be applied. Table 18.7 provides a brief description of the ladder of power transformations.

Box and Cox (1964) developed algorithms for determining $d$ in a regression context. John Tukey and many of his colleagues devised exploratory data analysis (EDA) techniques (e.g., spread-by-level plots and stem-and-leaf plots) to determine the most appropriate value for $d$. Tukey (1977), however, conceded that although $d$ can take on any real value, square roots, logarithms, inverses, and inverses of powers were the most common and useful of the ladder of power transformations. It is beyond the scope of this chapter to fully discuss all options for data transformation. The following sections will focus on four of the most common data transformations used for improving normality discussed in texts and the literature: square root, logarithmic, inverse, and inverse of squares transformations. Table 18.8 shows the BDI-II scores transformed by each of these procedures. Readers looking for more information on data transformations might refer to Micceri (1989); Hoaglin, Mosteller, and Tukey (1983); and Tukey (1977).

**TABLE 18.6**    Results for trimmed and Winsorized data.

| BDITrim15A | Control Group = 0 | Treatment Group = 1 | Mean Difference |
|---|---|---|---|
| Mean | 43.80 | 36.00 | 7.80 |
| *SD | 2.59 | 5.10 | SE = 2.25 |
| Skew | 0.36 | 0.13 | $df$ = 9.30** |
| Kurtosis | −2.41 | −0.41 | $t$ = 3.47 |
| Sample Size | $n$ = 5 | $m$ = 7 | $p$ = .007 |
| **BDITrim15S** | | | |
| Mean | 44.50 | 37.17 | 7.33 |
| *SD | 2.88 | 4.45 | SE = 2.16 |
| Skew | 0 | 0.20 | $df$ = 10 |
| Kurtosis | −2.30 | 0.45 | $t$ = 3.39 |
| Sample Size | $n$ = 6 | $m$ = 6 | $p$ = .007 |
| **BDIWin15A** | | | |
| Mean | 44.71 | 36.00 | 8.71 |
| SD | 2.63 | 5.10 | SE = 2.17 |
| Skew | −0.67 | 0.13 | $df$ = 8.98** |
| Kurtosis | −1.15 | −0.41 | $t$ = 4.02 |
| Sample Size | $n$ = 7 | $m$ = 7 | $p$ = .002 |
| **BDIWin15S** | | | |
| Mean | 45.00 | 36.29 | 8.71 |
| SD | 2.94 | 4.68 | SE = 2.09 |
| Skew | −0.33 | 0.40 | $df$ = 12 |
| Kurtosis | −2.10 | −0.35 | $t$ = 4.17 |
| Sample Size | $n$ = 6 | $m$ = 6 | $p$ = .001 |

BDITrim15A = BDI 15% asymmetrically trimmed; BDITrim15S = BDI 15% symmetrically trimmed; BDIWin15A = BDI 15% asymmetrically Winsorized; BDIWin15S = BDI 15% symmetrically Winsorized. *SD is not a valid measure of variance, but for simplicity is used rather than a bootstrapped estimate. **Welch correction was used for unequal variances.

© Cengage Learning

**TABLE 18.7**    Ladders of power transformation.

| $d$ | Transform | Description |
|---|---|---|
| −2 | $Y^{-2} = 1/Y^2$ | Square and take reciprocal |
| −3/2 | $Y^{-1.5} = Y\sqrt{Y}/Y^3$ | |
| −1 | $Y^{-1} = 1/Y$ | Reciprocal or inverse |
| −1/2 | $Y^{-0.5} = 1/\sqrt{Y}$ | Take square root, then invert |
| 0 | $\ln(Y)$ | Logarithmic transformation |
| 1/2 | $Y^{0.5} = \sqrt{Y}$ | Square root transformation |
| 1 | $Y^1 = Y$ | Identity (original data) |
| 3/2 | $Y^{1.5} = Y^3/Y\sqrt{Y}$ | |
| 2 | $Y^2 = Y^2$ | Square |

© Cengage Learning

| | ID | Group | BDI | BDIsqrt | BDIlogn | BDIinv | BDIsqinv | RankBDI |
|---|----|-------|-----|---------|---------|--------|----------|---------|
| 1 | A | 0 | 62 | 7.8740 | 4.1271 | .0161 | .0003 | 14 |
| 2 | B | 0 | 48 | 6.9282 | 3.8712 | .0208 | .0004 | 13 |
| 3 | C | 0 | 47 | 6.8557 | 3.8501 | .0213 | .0005 | 12 |
| 4 | D | 0 | 46 | 6.7823 | 3.8286 | .0217 | .0005 | 11 |
| 5 | E | 0 | 43 | 6.5574 | 3.7612 | .0233 | .0005 | 9 |
| 6 | F | 0 | 42 | 6.4807 | 3.7377 | .0238 | .0006 | 8 |
| 7 | G | 0 | 41 | 6.4031 | 3.7136 | .0244 | .0006 | 7 |
| 8 | H | 1 | 44 | 6.6332 | 3.7842 | .0227 | .0005 | 10 |
| 9 | I | 1 | 39 | 6.2450 | 3.6636 | .0256 | .0007 | 6 |
| 10 | J | 1 | 38 | 6.1644 | 3.6376 | .0263 | .0007 | 5 |
| 11 | K | 1 | 37 | 6.0828 | 3.6109 | .0270 | .0007 | 4 |
| 12 | L | 1 | 34 | 5.8310 | 3.5264 | .0294 | .0009 | 3 |
| 13 | M | 1 | 31 | 5.5678 | 3.4340 | .0323 | .0010 | 2 |
| 14 | N | 1 | 29 | 5.3852 | 3.3673 | .0345 | .0012 | 1 |

**TABLE 18.8** Data for square root, logarithmic, and inverse transformations on the BDI-II data.

ID = identification code; group: 0 = control 1 = treatment; BDI = Beck Depression Inventory; BDIsqrt = square root of BDI; BDIlogn = natural (Naperian) log of BDI; BDIinv = inverse of BDI.

© Cengage Learning

### Square Root Transformation

When one applies a square root transformation, the square root of every value is taken. However, because one cannot take the square root of a negative number, if there are negative values for a variable, a constant must be added to move the minimum value of the distribution above 0, preferably to 1.00. Numbers of 1.00 and above behave differently than numbers between 0.00 and 0.99 when computing square roots. The square root of numbers above 1.00 always become smaller, 1.00 and 0.00 remain constant, and numbers between 0.00 and 1.00 always become larger (e.g., the square root of 4 is 2, but the square root of 0.40 is 0.63). Thus, if one applies a square root to a continuous variable that contains values between 0 and 1 as well as above 1, one is treating some numbers differently than others, which may not be desirable in some cases. Table 18.9 shows that after square root transformation, the treatment group still has lower BDIsqrt scores than the control group, and this difference is still statistically significant [$t(12) = 3.55$, $p = 0.004$]; the square root transformation, however, did not alleviate the skew of the residuals in the control group.

### Log Transformations

Logarithmic transformations are actually a class of transformations rather than a single transformation. In brief, a logarithm is the power (exponent) to which a base number must be raised to get the original number. Any given number can be expressed as $Y$ to the $q$ power in an infinite number of ways. For example, if one talks about base 10, 1 is 100, 100 is 102, 16 is 101.2, and so on. Thus, log10(100) = 2 and log10(16) = 1.2. Base 10, however, is not the only option for log transformations. Another common option is the Natural (or Naperian) Logarithm, where the constant $e$ (2.7182818) is the base. In this case, the natural log 100 is 4.605. As the logarithm of any number $\leq 0$ is undefined, if a variable contains values less than or equal to 0, a constant must be added to move the minimum value of the distribution, preferably to 1.00. Table 18.9 shows that after logarithmic transformation, the treatment group still has lower BDIlogn scores than the control group, and this difference is still statistically significant [$t(12) = 3.65$, $p = 0.003$]; the log transformation, however, did not alleviate the skew of the residuals in the control group.

| **TABLE 18.9** | Results for square root, logarithmic, and inverse transformations on the BDI-II data. | | |
|---|---|---|---|
| **BDI** | **Control Group = 0** | **Treatment Group = 1** | **Mean Difference** |
| Mean | 47.00 | 36.00 | 11.00 |
| SD | 6712 | 5.10 | SE = 3.31 |
| Skew | 1.92 | 0.13 | *df* = 12 |
| Kurtosis | 4.20 | −0.41 | *t* = 3.32 |
| Sample Size | *n* = 7 | *m* = 7 | *p* = .006 |
| **BDIsqrt** | | | |
| Mean | 6.802 | 5.9870 | 0.8532 |
| SD | 0.4967 | 0.4257 | SE = 0.2472 |
| Skew | 1.81 | −0.01 | *df* = 12 |
| Kurtosis | 3.81 | −0.53 | *t* = 3.45 |
| Sample Size | *n* = 7 | *m* = 7 | *p* = .005 |
| **BDIlogn** | | | |
| Mean | 3.8414 | 3.5748 | 0.2665 |
| * SD | 0.1392 | 0.1427 | SE = 0.0754 |
| Skew | 1.70 | −0.14 | *df* = 12 |
| Kurtosis | 3.41 | −0.61 | *t* = 3.52 |
| Sample Size | *n* = 7 | *m* = 7 | *p* = .004 |
| **BDIinv** | | | |
| Mean | 0.0216 | 0.0249 | −0.0066 |
| SD | 0.0028 | 0.0041 | SE = 0.0019 |
| Skew | −1.45 | 0.38 | *df* = 12 |
| Kurtosis | 2.57 | −0.66 | *t* = −3.57 |
| Sample Size | *n* = 7 | *m* = 7 | *p* = .004 |
| **BDIsqinv** | | | |
| Mean | 0.000475 | 0.000813 | −.00034 |
| SD | 0.000112 | 0.000234 | SE = 0.0001 |
| Skew | −1.18 | 0.60 | *df* = 8.61** |
| Kurtosis | 1.73 | −0.56 | *t* = 3.45 |
| Sample Size | *n* = 7 | *m* = 7 | *p* = .008 |

BDI = Beck Depression Inventory; BDIsqrt = square root of BDI; BDIlogn = natural (Naperian) log of BDI; BDIinv = inverse of BDI.

© Cengage Learning

There are good reasons to consider a range of bases. Cleveland (1984) argued that base 10, 2, and *e* should always be considered at a minimum. For example, in cases where there are extremes of range, base 10 is desirable, but when there are ranges that are less extreme, using base 10 will result in a loss of resolution, and using a lower base (*e* or 2) will serve. Note that higher bases tend to pull extreme values more drastically than lower bases. Interested readers are encouraged to consult Cleveland (1984).

### Inverse Transformation

Taking the inverse of a variable (*Y*) is computing $1/Y$. This makes very small numbers become very large and very large numbers become very small. This transformation has the effect of reversing the order of the scores. Thus, one may choose to reflect, or reverse, the distribution prior to applying an inverse transformation, although this is not necessary. To reflect, one multiplies a variable by –1. Then, once the inverse transformation is complete, the ordering of the values will be identical to the original data. Inverse transformation is suggested because it often can help stabilize variance. That is, when there is heteroscedasticity, inverse transformation can lead to more constant variance. As can be seen in Table 18.9, however, this may not be the case because the treatment group had more than twice as much variance as the control group ($\sigma^2_T/\sigma^2_C = 2.522$). Yet, the Levene test for heterogeneity of variance was not statistically significant [$F(1,12) = 2.35$, $p = 0.152$]. Furthermore, with equal sample sizes, heterogeneity of variance is less problematic. Therefore, a $t$-test (assuming equal variances) was computed [$t(12) = 3.68$, $p = 0.003$], which showed a statistically significant result. Again, the inverse transformation did not alleviate the skew of the residuals in the control group.

### Inverse of Squares Transformation

To make this transformation is to compute $1/Y^2$. Again, this makes very small numbers become very large and very large numbers become very small. Also, this transformation has the effect of reversing the order of your scores, and one may choose to reflect, or reverse, the distribution prior to applying an inverse transformation as explained previously. More important, if there are scores below 0, the ordering of the variable will not be preserved. For example, values of –2 and +2 will result in values of 0.25 after transformation. Thus, the researcher must add a constant so that all scores exceed 0.

As can be seen in Table 18.9, this transformation worsened the heterogeneity of variance problem in that the treatment group had more than four times as much variance as the control group (4.36). The Levene test for heterogeneity of variance was large and significant [$F(1,12) = 4.23$, $p = 0.062$]. Therefore, a $t$-test (with Welch correction for unequal variances) was computed [$t(8.61) = 3.45$, $p = 0.008$], which showed a statistically significant result. Again, the inverse of squares transformation did not alleviate the skew of the residuals in the control group.

## Issues of Interpretation of Transformed Variables

The values of the transformed variable are different from the original variable. If a variable with those values were subjected to a square root transformation, where the variable's old values were {0, 1, 2, 3, 4}, the new values are now {0, 1, 1.41, 1.73, 2}, and the intervals are no longer equal between successive values. These transformations change the relative distance between adjacent values that were previously equidistant (assuming interval or ratio measurement). In the untransformed variable, the distance between values would be an equal 1.0 distance between each increment (1, 2, 3, etc.). The action of the transformations, however, dramatically alters this equal spacing. For example, although the original distance between 1 and 2 had been 1.0, now it is 0.41, 0.30, 0.50, or 0.25, depending on the transformation. Thus, although the order of the variable has been retained, order is *all* that has been maintained. The spacing of the original variable has been eliminated. This is because of the differential effects of the transformations across the number line. If a variable had been measured on interval or ratio scales, it has now been reduced to ordinal (rank) data. Although this might not be an issue in some cases, there are some statistical procedures that assume interval or ratio measurement scales. It is worth noting that ranking the data is a nonlinear transformation that provides equal spacing between adjacent data points. Rank-based methods will be discussed in the following section.

Data transformations are valuable tools, with many benefits. However, they should be used appropriately and in an informed manner. Too many statistical texts gloss over this issue, leaving researchers ill prepared to use these tools appropriately. All of the transformations examined here reduce nonnormality by reducing the relative spacing of scores on one side of the distribution more than the scores on the other side. The very act of altering the relative distances between data points, which is how these transformations improve normality, raises issues in the interpretation of the data. If done correctly, all data points remain in the same relative order as prior to transformation. This allows researchers to continue to interpret results in terms of increasing scores. This might be undesirable if the original variables were meant to be substantively interpretable (e.g., annual income, years of age, grade, and GPA), as the variables become more complex to interpret because of the curvilinear nature of the transformations. Professional counselors must, therefore, be careful when interpreting results based on transformed data. Unfortunately, many statistical texts provide minimal instruction on the use of simple data transformations for the purpose of improving the normality of variables, and coverage of the use of other transformations or for uses other than improving normality is almost nonexistent.

The first recommendation is that professional counselors always examine and understand their data prior to performing statistical analyses. The second recommendation is to know the requirements of the data analysis technique to be used. The third recommendation is to use data transformations with care and never perform them unless there is a clear reason. Data transformations can alter the fundamental nature of the data, such as changing the measurement scale from interval or ratio to ordinal, creating curvilinear relationships, and complicating interpretation. As just discussed, there are many valid reasons for using data transformations, including improvement of normality, variance stabilization, and conversion of scales to interval measurement (see the introductory chapters of Bond & Fox, 2001, for an excellent introduction).

# Robust Alternatives and Nonparametric Inference

Nonparametric tests are applied under two kinds of conditions. First, nonparametric procedures can be applied when the data are categorical (e.g., nominal data) or count variables and thus are known not to follow a normal curve. In many cases, a contingency table analysis (i.e., chi-square test) is performed. For more advanced designs with categorical dependent variables, a variety of procedures exist. Logistic (dichotomous outcome) and multinomial (categorical outcome) regression are used when the dependent variable is regressed onto a set of continuous and/or categorical predictors. Loglinear models are often applied to more advanced ANOVA models. Poisson regression, which would subsume ANOVA models, is used when a count variable is regressed onto a set of continuous and/or categorical predictors. Generalized estimating equations (GEE) are used for longitudinal data. These procedures are beyond the scope of this chapter, but the interested reader should see Stokes, Davis, and Koch (2000).

Second, nonparametric procedures are applied when the data, although measured as continuous variables, are suspected to violate the normality assumption. For better or worse, this second use is less common than it once was, because most parametric tests have been shown to be relatively robust to violations of the normality assumption. That is, the probability of a type I error for parametric tests are relatively unaffected with violation to the normality assumption, when the sample size is "sufficiently large." What constitutes "sufficiently large" is debatable.

When error distributions (the distribution of $Y$ for each value of $X$) are normal, or at least symmetric, then parametric tests are more powerful than nonparametric tests. When error distributions are identically skewed, then nonparametric tests begin to show advantages in statistical power over their parametric counterparts (Beasley, 2000, 2002). In discussing the robustness of parametric tests, notice that violations can cause serious problems if sample sizes are small, especially in ANOVA design situations where the group sample sizes are not equal.

One form of nonparametric inference provides an approach to testing whether two or more samples differ in their distribution without assuming normality. This often is referred to as "fully nonparametric" inference (Akritas & Arnold, 1994). Another form of nonparametric inference provides a robust alternative to testing whether two or more samples differ in their level of central tendency (location) without assuming that the test statistic approximates a known statistical distribution under the null hypothesis.

## Kolmogorov–Smirnov Statistic

The Kolmogorov test was modified by Smirnov to serve as a test of the null hypothesis that two samples come from identical populations (Goodman, 1954). The test is given as

$$KS = \max\left|P[Y_1 < a] - P[Y_2 < a]\right|, \tag{18.3}$$

where KS is the **Kolmogorov–Smirnov test**, $P[Y_1 < a]$ is the cumulative probability of sample 1, and $P[Y_2 < a]$ is the cumulative probability of sample 2. This statistic can also be framed in terms of cumulative distribution functions. Thus, this statistic tests a "fully nonparametric" null hypothesis that is similar to the null hypotheses for the rank-based test method. Furthermore, Hajek (1969) showed that the $KS$ test can be expressed in terms of the ranks. An important consequence of the fact that the value of $KS$ depends only on the ranks of the observations is that its null distribution is determined by permutation distribution. The permutation distribution of $KS$, however, is cruder (i.e., has fewer possible $p$-values) than the permutation distribution for the rank-based test. Therefore, it is likely to be less powerful than the bootstrap, permutation, or rank-based methods. Furthermore, since the rank-based methods are especially sensitive to location difference, the $KS$ will tend to be less powerful under the particular alternative hypothesis that the treatment somehow increases (or decreases) the average level. For the BDI-II data, the *SPSS* NPAR TESTS module (with the KS option specified) was used and resulted in $KS = 1.604$, $p = 0.012$. This rejects the null hypothesis that the two groups have identical distributions, but, unfortunately, it does not characterize the difference in the two distributions.

## Resampling-Based Inference

For the sake of explication, consider an experimental design with $J = 2$ groups with sample sizes of $n$ and $m$. The null hypothesis for the parametric $t$-test is $H_0$: $(\mu_1 = \mu_2)$ or equivalently $(\mu_1 - \mu_2) = \mu_D = 0$. The basic idea behind resampling-based nonparametric methods is to *estimate* a referent (e.g., null) distribution of a test statistic ($t$) by constructing a corresponding "null statistic" ($t^*$) under the null hypothesis. Under the null hypothesis, it is reasoned that a large number of samples randomly drawn from the distribution of the null statistic ($t^*$) provides a good approximation to the actual null (referent) distribution of $t$. Thus, the null statistic ($t^*$) is computed from *multiple resamples of the actual data*, and the distribution of the $t^*$ values is used to estimate the referent distribution. Statistical inference is accomplished by comparing $t$ computed on the actual data to its estimated referent distribution, based on the distribution of $t^*$ calculated from multiple random resamples. More important, this methodology provides a **robust alternative** that allows for statistical inference without relying on distributional assumptions or asymptotic theory (these concepts will be explained in the next section). The performance of such methods depends on how well the distribution of $t^*$ approximates the actual null (referent) distribution. There are two major approaches to estimating a null referent distribution using resampling: permutation and bootstrap. For an excellent introduction to resampling-based inference, see Good (2000) and Lunneborg (2000).

### Permutation-Based Nonparametric Methods

Permutation-based methods resample *without replacement* to create a referent distribution. With small sample sizes, it is not difficult to exhaust the number of unique permutations to construct an exact test. For the two-sample case, the number of possible permutations ($r$) is

$$r = \frac{(m+n)!}{n!m!} \tag{18.4}$$

For the current example,

$$r = \frac{14!}{7!7!} = \frac{14 * 13 * 12 * 11 * 10 * 9 * 8 * 7 * 6 * 5 * 4 * 3 * 2 * 1}{(7 * 6 * 5 * 4 * 3 * 2 * 1)(7 * 6 * 5 * 4 * 3 * 2 * 1)}$$

$$r = \frac{14 * 13 * 12 * 11 * 10 * 9 * 8}{(7 * 6 * 5 * 4 * 3 * 2 * 1)} = \frac{17,297,280}{5,040} = 3,432$$

The minimal possible two-tailed $p$-value for two-sample permutation-based tests is $p = 2/r$ (Table 18.10). For unequal sample sizes, $p = 1/r$. This difference is because the empirical distribution of a test statistic is symmetric for equal sample sizes but may be asymmetric for unequal sample sizes. Thus, the minimal possible two-tailed $p$-value for two-sample permutation-based tests is $p = 2/3432 = 0.00058275$. Table 18.11 shows the 24 most extreme permutations based on the BDI-II data. Specifically, $t^*$ is a $t$-test (assuming equal variances, but other statistics could be used) calculated on each permutation. Because a two-tailed test is of interest, the absolute value, $|t^*|$, is used. This is a nonparametric resampling-based method for constructing the tails of the referent distribution for the BDI-II scores. By comparing the actual $t$-test to the tail of the distribution of $|t^*|$, one can estimate a $p$-value, $p_{(PERM)}$. Notice that the $t$-test for the actual data falls on the 7th, 8th, 9th, and 10th most extreme permutations. The most common choice for computing $p$-values, which is used in Table 18.11, is the maximum of these ranks divided by $r$, $p_{(PERM)} = (10/3432) = 0.00291375$. Notice that in this particular instance, all of the $p_{(PERM)}$ are less than the $p$-values derived from the actual data. More important, however, these values of $p_{(PERM)}$ were calculated without any of the GLM assumptions (i.e., mean differences, standardized mean differences, or unequal variance $t$-tests

**TABLE 18.10**  Minimum two-tailed *p*-values for the Kolmogorov–Smirnov (KS), permutation, and bootstrap procedures.

| *n = m* | KS | Permutation | Bootstrap |
|---|---|---|---|
| 3 | .2000 | .10000000 | .01917808 |
| 4 | .0572 | .02857143 | .00027465 |
| 5 | .0158 | .00793651 | .00000225 |
| 6 | .0044 | .00216450 | .00000001 |
| 7 | .0012 | .00058275 | <.00000001 |

**TABLE 18.11** The 14 most extreme permutations of the BDI data ranked by $t^*$-test.

| Rank | Group 1 | | | | | | | | Group 2 | | | | | | $t^*$ | $\lvert t^* \rvert$ | Two-tailed $p_t$ | Two-tailed $p_{(PERM)}$ |
| | 1 | 2 | 3 | 4 | 5 | 6 | 7 | 8 | 9 | 10 | 11 | 12 | 13 | 14 | | | | |
|---|---|---|---|---|---|---|---|---|---|---|---|---|---|---|---|---|---|---|
| 1 | 62 | 48 | 47 | 46 | 44 | 43 | 42 | 41 | 39 | 38 | 37 | 34 | 31 | 29 | 3.884 | 3.884 | .00217211 | .00058275 |
| 2 | 41 | 39 | 38 | 37 | 34 | 31 | 29 | 62 | 48 | 47 | 46 | 44 | 43 | 42 | −3.884 | 3.884 | .00217211 | .00058275 |
| 3 | 62 | 48 | 47 | 46 | 44 | 43 | 41 | 42 | 39 | 38 | 37 | 34 | 31 | 29 | 3.682 | 3.682 | .00313838 | .00116550 |
| 4 | 42 | 39 | 38 | 37 | 34 | 31 | 29 | 62 | 48 | 47 | 46 | 44 | 43 | 41 | −3.682 | 3.682 | .00313838 | .00116550 |
| 5 | 62 | 48 | 47 | 46 | 44 | 43 | 41 | 43 | 39 | 38 | 37 | 34 | 31 | 29 | 3.496 | 3.496 | .00441513 | .00174825 |
| 6 | 43 | 39 | 38 | 37 | 34 | 31 | 29 | 62 | 48 | 47 | 46 | 44 | 42 | 41 | −3.496 | 3.496 | .00441513 | .00174825 |
| **7** | **62** | **48** | **47** | **46** | **44** | **43** | **39** | **42** | **41** | **38** | **37** | **34** | **31** | **29** | **3.324** | **3.324** | **.00606704** | **.00291375** |
| **8** | **42** | **41** | **38** | **37** | **34** | **31** | **29** | **62** | **48** | **47** | **46** | **44** | **43** | **39** | **−3.324** | **3.324** | **.00606704** | **.00291375** |
| **9** | **62** | **48** | **47** | **46** | **43** | **42** | **41** | **44** | **39** | **38** | **37** | **34** | **31** | **29** | **3.324** | **3.324** | **.00606704** | **.00291375** |
| **10** | **44** | **39** | **38** | **37** | **34** | **31** | **29** | **62** | **48** | **47** | **46** | **43** | **42** | **41** | **−3.324** | **3.324** | **.00606704** | **.00291375** |
| 11 | 62 | 48 | 47 | 46 | 44 | 43 | 38 | 42 | 41 | 39 | 37 | 34 | 31 | 29 | 3.164 | 3.164 | .00816481 | .00407925 |
| 12 | 42 | 41 | 39 | 37 | 34 | 31 | 29 | 62 | 48 | 47 | 46 | 44 | 43 | 38 | −3.164 | 3.164 | .00816481 | .00407925 |
| 13 | 62 | 48 | 47 | 46 | 44 | 42 | 39 | 43 | 41 | 38 | 37 | 34 | 31 | 29 | 3.164 | 3.164 | .00816481 | .00407925 |
| 14 | 43 | 41 | 38 | 37 | 34 | 31 | 29 | 62 | 48 | 47 | 46 | 44 | 42 | 39 | −3.164 | 3.164 | .00816481 | .00407925 |
| 15 | 62 | 48 | 47 | 46 | 44 | 41 | 39 | 43 | 42 | 38 | 37 | 34 | 31 | 29 | 3.014 | 3.014 | .01078472 | .00699301 |
| 16 | 43 | 41 | 39 | 37 | 34 | 31 | 29 | 62 | 48 | 47 | 46 | 44 | 42 | 38 | 3.014 | 3.014 | .01078472 | .00699301 |
| 17 | 42 | 41 | 39 | 38 | 34 | 31 | 29 | 62 | 48 | 47 | 46 | 44 | 43 | 37 | 3.014 | 3.014 | .01078472 | .00699301 |
| 18 | 62 | 48 | 47 | 46 | 44 | 43 | 37 | 42 | 41 | 39 | 38 | 34 | 31 | 29 | −3.014 | 3.014 | .01078472 | .00699301 |
| 19 | 46 | 39 | 38 | 37 | 34 | 31 | 29 | 62 | 48 | 47 | 46 | 43 | 42 | 41 | 3.014 | 3.014 | .01078472 | .00699301 |
| 20 | 62 | 48 | 47 | 46 | 44 | 42 | 38 | 43 | 41 | 39 | 37 | 34 | 31 | 29 | −3.014 | 3.014 | .01078472 | .00699301 |
| 21 | 44 | 41 | 39 | 37 | 34 | 31 | 29 | 62 | 48 | 47 | 44 | 43 | 42 | 39 | −3.014 | 3.014 | .01078472 | .00699301 |
| 22 | 43 | 42 | 38 | 37 | 34 | 31 | 29 | 62 | 48 | 47 | 46 | 43 | 41 | 39 | 3.014 | 3.014 | .01078472 | .00699301 |
| 23 | 62 | 48 | 47 | 46 | 43 | 42 | 39 | 44 | 44 | 38 | 37 | 34 | 31 | 29 | −3.014 | 3.014 | .01078472 | .00699301 |
| 24 | 62 | 48 | 47 | 44 | 43 | 42 | 41 | 46 | 39 | 38 | 37 | 34 | 31 | 29 | −3.014 | 3.014 | .01078472 | .00699301 |

*Note:* $t^*$ is the $t$-test, assuming equal variances calculated on each permutation; $\lvert t^* \rvert$ is the absolute value of $t^*$; $p_t$ is $p$-value based on the $t$-distribution with $df = 12$; $p_{(PERM)} = \mathrm{Max}(\mathrm{Rank}[\lvert t^* \rvert])/r$, where $r = 3432$ from Equation 19.4.

© Cengage Learning

would yield the same or extremely similar results) or reference to the *t*-distribution. This is why the permutation test is referred to as a "distribution-free" test. Because of the CLT, however, the permutation distribution will approximate the *t*-distribution as the sample size becomes large.

### Nonparametric Bootstrap

Nonparametric bootstrap tests are similar to the permutation approach, except the resamples are generated by drawing *with replacement* from the data (Efron & Tibshirani, 1993). The bootstrap is a method to "nonparametrically" produce the referent distribution and compute *p*-values. It is specified by a test-statistic (*t*) computed from the actual data and compared to many bootstrap test statistics (*t\**) computed from many bootstrap resamples randomly drawn with replacement from each group separately. Beasley et al. (2004) showed that the minimum *p*-value for a pivotal bootstrap statistic for the difference in two group means (e.g., *t*-test) is

$$\text{Min}[p_{(\text{BOOT})}] = 2(mn + 1)/m^m n^n + 1). \tag{18.5}$$

For the BDI-II data with $n = m = 7$ the minimum bootstrap *p*-value is less than 0.00000001.

The major difference between bootstrap and permutation methods is that bootstrap methods resample *with replacement*, so that the same data value can be in a resample twice (or more). In fact, it is possible in the BDI-II example, although very unlikely, for a bootstrap resample to have all 62's in one group and all 29's in the other group. This is why the total number of resamples is larger for bootstrap methods than for permutation methods. In turn, this is why the *p*-values are smaller for bootstrap methods than for permutation methods.

For small sample sizes (*m* or $n \leq 7$), the bootstrap resamples are generated by means of exhaustive enumeration rather than by random sampling with replacement via simulation, which is the standard approach in the nonparametric bootstrap (Fisher & Hall, 1991). In this situation, bootstrap samples are generated randomly a large number of times, and the assumption is that a large number of random bootstrap samples will adequately reflect the actual bootstrap distribution. In this case, however, the bootstrap *p*-value is a random variable rather than a fixed entity. The most common number of resamples drawn is 10,000, thus yielding a minimum bootstrap *p*-value = 0.0001, which is adequate for most behavioral researchers.

Table 18.10 shows the minimum two-tailed *p*-values for the *KS* test, Bootstrap-based *t*-test, and the Permutation test for several two-group balanced designs with small sample sizes. When sample sizes are larger, these methods often rely on asymptotic theory and use a known probability distribution (e.g., chi-square) as a referent distribution. For more complicated test statistics, however, the approximation of the estimated referent distribution to a known probability distribution is often questionable, even with larger sample sizes.

## Rank-Based Approach

A commonly used nonparametric approach involves ranking the data (from 1 to *N*) and computing the appropriate test statistics, which is the basis for the **Wilcoxen Rank Sum test** (*WRS*; Wilcoxen, 1945), the **Mann–Whitney *U* statistic** (Mann & Whitney, 1947), as well as many other rank-based methods. Ranks may be considered preferable to the actual data (Cliff, 1996). For example, if the numbers assigned to the observations have no meaning by themselves but attain meaning only in an ordinal comparison with the other observations, the actual data contain no more information than the ranks contain. Rank-transformed data are equally spaced and provide a robust adjustment in that ranks are less sensitive to outliers. Also, even if the numbers have meaning but the distribution's function is not normal, the probability theory for the test statistics cannot be derived if the distribution function is unknown. Yet, the probability theory of statistics based on ranks is relatively straightforward and does not depend on the distribution of the data in many cases (Bradley, 1968).

The referent distribution for the *WRS* is based on all unique combinations of ranks for one of the two groups and is identical to a permutation test applied to ranked data. Thus, it has a bounded distribution, especially with smaller samples. Therefore, in many cases (when there are no extreme outliers in small samples), the permutation test just described will result in the same *p*-value as the rank-based method, especially in the tails of the distribution. Table 18.12 shows the 24 most extreme permutations based on the ranked BDI-II data, which illustrates the similarity of the two procedures under these circumstances. The null distributions of the two methods will differ toward the middle of the distribution where the outlier of case A (BDI $= 62$) will have more influence on a *t*-test than will a Rank(BDI) $= 14$ on *WRS*.

*WRS* generalizes to the $J > 2$ groups situation and thus can also be performed by an ANOVA approach where the Between-Groups Rank Sum of Squares are computed and divided by the known Total Rank Sum of Squares to create the Kruskal–Wallis test statistic (*KW*) that approximates $\chi^2$ with $df = J - 1$ asymptotically (Kruskal & Wallis, 1952). When there are only $J = 2$ groups, *KW* is functionally equivalent to the *WRS* and Mann-Whitney *U* tests (Hollander & Wolfe, 1973). Thus, for the rest of the chapter, we will refer to *KW* as the rank-based method for group comparisons.

Table 18.8 showed the ranks of the BDI-II data. Table 18.13 shows the results of an ANOVA performed on the ranks (Conover, 1980). The descriptive statistics show that ranking reduced the skewness of the residuals, especially in the control group. Although Zimmerman (1998) noted that ranks can "inherit" the heterogeneity of variance in the original data, this was not the case for the ranks of BDI-II. Of most interest, however, the control group has a mean rank of 10.5714, whereas the treatment group had a mean rank of 4.4286. The *KW* statistic was computed using the SPSS NPAR TESTS module (with the K-W option specified), which resulted in *KW* = 7.547. Used as a chi-square approximate, the value of *KW* = 7.547 is comparable to a chi-square distribution with $df = 1$, which results in an approximate *p*-value of $p_{(APPROX)} = 0.00601121$. The *SPSS* NPAR TESTS module will also calculate an exact permutation-based *p*-value, $p_{(EXACT)} = 0.004079254$. To illustrate, notice in Table 18.12 that the *KW*-statistic for the actual ranked data falls on the 10th, 11th 12th, and 14th most extreme permutations. Again *p*-values are computed by dividing the maximum of these ranks by *r*, $p_{(PERM)} = (14/3432) = 0.004079254$.

Table 18.13 also shows that the *KW* statistic is functionally related to the ANOVA performed on ranks. Thus, *KW* can also be calculated by an ANOVA approach where the Between-Groups Rank Sum of Squares are computed and divided by the known Total Variance among ranks to create a test statistic *KW* that approximates $\chi^2$ with $df = J - 1$ asymptotically (Kruskal & Wallis, 1952):

$$KW = \frac{\sum_{j=1}^{J} n_j(\overline{R}_j - [(N+1)/2])2}{(N[N+1])/12}. \tag{18.6}$$

To elaborate, the grand mean of the ranks is always equal to $(N+1)/2$; thus, the numerator of Equation 18.6 is the Between-Groups Rank Sum of Squares. Further, variance of

**TABLE 18.12**  The 14 most extreme permutations of the ranked BDI-II data ranked by *t\**-test.

| Resample Rank | Group 1 | | | | | | | Group 2 | | | | | | | KW* | Two-tailed $p_{(APPROX)}$ | Two-tailed $p_{(PERM)}$ |
|---|---|---|---|---|---|---|---|---|---|---|---|---|---|---|---|---|---|
| | 1 | 2 | 3 | 4 | 5 | 6 | 7 | 8 | 9 | 10 | 11 | 12 | 13 | 14 | | | |
| 1 (1.5) | 14 | 13 | 12 | 11 | 10 | 9 | 8 | 7 | 6 | 5 | 4 | 3 | 2 | 1 | 9.800 | .00174512 | .0058275 |
| 2 (1.5) | 7 | 6 | 5 | 4 | 3 | 2 | 1 | 14 | 13 | 12 | 11 | 10 | 9 | 8 | 9.800 | .00174512 | .0058275 |
| 3 (3.5) | 14 | 13 | 12 | 11 | 10 | 9 | 7 | 8 | 6 | 5 | 4 | 3 | 2 | 1 | 9.016 | .00267579 | .00116550 |
| 4 (3.5) | 8 | 6 | 5 | 4 | 3 | 2 | 1 | 14 | 13 | 12 | 11 | 10 | 9 | 7 | 9.016 | .00267579 | .00116550 |
| 5 (6.5) | 14 | 13 | 12 | 11 | 10 | 9 | 6 | 8 | 7 | 5 | 4 | 3 | 2 | 1 | 8.265 | .00404098 | .00233100 |
| 6 (6.5) | 8 | 7 | 5 | 4 | 3 | 2 | 1 | 14 | 13 | 12 | 11 | 10 | 9 | 6 | 8.265 | .00404098 | .00233100 |
| 7 (6.5) | 14 | 13 | 12 | 11 | 10 | 8 | 7 | 9 | 6 | 5 | 4 | 3 | 2 | 1 | 8.265 | .00404098 | .00233100 |
| 8 (6.5) | 9 | 6 | 5 | 4 | 3 | 2 | 1 | 14 | 13 | 12 | 11 | 10 | 8 | 7 | 8.265 | .00404098 | .00233100 |
| **9 (11.5)** | **14** | **13** | **12** | **11** | **10** | **9** | **5** | **8** | **7** | **6** | **4** | **3** | **2** | **1** | **7.547** | **.00601121** | **.00407925** |
| **10 (11.5)** | **8** | **7** | **6** | **4** | **3** | **2** | **1** | **14** | **13** | **12** | **11** | **10** | **9** | **5** | **7.547** | **.00601121** | **.00407925** |
| **11 (11.5)** | **14** | **13** | **12** | **11** | **10** | **8** | **6** | **9** | **7** | **5** | **4** | **3** | **2** | **1** | **7.547** | **.00601121** | **.00407925** |
| **12 (11.5)** | **9** | **7** | **5** | **4** | **3** | **2** | **1** | **14** | **13** | **12** | **11** | **10** | **8** | **6** | **7.547** | **.00601121** | **.00407925** |
| **13 (11.5)** | **14** | **13** | **12** | **11** | **9** | **8** | **7** | **10** | **6** | **5** | **4** | **3** | **2** | **1** | **7.547** | **.00601121** | **.00407925** |
| **14 (11.5)** | **10** | **6** | **5** | **4** | **3** | **2** | **1** | **14** | **13** | **12** | **11** | **9** | **8** | **7** | **7.547** | **.00601121** | **.00407925** |
| 15 (19.5) | 14 | 13 | 12 | 11 | 10 | 9 | 4 | 8 | 7 | 6 | 5 | 3 | 2 | 1 | 6.861 | .00880862 | .00699301 |
| 16 (19.5) | 11 | 6 | 5 | 4 | 3 | 2 | 1 | 14 | 13 | 12 | 10 | 9 | 8 | 7 | 6.861 | .00880862 | .00699301 |
| 17 (19.5) | 14 | 13 | 12 | 11 | 10 | 8 | 5 | 9 | 7 | 6 | 4 | 3 | 2 | 1 | 6.861 | .00880862 | .00699301 |
| 18 (19.5) | 10 | 7 | 5 | 4 | 3 | 2 | 1 | 14 | 13 | 12 | 11 | 9 | 8 | 6 | 6.861 | .00880862 | .00699301 |
| 19 (19.5) | 14 | 13 | 12 | 11 | 10 | 7 | 6 | 9 | 8 | 5 | 4 | 3 | 2 | 1 | 6.861 | .00880862 | .00699301 |
| 20 (19.5) | 9 | 8 | 5 | 4 | 3 | 2 | 1 | 14 | 13 | 12 | 11 | 10 | 7 | 6 | 6.861 | .00880862 | .00699301 |
| 21 (19.5) | 14 | 13 | 12 | 11 | 9 | 8 | 6 | 10 | 7 | 5 | 4 | 3 | 2 | 1 | 6.861 | .00880862 | .00699301 |
| 22 (19.5) | 9 | 7 | 6 | 4 | 3 | 2 | 1 | 14 | 13 | 12 | 11 | 10 | 8 | 5 | 6.861 | .00880862 | .00699301 |
| 23 (19.5) | 14 | 13 | 12 | 10 | 9 | 8 | 7 | 11 | 6 | 5 | 4 | 3 | 2 | 1 | 6.861 | .00880862 | .00699301 |
| 24 (19.5) | 8 | 7 | 6 | 5 | 3 | 2 | 1 | 14 | 13 | 12 | 11 | 10 | 9 | 4 | 6.861 | .00880862 | .00699301 |

*Note: KW\* is the Kruskal-Wallis test calculated on each permutation, $p_{(APPROX)}$ is p-value based on the $\chi^2$-distribution with $df = 1$; $p_{(PERM)} = \text{Max(Rank}[KW*])/r$, where $r = 3432$ from Equation 19.4.*

| TABLE 18.13 | *t*-Test and ANOVA *F*-test performed on the ranks of BDI-II. | | |
|---|---|---|---|
| **BDI** | **Control Group = 0** | **Treatment Group = 1** | **Mean Difference** |
| Mean | 47.00 | 36.00 | 11.00 |
| SD | 7.12 | 5.10 | SE = 3.22 |
| Skew | 1.92 | 0.13 | *df* = 12 |
| Kurtosis | 4.20 | −0.41 | *t* = 3.41 |
| Sample Size | *n* = 7 | *m* = 7 | *p* = .005 |
| **RankBDI** | | | |
| Mean | 10.5714 | 4.4286 | 6.2857 |
| SD | 2.6367 | 2.9921 | SE = 1.4534 |
| Skew | −0.11 | 1.04 | *df* = 12 |
| Kurtosis | −1.64 | 1.28 | *t* = 4.33 |
| Sample Size | *n* = 7 | *m* = 7 | *p* = .001 |

BDI = Beck Depression Inventory, 2nd edition; RankBDIsqrt = Rank of BDI.

**ANOVA Table**

| SOURCE | Sum of Squares | df | Mean Square | F | Sig. |
|---|---|---|---|---|---|
| Between Groups | 138.071 | 1 | 132.071 | 16.608 | .002 |
| Within Groups | 95.429 | 12 | 7.393 | | |
| Total | 227.500 | 13 | 17.500 | | |

$$SS_{BETWEEN} = \Sigma n_\varphi (\bar{R}_\varphi - \bar{R}_*)^2 = \Sigma n(\bar{R}_j - [(N+1)/2])^2$$

$$SS_{BETWEEN} = 7(10.5714 - 7.5)^2 + 7(4.4286 - 7.5)^2 = 138.071$$

$$VAR_{TOTAL} = SS_{TOTAL}/(N-1) = N(N+1)/12 = 17.5$$

$$KW = \frac{\sum_{j=1}^{J} n_j (\bar{R}_j - [(N+1)/2])^2}{(N[N+1]/12} = \frac{SS_{BETWEEN}}{SS_{TOTAL}/df_{TOTAL}} = \frac{(df_{TOTAL})SS_{BETWEEN}}{SS_{TOTAL}} = \frac{(N-1)SS_{BETWEEN}}{SS_{TOTAL}}$$

$eta^2 = SS_{BETWEEN}/SS_{TOTAL} = (138.071/227.5) = 0.581$.

**Thus:** $(N-1)eta^2 = (13(.581)) = 7.547 = KW$.

© Cengage Learning

untied ranks is always equal to $N(N+1)/12$. The *KW* statistic divided by $N-1$ is equivalent to an eta-squared or $R^2$ computed form and ANOVA table (Table 18.13).

# Null Hypothesis for Rank-Based Statistics

With the assumption that the error components are independent, have a constant variance, and are sampled from a normal distribution ($NID(0, \sigma^2)$), the parametric test has "assumed away" everything but differences in location, which allows the parametric test to focus on a single parameter. The constant variance (homoscedasticity) assumption leads to the expectation that the groups will have identical variances. The normality assumption excludes differences in skew and kurtosis. All that can be left are differences in location. Assuming normality, the mean is the maximum likelihood estimate of location, and a parametric test is the most powerful statistical test. The $NID(0, \sigma^2)$ assumption simply allows the researcher to focus on a single parameter. Thus, the null hypothesis is that the groups have identical means, and by assuming $NID(0, \sigma^2)$, the null hypothesis actually involves sampling from identical normal distributions.

To test a null hypothesis for a two-sample design, rank-based approaches can be used to relax the normality assumptions by assuming that the error components for each group have constant variance and are random variables from ***Identical***, independent distributions [i.e., $IID(0, \sigma^2)$], not necessarily normally distributed. All that can be left are differences (shifts) in location; without assuming normality, however, the mean may not be the most powerful measure of location. If $IID(0, \sigma^2)$ is assumed, then rank-based tests evaluate a *shift* model. This provides a robust alternative to parametric procedures for testing hypotheses, allowing direct inference concerning location parameters (Akritas, Arnold, & Brunner, 1997).

The asymptotic relative efficiency (ARE) of the rank-based *KW* test (equation 18.7) is comparable to the parametric *F*-test; the contrary, however, does not hold. If the errors are $NID(0, \sigma^2)$, the ARE of the *KW* compared to the *F*-test is 0.955. If the two populations differ only in their location parameters (i.e., $IID(0, \sigma^2)$), the ARE is never lower than 0.864 but may be as high as infinity (Hodges & Lehmann, 1963). Thus, the rank-based *KW* test is often much more powerful than the parametric independent samples *t*-test, especially when error distributions are identically distributed with extreme skew. Therefore, rank-based tests can be "safer to use" in many situations (Conover, 1980).

Rank-based approaches, however, may not provide a robust alternative if simply applied because of *any* violation of model assumptions. For example, Zimmerman (1996) demonstrated that rank transformed scores can inherit the heterogeneity of variance in the original data, although this was not case for the BDI-II data. This leads to inflated type I error rates when using *KW* as a robust alternative for testing differences in location parameters when the groups differ in sample sizes, variance, or shape (Brunner & Munzel, 2000; Wilcox, 1993; Zimmerman, 1996). Based on the Welch (1947) correction, Brunner and Munzel (2000) developed a test for location differences when groups differ in variance; it does not, however, provide control of type I error rates for sample sizes less than 50. With sample sizes below 50, however, parametric tests may be valid because of the CLT.

Thus, if the two groups have identically skewed distribution with the same variance, then any differences would be due to differences in location. Parametric tests are valid in terms of type I error rates in most, but not all cases. Therefore, the rank-based tests simply relax the normality assumption while retaining the others. By ranking the data, the skewed data becomes more symmetric, which under the CLT will lead to valid inference. In this sense, it could be labeled a robust alternative because it leads to appropriate type I error rates even though the normality assumption was violated. Although a rank-based test will be sensitive to differences in other distributional properties (shape and spread), its power is driven by differences in mean ranks (similar to medians). Although the difference in mean ranks is not a parameter that defines the parent distribution, a rank-based test may be considered a robust alternative because it is testing a null hypothesis similar in concept to the parametric null.

## Fully Nonparametric Inference

Strictly speaking, the most commonly used parametric procedures test differences in location (e.g., means) because other distributional differences are assumed not to exist [i.e., $NID(0, \sigma^2)$]. Thus, to test hypotheses concerning shifts in location parameters, the assumptions of independence, homogeneity of variance, and identical shape must still exist. Specifically, credible inferences about means require the assumption that the population distributions are symmetric (Koch, 1969), whereas credible inferences concerning location parameters in general require the assumption that the population distributions are of identical shape but not necessarily symmetric [i.e., $IID(0, \sigma^2)$]. This frequently overlooked detail is a major reason that there was so much attention given to rank-based procedures as tests of "stochastic homogeneity" (Vargha & Delaney, 1998), "distributional equivalence" (Beasley, 2000; Agresti & Pendergast, 1986), or "fully nonparametric hypotheses" (Akritas & Arnold, 1994). Therefore, without assuming $IID(0, \sigma^2)$, rank-based methods are "**fully nonparametric**" tests and are *not* viewed as *robust alternatives* to normal theory methods for testing differences in means. Rather, statistically significant fully nonparametric tests may be attributed to differences among any distributional characteristic (e.g., location, dispersion, and shape).

As a departure from parametric models that test differences among means, general "fully nonparametric" models, which specify only that observations in different groups are governed by different distribution functions, have been developed for a variety of experimental designs (Akritas & Arnold, 1994; Brunner & Langer, 2000). Specifically, fully nonparametric means that these methods make no assumptions about the distribution of the error term (e.g., normality; constant variance). Thus, a sufficiently large test statistic indicates that the two groups significantly differ in their distribution. Cliff (1996) and others contend that if a test statistic becomes large enough to become a "significant result" when the normality or homoscedasticity assumptions are not met, even though population means are identical, then it is still a valuable result to educational and behavioral researchers.

Strictly speaking, fully nonparametric procedures (e.g., *KS*, *WRS*, and *KW*) test the null hypothesis that both samples are generated from identical probability distributions:

$$H_{0(k)} : G(Y_1) = H(Y_2), \tag{18.7}$$

where $G$ and $H$ are distribution functions for the two independent samples. As previously mentioned, by assuming $NID(0, \sigma^2)$ or $IID(0, \sigma^2)$, differences in probability distributions can only be because of shifts in location parameters (i.e., the means). Hypotheses of this form reduce the risk of drawing incorrect conclusions about the likely sources of the significant effect but do so at the cost of not being able to characterize precisely (i.e., focus on a single parameter) how population distributions differ. Because rank-based methods are based on test statistics that employ differences in mean ranks, they are most sensitive to differences in location (Bradley, 1968). A significant result, however, may also be attributable to difference in location, spread, or shape (Wilcox, 1993). Therefore, even if assumptions concerning identical distributions and homogeneous variances are not tenable, the researcher may still conclude that one group is stochastically dominant over the other group (Vargha & Delaney, 1998).

# Conclusion

Nonparametric tests of inference are used to analyze nominal, ordinal, and substantially skewed data sets. The chi-square statistic is a commonly used test of the null hypothesis of proportion or count equivalence between or among independent categorical data. In choosing data transformations or nonparametric alternatives to parametric tests, several issues should be considered. The beauty of parametric linear models is that a wide range of research designs can be analyzed. Rank methods and most other nonparametric methods generalize to multiple group experiments. For more complex designs that involve regression models, multiple factors, and potential interaction terms, issues in using data transformation and nonparametric procedures become more complicated. It is possible that an interaction or main effect that is present in the original data "disappears" when the data are transformed. It is also possible that the transformation can "create" an interaction effect. In fact, Salter and Fawcett (1993) demonstrated that some main effect structures with no interaction in factorial ANOVA designs can create an interaction in the ranks. Thus, they proposed an aligned rank test for factorial designs, which was adapted for repeated measures designs (Beasley, 2002). Although rank-based (Headrick & Rotou, 2001) and ordinal (Long & Cliff, 1997) regression procedures have been developed and investigated, such interpretational issues only become more complex in regression models.

Data transformations and nonparametric alternatives are often used so that model assumptions are more tenable or more relaxed. This works well when the original data, transformed data, and nonparametric procedure lead to the same conclusion and interpretation. Data transformations, however, can alter the fundamental nature of the data and the null hypothesis being tested, thus complicating interpretation. If a data transformation drastically changes the interpretation of the results, it begs the question of which results (the original or transformed) are more valid or believable. Data transformations often make reviewers and consumers skeptical because it conveys the suspicion that the data were manipulated to gain the desired results. Thus, when there is disagreement, the researcher is left in a quandary. In such cases, all analyses should be considered, but it is still up to the researcher to decide which results to interpret and report. Often researchers are asked to discuss the difference between the results with and without the transformation. There are no easy answers in these situations. It is vital for the data analyst to properly justify any data transformation or alternate procedure, especially when it results in conclusions that differ from those obtained with original untransformed data.

*Now go to the Student Workbook found on cengagebrain.com that accompanies this text for additional application and review activities.*

# An Overview of Multivariate Statistical Analyses

## CHAPTER 19

This chapter introduces the reader to multiple regression and multivariate analysis of variance with descriptive discriminant analysis. The focus is on conceptual understanding, methodological issues, and applications illustrated with the use of *SPSS*. This chapter introduces additional methods of multivariate analysis for research in counseling, including exploratory and confirmatory factor analysis, and brief notes on other multivariate methods, such as predictive discriminant analysis, canonical correlations, and structural equation modeling.

## The Concept of Multiple Regression

Simple linear regression is based on a linear relationship between a criterion variable ($Y$) and a single predictor ($X$) (see Chapter 17). With **multiple regression**, two or more predictor variables are used to predict the criterion variable, $Y$. For example, the multiple regression model with two predictors, $X_1$ and $X_2$, is

$$\hat{Y} = b_1 X_1 + b_2 X_2 + a, \tag{19.1}$$

where $\hat{Y}$ ($Y$ hat) denotes the predicted $Y$ values, $b_1$ and $b_2$ are regression coefficients, and $a$ is the intercept. (Some textbooks use the notation $Y'$ for the predicted $Y$ score.)

The logic of simple linear regression carries over into multiple regression. Using more than one predictor, however, leads to additional assumptions. In the multiple regression model with two predictors (Equation 19.1), for example, the prediction of $Y$ is affected not only by the correlation between $Y$ and each of the predictors, $X_1$ and $X_2$, but also by the correlation between $X_1$ and $X_2$. It is assumed that the relationship between $Y$ and $X_1$ is the same for any fixed value of $X_2$ and, conversely, the relationship between $Y$ and $X_2$ is the same for any fixed value of $X_1$. Graphically, the predicted $Y$ values ($\hat{Y}$) fall on a regression plane that cuts through a three-dimensional space that is determined by the perpendicular axis of $X_1$, $X_2$, and $Y$. As with simple linear regression, prediction *error* in multiple regression is the difference between actual and predicted $Y$ values: $e = Y - \hat{Y}$. The "best fit" for a sample of observations, used to develop a multiple regression model with two predictors, is the plane that produces that smallest sum of squared errors, $\Sigma e^2$, referred to as *regression plane* (e.g., see Figure 19.1, where the predicted $Y$ score for $X_1 = 1$ and $X_2 = 5$ is $Y' = 10$).

**Figure 19.1**

Regression plane for predicting $Y$ from $X_1$ and $X_2$.

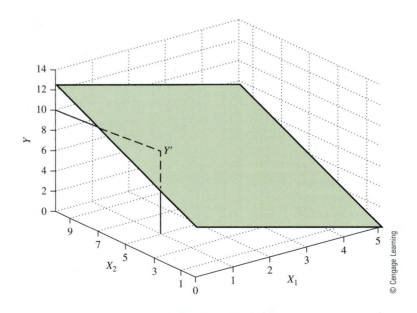

© Cengage Learning

The interpretation of the slope for a given predictor in multiple regression is similar to its interpretation in simple linear regression but under the assumption that the values of the other predictors are fixed. For example, the slope $b_1$ in equation 19.1 indicates the change in the predicted $Y$ score ($\hat{Y}$), associated with a unit change in $X_1$, assuming that the value of $X_2$ does not change. Similarly, the slope $b_2$ indicates the change in $\hat{Y}$, associated with a unit change in $X_2$, assuming that the value of $X_1$ does not change.

Suppose the regression equation for the prediction of test performance ($TPF$) from verbal ability ($VA$) and anxiety ($ANX$) is $T\hat{P}F = 0.25(VA) - 0.20(ANX) + 10$. For a person with a score of 20 on verbal ability and a score of 5 on anxiety, the predicted test performance is $T\hat{P}F = 0.25(20) - 0.20(5) + 10 = 14$. The positive regression coefficient ($b_1 = 0.25$) shows that there is a positive correlation between test performance and verbal ability for any fixed value of anxiety. It also shows that when a person's score on verbal ability increases by one unit, with no changes in the score on anxiety, the predicted test performance will increase by 0.25. Conversely, the negative regression coefficient ($b_2 = -0.20$) shows that there is a negative correlation between test performance and anxiety for any fixed value of verbal ability. When the anxiety score increases by one unit, with no changes in the verbal ability score, the predicted score on test performance will decrease by 0.20.

The point made in Chapter 17 that correlation (or simple regression prediction) does not necessarily mean causation holds for multiple regression predictions as well. Understanding the difference between predictive and explanatory (causal) research is crucial for valid applications of multiple regression analysis and interpretation of its results. The emphasis in predictive research is on practical applications of accurate predictions, whereas the focus in explanatory research is on causal explanations and conceptual understanding of relationship between variables. In this chapter, the multiple regression analysis is discussed in light of its predictive applications (not causal explanations). It is important, however, to keep in mind that results in predictive research can provide insights that may lead to causal explanations and, conversely, the chances of good prediction increase when the selection of predictor variables is based on their theoretical relationship with the criterion variable.

# Multiple Correlation and Coefficient of Determination

The Pearson $r$ between the actual and predicted $Y$ scores ($r_{Y\hat{Y}}$) is called the **coefficient of multiple correlation** between $Y$ and the predictors. The multiple correlation is denoted **R**, with a subscript when necessary to specify the predictors used to obtain the predicted scores ($\hat{Y}$). For example, $R_{Y.12}$ (read "$Y$ **dot** one two") is the designation when $Y$ is predicted from $X_1$ and $X_2$, and $R_{Y.123}$ is the designation, when $Y$ is predicted from $X_1$, $X_2$, and $X_3$. The squared multiple correlation ($R^2$), referred to as *coefficient of determination*, indicates the proportion of the variance in $Y$ associated with the variance in all predictors together. With the illustration in Figure 19.2, $R^2$ indicates what proportion is the shared variance ($A + B + C$) of the total variance in $Y$—that is, $R^2 = (A + B + C)/Y$. The $SSE$ part is the sum of squared errors, $SSE = \Sigma(Y - \hat{Y})^2$, in the prediction of $Y$ from $X_1$ and $X_2$. The total variability in $Y$ (bold circle) is represented with the sum of squares total: $SS_{Total} = \Sigma(Y - \overline{Y})^2$. Evidently, the sum of squares owing to regression is $SS_{Reg.} = A + B + C = SS_{Total} - SSE$. Thus, the coefficient of determination, $R^2 = SS_{Reg}/SS_{Total}$, shows what proportion of the total variability in $Y$ is because of regression. This relationship is expressed in Equation 19.2.

**Figure 19.2**

Variance in *Y* shared with $X_1$ and $X_2$.

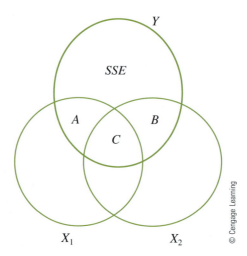

The coefficient of determination ($R^2$) indicates the proportion of individual differences on the criterion variable (*Y*) associated with individual differences on the predictors:

$$R^2 = \frac{SS_{\text{Total}} - SSE}{SS_{\text{Total}}} = \frac{SS_{\text{Reg}}}{SS_{\text{Total}}} = \frac{\text{Sum of squares due to regression}}{\text{Total sum of squares}} \qquad (19.2)$$

The interpretation of part A (or part B) in Figure 19.2 relates to the concept of *part correlation* discussed in Chapter 17. Specifically, the squared part correlation between *Y* and $X_1$, controlling for $X_2$, shows what proportion is part A from the total variance in *Y*—that is, $r^2_{Y(1.2)} = A/SS_{\text{Total}}$. As shown in Example 19.1, multiple regression analysis with *SPSS* provides information about the partial and part correlations between the criterion variable (*Y*) and any predictor, controlling for the other predictors.

## Example 19.1

The purpose of this example is to describe the steps in using *SPSS* for multiple regression analysis and provide interpretations of results with the *SPSS* output to facilitate the understanding of multiple regression concepts. Specifically, multiple regression analysis is used to predict task involvement (*Y*) from motivation ($X_1$) and self-reliance ($X_2$). The scores for $X_1$, $X_2$, and *Y* are tabulated in the first three columns of the *SPSS* Data Editor provided in Figure 19.3. The additional two columns, "pred_y" and "error," are the predicted *Y* value, $\hat{Y}$, and prediction error, $Y - \hat{Y}$, respectively, obtained with the *SPSS* multiple regression analysis. The same data were also used in Chapter 17 to illustrate correlations (Equation 17.1) and simple linear regression (Figure 17.8).

The variables named **X1**, **X2**, and **Y** in the *SPSS* Data Editor were labeled "motivation," "self-reliance," and "task involvement," respectively (to get the **Label** box, click on **Variable View**). To conduct the multiple regression analysis, follow these steps:

1. Click **Analyze**, click **Regression**, and click **Linear**.

2. Click **Y**, and then click ▶ to move **Y** into the **Dependent** box.

3. Hold down the **Ctrl** key, click on **X1** and **X2**, and then click ▶ to move them into the **Independent(s)** box.

4. Click **Statistics**. In the **Linear Regression: Statistics** dialog box that shows up, the default options **Estimates** and **Model fit** should already be selected.

5. Select **Part and partial correlations**.

6. Click **Continue**.

**Figure 19.3**

*SPSS* data file with $X_1$, $X_2$, and $Y$, as well as results for $\hat{Y}$ and error, $Y - \hat{Y}$.

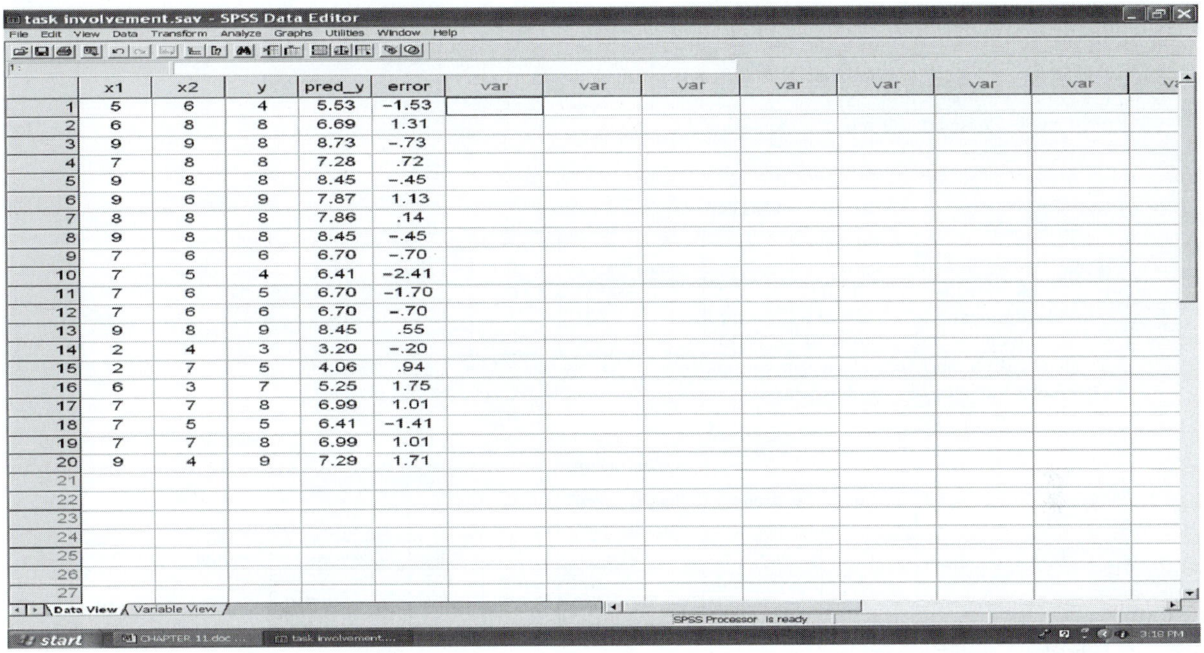

| | x1 | x2 | y | pred_y | error |
|---|---|---|---|---|---|
| 1 | 5 | 6 | 4 | 5.53 | -1.53 |
| 2 | 6 | 8 | 8 | 6.69 | 1.31 |
| 3 | 9 | 9 | 8 | 8.73 | -.73 |
| 4 | 7 | 8 | 8 | 7.28 | .72 |
| 5 | 9 | 8 | 8 | 8.45 | -.45 |
| 6 | 9 | 6 | 9 | 7.87 | 1.13 |
| 7 | 8 | 8 | 8 | 7.86 | .14 |
| 8 | 9 | 8 | 8 | 8.45 | -.45 |
| 9 | 7 | 6 | 6 | 6.70 | -.70 |
| 10 | 7 | 5 | 4 | 6.41 | -2.41 |
| 11 | 7 | 6 | 5 | 6.70 | -1.70 |
| 12 | 7 | 6 | 6 | 6.70 | -.70 |
| 13 | 9 | 8 | 9 | 8.45 | .55 |
| 14 | 2 | 4 | 3 | 3.20 | -.20 |
| 15 | 2 | 7 | 5 | 4.06 | .94 |
| 16 | 6 | 3 | 7 | 5.25 | 1.75 |
| 17 | 7 | 7 | 8 | 6.99 | 1.01 |
| 18 | 7 | 5 | 5 | 6.41 | -1.41 |
| 19 | 7 | 7 | 8 | 6.99 | 1.01 |
| 20 | 9 | 4 | 9 | 7.29 | 1.71 |

**7.** Click **Save**. In the **Linear Regression: Save** dialog box, select **Unstandardized** in the Predicted Values (left) panel and **Unstandardized** in the Residuals (right) panel.

**8.** Click **Continue**.

**9.** Click **OK**.

The *SPSS* output with these steps (without steps 7 and 8) is shown in Figure 19.4. Steps 7 and 8 are optional; they are used with *SPSS* for multiple regression to save the predicted $Y$ values and prediction errors (residuals), with default names "pre_1" and "res_1," respectively. For readability, these two resulting variables were renamed here to "pred_y" and "error," respectively (Figure 19.3). Description and interpretation of results in the *SPSS* output (Figure 19.4) follow:

**1.** The Model Summary table provides the estimates for (a) *multiple correlation*, $R = .766$, (b) *coefficient of determination*, $R^2 = .587$, and it's adjusted for the population value, $R^2_{\text{Adj.}} = .539$, and (c) the *standard error of estimate*, $SEE = 1.277$ (see Chapter 17 for its counterpart in simple linear regression, $s_{Y.X}$). As the multiple correlation is the Pearson $r$ between actual and predicted $Y$ values, $R = .766$ is the correlation between the variables Y and "pre_y" in Figure 19.3. Its squared value, $R^2 = .587$, indicates that 58.7 percent of the individual differences in task involvement ($Y$) are accounted for by individual differences in motivation ($X_1$) and self-reliance ($X_2$).

**2.** The ANOVA table provides information about the statistical significance of $R^2$. Specifically, the reported $F$ statistic is used to test the null hypothesis that the coefficient of determination equals zero for the study population, $H_0$: $R^2_{\text{pop}} = 0$. In this case, $H_0$ is rejected at the $\alpha = .05$ (even .01) level of statistical significance, $F(2, 17) = 12.095$, $p = .001$. Thus, the regression prediction of task involvement from motivation and self-reliance is statistically significant. The Sum of Squares column provides information that is interpretable with Figure 19.2. Specifically, (a) Regression = sum of

**Figure 19.4**

Selected *SPSS* output with multiple linear regression analysis.

**Model Summary**

| Model | R | R Square | Adjusted R Square | Std. Error of the Estimate |
|---|---|---|---|---|
| 1 | .766[a] | .587 | .539 | 1.277 |

a. Predictors: (Constant), self-reliance, motivation

**ANOVA**[b]

| Model | | Sum of Squares | df | Mean Square | F | Sig. |
|---|---|---|---|---|---|---|
| 1 | Regression | 39.465 | 2 | 19.732 | 12.095 | .001[a] |
| | Residual | 27.735 | 17 | 1.631 | | |
| | Total | 67.200 | 19 | | | |

a. Predictors: (Constant), self-reliance, motivation
b. Dependent Variable: task involvement

**Coefficients**[a]

| Model | | Unstandardized Coefficients | | Standardized Coefficients | t | Sig. | Correlations | | |
|---|---|---|---|---|---|---|---|---|---|
| | | B | Std. Error | Beta | | | Zero-order | Partial | Part |
| 1 | (Constant) | .879 | 1.342 | | .655 | .521 | | | |
| | motivation | .585 | .152 | .642 | 3.859 | .001 | .729 | .683 | .601 |
| | self-reliance | .288 | .191 | .251 | 1.508 | .150 | .475 | .343 | .235 |

a. Dependent Variable: task involvement

squares due to regression $= SS_{Reg} = A + B + C = 39.465$; (b) Residual $=$ sum of squared errors: $SSE = 27.735$; and (c) Total $=$ total sum of squares, $SS_{Total} = 67.200$ (given these results, one can calculate $R^2$ using equation 19.2).

3. The Coefficients table (Figure 19.2) provides information to (a) develop the regression equation, (b) test the regression coefficients for statistical significance, (c) compare the predictors on their relative importance for the prediction, and (d) evaluate correlations (Pearson *r*, partial, and part) between the criterion variable and each predictor. Specifically, with the **B**-values in the Unstandardized Coefficients column, the regression equation for the prediction of task involvement ($Y$) from motivation ($X_1$) and self-reliance ($X_2$) is $\hat{Y} = 0.585 \, X_1 + 0.288 \, X_2 + 0.879$.

The *p* values (Sig. column) for statistical significance of the regression coefficients indicate that the regression coefficient for $X_1$ ($b_1 = 0.585$) is statistically significant at the .05 level ($p = .001$). In the context of Figure 19.2, this means that part A $\neq$ 0; that is, the unique contribution of motivation ($X_1$) in predicting task performance ($Y$), while controlling for self-reliance ($X_2$), is statistically significant. The magnitude of this unique predictive contribution is estimated by the squared part (semipartial) correlation between $Y$ and $X_1$: $r^2_{Y(1.2)} = (.601)^2 = .3612$. In other words, 36.12 percent of the variance in task performance is uniquely accounted for by motivation. The regression coefficient for $X_2$, however, is not statistically significant at the .05 level ($p = .150$). Related to Figure 19.2, this means that part B $= 0$ for the population; that is, self-reliance does not contribute to the prediction of task involvement over and above the prediction provided by motivation.

The Zero-Order Correlations are, in fact, the Pearson *r* between the criterion variable ($Y$) and each predictor. For example, the Pearson correlation between task involvement ($Y$) and motivation ($X_1$) is $r_{Y1} = .729$. Likewise, the Pearson correlation between task involvement ($Y$) and self-reliance ($X_2$) is $r_{Y2} = .475$. The Standardized Coefficients (beta) indicate the relative importance of the predictors in terms of their unique contribution in predicting $Y$. Specifically, the larger the absolute value of beta, the more important the predictor. The same information is provided also by the absolute value of the part correlations. In this example, motivation (beta = .642) is more important than self-reliance (beta = .251) in predicting task involvement; compare also the part correlations for the two predictors. Motivation (part = .601) is more important than self-reliance (part = .235) in predicting task involvement.

# Comparison of Full and Restricted Regression Models

In multiple regression analysis, more is not necessarily better. If two variables can predict about the same amount of variance as four variables, the two-variable model is more practical and cost efficient (e.g., the expense of collecting data on two variables may be half that of collecting data on four variables). Consider the multiple regression model for predicting $Y$ from $X_1$, $X_2$, $X_3$, and $X_4$:

$$\hat{Y} = b_1X_1 + b_2X_2 + b_3X_3 + b_4X_4 + a. \tag{19.3}$$

After removing the predictors $X_3$ and $X_4$, the resulting multiple regression model is

$$\hat{Y} = b_1X_1 + b_2X_2 + a. \tag{19.4}$$

If $R_1^2$ is the coefficient of determination with the model in Equation 19.3, referred to as **full model**, and $R_2^2$ is the coefficient of determination with the model in Equation 19.4, referred to as **restricted model**, the question is whether the difference $\Delta R^2 = R_1^2 - R_2^2$ is statistically significant—that is, to test the null hypothesis $H_0: \Delta R_{\text{pop.}}^2 = 0$. A failure to reject $H_0$ would indicate that the full and restricted regression models are equally effective in predicting $Y$ (i.e., account for the same proportion of variance in $Y$). In such a case, the predictive contribution of $X_3$ and $X_4$, over and above that provided by $X_1$ and $X_2$, is not statistically significant. Thus, it would be much better to use the more parsimonious restricted model (e.g., to save costs on collecting data for $X_3$ and $X_4$). This is a critical concept in the efficient use of multiple regression.

In general, if the full model has $k_1$ predictors and the restricted model $k_2$ predictors (selected from the predictors in the full model), the statistic for testing $H_0: \Delta R_{\text{pop.}}^2 = 0$ is

$$F = \frac{(R_1^2 - R_2^2)/(k_1 - k_2)}{(1 - R_1^2)/(n - k_1 - 1)}, \tag{19.5}$$

where $n$ is the sample size. The distribution of this statistic, assuming that $H_0$ is true, is the $F$ distribution with degrees of freedom: $k_1 - k_2$ in the numerator and $n - k_1 - 1$ in the denominator.

For example, suppose that $R_1^2 = .663$ for a full regression model with five predictors and $R_1^2 = .645$, for a restricted regression model with three predictors (selected from the five predictors in the full model). Given also that the sample size is $n = 81$, the $F$ statistic for testing $H_0 : \Delta R_{\text{pop.}}^2 = 0$ in this case is

$$F = \frac{(.663 - .645)/(5 - 3)}{(1 - .663)/(81 - 5 - 1)} = 2.003.$$

This $F$ statistic is compared to a critical value, $F_{\text{cv}} = 3.126$, found in the $F$-distribution table (Table 16.8) with degrees of freedom $5 - 3 = 2$ for the numerator and $81 - 5 - 1 = 75$ for the denominator, at $\alpha = .05$ level of significance. As the computed $F$ statistic (2.003) does not exceed the $F$ critical value (3.126), the null hypothesis is not rejected. The conclusion is that the restricted model with three predictors is as effective as the full model with five predictors in predicting the criterion variable ($Y$). In fact, the $F$ statistic obtained from Equation 19.5 with $R_2^2 = 0$ and $k_2 = 0$ can be used to test the full multiple regression model for statistical significance. Although it is sometimes important to understand the equations and logic behind model comparisons, Example 19.2 demonstrates that *SPSS* can provide these comparisons quite simply.

## Example 19.2

The purpose of this example is to illustrate the comparison of full and restricted regression models using *SPSS*. The model conducted first is a restricted model (Model 1). Then a full model (Model 2) is conducted. Model 2 includes all predictors from Model 1 and some additional predictors. With this, equation 19.4 represents (in general) Model 1, whereas equation 19.3 represents Model 2. The *SPSS* output reports the change in $R^2$ from Model 1 to Model 2 and information about its statistical significance. The data come from a study on predicting *mental health* ($Y$; **mh**) from *social functioning* ($X_1$; **sf**); *physical functioning* ($X_2$; **pf**); *health perception* ($X_3$; **hp**); and *body pain* ($X_4$; **bp**), using a random sample of 81 participants (only the first 24 cases can be seen in Figure 19.5).

To compare Model 1 (restricted) and Model 2 (full) using *SPSS*, follow these steps:

1. Click **Analyze**, click **Regression**, and click **Linear**.

2. Click **Reset** to clear the dialog box (if there is some previous information).

### Figure 19.5

*SPSS* data file with five variables: **mh** = mental health, **sf** = social functioning, **pf** = physical functioning, **hp** = health perception, **bp** = body pain.

© Cengage Learning

3. Click **mh**, and click ▶ to move it to the Dependent box.

4. Hold down the **Ctrl** key, click **sf** and **pf**, and click ▶ to move them to the Independent box. This is the set of (two) predictors with Model 1.

5. Click **Next**.

6. Hold down the **Ctrl** key, click **hp** and **bp**, and then click ▶ to move them to the Independent box.

7. Click **Statistics**. The options **Estimates** and **Model fit** should already be selected by default, so click **R Squared Change**, **Descriptives**, and **Part and partial correlations**.

8. Click **Continue**.

9. Click **OK**.

The *SPSS* output is provided in Figure 19.6 (for space consideration, the descriptive statistics and the correlation matrix are not presented). The results in the Model Summary table show that the two predictors in Model 1 account for a statistically significant amount of the variance in mental health (Y), $R^2 = .609$, $F(2, 78) = 60.618$, $p = .000$.

**Figure 19.6**

*SPSS* multiple regression results for *Model 1* (restricted) and *Model 2* (full).

**Model Summary**

| Model | R | R Square | Adjusted R Square | Std. Error of the Estimate | Change Statistics R Square Change | F Change | $df_1$ | $df_2$ | Sig. F Change |
|---|---|---|---|---|---|---|---|---|---|
| 1 | .780[a] | .609 | .598 | 12.886 | .609 | 60.618 | 2 | 78 | .000 |
| 2 | .786[b] | .617 | .597 | 12.905 | .009 | .885 | 2 | 76 | .417 |

a. Predictors: (Constant), Physical functioning, Social functioning

b. Predictors: (Constant), Physical functioning, Social functioning, Body pain, Health perception

**ANOVA** [c]

| Model | | Sum of Squares | df | Mean Square | F | Sig. |
|---|---|---|---|---|---|---|
| 1 | Regression | 20129.858 | 2 | 10064.929 | 60.618 | .000 [a] |
| | Residual | 12951.030 | 78 | 166.039 | | |
| | Total | 33080.889 | 80 | | | |
| 2 | Regression | 20424.745 | 4 | 5106.186 | 30.663 | .000 [b] |
| | Residual | 12656.144 | 76 | 166.528 | | |
| | Total | 33080.889 | 80 | | | |

a. Predictors: (Constant), Physical functioning, Social functioning

b. Predictors: (Constant), Physical functioning, Social functioning, Body pain, Health perception

c. Dependent Variable: Mental health

**Coefficients**[a]

| Model | | Unstandardized Coefficients B | Std. Error | Standardized Coefficients Beta | t | Sig. | Correlations Zero-order | Partial | Part |
|---|---|---|---|---|---|---|---|---|---|
| 1 | (Constant) | −22.065 | 9.280 | | −2.378 | .020 | | | |
| | Social functioning | .774 | .083 | .688 | 9.281 | .000 | .752 | .724 | .658 |
| | Physical functioning | .271 | .092 | .218 | 2.947 | .004 | .420 | .317 | .209 |
| 2 | (Constant) | −23.240 | 9.697 | | −2.397 | .019 | | | |
| | Social functioning | .699 | .110 | .621 | 6.347 | .000 | .752 | .589 | .450 |
| | Physical functioning | .257 | .093 | .207 | 2.776 | .007 | .420 | .303 | .197 |
| | Health perception | .136 | .102 | .122 | 1.327 | .189 | .555 | .150 | .094 |
| | Body pain | −9.70E-03 | .084 | −.010 | −.115 | .908 | .394 | −.013 | −.008 |

a. Dependent Variable: Mental health

© Cengage Learning

The change in $R^2$ from Model 1 to Model 2, however, is not statistically significant, $R^2$ change = .009, $F(2, 76) = 0.885$, $p = .417$. Thus, health perception and body pain do not account for a statistically significant proportion of the variance in mental health ($Y$) over and above the proportion accounted for by social functioning and physical functioning. An implication for predicting mental health for the study population is that it would be better to use the more parsimonious Model 1, with social functioning and physical functioning as predictors. This will also likely reduce the costs and participant time associated with the data collection in the future.

Following the description and interpretation of results in the table's Model Summary, ANOVA, and Coefficients, provided with Example 19.1, one can interpret the results with the *SPSS* output in Figure 19.6, separately for Model 1 and Model 2. As an illustration, notice that the part correlation between mental health ($Y$) and social functioning ($X_1$) is .658 with Model 1 and .450, with Model 2. This is because when Model 1 is used, only physical functioning ($X_2$; **pf**) is removed from social functioning ($X_1$; **sf**) and the resulting part correlation between $Y$ and $X_1$ is: $r_{Y(1.2)} = .658$. With Model 2, however, physical functioning ($X_2$), health perceptions ($X_3$), and body pain ($X_4$) are removed from social functioning ($X_1$), so the part correlation between $Y$ and $X_1$ is $r_{Y(1.234)} = .450$.

# Multicollinearity

**Multicollinearity** occurs when there are (moderate to high) correlations among the predictors. There are three major problems related to multicollinearity in multiple linear regression. First, when the correlation between predictors increases, the proportion of the variance in the criterion variable ($Y$) uniquely accounted for by these predictors decreases. Thus, it is difficult to determine the relative importance of individual predictors in the presence of multicollinearity, as the effects of the predictors are confounded due to the correlations among the predictors. In Figure 19.2, for example, the multicollinearity among the two predictors is represented by part $C$. Imagine that as circles $X_1$ and $X_2$ increasingly overlap, part $C$ gets larger at the expense of parts $A$ and $B$. This is a helpful way to visualize how the increase in multicollinearity leads to smaller unique contributions of $X_1$ and $X_2$ in predicting $Y$ (or, equivalently, smaller squared part correlations $r^2_{Y(1.2)}$ and $r^2_{Y(2.1)}$, as they are proportion measures for parts $A$ and $B$, respectively). Second, when the predictors are highly correlated, changes (increase/decrease) in one predictor are naturally associated with changes in the other predictors. Therefore, when multicollinearity exists, it is not quite realistic to interpret the regression coefficient for a predictor as representing its effect while holding the other predictors constant. Finally, the higher the multicollinearity, the larger the standard errors of the regression coefficients and, therefore, the lower the accuracy of the prediction with future samples.

Given these difficulties for estimating and interpreting regression coefficients when the predictors are correlated, it is important to know the degree to which multicollinearity exists. If one regresses one predictor—say, $X_j$—on the remaining predictors (i.e., using $X_j$ as a criterion variable in a multiple linear regression), the resulting coefficient of multiple determination ($R^2_j$) will show the degree to which $X_j$ correlates with the other predictors. Conversely, the difference $1 - R^2_j$, called **tolerance** of $X_j$, will indicate the degree of nonredundancy between $X_j$ and the remaining predictors. The tolerance may take on values from 0.00 to 1.00. The closer the tolerance to 1.00, the lower the multicollinearity caused by predictor $X_j$. Likewise, the closer the tolerance is to 0.00, the higher the multicollinearity. The reciprocal of the tolerance, $1/(1 - R^2_j)$, is referred to as **variance** inflation factor (*VIF*) for $X_j$. Evidently, *VIF* can take on values of 1.00 (when $R_j^2 = 0$) and higher. The closer the *VIF* value for a given predictor to 1.00, the lower the multicollinearity caused by this predictor. A rule of thumb is that a predictor with *VIF* greater than 10 should be a concern regarding its contribution to multicollinearity. The "inflation" effect of the *VIF* on the variance of the regression coefficient $b_j$ (for the predictor $X_j$) can be seen from the statistical formula

$$\mathrm{Var}(b_j) = \frac{s_e^2}{(n-1)s_j^2} \times \frac{1}{1 - R_j^2}, \tag{19.6}$$

where $n$ is the sample size, $s_e^2$ is the error variance (squared standard error of estimate), and $s_j^2$ is the variance of the predictor $X_j$. Clearly, the smallest variance for the regression coefficient $b_j$ (thus, its smallest standard error) is achieved when $R_j^2 = 0$ (or, equivalently, $VIF_j = 1$). This will occur when the predictor $X_j$ is orthogonal to the remaining predictors (i.e., does not correlate with any of them). This is important to keep in mind when making decisions related to selection of predictors in multiple linear regression analysis.

## Example 19.3

This example illustrates the *SPSS* output for tolerance and variance inflation factor (*VIF*) using the multiple regression with Model 2 in Example 19.2: mental health (*Y*) regressed on social functioning (**sf**), physical functioning (**pf**), health perceptions (**hp**), and body pain (**bp**). To run the *SPSS* multiple regression for this purpose, follow these steps:

1. Click **Analyze**, click **Regression**, and click **Linear**.
2. Click **Reset** to clear the dialog box.
3. Click **mh**, and click ▶ to move it to the Dependent box.
4. Hold down the **Ctrl** key, click **sf**, **pf**, **hp**, and **bp**, and then click ▶ to move them to the Independent box.
5. Click **Statistics**. The options Estimates and Model fit should already be selected by default, so click **Part and partial correlations**, and click **Collinearity diagnostics**.
6. Click **Continue**.
7. Click **OK**.

Figure 19.7 includes only the Coefficients table from the resulting *SPSS* output. The other two tables, Model Summary and ANOVA, are not included because they are provided with the results for Model 2 in Figure 19.6.

The examination of the Collinearity Statistics column shows that, overall, there should not be a serious concern about multicollinearity (e.g., all *VIFs* < 2). Physical functioning is the predictor least contributing (almost none) to multicollinearity (Tolerance = .903, *VIF* = 1.108). It is interesting to note that the predictor most contributing to multicollinearity, social functioning (Tolerance = .526, *VIF* = 1.900), is at the same time the most important predictor in terms of unique contribution to the prediction of mental health (beta = .621). Clearly, it would be a mistake to exclude social functioning from the regression model based solely on its relatively lower performance on multicollinearity. To check this, notice that the coefficient of determination with all four predictors is $R^2 = .617$, but it drops down to $R^2 = .415$, after excluding social functioning from the regression model. Using the procedure described in model comparison above, one can test the $R^2$ change for statistical significance to determine whether keeping social functioning in the multiple regression model would make a difference in predicting mental health ($n = 81$).

**Figure 19.7**

Selected *SPSS* output with multiple regression for the prediction of mental health ($Y$) from social functioning ($X_1$), physical functioning ($X_2$), health perception ($X_3$), and body pain ($X_4$).

**Coefficients**[a]

| Model | Unstandardized Coefficients | | Standardized Coefficients | $t$ | Sig. | Correlations | | | Collinearity Statistics | |
|---|---|---|---|---|---|---|---|---|---|---|
| | B | Std. Error | Beta | | | Zero-order | Partial | Part | Tolerance | *VIF* |
| 1  (Constant) | −23.240 | 9.697 | | −2.397 | .019 | | | | | |
|    Social functioning | .699 | .110 | .621 | 6.347 | .000 | .752 | .589 | .450 | .526 | 1.900 |
|    Physical functioning | .257 | .093 | .207 | 2.776 | .007 | .420 | .303 | .197 | .903 | 1.108 |
|    Health perception | .136 | .102 | .122 | 1.327 | .189 | .555 | .150 | .094 | .596 | 1.679 |
|    Body pain | −9.70E-03 | .084 | −.010 | −.115 | .908 | .394 | −.013 | −.008 | .714 | 1.401 |

a. Dependent Variable: Mental health

# Cross-Validation

When a multiple regression equation is developed from a given data set, the question is how well this equation works for prediction with future samples. The sample initially used to develop a multiple regression equation is referred to as screening sample. The regression coefficients obtained with the screening sample are aimed at maximizing the coefficient of multiple correlation, $R$ (the correlation between the actual and predicted $Y$ scores, $r_{Y\hat{Y}}$). Thus, the coefficient of multiple determination produced with the screening sample is always greater than its counterpart produced by the original regression equation applied for any other (calibration) sample, $R^2_{cal}$. The $R^2$ shrinkage is estimated with the difference $\varepsilon = R^2_{scr} - R^2_{cal}$. If the researchers decide that the shrinkage is acceptably small, and $R^2$ is sufficiently large, the regression equation based on the original (screening) sample can be used for predictions with future samples.

The estimation of $R^2$ shrinkage is called **cross-validation**. When the shrinkage is small, one can combine the screening and calibration samples and use the regression equation obtained for the combined sample in future predictions. The coefficients in the regression equation for the combined sample are more stable because the number of participants in the combined sample is greater than those in either the screening or calibration sample. If it is difficult to obtain a second (i.e., calibration) sample, and the original sample is sufficiently large, one can randomly split the original sample into two (screening and calibration) subsamples.

The amount of $R^2$ shrinkage depends, among other things, on the ratio of sample size to number of predictors ($n/k$). Other things being equal, the larger this ratio, the better the regression equation will cross-validate in applications with future samples. According to a recommended rule (Stevens, 2009), about 15 participants per predictor are needed for a multiple regression equation to predict well with future samples. For example, it has been demonstrated that with a 15/1 ratio, the $R^2$ shrinkage is small (less than .05), with a probability of .90, if the coefficient of determination for the population is $R^2_{pop} = .50$.

# Statistical Power, Effect Size, and Sample Size

Let $P$ denote the statistical *power* of a test—that is, the probability of rejecting the null hypothesis when it is indeed false. For the null hypothesis $H_0$: $R^2_{pop} = 0$, the power of the test, $P$, depends on the level of significance ($\alpha$), sample size ($n$), number of predictors ($k$), and *effect size*:

$$ES = R^2_{pop}/(1 - R^2_{pop}).\qquad(19.7)$$

The following sample size formula is for prespecified $P$, $\alpha$, and $ES$ values:

$$n = \frac{L}{ES} + k + 1,\qquad(19.8)$$

where $L$ is a parameter reported in Cohen's statistical power tables as depending on $P$, $\alpha$, and $k$ (Cohen, 2003; see Table 19.1).

**TABLE 19.1** $L$ Values (for $\alpha = .05$) for sample size in multiple regression.

| | | | | | Power | | | | | | |
|---|---|---|---|---|---|---|---|---|---|---|---|
| **K** | .10 | .30 | .50 | .60 | .70 | .75 | .80 | .85 | .90 | .95 | .99 |
| 1 | .43 | 2.06 | 3.84 | 4.90 | 6.17 | 6.94 | 7.85 | 8.98 | 10.51 | 13.00 | 18.37 |
| 2 | .62 | 2.78 | 4.96 | 6.21 | 7.70 | 8.59 | 9.64 | 10.92 | 12.65 | 15.44 | 21.40 |
| 3 | .78 | 3.30 | 5.76 | 7.15 | 8.79 | 9.77 | 10.90 | 12.30 | 14.17 | 17.17 | 23.52 |
| 4 | .91 | 3.74 | 6.42 | 7.92 | 9.68 | 10.72 | 11.94 | 13.42 | 15.41 | 18.57 | 25.24 |
| 5 | 1.03 | 4.12 | 6.99 | 8.59 | 10.45 | 11.55 | 12.83 | 14.39 | 16.47 | 19.78 | 26.73 |
| 6 | 1.13 | 4.46 | 7.50 | 9.19 | 11.14 | 12.29 | 13.62 | 15.26 | 17.42 | 20.86 | 28.05 |
| 7 | 1.23 | 4.77 | 7.97 | 9.73 | 11.77 | 12.96 | 14.35 | 16.04 | 18.28 | 21.84 | 29.25 |
| 8 | 1.32 | 5.06 | 8.41 | 10.24 | 12.35 | 13.59 | 15.02 | 16.77 | 19.08 | 22.74 | 30.36 |
| 9 | 1.40 | 5.33 | 8.81 | 10.71 | 12.89 | 14.17 | 15.65 | 17.45 | 19.83 | 23.59 | 31.39 |
| 10 | 1.49 | 5.59 | 9.19 | 11.15 | 13.40 | 14.72 | 16.24 | 18.09 | 20.53 | 24.39 | 32.37 |
| 11 | 1.56 | 5.83 | 9.56 | 11.58 | 13.89 | 15.24 | 16.80 | 18.70 | 21.20 | 25.14 | 33.29 |
| 12 | 1.64 | 6.06 | 9.90 | 11.98 | 14.35 | 15.74 | 17.34 | 19.28 | 21.83 | 25.86 | 34.16 |
| 13 | 1.71 | 6.29 | 10.24 | 12.36 | 14.80 | 16.21 | 17.85 | 19.83 | 22.44 | 26.55 | 35.00 |
| 14 | 1.78 | 6.50 | 10.55 | 12.73 | 15.22 | 16.67 | 18.34 | 20.36 | 23.02 | 27.20 | 35.81 |
| 15 | 1.84 | 6.71 | 10.86 | 13.09 | 15.63 | 17.11 | 18.81 | 20.87 | 23.58 | 27.84 | 36.58 |
| 16 | 1.90 | 6.91 | 11.16 | 13.43 | 16.03 | 17.53 | 19.27 | 21.37 | 24.13 | 28.45 | 37.33 |
| 18 | 2.03 | 7.29 | 11.73 | 14.09 | 16.78 | 18.34 | 20.14 | 22.31 | 25.16 | 29.62 | 38.76 |
| 20 | 2.14 | 7.65 | 12.26 | 14.71 | 17.50 | 19.11 | 20.96 | 23.20 | 26.13 | 30.72 | 40.10 |
| 22 | 2.25 | 8.00 | 12.77 | 15.30 | 18.17 | 19.83 | 21.74 | 24.04 | 27.06 | 31.77 | 41.37 |
| 24 | 2.36 | 8.33 | 13.02 | 15.87 | 18.82 | 20.53 | 22.49 | 24.85 | 27.94 | 32.76 | 42.59 |
| 28 | 2.56 | 8.94 | 14.17 | 16.93 | 20.04 | 21.83 | 23.89 | 26.36 | 29.60 | 34.64 | 44.87 |
| 32 | 2.74 | 9.52 | 15.02 | 17.91 | 21.17 | 23.04 | 25.19 | 27.77 | 31.14 | 36.37 | 46.98 |
| 36 | 2.91 | 10.06 | 15.82 | 18.84 | 22.23 | 24.18 | 16.41 | 29.09 | 32.58 | 38.00 | 48.96 |
| 40 | 3.08 | 10.57 | 16.58 | 19.71 | 23.23 | 25.25 | 27.56 | 30.33 | 33.94 | 39.54 | 50.83 |
| 50 | 3.46 | 11.75 | 18.31 | 21.72 | 25.53 | 27.71 | 30.20 | 33.19 | 37.07 | 43.07 | 55.12 |
| 60 | 3.80 | 12.81 | 19.88 | 23.53 | 27.61 | 29.94 | 32.59 | 35.77 | 39.89 | 46.25 | 58.98 |
| 70 | 4.12 | 13.79 | 21.32 | 25.20 | 29.52 | 31.98 | 34.79 | 38.14 | 42.48 | 49.17 | 62.53 |
| 80 | 4.41 | 14.70 | 22.67 | 26.75 | 31.29 | 33.88 | 36.83 | 40.35 | 44.89 | 51.89 | 65.83 |
| 90 | 4.69 | 15.56 | 23.93 | 28.21 | 32.96 | 35.67 | 38.75 | 42.14 | 47.16 | 54.44 | 68.92 |
| 100 | 4.95 | 16.37 | 25.12 | 29.59 | 34.54 | 37.36 | 40.56 | 44.37 | 49.29 | 56.85 | 71.84 |

*Note:* $k$ = number of predictors; $k = 1$ is the case of simple linear regression.

Effect size enables researchers to decide *a priori* (i.e., before a study) what $R^2_{pop}$ will be necessary for both statistical and practical significance. Suppose that $R^2_{pop}$ as small as .20 is of interest for a multiple regression equation with five predictors ($k = 5$). How many participants are necessary to attain a power of .90 to detect the prespecified $R^2_{pop} = .20$ at the .05 level of significance? For $P = .90$, $k = 5$, and $\alpha = .05$, the Cohen's table for $L$ values (Table 19.1) provides $L = 16.47$. With $R^2_{pop} = .20$, the effect size is $ES = .20/(1 - .20) = .25$. Using Equation 19.8, we obtain the sample size $n = 16.47/.25 + 5 + 1 = 71.88$ ($\approx 72$). Thus, a sample of 72 participants is necessary to reject $H_0$: $R^2_{pop} = 0$ at the .05 level of significance and a power of .90, given that the actual $R^2_{pop}$ is as small as .20.

It is important to note that a sample size based on statistical power method does not necessarily guarantee stable regression coefficients. That is, obtaining a desired statistical power does not necessarily mean that the regression equation will provide accurate prediction with future samples. Therefore, along with sample size, effect size, and statistical power, other factors related to accuracy of prediction with multiple regression (e.g., multicollinearity, cross-validation, and data outliers) should also be taken into account.

# Outliers and Influential Data Points

The estimates of multiple regression parameters are sensitive to extreme observations ("outliers"). Therefore, it is important to examine the data for outliers and data points that have undue effect on the estimates ("influential data points"). One possible cause of outliers is data errors (e.g., data recording and data entry). Outliers not related to data errors may also occur when there are observations that represent extreme (large or small) magnitudes on variables involved in the regression model. Suppose that a researcher predicts "physical health" using a random sample of individuals that happens to include several people with chronic illnesses. The observations for the persons with chronic illnesses may be outliers, but they are not erroneous. Such observations require a special examination to build a better model and to better understand the phenomenon of physical health. The decision whether to delete an outlier from a data set should be based on criteria established in advance. Presenting results obtained with and without outliers and/or influential data points may enhance the researcher's final conclusions.

Fortunately, *SPSS* (and other major statistical packages) provide indices for detecting outliers and influential data points. Among the indices available with the *SPSS* multiple regression analysis, the following are the three most recommended procedures:

1. *Studentized deleted residual.* This index is used to detect outliers on *Y*. For any observation, the studentized deleted residual (*sdr*) is calculated for the sample, with this observation excluded ("deleted"). As the *sdr* index follows a Student *t* distribution, there should be a "red flag" for an outlier on *Y* when the studentized deleted residual for an observation is greater than 3.00 in absolute value—that is, $|sdr| > 3.00$.

2. *Leverage value.* This index is used to detect outliers on *X*—that is, observations with extreme (high or small) values on some predictors. A leverage value, denoted $h_{jj}$, is considered large when it exceeds $3(k + 1)/n$, where $k$ is the number of predictors and $n$ is the sample size. For example, with $n = 100$ and $k = 4$, a leverage greater than $3(5)/100 = 0.15$ is large.

3. *Cook's distance.* This index is used to detect influential data points. It should be noted that an observation may not be an outlier but may still influence the estimates

of the regression coefficients, thus causing problems with the accuracy of prediction with future samples. The *Cook's distance* (*CD*), proposed by Cook (1977), considers the effect of deleting an observation on the residual of all observations. It measures the impact of a specific observation on the estimates of regression parameters; the calculation of the *CD* involves the sum of squared differences between the predicted *Y* scores obtained with, and then without, the specific observation. All *CD* values are positive, but a *CD* value greater than 1.00 is considered large (i.e., $CD > 1.00$ indicates an influential data point).

## Example 19.4: Detecting Outliers and Influential Data Points

The purpose of this example is to illustrate some indices for detecting outliers or influential data points reported with the *SPSS* multiple regression output. The multiple regression in Example 19.3 is used again, and so steps 1–6 should be done to use the *SPSS* multiple regression with the data in Figure 19.5. In addition, to obtain information about outliers and influential data points, insert the following two steps right after step 6 in Example 19.3:

- Click **Save**. In the **Linear Regression: Save** dialog box, (a) select **Cook's**, select **Leverage values**, from the Distances box (left panel); and (b) select **Standardized** deleted from the Residuals box (right panel).

- Click **Continue**.

As a result, three additional variables appear in the *SPSS* Data Editor: **sdr_1** (studentized deleted residual), **coo_1** (Cook's distance), and **leve_1** (leverage value). The Residuals Statistics table (Figure 19.8), provided with the *SPSS* output, includes descriptive statistics for all residual statistics available in the Linear Regression: Save box (of which we selected only Cook's, Leverage values, and Standardized deleted).

In the Residuals Statistics table, both the minimum and maximum values for Stud. Deleted Residual (*sdr*) are greater than 3.00 in absolute value (−3.162 and 3.054, respectively), thus indicating the presence of at least two outliers on *Y*. The outliers on *Y* can be identified by selecting cases that satisfy the condition $|sdr\_1| > 3.00$ for the values in the column named **sdr_1** in the *SPSS* Data Editor. Further, the maximum value for the Cook's distance (1.577) is greater than 1.00, thus indicating that there is at least one influential data point. The influential data points can be identified by selecting cases

**Figure 19.8**

Residual statistics with the multiple regression for predicting mental health from social functioning, physical functioning, health perception, and body pain.

### Residuals Statistics[a]

| | Minimum | Maximum | Mean | Std. Deviation | N |
|---|---|---|---|---|---|
| Predicted Value | 25.85 | 85.03 | 67.70 | 15.978 | 81 |
| Std. Predicted Value | −2.620 | 1.085 | .000 | 1.000 | 81 |
| Standard Error of Predicted Value | 1.708 | 8.834 | 2.969 | 1.218 | 81 |
| Adjusted Predicted Value | 19.02 | 85.08 | 68.00 | 16.429 | 81 |
| Residual | −31.25 | 34.15 | .00 | 12.578 | 81 |
| Std. Residual | −2.422 | 2.647 | .000 | .975 | 81 |
| Stud. Residual | −2.990 | 2.899 | −.010 | 1.038 | 81 |
| Deleted Residual | −52.93 | 40.98 | −.30 | 14.489 | 81 |
| Stud. Deleted Residual | −3.162 | 3.054 | −.015 | 1.060 | 81 |
| Mahal. Distance | .413 | 36.502 | 3.951 | 5.327 | 81 |
| Cook's Distance | .000 | 1.577 | .036 | .179 | 81 |
| Centered Leverage Value | .005 | .456 | .049 | .067 | 81 |

a. Dependent Variable: Mental health

© Cengage Learning

that satisfy the condition **coo_1 > 1.00** (i.e., *CD* > 1.00) for the values in the column named **coo_1** in the *SPSS* Data Editor. To decide whether the maximum value of the Centered Leverage Value (i.e., $h_{jj}$) is a "red flag" for the presence of (at least one) outlier on *X*, we compare this value (0.456) to $3(k + 1)/n = 3(4 + 1)/81 = 0.1852$; (with the data in this example, $n = 81$, $k = 4$). Because the maximum leverage value (0.456) exceeds the "cutoff" value (0.1852), it would be necessary to trace cases for outliers on *X* in the column named **leve_1** in the *SPSS* Data Editor.

# Interaction in Multiple Regression

As described earlier, the interpretation of any regression coefficient (*b*) is based on the assumption that the relationship between the criterion variable (*Y*) and the predictor ($X_j$) is the same for any fixed value of the other predictors. If this assumption is not true, there is an interaction between $X_j$ and the other predictors. To test for interaction between any two predictors, $X_j$ and $X_m$, one can add their product, $X_j X_m$, to the set of predictors in the regression equation. For example, to test for interaction between $X_1$ and $X_2$ in a regression equation with two predictors (Equation 19.1), the product $X_1X_2$ is added as a third predictor, thus obtaining the regression equation

$$\hat{Y} = b_1X_1 + b_2X_2 + b_3(X_1X_2) + a. \tag{19.9}$$

In Equation 19.9, the values of the third predictor, $X_3 = X_1X_2$, are obtained by multiplying the values of $X_1$ and $X_2$. If the regression coefficient $b_3$ is not statistically significant, there is no statistical interaction between $X_1$ and $X_2$.

The unique predictive effect of $X_1$ and $X_2$, with Equation 19.9, will always be lower than their unique predictive effect with Equation 19.1 (that is, before including their product as a predictor). This is because $X_1$ and $X_2$ are both highly correlated with their product ($X_1X_2$), which increases their multicollinearity, thus decreasing their unique predictive effect. In fact, it does not make much sense to interpret the unique predictive effect of predictors in the presence of interaction between them. It would be better, for example, to divide the sample into groups by score levels on one predictor (e.g., low, medium, and high) and to determine the predictive effect of the other predictor for each group separately. Or it might be useful to develop separate regression equations for fixed values of one of the predictors. The presence or absence of interaction between two predictors, however, does not depend on the level of correlation (multicollinearity) between them.

## Example 19.5: Exploring the Interaction Between Predictors

The purpose of this example is to test for interaction between two predictors, motivation ($X_1$) and self-reliance ($X_2$), in the prediction of task involvement (*Y*), using *SPSS* with the data in Example 19.1. To obtain the values for the product $X_1X_2$ in *SPSS* follow these steps:

1. In the *SPSS* Data Editor box, click **Transform**, and click **Compute**.

2. In the **Compute Variable** dialog box, type the name of the product variable, **X1X2**, in the **Target** *Variable* box, and type **X1\*X2** in the **Numeric Expression** box.

3. Click **OK**.

In step 2, **X1X2** is the name of the product variable, whereas **X1\*X2** is an algebraic expression for the values of this variable, obtained by multiplying the values of **X1** and **X2**. For the purpose of this example, Figure 19.9 shows only the **Coefficients** table from

**Figure 19.9**

Testing the product X1X2 for statistical significance to determine possible interaction between motivation (X1) and self-reliance (X2) in predicting task involvement (Y).

**Coefficients**[a]

| | | Unstandardized Coefficients | | Standardized Coefficients | | |
|---|---|---|---|---|---|---|
| Model | | B | Std. Error | Beta | $t$ | Sig. |
| 1 | (Constant) | −2.270 | 3.896 | | −.583 | .568 |
| | motivation | 1.039 | .549 | 1.140 | 1.893 | .077 |
| | self-reliance | .823 | .650 | .717 | 1.266 | .224 |
| | X1X2 | −7.53E-02 | .087 | −.804 | −.862 | .402 |

a. Dependent Variable: Task involvement

© Cengage Learning

the *SPSS* output for the multiple regression with three predictors: motivation (**X1**), self-reliance (**X2**), and their product (**X1X3**).

The results in Figure 19.9 show that the regression coefficient for the predictor **X1X2** (the product of **X1** and **X2**) is not statistically significant ($p = .402$). Thus, we can conclude that there is no statistically significant interaction between motivation (**X1**) and self-reliance (**X2**) in predicting task involvement (*Y*). Note that the regression coefficient for motivation is not statistically significant ($p = .077$), but it is statistically significant ($p = .001$) when product **X1X2** is not included in the regression equation. As alluded to earlier, this should not be a surprise, given that the high correlation between any predictor and its product with another predictor increases the multicollinearity for this predictor.

# Selection of Predictors in Multiple Regression

Given a set of potential predictors, how many and which predictors to select depends on various (practical, theoretical, statistical, or circumstantial) considerations. It is methodologically sound that researchers specify criteria for "best" set of predictors before conducting a regression analysis. Particular attention should be paid to errors that occur when relevant predictors are omitted or irrelevant predictors are included into the regression equation. Such errors are referred to as *specification errors*. Caution is required when predictors are deleted from the equation (e.g., with the purpose of reducing multicollinearity) because the removal of relevant predictors is a serious specification error. Described in this section are five approaches to statistical selection of predictors in multiple regression: forward, backward, stepwise, blockwise, and hierarchical selection.

## Forward Selection

The first step in forward selection consists of selecting the predictor that has the highest zero-order (Pearson $r$) correlation with the criterion variable, *Y*. At any subsequent step, the predictor producing the greatest increment in $R^2$ (i.e., the highest squared part correlation with *Y*) enters the equation if it meets the criterion of inclusion (e.g., statistical significance at the .05 level). If not, the procedure terminates. A major drawback of the forward selection is that once a predictor enters the equation, it stays in the equation, although it might have lost its initial importance with new predictors added to the equation.

## Backward Selection

The backward selection begins with all predictors in the equation and removes them one at a time until the final equation is obtained. At each step, the predictor that produces the smallest increment $R^2$ (i.e., the smallest squared part correlation with *Y*) is selected and tested for removal (e.g., removed if its squared part correlation with *Y* is not statistically significant at the .05 level).

## Stepwise Selection

The stepwise selection combines the methods of forward selection and backward elimination. It works as a forward selection, but at each step the predictors that are in the equation are reexamined for possible backward elimination. In this way, predictors that were suitable to enter the equation at previous steps, but lost much of their predictive power when additional predictors were added, may be removed from the regression equation. This is an important advantage of the stepwise selection over the forward selection.

## Blockwise Selection

In blockwise selection, predictors are grouped in "blocks" (e.g., Block 1–demographic variables, Block 2–academic performance, and Block behavioral variables). The assignment of variables to blocks and the order of the blocks is based on some theoretical and/or empirical considerations. First, a stepwise selection is conducted for the predictors in the first block. With the other blocks, one at a time, a stepwise selection is conducted for the predictors in each block and the predictors that have survived the immediately preceding stepwise selection.

## Hierarchical Regression

In hierarchical regression, intact blocks (meaningful units) of predictors are forced into the regression equation, one at a time, to determine their unique contribution ($R^2$ change) to the prediction of the criterion variable, *Y*. Also, forcing some blocks (e.g., treatment variables) into the equation and conducting blockwise selection on others is a very useful combination in many research applications of multiple regression.

As an example from research in rehabilitation counseling, Enright (1996) used a hierarchical regression analysis in predicting career indecision from self-doubting career beliefs, disability status, age, and gender. The decision of using these four predictors stemmed from past research and preliminary analysis of predictive relationships between the criterion (career indecision) and potential predictors. The hierarchical regression included two steps: (1) a multiple regression model was conducted with three predictors: age, gender, and self-doubting career belief; and (2) a multiple regression analysis was conducted with these three predictors and the fourth predictor (disability status). The $R^2$ change from step 1 to step 2 was used to determine the significance of the prediction effect of disability status, over and above the combined prediction effect of age, gender, and self-doubting career belief. These two-step procedures were conducted for two different measures of career indecision: the *Career Decision Scale* and the *Vocational Identity Scale*. Additional regressions were performed to test the significance of interaction effects. The results from these tests strengthened the conclusions about the prediction of career indecision.

# Multivariate Analysis of Variance (MANOVA)

**Multivariate analysis of variance (MANOVA)** is employed when two or more groups are compared on a set of two or more dependent variables. For example, one can compare three groups of people categorized by disability type (e.g., blindness, spinal cord injury, and mental illness) on a set of three dependent variables that measure psychological adjustment (e.g., acceptance of disability, personal control, and self-efficacy). With this design, disability type is the independent variable, whereas the three variables of psychological adjustment are dependent variables. As a real-data example (Vaughan & Kinnier, 1996), adults with HIV disease were randomly assigned to one of three conditions: a life interview group, a traditional support group, and a waiting list group. The three groups (three levels of the independent variable "intervention condition") were compared on six (pretest-posttest) psychological measures of optimism, self-esteem, purpose in life, coping ability, psychological distress, and death anxiety. It is important to emphasize that decisions about using (a) MANOVA to compare groups on a set of dependent variables or (b) separate univariate analyses of variance (multiple ANOVAs) to compare groups on each dependent variable separately should be governed by the nature of the research question. The next sections reveal the rationale behind a choice between MANOVA and separate ANOVAs and illustrate MANOVA applications using *SPSS*.

# The Logic Behind MANOVA

Suppose that three groups, representing three treatment conditions, are compared on a single dependent variable, and the null hypothesis is that the means of the populations to which the groups belong are equal:

$$H_0 : \mu_1 = \mu_2 = \mu_3. \tag{19.10}$$

In the framework of univariate analysis of variance (ANOVA), this null hypothesis is tested with the $F$ statistic ($F = MS_B/MS_w$), where $MS_B$ (mean squares between) is the variance between the group means, and $MS_w$ (mean squares within) is the variance within the groups.

Suppose now that three groups are compared on a set of two dependent variables, $Y_1$ and $Y_2$. The null hypothesis in this case is that the three population means are equal on both $Y_1$ ($\mu_{11} = \mu_{12} = \mu_{13}$) and $Y_2$ ($\mu_{21} = \mu_{22} = \mu_{23}$), where the first part of the subscript indicates the (dependent, pretest, or posttest) variable and the second part, the group. In matrix algebra, this multivariate null hypothesis translates into "the population mean vectors are equal":

$$H_0 : \begin{pmatrix} \mu_{11} \\ \mu_{21} \end{pmatrix} = \begin{pmatrix} \mu_{12} \\ \mu_{22} \end{pmatrix} = \begin{pmatrix} \mu_{13} \\ \mu_{23} \end{pmatrix}. \tag{19.11}$$

Among the several statistics available for testing the multivariate null hypothesis, the most widely used is **Wilk's** $\Lambda$, where $\Lambda$ (*lambda*) is the ratio "within-group variability to total variability," denoted in matrix algebra as: $\Lambda = |W| / |T|$. The numerator, $|W|$, is a number (determinant) for the multivariate analog of the "within" variability in univariate ANOVA, whereas the denominator, $|T|$, is a number (determinant) for the multivariate analog to the "total" (between + within) variability in univariate ANOVA. Thus, $W$ is a matrix of the "sum of squares and cross products" for the set of dependent variables across all groups, whereas its determinant, ($|W|$), is a number called the generalized within variance for the set of variables. Similarly, $T$ is the "total" variance−covariance matrix and its determinant ($|T|$) is a number called generalized total variance for the set of variables; $T$ is the sum of "between-group" and "within-group" variability: $T = B + W$.

Ideally, $\Lambda = 0$ occurs when $|W| = 0$—that is, when the "within" (or "error") variance is zero (i.e., the total variance is accounted for by group differences). In the worst-case scenario, $\Lambda = 1$, which occurs when $|W| = |T|$ (i.e., the total variance is "within" [error] variance). Given this, $\Lambda$ value may be viewed as an *effect size* produced by differentiation among the groups being compared. Just keep in mind that the closer Wilk's $\Lambda$ is to zero, the larger the effect size for the differences between the groups on the set of dependent variables.

# MANOVA Versus Separate ANOVAs

It is important to emphasize that *Wilk's lambda* in MANOVA takes into account the correlations among the dependent variables, whereas such correlations are ignored when the groups are compared on each dependent variable separately using multiple ANOVAs. Also, a statistically significant *Wilk's lambda* does not necessarily mean that the groups differ on separate dependent variables. Rather, it indicates that the groups differ on some combination (linear composite) of dependent variables that have a common substantive meaning. Therefore, *Wilk's lambda* does not provide information about the overall type I error rate produced by using separate ANOVAs. It may even happen that *Wilk's lambda* is statistically significant, yet none of the univariate ANOVA test statistics is statistically significant. Conversely, a statistically nonsignificant *Wilk's lambda* may be followed by a statistically significant result for some univariate ANOVAs. Thus, conducting MANOVA as a preliminary step to using univariate ANOVAs is unnecessary (if not misleading). A misunderstanding on this matter is, however, still manifested in numerous applications of MANOVA in behavioral research. In fact, MANOVA and separate univariate ANOVAs address different research questions and provide different information about the data and their interpretation. The nature of the research question(s) should guide researchers in their choice (and proper applications) of MANOVA versus separate ANOVAs. Also, the results from the initial analysis may suggest the investigation of additional (refining) research questions that involve appropriate statistical methods (e.g., *t*-tests, discriminant analysis, and factor analysis).

# Univariate Research Questions

Using univariate ANOVAs is appropriate when the researcher wants to know the individual dependent variables on which the compared groups differ. One scenario in which this is the right question to ask is when the dependent variables are conceptually independent of one another, such as when one is a measure of anxiety and the other of oppositional behavior. In this case, it is not expected that some linear composite of dependent variables will reveal an underlying construct. Therefore, MANOVA is not necessary to compare the groups on this construct. Another situation in which using univariate ANOVAs is appropriate occurs when the researcher wants to examine relationships between the grouping variable (e.g., treatment condition) and individual dependent variables, either for exploratory purposes or to compare the results with previous studies on such relationships. For example, the effectiveness of a token economy behavior modification procedure, compared to other (control) methods, on altering oppositional behavior and anxious behavior (two dependent variables) would be best explored using two separate univariate ANOVAs.

As noted earlier, it is a common misconception that if the MANOVA statistic (*Wilk's lambda*) is statistically significant, this will maintain the overall probability of type I error (i.e., falsely reject the null hypothesis), with univariate ANOVAs at the adopted level of significance (e.g., $\alpha = 0.05$). Instead of following a significant MANOVA, one can maintain the overall (familywise) level of significance for univariate

ANOVAs by conducting each of them at a level lower than $\alpha$. Specifically, using the Bonferroni adjustment, one should use for each ANOVA a level of significance equal to $\alpha/k$, where $k$ is the number of univariate ANOVAs. For example, for the comparison of groups on four dependent variables ($k = 4$), each separate univariate ANOVA should be tested at the level of significance 0.0125 (i.e., 0.05/4) to maintain the familywise level of significance at 0.05. Also, it should be kept in mind that univariate ANOVAs ignore correlations among the dependent variables, thus opening the door for analysis and interpretation of redundant information.

# MANOVA Research Questions

Comparing groups on separate dependent variables through the use of separate univariate ANOVAs does not allow researchers to address broader and more insightful questions that involve relationships between the dependent variables. Such questions can be answered by using MANOVA, which would allow researchers to view substantive relationships from new perspectives. For example, the researcher may want to know (a) which subsets of dependent variables (if any) account for group separation, (b) what are the underlying constructs for such subsets, and (c) what is the relative contribution of individual dependent variables to group separation.

A significant omnibus MANOVA (statistically significant *Wilk's lambda*) means that the groups differ on some linear combination(s) of the dependent variables. Such linear combinations (linear composites) are referred to as **linear discriminant functions (LDFs)**. Thus, *LDF* is a latent construct that discriminates (separates) the groups. With $m$ groups and $k$-dependent variables, the numbers of possible *LDF*s is the smaller number of ($m - 1$) and $k$. For example, with three groups compared on four variables, there are two possible *LDF*s ($m - 1 = 3 - 1 = 2$; $k = 4$). Information about the *LDF*s and how they discriminate the groups is provided with discriminant analysis following a statistically significant *Wilk's lambda*.

As a point of comparison, note that the predicted $Y$ score ($\hat{Y}$) in multiple regression is a linear combination of the predictors ($\hat{Y} = b_1X_1 + b_2X_2 + \cdots + b_kX_k + a$) that maximally correlates with the observed $Y$ score ($r_{Y\hat{Y}} = \text{max}$), whereas the linear discriminant function (*LDF*) in discriminant analysis is a linear combination of dependent variables that maximally discriminates (separates) the groups.

# Assumptions in MANOVA

The statistical assumptions in MANOVA are closely related to those in ANOVA:

1. The participants are randomly sampled from the target population.
2. The observations (e.g., scores on a psychological inventory) are statistically independent of one another.
3. The dependent variables have a multivariate normal distribution within each group.
4. All groups have the same variance on each dependent variable.
5. The correlation between any two dependent variables must be the same in all groups.

It is difficult, if not impossible, that all assumptions be met precisely in practical applications of MANOVA. In particular, violation of any of the first two assumptions may jeopardize the validity of the MANOVA results. The violation of the second assumption may occur, for example, when the participants in a treatment condition work in small groups and interact with each other. Although MANOVA is robust to a large extent to violation of the last three assumptions, some caution is necessary. The third assumption is difficult to test, but for practical purposes, one can just test the normality of each dependent variable in each group separately (e.g., using *SPSS*; see Chapter 15, Figure 15.35). The violation of normality has little effect on the type I error rates, but serious departures from normality may reduce the statistical power of MANOVA test statistics (e.g., *Wilk's lambda*).

Taken together, the last two assumptions are equivalent to the assumption that all groups have the same within-group population covariance matrix. A test for homogeneity of covariance matrices, referred to as **Box's M**, is available with *SPSS* (and other major statistical packages). Box's M, however, is not dependable when the normality assumption is not met. The assumption of homogeneity of covariance matrices (assumptions 4 and 5 together) is taken care of relatively well with a balanced MANOVA design (the groups have equal sample size). This, however, is not the case with sharply unequal group sizes. Specifically, the omnibus MANOVA test becomes (a) "liberal" (i.e., makes it unduly easy to reject the null hypothesis) when the larger sample sizes are associated with the smaller variances, and (b) "conservative" (i.e., makes it unduly difficult to reject the null hypothesis) when the larger sample sizes are associated with the larger variances. An approach to dealing with this problem is to transform the original scores on the dependent variables. For example, if the scores on a dependent variable are proportions, one can stabilize the group variance on this variable by using the "square root" transformation (i.e., replacing each score by its square root value). For more information on transformations related to MANOVA assumptions, the reader is referred to Stevens (2009).

# MANOVA with Discriminant Analysis

As noted earlier, a statistically significant *Wilk's lambda* for the omnibus MANOVA test indicates that there is at least one linear combination of the dependent variables (linear discriminant function [*LDF*]) that maximally separates the groups. Specifically, the *LDF*s maximize the "between-to-within-group variability" ratio, $B/W$, where $B$ and $W$ are the multivariate analogs of "sum of squares between" ($SS_B$) and "sum of squares within" ($SS_W$), respectively, in univariate ANOVA. As $B$ is a measure of the differential effect of the grouping variable (e.g., treatment conditions), the larger the $B/W$ ratio, the larger the group separation.

Notice that the *LDF*s are determined in decreasing order of their contribution to the group separation, and they are orthogonal (uncorrelated) because, after an *LDF* is determined, its contribution to the group separation is "partialled out," so the next (less contributing) *LDF* is the one that maximizes the remaining (residualized) $B/W$ ratio. At each step, an *LDF* is tested for statistical significance by a chi-square statistic, with degrees of freedom equal to $(p - d)[k - (d + 1)]$, where $k$ = number of groups, $p$ = number of dependent variables, and $d$ = number of statistically significant *LDF*s determined at the previous steps.

## Example 19.6

The purpose of this example is to illustrate MANOVA, with discriminant analysis, using *SPSS*. The data come from an employment preparation survey for persons with multiple sclerosis. The research question in this example is "What aspects of quality of life separate persons from the study population who have different marital status (single, married, and divorced)?" The relative importance of individual dependent variables to the separation among the three groups of marital status (the independent variable) is also of interest. For the purposes of this example, six dependent variables related to "quality of life" in the survey were used: social life and experiences ($Y_1$); family life and experiences ($Y_2$); hobbies and recreational experiences ($Y_3$); educational and intellectual development ($Y_4$); experience of daily living ($Y_5$); and expectations and hopes for the future ($Y_6$).

The Pearson correlations between all pairs of these six dependent variables were statistically significant and varied from 0.48 to 0.68. Evidently, MANOVA is appropriate because the research question relates to differences among three groups (single, married, and divorced) on aspects of quality of life that may emerge as linear composites of six substantively related dependent variables ($Y_1, \ldots, Y_6$).

The *SPSS* syntax for conducting MANOVA, with a subsequent discriminant analysis, and *post hoc* comparisons of the groups on individual dependent variables (also of interest in this example) is provided with Table 19.2. To run the *SPSS* syntax, follow these steps:

1. In the *SPSS* Data Editor, click **File**, click **New**, and click **Syntax**.

2. In the *SPSS* Syntax Editor, type the syntax in Table 19.2.

3. In the *SPSS* Syntax Editor, click **Run**, click **All**.

Notice that another option for step 3 is to run the syntax in "steps": (a) MANOVA— select (highlight) syntax lines 1–2, click **Run**, click **Selection**; (b) Discriminant Analysis—select syntax lines 3–6, click **Run**, click **Selection**; and (c) *t*-tests for pairwise group comparisons—select the last six syntax lines (7–12), click **Run**, click **Selection**.

The *Wilk's lambda* ($\Lambda = 0.89$) was found to be statistically significant, $F(12, 2396) = 11.30$, $p < .001$. At this point, we can only conclude that there is a statistically significant difference between at least two (out of three) groups on some linear composite(s) of the six dependent variables that represent aspects of quality of life. The normality assumption, which is important primarily for the correctness of the Box's M statistic, was supported

**TABLE 19.2** *SPSS* syntax for MANOVA, subsequent discriminant analysis, and *post hoc* comparisons of three groups on six individual dependent variables.

```
MANOVA y1 y2 y3 y4 y5 y6 BY group(1,3)/
    PRINT CELLINFO(MEANS) HOMOGENEITY(COCHRAN, BOXM)/.

DISCRIMINANT GROUPS = group(1,3)/
    VARIABLES = y1 TO y6/
    METHOD = WILKS/FIN=0/FOUT=0/
    STATISTICS = FPAIR/.

T-TEST GROUPS = group(1,2)/
    VARIABLES = y1 TO y6.

T-TEST GROUPS = group(1,3)/
    VARIABLES = y1 TO y6.

T-TEST GROUPS = group(2,3)/
    VARIABLES = y1 TO y6.
```

to a large extent by the normality (P-P plot) test, provided in *SPSS*, for each dependent variable within each group. The Box's M value (156.42) was statistically significant, $\chi^2(42) = 155$, $p < .01$, thus indicating that the assumption of homogeneity of variance–covariance matrices is not met. The results with the univariate tests (which are not reported here), however, showed that the homogeneity of variance assumption was met for each individual dependent variable. With this knowledge, one can proceed with the analysis in this illustrative example, but in a real study, one also may use data transformations to improve the homogeneity of the variance–covariance matrices. (A discussion of data transformations is provided in Chapter 18.)

As a next step, the discriminant analysis in *SPSS* was used to determine which specific dependent variables define linear discriminant functions (*LDFs*) that represent aspects of quality of life separating the groups. Results from the *SPSS* output for the discriminant analysis, produced with the syntax in Table 19.2 (lines 3–6), are provided in Figure 19.9. As three groups are being compared on a set of six dependent variables, there are two possible *LDFs* (i.e., the smaller number of [3 − 1] and 6). The results in the Eigenvalues table show that the first linear discriminant function (*LDF*1) accounts for 91.5 percent of the total (between association) variance for the set of dependent variables across the groups. The remaining 8.5 percent of this variance are accounted for by the second linear discriminant function (*LDF*2). As noted earlier, the *LDFs* are orthogonal (uncorrelated) and ordered from most to least important.

The result in the **Wilk's lambda** table of Figure 19.10 indicates that the *Wilk's lambda* (.896) for the first linear discriminant functions (*LDF*1) is statistically significant ($\chi^2(12) = 132.214$, $p = .000$). The *Wilk's lambda* (.990) for the second linear discriminant functions (*LDF*2) is also statistically significant ($\chi^2(12) = 11.721$, $p = .039$). Examination of the Structure Matrix table of Figure 19.10 clearly indicates that the dependent variables $Y_2$, $Y_1$, and $Y_5$ correlate (in this order of correlation magnitudes) with *LDF*1, whereas $Y_6$, $Y_4$, and $Y_3$ correlate with *LDF*2. To determine possible redundancy in these correlations, we examine the Standardized Canonical Discriminant Function Coefficients table of Figure 19.10. The comparison of the standardized coefficients for $Y_2$, $Y_1$, and $Y_5$ in the column for *LDF*1 shows that $Y_5$ provides redundant information about *LDF*1 because its standardized coefficient (0.111) is much smaller than this for $Y_2$ (0.883) and $Y_1$ (0.452). Therefore, the meaning of *LDF*1 is determined by examining the conjoint meaning of $Y_2$ ("family life and experiences") and $Y_1$ ("social life and experiences"), with a leading role of $Y_2$ due to its very strong correlation with *LDF*1. Given this, we use the label "family and social life" for the first aspect of "quality of life," represented by *LDF*1. On the other side, the values of the standardized coefficients for $Y_6$ (0.777), $Y_4$ (.344), and $Y_3$ (0.431) do not indicate redundancy among these dependent variables in defining *LDF*2. Given this, we use the label "Education and hopes for the future" for the second aspect of "quality of life," represented by *LDF*2.

Two aspects of quality of life, "family and social life" (*LDF*1) and "education and hopes for the future" (*LDF*2) were identified that separate the three groups of marital status for persons with multiple sclerosis. The group means, called "group centroids," are provided in the Functions at Group Centroids table in the *SPSS* output (Figure 19.10) and graphically represented with Figure 19.11.

The omnibus null hypothesis in MANOVA states that the group centroids are equal for the study population. As shown in Figure 19.10, the three groups in this example are separated by two aspects of quality of life, with the strongest separation between "single" and "married" on the first aspect, "family and social life" (*LDF*1). The largest separation on the second aspect, "education and hopes for the future" (*LDF*2), is between the groups "single" and "divorced." Notice also that the group "married" is on the positive

**Figure 19.10**

*SPSS* output with the discriminant analysis for the comparison of three groups (single, married, and divorced) on a set of six dependent variables ($Y_1, \ldots, Y_6$).

**Eigen values**

| Function | Eigenvalue | % of Variance | Cumulative % | Canonical Correlation |
|---|---|---|---|---|
| 1 | .106[a] | 91.5 | 91.5 | .309 |
| 2 | .010[a] | 8.5 | 100.0 | .099 |

a. First 2 canonical discriminant functions were used in the analysis.

**Wilk's Lambda**

| Test of Function(s) | Wilk's Lambda | Chi-square | df | Sig. |
|---|---|---|---|---|
| 1 through 2 | .896 | 132.214 | 12 | .000 |
| 2 | .990 | 11.721 | 5 | .039 |

**Standardized Canonical Discriminant Function Coefficients**

| | Function 1 | Function 2 |
|---|---|---|
| Y1 | .452 | −1.245 |
| Y2 | .883 | .413 |
| Y3 | −.523 | .431 |
| Y4 | −.257 | .344 |
| Y5 | .111 | −.117 |
| Y6 | .079 | .777 |

**Structure Matrix**

| | Function 1 | Function 2 |
|---|---|---|
| Y2 | .881* | .337 |
| Y1 | .675* | −.073 |
| Y5 | .442* | .313 |
| Y6 | .463 | .591* |
| Y4 | .221 | .469* |
| Y3 | .216 | .432* |

Pooled within-group correlations between discriminating variables and standardized canonical discriminant functions. Variables ordered by absolute size of correlation within function.

*Largest absolute correlation between each variable and any discriminant function

**Functions at Group Centroids**

| GROUP | Function 1 | Function 2 |
|---|---|---|
| Single | −.502 | .204 |
| Married | .236 | 6.101 E-03 |
| Divorced | −.406 | −.141 |

Unstandardized canonical discriminant functions evaluated at group means

direction, whereas the other two groups are on the negative direction of "family and social life" (*LDF*1). In fact, the "divorced" group is on the negative directions of both aspects of quality of life (*LDF*1 and *LDF*2). [Note: The sample sizes of the groups are 171 (single), 835 (married), and 274 (divorced).]

The relative importance of a given dependent variable (which also is of interest in this example) is determined by the magnitude of its "*F*-to-remove" statistic, which indicates the impact of this dependent variable (if deleted) on the decrease of the group separation. The values of the *F*-to-remove statistics are provided in Table 19.3, along with the results from the tables Structure Matrix and Standardized Canonical Discriminant Function Coefficients in Figure 19.10. The *F*-to-remove statistic for $Y_1$ (23.802) is much higher than the values of this statistic for all other dependent variables. Thus, $Y_1$ ("social life and experiences") is the most important contributor to the separation of persons

**Figure 19.11**

Group centroids for three groups (single, married, divorced) separated by two linear discriminant functions: *LDF*1 = "family and social life" and *LDF*2 = "education and hopes for the future."

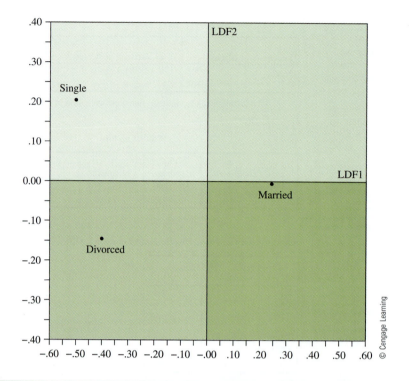

**TABLE 19.3**    Statistics of six "quality of life" variables related to two linear discriminant functions, *LDF1* and *LDF2*.

| VARIABLE | Correlation Coefficients | | Standardized Coefficients | | F-TO-REMOVE |
|---|---|---|---|---|---|
| | *LDF*1 | *LDF*2 | *LDF*1 | *LDF*2 | |
| $Y_1$ | .881* | .337 | 0.452 | −1.245 | 23.802 |
| $Y_2$ | .675* | −.073 | 0.883 | 0.413 | 7.483 |
| $Y_3$ | .442* | .313 | −0.523 | 0.431 | 8.021 |
| $Y_4$ | .463 | .591* | −0.257 | 0.344 | 2.332 |
| $Y_5$ | .221 | .469* | 0.111 | −0.117 | 1.861 |
| $Y_6$ | .216 | .432* | 0.079 | 0.777 | 0.357 |

*Note:* $Y_1$ = social life and experiences, $Y_2$ = family life and experiences, $Y_3$ = hobbies and recreational experiences, $Y_4$ = educational and intellectual development, $Y_5$ = experience of daily living, and $Y_6$ = expectations and hopes for the future; (* $p < .05$).
© Cengage Learning

with multiple sclerosis by their marital status. Conversely, the very small *F*-to-remove values for $Y_6$ (0.357) indicates that "experience and hopes for the future" has a negligible contribution to the multivariate group separation.

The *SPSS* output for MANOVA syntax in Table 19.2 (the last six lines) provides pairwise group comparisons. The results from these comparisons (which are not reported here for space consideration) showed, for example, that there was a statistically significant difference between the first two groups ("single" and "married") on each of the six dependent variables. One may wish to investigate other group contrasts—for example, to compare group "married" versus the other two groups together. More information on using *SPSS* in multivariate comparisons planned *a priori* is provided in the next section.

# MANOVA with Planned Comparisons

A question of interest with MANOVA applications may relate to some multivariate comparisons among groups that researchers have planned in advance. For example, in comparing four groups, the first two of which are variations of an experimental treatment and the other two control variations, on a set of two dependent variables (e.g., anxiety and depression), one may wish to compare (1) the two experimental groups versus the two control groups, (2) the two experimental groups, and (3) the two control groups. The null hypotheses associated with these three questions (in this order) are

$$H_{01} : \frac{\mu_1 + \mu_2}{2} = \frac{\mu_3 + \mu_4}{2}, \quad H_{02} : \mu_1 = \mu_2, \quad \text{and} \quad H_{03} : \mu_3 = \mu_4.$$

Representing $H_{01}$ in a "standard" form ($H_{01}: \mu_1 + \mu_2 - \mu_3 - \mu_4 = 0$), the coefficients for the group means provide the coding for this planned comparison (*contrast*), $\Psi_1$: 1 1 −1 −1. Similarly, the coefficients for the group means in the standard form of the second null hypothesis [$H_{02}: \mu_1 - \mu_2 + 0(\mu_3) + 0(\mu_4) = 0$] provide the coding for the contrast in this case, $\Psi_2$: 1 − 1 0 0. Finally, the coefficients for the group means in the standard form of the third null hypothesis [$H_{03}: 0(\mu_1) + 0(\mu_2) + \mu_3 - \mu_4 = 0$] provide the coding for the third contrast, $\Psi_3$: 0 0 1 −1. Notice that, for any two contrasts, the sum of the products of their coefficients is zero (e.g., $\Psi_1 \Psi_2 = (1)(1) + (1)(-1) + (-1)(0) + (-1)(0) = 0$); [**Check:** Show that $\Psi_1 \Psi_3 = 0$ and $\Psi_2 \Psi_3 = 0$].) This indicates that, if used with a balanced MANOVA design, the contrasts $\Psi_1$, $\Psi_2$, and $\Psi_3$ will be *orthogonal* (i.e., uncorrelated).

The advantage of having orthogonal contrasts in MANOVA is analogous to that of orthogonal predictors in multiple regression analysis; that is, the total contribution of each contrast to the multivariate between-groups variability is unique (i.e., not confounded with the contribution of other contrasts). Correlated contrasts may occur when (a) the sum of coefficient products is not equal to zero or (b) the compared groups do not have equal sample sizes. In such case, the unique contribution of each contrast is determined by partialing out its correlation with the other contrasts.

## Example 19.7

The purpose of this example is to illustrate how to test orthogonal contrasts for statistical significance using *SPSS*. Specifically, the preceding contrasts, $\Psi_1$, $\Psi_2$, and $\Psi_3$, are tested for statistical significance on a set of two dependent variables, $Y_1$ and $Y_2$, with a balanced design ($n_1 = n_2 = n_3 = n_4 = 50$). Table 19.4 provides the *SPSS* syntax, where y1 and y2 denote the dependent variables, and group denotes the grouping (independent) variable. Recall that the notations should match the names given to these variables in the *SPSS* Data Editor. The coefficients for the contrasts are enclosed in parentheses after SPECIAL

**TABLE 19.4**   *SPSS* syntax for MANOVA with planned orthogonal contrasts for the comparison of four groups on a set of two dependent variables.

```
MANOVA y1 TO y2 BY group(1,4)
    /CONTRAST(group) = SPECIAL(1 1 1 1    1 1 −1 −1    1 −1 0 0    0 0 1 −1)
    /PARTITION(group)
    /DESIGN = group(1), group(2), group(3)
    /PRINT = CELLINFO(MEAN, COV, COR)/.
```

**Figure 19.12**

Selected *SPSS* output for multivariate and univariate tests of significance for contrast $\Psi_1: \mu_1 + \mu_2 - \mu_3 - \mu_4$.

EFFECT .. **GROUP(1)**

**Multivariate Tests of Significance** (S = 1, M = 0, N = 96 1/2)

| Test Name | Value | Exact F | Hypoth. DF | Error DF | Sig. of F |
|---|---|---|---|---|---|
| Pillais | .38787 | 61.78019 | 2.00 | 195.00 | .000 |
| Hotellings | .63364 | 61.78019 | 2.00 | 195.00 | .000 |
| **Wilk's** | **.61213** | 61.78019 | 2.00 | 195.00 | **.000** |
| Roys | .38787 | | | | |

Note: F statistics are exact.

- - - - - - - - - - - - - - - - - - - - - - - - - - - - - - - - - - - - -

EFFECT .. GROUP(1) (Cont.)

**Univariate F-tests** with (1,196) D. F.

| Variable | Hypoth. SS | Error SS | Hypoth. MS | Error MS | F | Sig. of F |
|---|---|---|---|---|---|---|
| **Y1** | 194.95226 | 307.75674 | 194.95226 | 1.57019 | 124.15859 | **.000** |
| **Y2** | 28.95757 | 74.45307 | 28.95757 | .37986 | 76.23170 | **.000** |

in the subcommand CONTRAST: The first four 1's indicate that there are four groups in this case, followed by the coding for the contrasts $\Psi_1$, $\Psi_2$, and $\Psi_3$, respectively. The part of the *SPSS* syntax given in bold (for reference purposes) is not case sensitive and does not change with different orthogonal contrasts. Of course, what may change is the coding coefficients and notations for the dependent and grouping variables.

The results in the selected *SPSS* output (Figure 19.12) are for the first contrast ($\Psi_1$), which is indicated by the notation GROUP(1). The results for $\Psi_2$ and $\Psi_3$, denoted GROUP(2) and GROUP(3) in the *SPSS* output, are not provided here. The results for $\Psi_1$ show that this contrast is statistically significant (a) on the set of two dependent variables, as indicated by the multivariate test (*Wilk's lambda* = 0.61, $F(2, 195)$ = 61.78, $p$ = .000), and (b) on each dependent variable separately, as indicated by the univariate $F$-tests for $Y_1$ [$F(1, 196)$ = 124.16, $p$ = .000, and $Y_2$, $F(1, 196)$ = 76.23, $p$ = .000]. As $H_{01}$ is rejected at both the multivariate and univariate levels, we can conclude that the joint effect of groups of the two experimental conditions (groups 1 and 2) is different from the joint effect of the two control conditions (groups 3 and 4) on the set of two dependent variables, as well as on each of them separately. The results for $\Psi_2$ and $\Psi_3$ (which are not reported here) showed that these two contrasts are also statistically significant at both multivariate and univariate levels. Information on the power for the multivariate and univariate tests, at the .05 level of significance, is obtained with the following subcommand in MANOVA syntax: PRINT = CELLINFO(MEANS) SIGNIF(EFSIZE)/POWER/.

## Example 19.8

Suppose now that one wants to test the following null hypotheses for the four groups and two dependent variables in Example 19.7:

$$H_{01} : \frac{\mu_1 + \mu_2 + \mu_3}{3} = \mu_4, \quad H_{02} : \frac{\mu_1 + \mu_4}{2} = \frac{\mu_2 + \mu_3}{2}; \quad \text{and} \quad H_{03} : \mu_1 = \mu_4.$$

**TABLE 19.5**  *SPSS* syntax for MANOVA with planned correlated contrasts for the comparison of four groups on a set of two dependent variables.

**MANOVA** *y1* **TO** *y2* **BY** group(1,4)
    **/METHOD = SEQUENTIAL**
    **/CONTRAST**(group) = **SPECIAL**(1 1 1 1    1 1 1 −3    1 1 −1 −1    1 0 0 −1)
    **/PARTITION**(group)
    **/DESIGN** = group(1), group(2), group(3)
    /DESIGN = group(2), group(3), group(1)
    **/DESIGN** = group(3), group(1), group(2).

© Cengage Learning

The standard form for the first null hypothesis is $H_{01}: \mu_1 + \mu_2 + \mu_3 - 3\mu_4 = 0$, thus providing the coefficients for the first contrast, $\Psi_1$: 1 1 1 −3. Similarly, the standard forms for $H_{02}$ and $H_{03}$ provide the coefficients for the contrasts $\Psi_2$: 1 1 −1 −1 and $\Psi_3$: 1 0 0 −1, respectively. Although the sample sizes of the four groups are equal, the contrasts $\Psi_1$ and $\Psi_2$ are correlated because the sum of the products of their coefficients is not zero: $(1)(1) + (1)(1) + (1)(-1) + (-3)(-1) = 4$. Similarly, one can see that $\Psi_1$ correlates with $\Psi_3$, and $\Psi_2$ correlates with $\Psi_3$. Therefore, to determine the unique contribution of a contrast ($\Psi_1$, $\Psi_2$, or $\Psi_3$), one needs to partial out its correlation with the other contrasts. In *SPSS*, this can be achieved with the syntax in Table 19.5.

With the subcommand METHOD = SEQUENTIAL, each contrast is adjusted only for all contrasts to the left of it in any DESIGN subcommand that follows. Also, group(1), group(2), and group(3) in a DESIGN subcommand stand for the contrasts $\Psi_1$, $\Psi_2$, or $\Psi_3$, respectively. It is clear then that the purpose of using three DESIGN subcommands in the syntax is to adjust each contrast for its correlation with any other two contrasts. The results in the *SPSS* output in Figure 19.13 are obtained with the second DESIGN subcommand (design 2): DESIGN = group(2), group(3), group(1), where group(1) ($\Psi_1$) is adjusted for its correlation with the contrasts to the left of it, group(2) and group(3) ($\Psi_2$ and $\Psi_3$), respectively. These results show that the unique contribution of $\Psi_1$ is statistically significant (a) on the set of two dependent variables, as indicated by the multivariate test (*Wilk's lambda* = 0.45, $F(2, 195) = 119.51$, $p = .000$); and (b) on each dependent variable separately, as indicated by the univariate *F*-tests for $Y_1$ [$F(1, 196) = 239.95$, $p = .000$], and $Y_2$ [$F(1, 196) = 159.54$, $p = .000$]. The same holds for the unique contributions of $\Psi_2$ and $\Psi_3$, as indicated by the results (not provided here) in the *SPSS* output for design 1 and design 3 (third and first DESIGN subcommands, respectively).

# Sample Size with MANOVA

Determining (*a priori*) an appropriate sample size with MANOVA applications is not a simple matter. It depends on the number of groups, number of dependent variables, effect size, power of the test, and level of statistical significance (e.g., $\alpha = .05$ or .01). Using too many dependent variables is not recommended because the power of the test tends to decrease when the number of dependent variables increases, meaning that larger sample sizes would be required to maintain a desired test power. Also, small differences on a large number of dependent variables, without any strong substantive role, may obscure differences on fewer, yet substantively important, dependent variables. Further, problems related to reliability of scores on dependent variables may accumulate when

**Figure 19.13**

Selected *SPSS* output for multivariate and univariate tests of significance for the unique contribution of contrast $\Psi_1$: $\mu_1 + \mu_2 + \mu_3 - 3\mu_4$ (adjusted for its correlation with other two contrasts, $\Psi_2$, and $\Psi_3$).

```
* * * * A n a l y s i s   o f   V a r i a n c e -- design 2 * *
```

EFFECT .. **GROUP(1)**

**Multivariate Tests of Significance** (S = 1, M = 0, N = 96 1/2)

| Test Name | Value | Exact F | Hypoth. DF | Error DF | Sig. of F |
|-----------|-------|---------|------------|----------|-----------|
| Pillais | .55072 | 119.51395 | 2.00 | 195.00 | .000 |
| Hotellings | 1.22578 | 119.51395 | 2.00 | 195.00 | .000 |
| **Wilk's** | **.44928** | 119.51395 | 2.00 | 195.00 | **.000** |
| Roys | .55072 | | | | |

Note: F statistics are exact.

- - - - - - - - - - - - - - - - - - - - - - - - - - - - - - - - - - - -

EFFECT .. GROUP(1) (Cont.)

**Univariate F-tests** with (1,196) D. F.

| Variable | Hypoth. SS | Error SS | Hypoth. MS | Error MS | F | Sig. of F |
|----------|-----------|----------|-----------|----------|---|-----------|
| **Y1** | 376.77035 | 307.75674 | 376.77035 | 1.57019 | 239.95247 | **.000** |
| **Y2** | 60.60192 | 74.45307 | 60.60192 | .37986 | 159.53641 | **.000** |

the number of such variables increases. Therefore, when a large number of dependent variables is initially available, researchers may consider reducing it by selecting dependent variables with important empirical or theoretical roles for the study question(s). Or if items of an instrument (e.g., test or survey) are used as dependent variables, it might be better to use subscales (underlying constructs) of the instrument instead of the individual items, thus obtaining fewer, yet more meaningful, dependent variables.

Tables on determining sample size for MANOVA applications are provided in Stevens (2009) for prespecified number of groups, number of dependent variables, effect size, test power, and level of statistical significance ($\alpha$). As a short illustration for studies with three to five groups, rough estimates for a sample size needed to maintain a power of .70, at the .05 level of significance, is (a) $n \approx 16$, with a very large effect size; (b) $n \approx 31$, with a large effect size; (c) $n \approx 54$, with a medium effect size; and (d) $n \approx 120$, with a small effect size. Recall that the univariate effect size (*ES*) shows the distance of separation between the population means in standard deviation units: $ES = (\mu_1 - \mu_2)/\sigma$, where $\sigma$ is the common standard deviation for the compared populations. According to a rule of thumb proposed by Cohen (1988), an effect size close to .20 is small, an effect size close to .50 is medium, and an effect size close to .80 is large. (See Chapters 4 and 16 for a discussion of effect size.)

# Factor Analysis and Other Multivariate Methods

Suppose that five variables are used as predictors in a multiple regression for predicting academic achievement: $X_1$ = reading comprehension, $X_2$ = word identification, $X_3$ = mathematics computational skills, $X_4$ = logical reasoning, and $X_5$ = analytic skills. Also, assume that $X_1$ and $X_2$ are highly correlated, but they do not correlate well with $X_3$, $X_4$, and $X_5$. Conversely, $X_3$, $X_4$, and $X_5$ are highly correlated among themselves but not with $X_1$ and $X_2$. With this, two factors emerge from the set of five variables: $F_1 = $ *reading ability* factor formed by $X_1$ and $X_2$, and $F_2 = $ *logical-mathematical ability* factor formed by $X_3$, $X_4$, and $X_5$. It would be better then to use $F_1$ and $F_2$ as predictors of academic achievement, thus reducing the number of predictor variables and avoiding multicollinearity problems. This is a primary application of useful statistical procedures known as factor analysis.

In general, methods of **factor analysis** are used to determine (a) how many factors underlie the set of variables, (b) which variables form which factor, (c) the correlation between each variable and each factor, (d) the scores of each individual on the factors, and (e) the correlations (if any) among the factors. As an example, Erford, Balcolm, and Moore-Thomas (2007) used factor analysis to examine the underlying structure of a 40-item teacher and parent rating scale called the *Screening Test for Emotional Problems* (STEP). One can imagine that making sense out of the responses of a mother or teacher to 40 different questions may be somewhat difficult, requiring complex and sophisticated interpretation regarding the relationships between and among the 40 variables. Factor analysis helps to simplify this process somewhat by sorting the items into groupings called factors. In the STEP example, Erford et al. determined that the 40 items actually comprised four underlying factors: academic problems, anxiety/depression, social problems, and behavior problems. Each factor comprised of between 5 and 14 items and could be interpreted on its own as a separate construct composed of those individual variables. One can see how it is far easier to interpret the results of four bits of information compared to 40 bits of information. As such, factor analysis takes a large amount of information (variables), analyzes the relationships among the variables, and identifies underlying factors that help simplify interpretation of the variables. It is important to distinguish between two fundamentally different approaches to factor analysis: exploratory factor analysis and confirmatory factor analysis.

## Exploratory Factor Analysis

An **exploratory factor analysis** (EFA) is typically used when researchers do not have enough theoretical and/or empirical information to hypothesize how many factors underlie the set of observable variables and which variables form which factor. An EFA defines factors through a mathematical procedure that usually maximizes the total variance in the observed variables accounted for by the factors. There are several types of EFA procedures, each with different purposes and yielding somewhat different results. Under the commonly used **principal factor methods** in the EFA, the first factor extracted from the correlation matrix between the observed variables is a weighted linear combination of all observed variables that produces the highest squared correlation between the variables and the factor. The second factor extracted is uncorrelated with the first factor because it maximizes the variance extracted from the residual matrix after the first factor has been removed. The process continues until all factors meeting a prespecified statistical criterion are extracted.

The principal factor method is referred to as **principal component analysis** when the observed score of an individual $i$ on a variable $v$ ($X_{iv}$) is reproduced with no error by a linear combination of the factor scores for this individual. In the example of the five variables and two factors, the score of an individual ($i$) on any variable ($v$) is reproduced with

$$X_{iv} = w_{v1}F_{1i} + w_{v2}F_{2i}, \tag{19.12}$$

where $w_{v1}$ and $w_{v2}$ are the "weights" for variable $v$ on factors $F_1$ and $F_2$, respectively, and $F_{1i}$ and $F_{2i}$ are the scores of individual $i$ on $F_1$ and $F_2$, respectively ($v = 1, \ldots, 5$). The model with Equation 19.12 is referred to as the full component model. Thus, the principal component analysis is the principal factor method under the full component model.

With another model, called common factor model, the term $w_{vu}U_{iv}$ is added in Equation 19.12 to reflect the assumption that there is a "unique" factor ($U_v$) for each variable $v$. The principal factor method under the common factor model is referred to as principal axis analysis.

Note that the weights for an observed variable are referred to as **pattern coefficients**, whereas the correlations between a factor and all observed variables are referred to as **structure coefficients** for that factor. When the factors are **orthogonal** (uncorrelated), the pattern coefficients equal the structure coefficients. Recall that when the predictor variables in multiple regression are orthogonal, the standardized regression coefficients equal the correlation coefficients between the predictors and the criterion.

The structure coefficients are used to determine which variables form which factors, thus allowing the investigator to interpret and label the factors. Because the initially extracted factors are usually difficult to interpret, they are transformed by rotation. A rotated factor is a linear combination of the initial factors and is much easier to interpret. In fact, the rotated factors explain the same amount of the total variance of the observed variables, but they divide it up in a way that is more useful for their interpretation. With a frequently used rotation, called "varimax," the variance of the squared structure coefficients across all factors is maximized. Varimax is an orthogonal rotation because it assumes that the factors are uncorrelated. The varimax rotation is inappropriate when there is a tendency that a single general factor underlies the set of observed variables. For example, it is inappropriate to apply varimax to test items with high internal consistency (e.g., indicated by a high Cronbach's alpha coefficient) because high internal consistency means that there is a general factor underlying the test items.

When correlated factors are expected, an oblique rotation (e.g., promax) should be used instead. Both orthogonal and oblique rotations are available with the EFA in *SPSS*. It is important to emphasize that models involving different assumptions do produce different results, but this should not be a concern unless such results lead to interpretations that are sufficiently different to alter the theory. An EFA without any theory or substantive rationale for selecting the observed variables should be undertaken with extreme caution, if at all. Factor analysis is best pursued for specific empirical and theoretical verification purposes, not for the purpose of "building" or "discovering" a theory.

## Example 19.9: Exploratory Factor Analysis

The purpose of this example is to illustrate the use of *SPSS* in EFA when the factors are hypothesized to be orthogonal (i.e., uncorrelated). The data set consists of the responses of 30 participants on four survey questions on a 5-point Likert-type scale (Figure 19.14). To perform an EFA using the principal component method with varimax rotation in *SPSS*, follow these steps:

1. Click **Analyze**, click **Data Reduction**, and click **Factor**.
2. Click Reset to clear the dialog box (if there is some previous information).
3. Hold down the **Ctrl** key, click *q1*, *q2*, *q3*, and *q4*, and then click ▶ to move them to the Variables box.
4. Click **Extraction**. The option **Principal Components** in the Method box should already be selected by default, so click on **Continue**.

**Figure 19.14**

SPSS data set with the responses of 30 subjects on four survey questions.

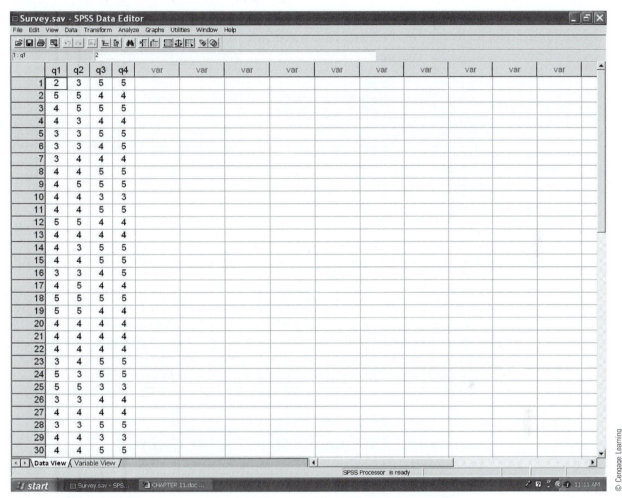

5. Click **Rotation**, select **Varimax**, and click **Continue**.

6. Click **Options**, select **Sorted by size**, and click **Continue**. (This will sort the variables associated with a given factor by the size of their structure coefficients.)

7. Click on **OK**.

The selected SPSS output is provided in Figure 19.15. As the results in the Total Variance Explained table indicate, two factors emerged: the first factor explaining 48.007 percent and the second factor explaining an additional 41.644 percent of the total variance of the four survey questions. The two factors together explain 89.651 percent of the total variance. The factor structure coefficients (loadings) are provided with the Rotated Component Matrix table. The third and fourth questions (q3 and q4, respectively) of the survey form the first factor, whereas the first two questions (q1 and q2, respectively) form the second factor. This is indicated by the high correlations for q3 and q4 with the first factor (.983 and .960, respectively) and their negligible correlations with the second factor (−.0722 and −.216, respectively). Conversely, there are high correlations for

**Figure 19.15**

Selected *SPSS* output with the factor analysis of four survey questions using the principal components analysis with varimax rotation.

**Factor Analysis**

**Total Variance Explained**

| Component | Initial Eigen values | | | Rotation Sums of Squared Loadings | | |
|---|---|---|---|---|---|---|
|  | Total | % of Variance | Cumulative % | Total | % of Variance | Cumulative % |
| 1 | 2.319 | 57.968 | 57.968 | 1.920 | 48.007 | 48.007 |
| 2 | 1.267 | 31.683 | 89.651 | 1.666 | 41.644 | 89.651 |
| 3 | .352 | 8.805 | 98.456 |  |  |  |
| 4 | 6.176E-02 | 1.544 | 100.000 |  |  |  |

Extraction Method: Principal Component Analysis.

**Rotated Component Matrix**[a]

|  | Component | |
|---|---|---|
|  | 1 | 2 |
| Q3 | .983 | −7.22E-02 |
| Q4 | .960 | .216 |
| Q2 | −.115 | .902 |
| Q1 | −.143 | .895 |

Extraction Method: Principal Component Analysis.
Rotation Method: Varimax with Kaiser Normalization.
a. Rotation converged in 3 iterations.

$q2$ and $q1$ with the second factor (.902 and .895, respectively) and negligible correlations with the first factor (−.115 and −.143, respectively). Evidently, there is a clear structure of two factors underlying the set of four survey questions. The interpretation of these two factors would depend on the substantive meaning of the survey questions: $q3$ and $q4$ for the interpretation of the first factor and $q2$ and $q1$ for the interpretation of the second factor.

## Example 19.10: Exploratory Factor Analysis

Erford et al. (2007) reported an EFA of responses to the *Screening Test for Emotional Problems* (STEP) of teachers and mothers (separately analyzed) of 470 students aged 5–18 years with emotional problems. The data were initially analyzed using a principal axis factoring (PAF) method without rotation (Thompson, 1989) so that the resulting eigenvalue curve (Figure 19.16) could be "eyeballed" using a "scree" test (Cattell, 1966) to determine the likely number of factors that will emerge from the rotated analyses to follow (e.g., where the curve begins to flatten). Scree analysis indicated the likely presence of between three and six factors, so sequential PAFs were run and the criteria set for these numbers of factors. Also, the analyses were rotated to the "promax" criterion because it was assumed that the built in factors were correlated, not uncorrelated (orthogonal). After analyzing the resulting pattern and structure coefficients, it was determined that the four-factor solution was the most parsimonious (e.g., explained best how the model fit the data), accounting for more than 45 percent of the item-factor variance. The resulting structure coefficients for the teacher data are presented in Table 19.6.

Although these results are a bit more complicated than the previous example of academic achievement, interpretation is conducted in a similar manner. An item-factor correlation of .30 is considered significant. Notice how under the Poor Socialization factor, the coefficients in structure coefficients column (factor) 4 are all $\geq.30$, and the items (#2, 17, 22, 24, 27, 37) appear rationally related to social skills and social problems. One

**Figure 19.16**

Scree analysis of STEP teacher eigenvalues.

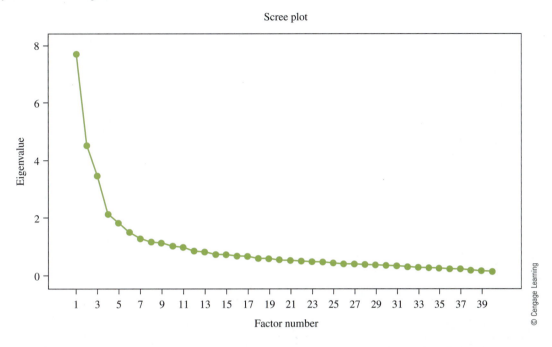

**TABLE 19.6**   PAF with promax rotation for the STEP teacher sample.

| Factors/Items | Structure Coefficients | | | | |
|---|---|---|---|---|---|
| | **1** | **2** | **3** | **4** | $h^2$ |
| *Factors/Items* | | | | | |
| *Factor: Anxiety/Depression* | | | | | |
| 4. Pessimistic, negative. | .43 | .17 | **.56** | .37 | .48 |
| 5. Easily upset by personal or school experiences. | .40 | .12 | **.52** | .36 | .45 |
| 9. Speaks of self as dumb or inferior. | .13 | .18 | **.44** | .29 | .44 |
| 10. Becomes visibly upset when nervous (shaking, trembling, dizzy). | .18 | .09 | **.41** | .50 | .40 |
| 14. Feels sad, depressed. | .14 | .18 | **.71** | .38 | .57 |
| 15. Has unrealistic fears (e.g., dark, heights, thunder, being alone). | .20 | .08 | **.41** | .44 | .39 |
| 19. Cries for no apparent reason, or has an inappropriate response to personal or school situations. | .24 | .00 | **.35** | .42 | .37 |
| 20. Must do things perfectly. | .13 | −.19 | .29 | .40 | .30 |
| 25. Develops headaches, stomachaches, etc., as a reaction to stressful situations. | .17 | .12 | **.58** | .29 | .54 |
| 29. Feels worthless, helpless or hopeless. | .18 | .14 | **.60** | .43 | .55 |
| 30. Talks about worries or fears regarding school, home, or personal situations. | .17 | .10 | **.50** | .16 | .34 |
| 34. Dramatic mood swings (usually between euphoria, anxiety, and depression). | .46 | .02 | **.62** | .24 | .49 |
| 35. Anxious, fearful. | .22 | .10 | **.59** | .57 | .54 |
| 39. Speaks or writes notes of potential self-harm (e.g., I wish I were dead, I may as well kill myself). | .22 | .01 | **.49** | .29 | .35 |
| 40. Complains of body aches or other problems (e.g., stomachaches, headaches, muscle aches, nausea). | .25 | .16 | **.66** | .32 | .57 |

*(Continued)*

**TABLE 19.6**  *continued*

| | Structure Coefficients | | | | |
|---|---|---|---|---|---|
| | 1 | 2 | 3 | 4 | $h^2$ |
| *Factor: Inappropriate Behavior* | | | | | |
| 3. Tells lies. | **.52** | .36 | .26 | .03 | .47 |
| 7. Makes derogatory comments to adults or children. | **.76** | .15 | .32 | .16 | .60 |
| 8. Steals things that belong to others. | **.41** | .28 | .11 | .04 | .40 |
| 12. Threatens others (verbally or physically). | **.79** | .20 | .29 | .09 | .68 |
| 18. Does not obey home or school rules. | **.71** | .34 | .31 | −.06 | .55 |
| 23. Becomes violent (fights with others or becomes physically and emotionally out of control). | **.75** | .08 | .30 | .08 | .66 |
| 28. Vandalizes or destroys the property of others. | **.53** | .18 | .21 | .16 | .37 |
| 32. Doesn't care about hurting the feelings of others. | **.74** | .15 | .27 | .15 | .56 |
| 38. Expresses inappropriate sexually related thoughts or behaves in an inappropriate sexually related manner. | **.32** | .07 | .22 | .03 | .18 |
| | | | | | |
| *Factor: Academic Performance* | | | | | |
| 1. Has trouble learning at school. | .21 | **.79** | .23 | .12 | .65 |
| 6. Displays inconsistent daily school performance. | .49 | **.46** | .41 | .09 | .46 |
| 11. Fails tests and quizzes. | .22 | **.81** | .22 | .00 | .65 |
| 16. Is currently failing at least one major subject area (e.g., reading, math, written language, spelling). | .29 | **.60** | .21 | −.05 | .61 |
| 21. Fails to grasp concepts being taught. | .14 | **.77** | .08 | .12 | .68 |
| 26. Performs schoolwork or homework at a failing level. | .32 | **.78** | .23 | −.04 | .70 |
| 31. Has difficulty understanding written or verbal directions for schoolwork. | .10 | **.66** | .10 | .19 | .61 |
| 36. Needs a lot of help from adults to complete school assignments. | .22 | **.70** | .14 | .15 | .54 |
| | | | | | |
| *Factor: Poor Socialization* | | | | | |
| 2. Usually plays alone, prefers to be alone. | −.04 | .05 | .25 | **.67** | .51 |
| 17. Has few friends. | .12 | .17 | .33 | **.65** | .56 |
| 22. Is not accepted by other children because of behavior. | .32 | .21 | .28 | **.62** | .53 |
| 24. Shows little or no emotion (e.g., no animation in facial expressions, does not respond to emotion-invoking situations). | .11 | .12 | .17 | **.30** | .23 |
| 27. Avoids talking to students or adults. | .11 | .09 | .29 | **.56** | .48 |
| 37. Withdraws from others. | .07 | .02 | .38 | **.61** | .51 |
| | | | | | |
| Other items | | | | | |
| 13. Uses or possesses alcohol or other drugs. | .23 | .17 | .21 | −.34 | .38 |
| 33. Runs away from home or school. | .30 | .07 | .39 | −.02 | .28 |

*Note:* $h^2$ = communality (proportion of the variable's variance accounted for by all factors).

© Cengage Learning

interpretation for these results is that these six items load significantly on factor 4 and measure poor socialization, thus leading Erford et al. (2007) to name the factor Poor Socialization. The same is true for the items loading on the other three factors. Of course, decision-making processes underlying interpretation of factor structure are more complex than these simple examples, and interested readers are referred to Erford et al. (2007) for a more in-depth commentary on the STEP data analysis.

EFA is widely used in counseling research. Holcomb-McCoy and Day-Vines (2004) used a principal component analysis with the items of the revised version of the *Multicultural Counseling Competence and Training Survey (MCCTS-R)*. Instead of varimax (used for uncorrelated factors), they used an oblique analytic rotation called oblimin (which is somewhat different than promax) to take into account that the correlations among the three emerging factors—Multicultural Terminology, Multicultural Knowledge, and Multicultural Awareness—were relatively high (e.g., greater than .32). It should be noted, however, that instrument development and validation in counseling, education, and other behavioral fields should more often rely on (theory-driven) confirmatory factor analysis because, more often than not, the instrument is based on some theory or model.

## Confirmatory Factor Analysis

In contrast to EFA, in which factors are extracted mathematically and interpreted by the researchers, in **confirmatory factor analysis** (CFA) factors are defined directly through their hypothesized relations with observed variables (e.g., test items or survey questions). Based on theoretical considerations, CFA forces researchers to think about the reasons for selecting observed variables and the organization of the data ahead of time; thus, the process is more "theory-driven." With CFA, researchers decide *a priori* (e.g., ahead of time) (a) the number of factors, (b) which factors are (possibly) correlated, and (c) which variables relate to which factors.

Figure 19.17 provides a graphical representation (*path model*) of a hypothesized three-factor structure. The hypothesized factors, $F_1$ (*Motivation*), $F_2$ (*Performance*), and $F_3$ (*Anxiety*), are depicted by circles and the curved arrow connecting two circles indicate that the two factors represented by these circles are hypothesized to be correlated. Thus,

**Figure 19.17**

Three-factor hypothetical confirmatory model.

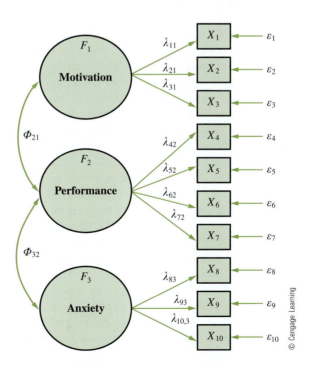

© Cengage Learning

it is hypothesized that there is a correlation between motivation and performance ($\Phi_{21}$) and between anxiety and performance ($\Phi_{32}$), but not between motivation and anxiety.

The observed variables (e.g., test items; $X_1$, $X_2$, ..., $X_{10}$) are represented by squares and connected to the factors by straight arrows. The coefficient $\lambda$ stands for a factor loading (i.e., a structure coefficient) that represents the direction (positive or negative) and strength of the relationship between a factor and an observed variable. In CFA, each observed variable has a measurement error term ($\varepsilon$), which means that the variance of the observed variable is not assumed to be fully explained by the factor(s) to which this variable relates. The relationship between the observed variables ($X$) to the factors ($F$) and measurement errors ($\varepsilon$) is provided with the equation

$$X = \lambda F + \varepsilon. \tag{19.13}$$

This equation is similar to a regression equation for the prediction of $X$ from $F$, with the difference being that here the "predictor" ($F$) is not an observed variable but a latent factor. Thus, the values of $\lambda$ and $\varepsilon$ cannot be obtained through typical regression analysis. Instead, they are estimated through the use of the correlation (or covariance) matrix of the observed variables. Statistical computer programs such as *EQS* (Bentler, 2006), *Mplus* (Muthen & Muthen, 2012), and *Amos* (Arbuckle, 2012) provide estimates of $\Phi$, $\lambda$, and other parameters of the confirmatory model, as well as statistics for its goodness-of-fit (i.e., the degree to which the model fits the data). Data that confirm the theory under study will yield reasonable goodness-of-fit indices; that is, the data confirm the test-item structure predicted by the model (theory).

Among the most widely used measures of goodness-of-fit for confirmatory models are the **chi-square ($\chi^2$) statistic**, **goodness-of-fit index (GFI)**, **comparative fit index (CFI)**, **root mean square error of approximation (RMSEA)**, and **standardized root mean squared residual (SRMSR)**. The chi-square statistic is used to test the null hypothesis that "the original covariance matrix for the population is equal to (i.e., is reproduced by) the covariance matrix obtained with the hypothesized confirmatory model." Therefore, contrary to the typical goal in hypothesis testing, the researcher would *not* want to reject the null hypothesis in this case. Thus, a reasonable model fit would be indicated if the chi-square statistic is *not* statistically significant (i.e., its $p$ value is greater than, say, .05). It is recommended, however, that the chi-square statistic be used more as a descriptive index rather than as a test statistic because of its sensitivity to the sample size. A close model fit is indicated with (a) GFI greater than .92, (b) CFI greater than .95, (c) RMSEA less than .06, and (d) SRMSR less than .08. A detailed discussion of model fit indices is provided by Bentler (2006).

CFA is used in research on counseling, education, and other behavioral fields primarily for development, revision, and validation of instruments. CFA is a part of a structural equation modeling (SEM) design for investigation of causal relationships and their change across time points. As an example, a CFA was used in developing the *Career-Related Parent Support Scale (CRPSS)* to confirm (theory-derived) relationships between hypothesized factors and items of the *CRPSS* (Turner, Alliman-Brissett, Lapan, Upidi, & Ergun, 2003). Specifically, four factors were hypothesized based on Bandura's (1977a, 1977b, 1997) theory of self-efficacy: $F_1$ = Instrumental Assistance (seven items: e.g., "My parents help me do my homework"), $F_2$ = Career-Related Modeling (seven items: e.g., "My parents have taken me to their work"), $F_3$ = Verbal Encouragement (six items: e.g., "My parents told me they expect me to finish school"), and $F_4$ = Emotional Support (seven items: e.g., "My parents praise me when I learn job-related skills").

As a second example, Erford and Hase (2006) performed a CFA on the responses of teachers of 348 students in kindergarten to grade five to the ACTeRS-2, a behavior rating scale used to measure attention, opposition, hyperactivity, and social skills (Ullman, Slea-tor, & Sprague, 2000). Output from the LISREL 8.5 analysis indicated the following:

> The overall goodness-of-fit index (GFI) was .93. In general, a minimally acceptable GFI is considered to be .90 (Clark et al., 1994). The CFI was .97. The root mean square error of approximation (RMSEA) was 0.030 (90 percent confidence interval for RMSEA was 0.020−0.039), and the standardized root mean square residual was 0.048. Thompson (2004) stated that, generally, models with CFI of .95 or higher and an RMSEA of ≤.06 demonstrate a reasonable fit. Thus, the tested model appears to fit the data reasonably well (Erford & Hase, 2006, pp. 100−101).

As a final aside, Jöreskog (1969) suggested that EFA can be useful in a framework of CFA for specific technical purposes (e.g., to obtain standard errors to determine if factor loadings are statistically significant). This, however, does not justify the approach of conducting EFA first, thus ignoring the theoretical conceptualization of relationships between factors and variables, and then "confirming" the exploratory findings with a CFA using the same data. It should be noted also that with the EFA on test items (e.g., tests of intelligence or achievement), some "artificial" factors may emerge because of differences primarily in item difficulty, not underlying constructs; that is, sometimes one factor of "easy" items will emerge, while another factor of "challenging" items emerges. In such a result, what each item was designed to measure (e.g., math calculation, math concepts, or problem-solving) is a less important contributing factor than how difficult an item is (e.g., easy or challenging).

# Other Multivariate Methods

## Predictive Discriminant Analysis

Descriptive discriminant analysis is used with MANOVA to provide information about the separation of groups on linear composites of dependent variables. Each linear composite is interpreted as a linear discriminant function (*LDF*) that maximizes the group separation. Thus, one application of discriminant analysis is for description of MANOVA results. Another purpose for using discriminant analysis is to classify participants into groups (i.e., to predict group membership). For example, Stevens (2009) illustrated the use of predictive discriminant analysis to classify kindergarten children into two levels (low risk and high risk) of reading problems based on the children's scores on three variables: word identification, word comprehension, and passage comprehension. Readily understandable examples of discriminant analysis exemplar studies are provided in Huberty and Olejnik (2006) and Stevens (2009).

## Canonical Correlation

Although MANOVA and discriminant analysis deal with linear composites within a set of variables, the analysis of canonical correlations deals with correlations between linear composites in two sets of variables. The linear composites of variables are referred to as canonical variates. As Stevens (2009, p. 471) noted, "Canonical correlation is appropriate if the wish is to parsimoniously describe the number and the nature of mutually independent relationships existing between two sets." Stevens described, for example, a study (Tetenbaum, 1975) that addresses the validity of student ratings of teachers. Specifically, the research question was whether in the process of rating a teacher, the students focused on the need-related aspects of the perceptual situation and based their judgment on those areas of the teacher's performance most relevant to their own needs. The canonical analysis applied in this study revealed that there were three statistically significant canonical correlations between the composites of 12 *need* variables and linear composites of the corresponding 12 *rating* variables (in general, the two sets do not necessarily have to contain the same number of variables). For example, the first pair of canonical variates (i.e., the pair of linear composites with the highest canonical correlation) showed a strong relationship between needs and ratings on the same latent continuum. The "positive" direction of this latent continuum is interpreted as ascendancy and its "negative" direction, as the intellectual striving needs of the students.

In general, the number of possible canonical correlations equals the smaller number of the variables in the two sets. For example, if the first set has nine variables and the second set seven variables, then there are seven possible pairs of canonical variates. The pairs of canonical variates are mutually independent. This means that (a) the canonical variates within each set are uncorrelated, and (b) any two canonical variates that belong to different pairs and different sets of variables are uncorrelated. Readily understandable examples of canonical correlation exemplars are provided in Stevens (2009).

## Structural Equation Modeling

**Structural equation modeling** is a versatile statistical framework for modeling causal relationships between variables and constructs. SEM also provides methods for testing differences between groups on a set of variables. Which method (SEM or MANOVA) is more appropriate in a particular study depends on the type of relationships between observed variables and constructs. MANOVA is more appropriate with an emergent variable system in which the construct "emerges" as a linear composite of observed variables that represent causal agents of the construct. For example, "stress" is a construct that emerges as a linear composite of observed dependent variables, such as relationships with parents, relationships with spouse, and demands of the workplace. Conversely, SEM is more appropriate with a latent variable system in which the construct has causal influence on the observed variables. For example, self-esteem is a construct that may have causal influence on the responses of alcohol abusers on particular questionnaire items during a rehabilitation process. An important advantage of using SEM over MANOVA is that SEM operates with error-free constructs, whereas MANOVA uses linear composites that are not free from measurement errors associated with the observed variables. Thus, using MANOVA with a latent variable system (i.e., when a construct has causal effects on observed variables) may provide inaccurate results about group differences on the construct of interest. Numerous readily understandable presentations of SEM methods are available in the literature (e.g., Byrne, 2001; Raykov & Marcoulides, 2000; Schumacker & Lomax, 2004).

# Conclusion

The general form of a multiple regression model for the prediction of a criterion variable ($Y$) from $k$ predictors ($k \geq 2$) is $\hat{Y} = b_1X_1 + b_2X_2 + \cdots + b_kX_k + a$. Important concepts related to multiple regression were reviewed, including multiple correlation, interpretation of the regression coefficient, standardized regression equations, the significance of the multiple regression model, the significance of the multiple regression coefficient, comparison of full and restricted models, multicollinearity, cross validation, statistical power method for sample size, outliers and influential data points, interactions, and selection of predictors.

Multivariate analysis of variance (MANOVA) is used to address complex phenomena and research questions in counseling. Univariate analysis of variance (ANOVA) often fails to provide sufficient information to address questions involving (two or more) substantively related variables. MANOVA is appropriate with research questions about group differences on linear composites of dependent variables. A linear composite (linear discriminant function, *LDF*) represents a weighted sum of the dependent variables. The omnibus null hypothesis in MANOVA states that the group centroids are equal for the study population. A statistically significant *Wilk's lambda* for the omnibus test in MANOVA indicates that there is at least one construct (*LDF*) that emerged as a linear composite of the dependent variable that maximally separates the groups. A subsequent discriminant analysis is needed to test such constructs for statistical significance, define them substantively, and determine their role in separating the groups.

This chapter also presented procedures and methods for conducting EFA and CFA, and brief notes on other multivariate methods, such as predictive discriminant analysis, canonical correlations, and structural equation modeling. Factor analysis is used to determine (a) how many factors underlie the set of variables, (b) which variables form which factor, (c) the correlation between each variable and each factor, (d) the scores of each individual on the factors, and (e) the correlations (if any) among the factors. Factor analysis should not be used to construct a theory. EFA is used when researchers do not have enough theoretical or empirical information to hypothesize the number of factors that underlie a set of items and which items form which factor. CFA is a theory-driven process which defines factors directly through their hypothesized relations with observed variables or items and allows researchers to determine the fit of the *a priori* model to some set of data. A number of indexes used to indicate model fit were presented.

Predictive discriminant analysis is used with MANOVA to provide information about the separation of groups on linear composites of dependent variables. Canonical correlation is used to describe the number and nature of mutually independent relationships that exist between two sets of variables. Finally, structural equation modeling is used to model causal relationships between variables and constructs and also provides methods for testing differences between groups on a set of variables. These multivariate methods are quite complex and should be studied thoroughly using advanced statistical texts and supervision.

*Now go to the Student Workbook found on cengagebrain.com that accompanies this text for additional application and review activities.*

# REFERENCES

Achenbach, T. M., & Rescorla, L. A. (2001). *Manual for the Achenbach system of Empirically Based Assessment (ASEBA)*. Burlington, VT: ASEBA.

Agresti, A., & Pendergast, J. (1986). Comparing mean ranks for repeated measures data. *Communications in Statistics A: Theory & Method, 15,* 1417–1433.

Ahern, K. J. (1999). Ten tips for reflexive bracketing. *Qualitative Health Research, 9,* 407–411.

Akritas, M. G., & Arnold, S. F. (1994). Fully nonparametric hypotheses for factorial designs I: Multivariate repeated-measures designs. *Journal of the American Statistical Association, 89,* 336–343.

Akritas, M. G., Arnold, S. F., & Brunner, E. (1997). Nonparametric hypotheses and rank statistics for unbalanced factorial designs. *Journal of the American Statistical Association, 92,* 258–265.

Alberto, P. A., & Troutman, A. C. (2004). *Applied behavior analysis for teachers* (6th ed.). Columbus, OH: Merrill Prentice Hall.

Allen, B. (2009). Are researchers ethically obligated to report suspected child maltreatment? A critical analysis of opposing perspectives. *Ethics & Behavior, 19,* 15–24. doi:10.1080/10508420802623641

American Counseling Association. (Ed.). (2009). *The American Counseling Association encyclopedia of counseling*. Alexandria, VA: Author.

American Counseling Association. (2014). *Code of ethics*. Retrieved from http://www.counseling.org/knowledge-center/ethics

American Psychiatric Association. (2013). *Diagnostic and statistical manual of mental and emotional disorders* (5th ed.). Washington, DC: Author.

American Psychological Association. (2010). *Publication manual of the American Psychological Association* (6th ed.). Washington, DC: Author.

American School Counselor Association. (2012). *The ASCA national model: A framework for school counseling programs* (3rd ed.). Alexandria, VA: Author.

Anderson, R. E., Tatum, R. L., & Black, W. C. (2006). *Multivariate data analysis* (6th ed.). Upper Saddle River, NJ: Prentice Hall.

Arbuckle, J. L. (2012). *Amos 21.0 user's guide*. Chicago, IL: SPSS.

Ary, D., Jacobs, L. C., Sorensen, C., & Walker, D. (2013). *Introduction to research in education* (9th ed.). Belmont, CA: Wadsworth.

Asmussen, K. J., & Creswell, J. W. (1995). Campus response to a student gunman. *Journal of Higher Education, 66,* 575–591.

Astramovich, R. L., & Coker, J. K. (2007). Program evaluation: The accountability bridge model for counselors. *Journal of Counseling and Development, 85,* 162–172.

Astramovich, R. L., Coker, J. K., & Hoskins, W. J. (2005). Training school counselors in program evaluation. *Professional School Counseling, 9,* 49–54.

Bachar, E. (1998). Psychotherapy—an active agent: Assessing the effectiveness of psychotherapy and its curative factors. *Israel Journal of Psychiatry and Related Sciences, 35,* 128–135.

Baer, D. M., Wolf, M. M., & Risley, T. R. (1968). Some current dimensions of applied behavior analysis. *Journal of Applied Behavior Analysis, 1,* 91–92.

Baker, S. B., Swisher, J. D., Nadenichek, P. E., & Popowicz, C. L. (1984). Measured effects of primary prevention strategies. *Personnel and Guidance Journal, 62,* 459–464.

Baker, S. B., & Taylor, J. G. (1998). Effects of career education interventions: A meta-analysis. *Career Development Quarterly, 46,* 376–385.

Balkin, R. S., & Sheperis, C. J. (2011). Evaluating and reporting statistical power in counseling research. *Journal of Counseling & Development, 89,* 268–272.

Bandura, A. (1977a). Self-efficacy: Toward a unifying theory of behavioral change. *Psychological Review, 84,* 191–215.

Bandura, A. (1977b). *Social learning theory.* New York, NY: General Learning Press.

Bandura, A. (1997). *Self-efficacy: The exercise of control.* New York, NY: Freeman.

Barlow, D. H., & Hayes, S. C. (1979). Alternating treatment design: One strategy for comparing the effects of two treatments in a single subject. *Journal of Applied Behavior Analysis, 12,* 199–210.

Barsky, A. E. (2009). The legal and ethical context for knowing and using the latest child welfare research. *Child Welfare, 88,* 69–92.

Bauer, S. R., Sapp, M., & Johnson, D. (2000). Group counseling strategies for rural at-risk high school students. *The High School Journal, 83,* 41–50.

Beasley, T. M. (2000). Nonparametric tests for analyzing interactions among intra-block ranks in multiple group repeated measures designs. *Journal of Educational & Behavioral Statistics, 25,* 20–59.

Beasley, T. M. (2002). Multivariate aligned rank test for interactions in multiple group repeated measures designs. *Multivariate Behavioral Research, 37,* 197–226.

Beasley, T. M., Page, G. P., Brand, J. P. L., Gadbury, G. L., Mountz, J. D., & Allison, D. B. (2004). Chebyshev's inequality for non-parametric testing with small $N$ and $\alpha$ in microarray research. *Journal of the Royal Statistical Society, Series C: Applied Statistics, 53,* 95–108.

Beck, A. T., Steer, R. A., & Brown, G. K. (1996). *Manual for the Beck Depression Inventory— Second Edition (BDI-II).* San Antonio, TX: Psychological Corporation.

Benkofski, M., & Heppner, C. C. (1999). Program evaluation. In P. P. Heppner, D. M. Kivlighan, & B. E. Wampold (Eds.), *Research design in counseling* (pp. 488–513). Belmont, CA: Wadsworth.

Bennett, D. S., & Gibbons, T. A. (2000). Efficacy of child cognitive-behavioral interventions for antisocial behavior: A meta-analysis. *Child and Family Behavior Therapy, 22,* 1–15.

Bentler, P. M. (2006). *EQS6: Structural equations program manual.* Encino, CA: Multivariate Software.

Berg, B. L., & Lune, H. (2011). *Qualitative research methods for the social sciences* (8th ed.). Boston, MA: Pearson.

Best, J. W., & Kahn, J. V. (2006). *Research in education* (10th ed.). Upper Saddle River, NJ: Pearson.

Beutler, L. E., Frank, M., Schieber, S. C., Calvert, S., & Gaines, J. (1984). Comparative effects of group psychotherapies in a short-term inpatient setting: An experience with deterioration effects. *Psychiatry, 47*(1), 66–76.

Beutler, L. E., Machado, P. P. P., & Neufeldt, S. A. (1994). Therapist variables. In A. E. Bergin & S. L. Garfield (Eds.), *Handbook of psychotherapy and behavior change* (pp. 229–269). New York, NY: Wiley.

Blake, V., Joffe, S., & Kodish, E. (2011). Harmonization of ethics policies in pediatric research. *Journal of Law, Medicine & Ethics, 39,* 70–78. doi:10.1111/j.1748-720X.2011.00551.x

Bogdan, R. C., & Biklen, S. K. (2006). *Qualitative research in education: An introduction to theories and methods* (5th ed.). Boston, MA: Pearson.

Bond, T. G., & Fox, C. M. (2001). *Applying the Rasch model: Fundamental measurement in the human sciences.* Mahwah, NJ: Lawrence Erlbaum.

Borders, L. D., & Drury, S. M. (1992). Comprehensive school counseling programs: A review for policymakers and practitioners. *Journal of Counseling and Development, 70,* 487–498.

Borenstein, M., & Cohen, J. (1988). *Statistical power analysis: A computer program.* Hillsdale, NJ: Erlbaum.

Botvin, G. J., Schinke, S., & Orlandi, M. A. (1995). School-based health promotion: Substance abuse and sexual behavior. *Applied Prevention Psychology, 4,* 167–184.

Box, G. E. P., & Cox, D. R. (1964). An analysis of transformations. *Journal of the Royal Statistical Society B, 26,* 211–243.

Bradley, J. V. (1968). *Distribution-free statistical tests.* Englewood Cliffs, NJ: Prentice Hall.

Bratton, S. C., Ray, D., Rhine, T., & Jones, L. (2005). The efficacy of play therapy with children: A meta-analytic review of treatment outcomes. *Professional Psychology: Research and Practice, 36,* 376–390.

Brigman, G., & Campbell, C. (2003). Helping students improve academic achievement and school success behavior. *Professional School Counseling, 7,* 91–98.

Brott, P. E., & Myers, J. E. (1999). Development of a professional school counselor identity: A grounded theory. *Professional School Counseling, 2,* 339–348.

Brunner, E., & Langer, F. (2000). Nonparametric analysis of ordered categorical data in designs with longitudinal observations and small sample sizes. *Biometrical Journal, 42,* 663–675.

Brunner, E., & Munzel, U. (2000). The nonparametric Behrens-Fisher problem: Asymptotic theory and a small-sample approximation. *Biometrical Journal, 42,* 17–25.

Burstyn, J., & Stevens, R. (2001). Involving the whole school in violence prevention. In J. Burstyn, G. Bender, R. Castella, H. Gordon, D. Guerra, K. Luschen, R. Stevens, & K. Williams (Eds.), *Preventing violence in schools: A challenge to American democracy* (pp. 139–158). Mahwah, NJ: Lawrence Erlbaum.

Byrne, B. M. (2001). *Structural equation modeling with Amos.* Mahwah, NJ: Lawrence Erlbaum.

Campbell, C., & Brigman, G. (2005). Closing the achievement gap: A structured approach to group counseling. *The Journal for Specialists in Group Work, 30,* 67–82.

Campbell, C., & Dahir, C. A. (1997). *The national standards for school counseling programs.* Alexandria, VA: American School Counselor Association.

Campbell, D., & Stanley, J. (1963). *Experimental and quasi-experimental designs for research.* Boston, MA: Houghton Mifflin.

Capella, M. E. (2002). Inequities in the VR system: Do they still exist? *Rehabilitation Counseling Bulletin, 45,* 143–153.

Carver, C. S., Scheier, M. F., & Weintraub, J. K. (1989). Assessing coping strategies: A theoretically based approach. *Journal of Personality and Social Psychology, 56,* 267–283.

Casey, R. J., & Berman, J. S. (1985). The outcome of psychotherapy with children. *Psychological Bulletin, 98,* 388–400.

Catalano, R. F., Arthur, M. W., Hawkins, J. D., Berglund, L., & Olson, J. J. (1998). Comprehensive community- and school-based interventions to prevent antisocial behavior. In R. Loeber & D. P. Farrington (Eds.), *Serious and violent juvenile offenders: Risk factors and successful interventions* (pp. 248–283). Thousand Oaks, CA: Sage Publications.

Cattell, R. B. (1966). The "scree" test for the number of factors. *Multivariate Behavioral Research, 1,* 245–276.

Charmaz, K. (2005). Grounded theory in the 21st century: Applications for advancing social justice studies. In N. K. Denzin & Y. S. Lincoln (Eds.), *Handbook of qualitative research* (3rd ed., pp. 507–536). Thousand Oaks, CA: Sage.

Christenson, A., & Jacobson, N. S. (1993). Who (or what) can do psychotherapy: The status and challenge of nonprofessional therapies. *Psychological Science, 5*(1), 8–14.

Cleveland, W. S. (1984). Graphical methods for data presentation: Full scale breaks, dot charts, and multibased logging. *American Statistician, 38*(4), 70–80.

Cliff, N. (1996). *Ordinal methods for behavorial data analysis.* Mahwah, NJ: Erlbaum.

Cohen, J. (1988). *Statistical power analysis for the behavioral sciences* (2nd ed.). Hillsdale, NJ: Erlbaum.

Cohen, J. (1992). A power primer. *Psychological Bulletin, 112,* 155–159.

Cohen, J. (2003). *Applied multiple regression/correlation analysis for the behavioral sciences* (3rd ed.). Hillsdale, NJ: Lawrence Erlbaum.

Conners, C. K. (2007). *Manual for the Conners 3.* North Tonawanda, NY: Multi-Health Systems.

Conover, W. J. (1980). *Practical nonparametric statistics.* New York, NY: John Wiley & Sons.

Constantine, M. G. (2002). Racism attitudes, white racial identity attitudes, and multicultural competence in school counselor trainees. *Counselor Education and Supervision, 41,* 162–174.

Cook, R. D. (1977). Detection of influential observations in linear regression. *Technometrics, 19,* 15–18.

Cook, T. D., & Campbell, D. T. (1979). *Quasi-experimentation: Design and analysis issues for field settings.* Boston, MA: Houghton Mifflin.

Corbin, J., & Strauss, A. (2007). *Basics of qualitative research: Techniques and procedures for developing grounded theory* (3rd ed.). Thousand Oaks, CA: Sage.

Council on Accreditation of Counseling and Related Educational Programs. (CACREP). (2009). *2009 standards.* Alexandria, VA: Author.

Crane, R. D., & Hafen, M. (2002). Meeting the needs of evidence-based practice in family therapy: Developing the scientist-practitioner model. *Journal of Family Therapy, 24,* 113–124.

Creswell, J. W. (2012). *Educational research: Planning, conducting, and evaluating quantitative and qualitative research* (4th ed.). Upper Saddle River, NJ: Pearson.

Creswell, J. W. (2013). *Qualitative inquiry and research design: Choosing among five approaches* (3rd ed.). Thousand Oaks, CA: Sage.

Crits-Christoph, P., & Mintz, J. (1991). Implications of therapist effects for the design and analysis of comparative studies of psychotherapies. *Journal of Consulting and Clinical Psychology, 59*(1), 20–26.

Cuijpers, P. (1998). Psychological outreach programmes for the depressed elderly: A meta-analysis of effects and dropout. *International Journal of Geriatric Psychiatry, 13*(1), 41–48.

Danzinger, P. R., & Welfel, E. R. (2001). The impact of managed care on mental health counselors: A survey of perceptions, practices, and compliance with ethical standards. *Journal of Mental Health Counseling, 23,* 137–150.

DeLuca, R., & Holborn, S. (1992). Effects of a variable ratio reinforcement schedule with changing criteria on exercise in obese and nonobese boys. *Journal of Applied Behavioral Analysis, 25,* 671–679.

Denzin, N. K. (2009). *The research act: A theoretical introduction to sociological methods.* Piscataway, NJ: Aldine Transaction.

Denzin, N. K., & Lincoln, Y. S. (Eds.). (2011). *Handbook of qualitative research* (4th ed.). Thousand Oaks, CA: Sage.

Derogatis, L. R. (1993). *Brief Symptom Inventory: Administration, scoring and procedures manual* (4th ed.). Minneapolis, MN: NCS-Pearson Assessments.

Dobson, A. J. (2002). *An introduction to generalized linear models* (2nd ed.). Boca Raton, FL: Chapman Hall/CRC.

Doggett, R. A., Edwards, R. P., Moore, J. W., Tingstrom, D. H., & Wilczynski, S. M. (2001). An approach to functional assessment in general education classroom settings. *School Psychology Review, 30,* 313–328.

Draper, N. R., & Smith, H. (1998). *Applied regression analysis* (3rd ed.). New York: Wiley.

Durlack, J. A. (1995). *School-based prevention programs for children and adolescents.* Thousand Oaks, CA: Sage Publications.

Eaves, S., Emens, R., & Sheperis, C. J. (2008). Counselors in the managed care era: The efficacy of the data-based problem solver model. *Journal of Professional Counseling, Practice, Theory, & Research, 36*(2), 1–12.

Efron, B., & Tibshirani, R. J. (1993). *An introduction to the bootstrap.* New York, NY: Chapman & Hall.

Ekstrom, R. B., Elmore, P. B., Schafer, W. D., Trotter, T. V., & Webster, B. (2004). A survey of assessment and evaluation activities of school counselors. *Professional School Counseling, 8,* 24–30.

Elkin, I., Shea, M. T., Watkins, J. T., Imber, S. D., Sotsky, S., Collins, J. F., ... Parloss, M. B. (1989). National Institute of Mental Health Treatment of Depression Collaborative Research Program: General effectiveness of treatments. *Archives of General Psychiatry, 46,* 971–982.

Enright, M. S. (1996). The relationship between disability status, career beliefs, and career indecision. *Rehabilitation Counseling Bulletin, 40,* 134–151.

Erford, B. T. (1999). The comparative effectiveness of a modified time-out procedure for oppositional and defiant children. *The Professional School Counselor, 2,* 205–210.

Erford, B. T. (Ed.). (2010). *Professional school counseling: A handbook of theories, programs, and practices* (2nd ed.). Austin, TX: Pro-ed.

Erford, B. T. (Ed.). (2013). *Assessment for counselors* (2nd ed.). Boston, MA: Cengage.

Erford, B. T. (Ed.). (2015). *Transforming the school counseling profession* (4th ed.). Columbus, OH: Pearson Merrill.

Erford, B. T., Balcom, L., & Moore-Thomas, C. (2007). The Screening Test for Emotional Problems (STEP): Studies of reliability and validity. *Measurement and Evaluation in Counseling and Development, 39,* 209–225.

Erford, B. T., & Clark, K. (2011). Technical analysis of the Disruptive Behavior Rating Scale–Second Edition–Teacher Version. *Measurement and Evaluation in Counseling and Development, 44,* 3–15.

Erford, B. T., & Crockett, S. A. (2012). Annual review: Practice and research in career counseling and development-2011. *Career Development Quarterly, 60,* 290–332.

Erford, B. T., Erford, B. M., Lattanzi, G., Weller, J., Schein, H., Wolf, E., … Peacock, E. (2011). Counseling outcomes from 1990 to 2008 for school-age youth with depression: A meta-analysis. *Journal of Counseling & Development, 89,* 439–457.

Erford, B. T., & Hase, K. (2006). Reliability and validity of scores on the ACTeRS-2. *Measurement and Evaluation in Counseling and Development, 39,* 97–106.

Erford, B. T., Kress, V. E., Giguere, M., Cieri, D., & Erford, B. M. Counseling outcomes for youth with anxiety: 1990–2009. Unpublished manuscript.

Erford, B. T., Miller, E. M., Duncan, K., & Erford, B. M. (2010). Submission patterns: *Measurement and Evaluation in Counseling and Development* author and article characteristics from 1990–2009. *Measurement and Evaluation in Counseling and Development, 42,* 296–307.

Erford, B. T., Miller, E. M., Schein, H., McDonald, A., Ludwig, L., & Leishear, K. (2011). *Journal of Counseling & Development* publication patterns: Author and article characteristics from 1994–2009. *Journal of Counseling & Development, 89,* 73–80.

Erford, B. T., Moore-Thomas, C., & Wallace, L. L. (2010). Program accountability. In B. T. Erford (Ed.), *Professional school counseling: A handbook of theories, programs, and practices* (2nd ed., pp. 251–259). Austin, TX: pro-ed.

Erford, B. T., Paul, L. E., Oncken, C., Kress, V. E., & Erford, M. R. (in press). Counseling outcomes for youth with oppositional behavior: A meta-analysis. *Journal of Counseling & Development.*

Erford, B. T., Richards, T., Peacock, E. R., Voith, K., McGair, H., Muller, B., … Chang, C. Y. (2013). Counseling and guided self-help outcomes for clients with bulimia nervosa: A meta-analysis of clinical trials from 1980-2010. *Journal of Counseling & Development, 91,* 152–172.

Erford, B. T., Vitali, G., & Slosson, S. (1999). *Manual for the Slosson Intelligence Scale—Primary (SIT-P).* East Aurora, NY: Slosson Educational Publications.

Erford, B. T., & Wallace, L. L. (2010). Outcomes research on school counseling. In B. T. Erford (Ed.), *Professional school counseling: A handbook of theories, programs, and practices* (pp. 34–44). Austin, TX: PRO-ED.

Fassinger, R. E. (2005). Paradigms, praxis, problems, and promise: Grounded theory in counseling psychology research. *Journal of Counseling Psychology, 52,* 156–166.

Federal Interagency Forum on Child and Family Statistics. (2012). *America's children in brief: Key national indicators of well-being.* Washington, DC: U.S. Government Printing Office.

Fisher, N. I., & Hall, P. (1991). Bootstrap algorithms for small samples. *Journal of Statistical Planning and Inference, 27,* 157–169.

Fox, R. M., & Rubinoff, A. (1979). Behavioral treatment of caffenism: Reducing excessive coffee drinking. *Journal of Applied Behavior Analysis, 12,* 335–344.

Fraenkel, J. R., Wallen, N. E., & Hyun, H. (2011). *How to design and evaluate research in education* (8th ed.). Boston, MA: McGraw-Hill.

Frank, J. D. (1959). The dynamics of the psychotherapeutic relationship. *Psychiatry, 22,* 17–39.

Friedman, H. J. (1963). Patient-expectancy and symptom reduction. *Archives of General Psychiatry, 8,* 61–67.

Furlong, N., Lovelace, E., & Lovelace, K. (2000). *Research methods and statistics: An integrated approach.* Fort Worth, TX: Harcourt Brace.

Galassi, J. P., Crace, R. K., Martin, G. A., James, R. M., & Wallace, R. L. (1992). Client preferences and anticipations in career counseling: A preliminary investigation. *Journal of Counseling Psychology, 39,* 46–55.

Garfield, S. L. (1994). Research on client variables in psychotherapy. In A. E. Bergin & S. L. Garfield (Eds.), *Handbook of psychotherapy and behavior change* (3rd ed., pp. 190–228). New York, NY: Wiley.

Garis, J. W., & Niles, S. G. (1990). The separate and combined effects of SIGI and DISCOVER and a career planning course on undecided university students. *Career Development Quarterly, 39,* 261–274.

Gay, L. R., Mills, G. E., & Airasian, P. (2011). *Educational research: Competencies for analysis and applications* (10th ed.). Upper Saddle River, NJ: Pearson.

Gehart, D. R., & Lyle, R. R. (2001). Client experience of gender in therapeutic relationships: An interpretive ethnography. *Family Process, 40,* 443–458.

Gerber, S., & Terry-Day, B. (1999). Does peer mediation really work? *Professional School Counseling, 2,* 169–171.

Gerler, E. R. (1985). Elementary school counseling research and the classroom learning environment. *Elementary School Guidance and Counseling, 20,* 39–40.

Gladwell, M. A. (2008). *Outliers: The story of success.* New York, NY: Little, Brown and Company.

Glaser, B. G. (1978). *Theoretical sensitivity: Advances in the methodology of grounded theory.* Mill Valley, CA: Sociology Press.

Glaser, B. G., & Strauss, A. L. (1967). *The discovery of grounded theory: Strategies for qualitative research.* New York, NY: Aldine de Gruyter.

Glass, G. V. (1976). Primary, secondary, and meta-analysis of research. *Educational Researcher, 5,* 3–8.

Glass, G. V., & Hopkins, K. D. (2008). *Statistical methods in education and psychology* (3rd ed.). Upper Saddle River, NJ: Pearson.

Glense, C. (2010). *Becoming qualitative researchers: An introduction* (4th ed.). Upper Saddle River, NJ: Pearson.

Goldstein, A. P. (1960). Patients' expectancies and nonspecific therapy as a basis for (un)spontaneous remission. *Journal of Clinical Psychology, 16,* 399–403.

Gonzalez, J. E., Nelson, J. R., Gutkin, T. B., Saunders, A., Galloway, A., & Shwery, C. S. (2004). Rational emotive therapy with children and adolescents: A meta-analysis. *Journal of Emotional and Behavioral Disorders, 12,* 222–235.

Good, P. I. (2000). *Permutation tests: A practical guide to resampling methods for testing hypotheses* (2nd ed.). London, UK: Springer-Verlag.

Goodman, L. A. (1954). Kolmogorov-Smirnov tests for psychological research. *Psychological Bulletin, 51,* 160–168.

Gottfredson, D. C. (1997). School-based crime prevention. In L. W. Sherman, D. C. Gottfredson, D. MacKenzie, J. Eck, P. Reuter, & S. Bushway (Eds.), *Preventing crime: What works, what doesn't, what's promising: A report to the United States Congress* (pp. 5.1–5.71). Washington, DC: U. S. Department of Justice, Office of Justice Programs.

Gottfredson, D. C. (2001). *Schools and delinquency.* New York, NY: Cambridge University Press.

Gottfredson, D. C., Wilson, D. B., & Najaka, S. S. (2001). School-based crime prevention. In L. W. Sherman, D. P. Farrington, B. Welsh, & D. C. MacKenzie (Eds.), *Evidence-based crime prevention.* New York, NY: Harwood Academic.

Guba, E. G., & Lincoln, Y. S. (2005). Paradigmatic controversies, contradictions, and emerging influences. In N. K. Denzin & Y. S. Lincoln (Eds.), *The Sage handbook of qualitative research* (3rd ed., pp. 191–215). Thousand Oaks, CA: Sage.

Gysbers, N. C., & Henderson, P. (2012). *Developing and managing your school guidance program* (5th ed.). Alexandria, VA: American Counseling Association.

Hajek, J. (1969). *A course in nonparametric statistics.* San Francisco, CA: Holden-Day.

Hancock, B. (2002). *Trend focus for research and development in primary health care: An introduction to qualitative research.* Retrieved from http://faculty.cbu.ca/pmacintyre/course_pages/MBA603/MBA603_files/IntroQualitativeResearch.pdf

Hartung, P. J. (2010). Practice and research in career counseling and development—2009. *The Career Development Quarterly, 59,* 98–142.

Hawkins, J. D., Farrington, D. P., & Catalano, R. F. (1998). Reducing violence through the schools. In D. S. Elliott, B. A. Hamburg, & K. R. Williams (Eds.), *Violence in American schools* (pp. 188–216). New York, NY: Cambridge University Press.

Hayes, S. C., Barlow, D. H., & Nelson-Gray, R. O. (1999). *The scientist-practitioner: Research and accountability in the age of managed care.* Boston, MA: Allyn & Bacon.

Hays, D. G., Chang, C. Y., & Dean, J. K. (2004). White counselors' conceptualization of privilege and oppression: Implications for counselor training. *Counselor Education and Supervision, 43,* 242–257.

Hays, D. G., & Singh, A. (2012). *Qualitative inquiry in clinical and educational settings.* New York, NY: Guilford Press.

Headrick, T. C., & Rotou, O. (2001). An investigation of the rank transformation in multiple regression. *Computational Statistics and Data Analysis, 38,* 203–215.

Henry, W. P., Schacht, T. E., & Strupp, H. H. (1986). Structural analysis of social behavior: Application to a study of interpersonal process in differential psychotherapeutic outcome [Special issue: Psychotherapy research]. *Journal of Consulting and Clinical Psychology, 54,* 27–31.

Henry, W. P., Strupp, H. H., Butler, S. F., Schacht, T. E., & Binder, J. L. (1993). The effects of training in time-limited dynamic psychotherapy: Changes in therapist behavior. *Journal of Consulting and Clinical Psychology, 61,* 434–440.

Heppner, P. P., & Heppner, M. J. (2004). *Writing and publishing your thesis, dissertation, & research: A guide for students in the helping professions.* Belmont, CA: Brooks/Cole.

Heppner, P. P., Kivlighan, D. M., & Wampold, B. E. (2008). *Research design in counseling* (3rd ed.). Belmont, CA: Thomson Brooks/Cole.

Hill, C. E., Knox, S., Thompson, B. J., Williams, E. N., Hess, S. A., & Ladany, N. (2005). Consensual qualitative research: An update. *Journal of Counseling Psychology, 52,* 196–205.

Hill, C. E., Thompson, B. J., & Williams, E. N. (1997). A guide to conducting consensual qualitative research. *The Counseling Psychologist, 25,* 517–572.

Hinton, W. J., Sheperis, C. J., & Sims, P. (2003). Family-based approaches to juvenile delinquency: A review of the literature. *The Family Journal, 11,* 167–173.

Hoag, M. J., & Burlingame, G. M. (1997). Evaluating the effectiveness of child and adolescent group treatment: A meta-analytic review. *Journal of Clinical Child Psychology, 26,* 234–246.

Hoaglin, D. C., Mosteller, F., & Tukey, J. W. (1983). *Understanding robust and exploratory data analysis.* New York, NY: Wiley.

Hodges, J. L., & Lehmann, E. L. (1963). Estimates of location based on ranks. *Annals of Mathematical Statistics, 34,* 598–611.

Holcomb-McCoy, C., & Day-Vines, N. (2004). Exploring school counselor multicultural competence: A multidimensional concept. *Measurement and Evaluation in Counseling and Development, 37,* 154–162.

Hollander, M., & Wolfe, D. A. (1973). *Nonparametric statistical methods.* New York, NY: Wiley.

Horvath, A. O., & Symonds, B. D. (1991). Relation between working alliance and outcome in psychotherapy. A meta-analysis. *Journal of Counseling Psychology, 38*(2), 139–149.

Howard, K. I., Kopta, S. M., Krause, M. S., & Orlinsky, D. E. (1986). The dose-effect relationship in psychotherapy [Special issue: Psychotherapy research]. *American Psychologist, 41,* 159–164.

Huber, P. (2004). *Robust statistics.* New York, NY: Wiley.

Huberty, C. J., & Olejnik, S. (2006). *Applied MANOVA and discriminant analysis* (2nd ed.). Hoboken, NJ: John Wiley and Sons, Inc.

Hutchinson, D. S., & Razzano, L. (2005). Multifaceted perspectives on program evaluation for psychiatric rehabilitation services. *Psychiatric Rehabilitation Journal, 28,* 207–208.

In-Albon, T., & Schneider, S. (2007). Psychotherapy of childhood anxiety disorders: A meta-analysis. *Psychotherapy & Psychosomatics, 76*(1), 15–24. doi:10.1159/000096361

Jackson, J., & Daughhetee, C. (2015). Record keeping: What to include and what to leave out. In B. T. Erford (Ed.), *Clinical experiences in counseling.* Columbus, OH: Pearson.

Johnson, B., & Christensen, L. (2012). *Educational research: Quantitative, qualitative, and mixed approaches* (4th ed.). Boston, MA: Pearson Education, Inc.

Jöreskog, K. G. (1969). A general approach to confirmatory maximum likelihood factor analysis. *Psychometrika, 34*(2), 183–202.

Judd, C. M., & McClelland, G. H. (1989). *Data analysis: A model-comparison approach*. San Diego, CA: Harcourt Brace Jovanovich.

Kazdin, A. E. (1982). *Single-case research designs*. Oxford, UK: Oxford University Press.

Kazdin, A. E. (1991). Effectiveness of psychotherapy with children and adolescents [Special section: Clinical child psychology: Perspectives on child and adolescent therapy]. *Journal of Consulting and Clinical Psychology, 59*, 785–798.

Kazdin, A. E. (1993). Psychotherapy for children and adolescents: Current progress and future research direction. *American Psychologist, 48*, 644–657.

Kazdin, A. E. (1994). Methodology, design and evaluation in psychotherapy research. In A. E. Bergin & S. L. Garfield (Eds.), *Handbook of psychotherapy and behavior change* (3rd ed., pp. 19–71). New York, NY: Wiley.

Kazdin, A. E. (2011). Evidence-based treatment research: Advances, limitations, and next steps. *American Psychologist, 66*, 685–698.

Kazdin, A. E., Bass, D., Ayers, W. A., & Rodgers, A. (1990). Empirical and clinical focus of child and adolescent psychotherapy research. *Journal of Consulting and Clinical Psychology, 58*, 729–740.

Kennedy, C. H. (2005). *Single-case designs for educational research*. Boston, MA: Pearson Education.

Kennedy, C. H., & Souza, G. (1995). Functional analysis and treatment of eye poking. *Journal of Applied Behavior Analysis, 28*, 27–37.

Keselman, H. J., Wilcox, R. R., Kowalchuk, R. K., & Olejnik, S. (2002). Comparing trimmed and least squares means of two independent skewed populations. *Biometrical Journal, 44*, 478–489.

Kidd, S. A., & Kral, M. J. (2005). Practicing participatory action research. *Journal of Counseling Psychology, 52*, 187–195.

Kirk, R. E. (1995). *Experimental design: Procedures for the behavioral sciences* (3rd ed.). Pacific Grove, CA: Brooks/Cole Publishing Company.

Kiselica, M. S., Baker, S. B., Thomas, R. N., & Reddy, S. (1994). Effects of stress inoculation training on anxiety, stress, and academic performance among adolescents. *Journal of Counseling Psychology, 41*, 335–342.

Koch, G. G. (1969). Some aspects of the statistical analysis of "split-plot" experiments in completely randomized layouts. *Journal of the American Statistical Association, 64*, 485–506.

Kowalik, J., Weller, J., Venter, J., & Drachman, D. (2011). Cognitive behavioral therapy for the treatment of pediatric posttraumatic stress disorder: A review and meta-analysis. *Journal of Behavior Therapy and Experimental Psychiatry, 42*(1), 405–413. doi:10.1016/j.jbtep.2011.02.002

Kozol, J. (1991). *Savage inequalities*. New York, NY: Crown Publishers.

Kruskal, W. H., & Wallis, W. A. (1952). Use of ranks on one-criterion variance analysis. *Journal of the American Statistical Association, 48*, 907–911.

Lambert, M. J. (1976). Spontaneous remission in adult neurotic disorders: A revision and summary. *Psychological Bulletin, 83*(1), 107–119.

Lambert, M. J. (1989). The individual therapist's contribution to psychotherapy process and outcome [Special issue: Psychotherapy process research]. *Clinical Psychology Review, 9*, 469–485.

Lambert, M. J. (1991). Introduction to psychotherapy research. In L. E. Beutler & M. Crago (Eds.), *Psychotherapy research: An international review of programmatic studies* (pp. 1–23). Washington, DC: American Psychological Association.

Lambert, M. J., & Bergin, A. E. (1994). The effectiveness of psychotherapy. In A. E. Bergin & S. L. Garfield (Eds.), *Handbook of psychotherapy and behavior change* (3rd ed., pp. 143–189). New York, NY: Wiley.

Lambert, M. J., Masters, K. S., & Ogles, B. M. (1991). Outcome research in counseling. In C. E. Watkins & L. J. Schneider (Eds.), *Research in counseling* (pp. 51–83). Hillsdale, NJ: Erlbaum.

Lapan, R. T. (2001). Results-based comprehensive guidance and counseling programs: A framework for planning and evaluation. *Professional School Counseling, 4*, 289–299.

LeBlanc, M., & Ritchie, M. (2001). A meta-analysis of play therapy outcomes. *Counseling Psychology Quarterly, 14,* 149–163.

LeCompte, M. D., & Schensul, J. J. (2010). *Designing and conducting ethnographic research* (2nd ed.). Lanham, MD: Alta Mira Press.

Lee, R. S. (1993). Effects of classroom guidance on student achievement. *Elementary School Guidance and Counseling, 27,* 163–171.

Lenz, J. G., Reardon, R. C., & Sampson, J. P. (1993). Holland's theory and effective use of computer-assisted career guidance systems. *Journal of Career Development, 19,* 245–253.

Lewis, M. W., & Lewis, A. C. (1996). Peer helping programs: Helper role, supervisor training, and suicidal behavior. *Journal of Counseling and Development, 74,* 307–313.

Lilliefors, H. W. (1967). On the Kolmogorov-Smirnov test for normality with mean and variance unknown. *Journal of the American Statistical Association, 62,* 399–402.

Lipsey, M. W., & Derzon, J. H. (1998). Predictors of violent or serious delinquency in adolescence and early childhood: A synthesis of longitudinal research. In R. Loeber & D. P. Farrington (Eds.), *Serious and violent juvenile offenders: Risk factors and successful interventions* (pp. 86–105). Thousand Oaks, CA: Sage.

Littrell, J. M., Malia, J. A., & Vanderwod, M. (1995). Single session brief counseling in a high school. *Journal of Counseling and Development, 73,* 451–458.

Loesch, L. C. (2001). Counseling program evaluation: Inside and outside the box. In D. C. Locke, J. E. Myers, & E. L. Herr (Eds.), *The handbook of counseling* (pp. 513–525). Thousand Oaks, CA: Sage.

Long, J. D., & Cliff, N. (1997). Confidence intervals for Kendall's tau. *British Journal of Mathematical & Statistical Psychology, 50,* 31–41.

Lubin, B., Lubin, A. W., & Sargent, C. W. (1972). The group psychotherapy literature: 1972. *International Journal of Group Psychotherapy, 22,* 492–529.

Luborsky, L., McClellan, A. T., Woody, G. E., O'Brien, C. P., & Auerbach, A. (1985). Therapist success and its determinants. *Archives of General Psychiatry, 42,* 602–611.

Lunneborg, C. E. (2000). *Data analysis by resampling: Concepts and applications.* Pacific Grove, CA: Duxbury.

Lyons, L. C., & Woods, P. J. (1991). The efficacy of rational-emotive therapy: A quantitative review of the outcome research. *Clinical Psychology Review, 11,* 357–369.

Madison, D. S. (2011). *Critical ethnography: Method, ethics, and performance* (2nd ed.). Thousand Oaks, CA: Sage.

Mann, A. H., Jenkins, R., & Belsey, E. (1981). The twelve-month outcome of patients with neurotic illness in general practice. *Psychological Medicine, 11,* 535–550.

Mann, H. B., & Whitney, D. R. (1947). On a test of whether one of two random variables is stochastically larger than the other. *Annals of Mathematical Statistics, 18,* 50–60.

Marshall, C., & Rossman, G. B. (2011). *Designing qualitative research* (5th ed.). Thousand Oaks, CA: Sage.

Martin, D. J., Garske, J. P., & Davis, M. K. (2000). Relation of the therapeutic alliance with outcome and other variables: A meta-analytic review. *Journal of Consulting and Clinical Psychology, 68,* 438–450.

Maxwell, J. (2005). *Qualitative research design: An interactive approach* (2nd ed.). Thousand Oaks, CA: Sage.

McCulloch, C. E., & Searle, S. R. (2001). *Generalized, linear, and mixed models.* New York, NY: Wiley.

McRoberts, C., Burlingame, G. M., & Hoag, M. J. (1998). Comparative efficacy of individual and group psychotherapy: A meta-analytic perspective. *Group Dynamics: Theory, Research, and Practice, 2,* 101–117.

Merchant, N. (1997). Qualitative research for counselors. *Counseling and Human Development, 30,* 1–19.

Merriam, S. B. (Ed.). (2002). *Qualitative research in practice: Examples for discussion and analysis.* San Francisco, CA: Jossey-Bass.

Mertens, D. M. (2004). *Research methods in education and psychology: Integrating diversity with quantitative and qualitative approaches* (2nd ed.). Thousand Oaks, CA: Sage.

Micceri, T. (1989). The unicorn, the normal curve, and other improbable creatures. *Psychological Bulletin, 105,* 156–166.

Miles, M., & Huberman, M. (1994). *Qualitative data analysis.* Thousand Oaks, CA: Sage.

Mills, G. E. (2014). *Action research: A guide for teacher researcher* (5th ed.). Upper Saddle River, NJ: Merrill Prentice Hall.

Mitte, K. (2005). Meta-analysis of cognitive-behavioral treatments for Generalized Anxiety Disorder: A comparison with pharmacotherapy. *Psychological Bulletin, 131,* 785–795.

Mohl, P. C., Martinez, D., Ticknor, C., Huang, M., & Cordell, M. D. (1991). Early dropouts from psychotherapy. *Journal of Nervous and Mental Disease, 179,* 478–481.

Mohr, W. K. (2003). The substance of a support group. *Western Journal of Nursing Research, 25,* 676–692.

Moncher, F. J., & Prinz, R. J. (1991). Treatment fidelity in outcome studies. *Clinical Psychology Review, 11,* 247–266.

Monette, D. R., Sullivan, T. J., & DeJong, C. R. (2011). *Applied social research: A tool for the human services* (8th ed.). Belmont, CA: Brooks/Cole-Thomson Learning.

Moore, D. L. (2005). Expanding the view: The lives of women with severe work disabilities in context. *Journal of Counseling and Development, 83,* 343–348.

Moore, J. W., Tingstrom, D. H., Doggett, R. A., & Carlyon, W. D. (2001). Restructuring an existing token economy in a psychiatric facility for children. *Child and Family Behavior Therapy, 23,* 51–57.

Morrissette, P. J. (2000). The experiences of the rural school counselor. *Professional School Counseling, 3,* 197–207.

Muller, K. E., & Fetterman, B. A. (2002). *Regression and ANOVA: An integrated approach using SAS software.* Cary, NC: SAS Publishing.

Murray, L. K., & Kollins, S. H. (2000). Effects of methylphenidate on sensitivity to reinforcement in children diagnosed with Attention Deficit Hyperactivity Disorder: An application of the matching law. *Journal of Applied Behavioral Analysis, 33,* 573–592.

Muthen, L. K., & Muthen, B. O. (2012). *Mplus: Statistical analysis with latent variables. User's guide.* Los Angeles, CA: Muthen & Muthen.

Nagle, B., & Williams, N. (2013). *Methodology brief: Introduction to focus groups.* Retrieved from http://www.uncfsp.org/projects/userfiles/File/FocusGroupBrief.pdf

Nearpass, E. L. (1990). Counseling and guidance effectiveness in North American high schools: A meta-analysis of the research findings. *Dissertation Abstracts International, 50,* 1984A.

Niles, S. G., & Garis, J. W. (1990). The effects of a career planning course and a computer-assisted career guidance program (SIGI PLUS) on undecided university students. *Journal of Career Development, 16,* 237–248.

Noell, G. H., & Witt, J. C. (1998). When does consultation lead to intervention implementation? *Journal of Special Education, 33,* 29–35.

Okubo, Y., Yeh, C. J., Lin, P.-Y., Fujita, K., & Shea, J. M.-Y. (2007). The career decision-making process of Chinese American youth. *Journal of Counseling & Development, 85,* 440–449.

Oliver, L. W., & Spokane, A. R. (1988). Career intervention outcome: What contributes to client gain? *Journal of Counseling Psychology, 35,* 447–462.

Omizo, M. M., & Omizo, S. A. (1988). The effects of participation in group counseling on self-esteem and locus of control among adolescents from divorced families. *The School Counselor, 16,* 54–60.

Omizo, M. M., Omizo, S. A., & D'Andrea, M. J. (1992). Promoting wellness among elementary school children. *Journal of Counseling and Development, 71,* 194–198.

Orlinsky, D. E., Grawe, D., & Parks, B. K. (1994). Process and outcome in psychotherapy. In A. E. Bergin & S. L. Garfield (Eds.), *Handbook of psychotherapy and behavior change* (3rd ed., pp. 270–378). New York, NY: Wiley.

Orr, J. M., Sackett, P. R., & DuBois, C. L. Z. (1991). Outlier detection and treatment in I/O psychology: A survey of researcher beliefs and an empirical illustration. *Personnel Psychology, 44,* 473–486.

Osborne, J. (1990). Some basic existential-phenomenological research methodology for counselors. *Canadian Journal of Counseling, 24,* 79–91.

Pan, P. J. D., & Lin, C. W. (2004). Members' perceptions of leader behaviors, group experiences, and therapeutic factors in group counseling. *Small Group Research, 35,* 174–194.

Patten, M. (2009). *Understanding research methods* (7th ed.). Glendale, CA: Pyrczak Publishing.

Patton, M. Q. (2002). *Qualitative research and evaluation methods* (3rd ed.). Thousand Oaks, CA: Sage.

Paul, G. L. (1967). Strategy of outcome research in psychotherapy. *Journal of Consulting Psychology, 31,* 109–118.

Pearson, E. S., & Hartley, H. O. (1970). *Biometrika tables for statisticians* (3rd ed.). Cambridge, UK: Biometrika Trustees at the University Press.

Pedro-Carroll, J. L., & Alpert-Gillis, L. J. (1997). Preventive interventions for children of divorce: A developmental model for 5 and 6 year old children. *Journal of Primary Prevention, 18,* 5–23.

Pedro-Carroll, J. L., Sutton, S. E., & Wyman, P. A. (1999). A two-year follow-up of a preventive intervention for young children of divorce. *School Psychology Review, 28,* 467–476.

Perkins, D. V., Born, D. L., Raines, J. A., & Galka, S. W. (2005). Program evaluation from an ecological perspective: Supported employment services for persons with serious psychiatric disabilities. *Psychiatric Rehabilitation Journal, 28,* 217–224.

Phillips, E. L., & Fagan, P. J. (1982, August). *Attrition: Focus on the intake and first therapy interviews.* Paper presented at the 90th annual convention of the American Psychological Association, Washington, DC.

Polkinghorne, D. E. (2005). Language and meaning: Data collection in qualitative research. *Journal of Counseling Psychology, 52,* 137–145.

Ponterotto, J. G. (2002). Qualitative research methods: The fifth force in psychology. *The Counseling Psychologist, 30,* 394–406.

Ponterotto, J. G. (2005). Qualitative research in counseling psychology: A primer on research paradigms and philosophy of science. *Journal of Counseling Psychology, 52,* 126–136.

Prout, H. T., & DeMartino, R. A. (1986). A meta-analysis of school-based studies of psychotherapy. *Journal of School Psychology, 24,* 285–292.

Prout, S. M., & Prout, H. T. (1998). A meta-analysis of school-based studies of counseling and psychotherapy: An update. *Journal of School Psychology, 36,* 121–136.

Rathus, S. A., Nevid, J. S., & Fichner-Rathus, L. (2005). *Human sexuality in a world of diversity* (6th ed.). Boston, MA: Allyn & Bacon.

Raykov, T., & Marcoulides, G. A. (2000). *A first course in structural equation modeling.* Mahwah, NJ: Lawrence Erlbaum.

Reisetter, M., Korcuska, J. S., Yexley, M., Bonds, D., Nikels, H., & McHenry, W. (2004). Counselor educators and qualitative researchers: Affirming a research identity. *Counselor Education and Supervision, 44,* 2–16.

Reynolds, W. M. (2002). *Manual for the Reynolds Adolescent Depression Scale—Second Edition (RADS-2).* Lutz, FL: Psychological Assessment Resources.

Robinson, L. A., Berman, J. S., & Neimeyer, R. A. (1990). Psychotherapy for the treatment of depression: A comprehensive review of controlled outcome research. *Psychological Bulletin, 108,* 30–49.

Roid, G. H. (2003). *The Stanford-Binet Intelligence Scale—Fifth Edition (SB5).* Itasca, IL: Riverside Publishing.

Rongione, D., Erford, B. T., & Broglie, C. (2011). Alcohol and other drug counseling outcomes for school-aged youth: A meta-analysis of studies from 1990-2009. *Counseling Outcome Research and Evaluation, 2,* 1–17. doi:10.1177/2150137811400595

Rosenthal, R. (1968). An application of the Kolmogorov-Smirnov test for normality with estimated mean and variance. *Psychological Reports, 22,* 570.

Rowley, W. J., Stroh, H. R., & Sink, C. A. (2005). Comprehensive guidance and counseling programs' use of guidance curricula materials: A survey of national trends. *Professional School Counseling, 8,* 296–304.

Royse, D., Thyer, B. A., Padgett, D. K., & Logan, T. K. (2001). *Program evaluation: An introduction* (3rd ed.). Belmont, CA: Brooks-Cole.

Saldana, J. (2013). *The coding manual for qualitative researchers.* Belmont, CA: Sage.

Salter, K. C., & Fawcett, R. F. (1993). The ART test of interaction: A robust and powerful test of interaction in factorial models. *Communications in Statistics B: Simulation & Computation, 22,* 137–153.

Samplers, F., & Aber, L. (1998). Evaluations of school-based violence prevention programs. In D. S. Elliott, B. A. Hamburg, & K. R. Williams (Eds.), *Violence in American schools* (pp. 217–252). New York, NY: Cambridge University Press.

Scheffé, H. (1959). *The analysis of variance.* New York, NY: Wiley.

Scheid, T. L. (2003). Managed care and the rationalization of mental health services. *Journal of Health and Social Behavior, 44,* 142–161.

Schlossberg, S. M., Morris, J. D., & Lieberman, M. G. (2001). The effects of a counselor-led guidance intervention on students' behaviors and attitudes. *Professional School Counseling, 4,* 156–174.

Schumacker, R. E., & Lomax, R. G. (2004). *A beginner's guide to structural equation modeling.* Mahwah, NJ: Lawrence Erlbaum.

Sexton, T. L., & Whiston, S. C. (1991). A review of the empirical basis for counseling: Implications for practice and training. *Counselor Education and Supervision, 30,* 330–354.

Sexton, T. L., Whiston, S. C., Bleuer, J. C., & Walz, G. R. (1995). *A critical review of the counseling outcomes research: Technical Report submitted to the Human Development Foundation.* Alexandria, VA: American Counseling Association.

Sexton, T. L., Whiston, S. C., Bleuer, J. C., & Walz, G. R. (1997). *Integrating outcome research into counseling practice and training.* Alexandria, VA: American Counseling Association.

Shechtman, Z., & Perl-Dekel, O. (2000). A comparison of therapeutic factors in two group treatment modalities: Verbal and art therapy. *Journal for Specialists in Group Work, 25,* 288–304.

Sheperis, C. J. (2001). *The development of an instrument to measure racial identity in juvenile offenders.* Unpublished dissertation, The University of Florida, Gainesville, FL.

Sheperis, C. J., Doggett, T., & Henington, C. (2006). Behavioral assessment: Principles and applications. In B. T. Erford (Ed.), *Counselor's guide to clinical, personality, and behavioral assessment* (pp. 105–123). Boston, MA: Houghton Mifflin/Lahaska Press.

Shirk, S. R., & Karver, M. (2003). Prediction of treatment outcome from relationship variables in child and adolescent therapy: A meta-analytic review. *Journal of Consulting and Clinical Psychology, 71,* 452–464.

Siedman, I. (2006). *Interviewing as qualitative research: A guide for researchers in education and the social sciences* (3rd ed.). New York, NY: Teachers College Press.

Silverman, W. K., Pina, A. A., & Viswesvaran, C. (2008). Evidence-based psychosocial treatments for phobic and anxiety disorders in children and adolescents. *Journal of Clinical Child & Adolescent Psychology, 37*(1), 105–130. doi:10.1080/15374410701817907

Singh, A. A. (2006). *Resilience strategies of South Asian women who have survived child sexual abuse.* Unpublished doctoral dissertation, Georgia State University, Atlanta, Georgia.

Sink, C. A., & Stroh, H. R. (2003). Raising achievement test scores of early elementary school students through comprehensive school counseling programs. *Professional School Counseling, 6,* 350–364.

Skinner, B. F. (1956). A case history in scientific methods. *American Psychologist, 11,* 221–233.

Sophie, J. (1986). A critical examination of stage theories of lesbian identity development. *Journal of Homosexuality, 12,* 39–51.

Sprinthall, N. A. (1981). A new model for research in the service of guidance and counseling. *Personnel and Guidance Journal, 59,* 487–493.

Stage, S. A., & Quiroz, D. R. (1997). A meta-analysis of interventions to decrease disruptive classroom behavior in public education settings. *School Psychology Review, 26,* 333–369.

St. Clair, K. L. (1989). Middle school counseling research: A resource for school counselors. *Elementary School Guidance and Counseling, 23,* 219–226.

Steering Committee. (2002). Empirically supported therapy relationships: Conclusions and recommendations of the Division 29 task force. In J. C. Norcross (Ed.), *Psychotherapy relationships that work: Therapist contribution and responsiveness to patients* (pp. 441–443). Oxford, UK: Oxford University Press.

Stein, D. M., & Lambert, M. J. (1995). Graduate training in psychotherapy: Are therapy outcomes enhanced? *Journal of Consulting and Clinical Psychology, 63,* 182–196.

Sterling-Turner, H. E., Watson, T. S., & Moore, J. W. (2002). The effects of direct training and treatment integrity on treatment outcomes in school consultation. *School Psychology Quarterly, 17,* 47–77.

Stevens, J. P. (2009). *Applied multivariate statistics for the social sciences* (5th ed.). Mahwah, NJ: Lawrence Erlbaum.

Stokes, M. E., Davis, C. S., & Koch, G. G. (2000). *Categorical data analysis using the SAS system* (2nd ed.). Cary, NC: SAS Institute.

Strangor, C. (2011). *Research methods for the behavioral sciences* (4th ed.). Belmont, CA: Wadsworth.

Suzuki, L. A., Ahluwalia, M. K., Mattis, J. S., & Quizo, C. A. (2005). Ethnography in counseling psychology research: Possibilities for application. *Journal of Counseling Psychology, 52,* 206–214.

Svartberg, M., & Stiles, T. C. (1991). Comparative effects of short-term psychodynamic psychotherapy: A meta-analysis. *Journal of Consulting and Clinical Psychology, 59,* 704–714.

Swanson, J. L. (1995). The process and outcome of career counseling. In W. B. Walsh & S. H. Osipow (Eds.), *Handbook of vocational psychology: Theory, research, and practice* (pp. 217–259). Mahwah, NJ: Erlbaum.

Tedlock, B. (2011). Braiding narrative ethnography with memoir and creative nonfiction. In N. K. Denzin & Y. S. Lincoln (Eds.), *Handbook of qualitative research* (4th ed., pp. 331–340). Thousand Oaks, CA: Sage.

Tetenbaum, T. (1975). The role of student needs and teacher orientation in student ratings of teachers. *American Educational Research Journal, 12,* 417–433.

Thompson, B. (1989). Prerotation and postrotation eigenvalues shouldn't be confused: A reminder. *Measurement and Evaluation in Counseling and Development, 22,* 114–116.

Thompson, B. (1994). Guidelines for authors. *Educational and Psychological Measurement, 54,* 837–847.

Thompson, B. (1999). Journal editorial policies regarding statistical significance tests: Heat is to fire as p is to importance. *Educational Psychology Review, 11,* 157–169.

Thompson, R., & Littrell, J. M. (1998). Brief counseling for students with learning disabilities. *Professional School Counseling, 2,* 60–67.

Tilliski, L. (1990). A meta-analysis of estimated effect sizes for group versus individual versus control treatments. *International Journal of Group Psychotherapy, 40,* 215–224.

Tobler, N. S., & Stratton, H. H. (1997). Effectiveness of school-based drug prevention programs: A meta-analysis of the research. *Journal of Primary Prevention, 18,* 71–128.

Trask, E. V., Walsh, K., & DiLillo, D. (2011). Treatment effects for common outcomes of child sexual abuse: A current meta-analysis. *Aggression and Violent Behavior, 16*(1), 9–16. doi:10.1016/j.avb.2010.10.001

Trevisan, M. S. (2002). Enhancing practical evaluation training through long-term evaluation projects. *American Journal of Evaluation, 23,* 81–92.

Tukey, J. W. (1977). *Exploratory data analysis.* Reading, MA: Addison-Wesley.

Turner, S. L., Alliman-Brissett, A., Lapan, R. T., Upidi, S., & Ergun, D. (2003). The career-related parent support scale. *Measurement and Evaluation in Counseling and Development, 36*(2), 83–94.

Ullman, R. K., Sleator, E. K., & Sprague, R. (2000). *The ADD Comprehensive Teacher Rating Scale—2nd Edition.* Chicago, IL: MetriTech.

U. S. Congress. (2001). *No Child Left Behind Act of 2001 (H.R.1).* Washington, DC: Author.

Vargha, A., & Delaney, H. D. (1998). The Kruskal-Wallis test and stochastic homogeneity. *Journal of Educational & Behavioral Statistics, 23,* 170–192.

Vaughan, S. M., & Kinnier, R. T. (1996). Psychological effects of a life review intervention for persons with HIV disease. *Journal of Counseling and Development, 75,* 115–123.

Vaughn, M. G., & Howard, M. O. (2004). Adolescent substance abuse treatment: A synthesis of uncontrolled evaluations. *Research on Social Work Practice, 14,* 325–335. doi:10.1177/1049731504265834

Wakefield, J. C., & Kirk, S. A. (1996). Unscientific thinking about scientific practice: Evaluating the scientist-practitioner model. *Social Work Research, 20,* 83–95.

Wechsler, D. (2008). *Manual for the Wechsler Adult Intelligence Scale (WAIS-IV)* (4th ed.). San Antonio, TX: The Psychological Corporation.

Weissburg, R. P., Caplan, M., & Harwood, R. L. (1991). Promoting competent young people in competence-enhancing environments: A systems-based perspective on primary prevention. *Journal of Consulting and Clinical Psychology, 59,* 830–841.

Weisz, J. R., McCarty, C. A., & Valeri, S. M. (2006). Effects of psychotherapy for depression in children and adolescents: A meta-analysis. *Psychological Bulletin, 132,* 132–149. doi:10.1037/0033-2909.132.1.132

Weisz, J. R., Weiss, B., Alicke, M. D., & Klotz, M. L. (1987). Effectiveness of psychotherapy with children and adolescents: A meta-analysis for clinicians. *Journal of Consulting and Clinical Psychology, 55,* 542–549.

Weisz, J. R., Weiss, B., Han, S. S., Granger, D. A., & Morton, T. (1995). Effects of psychotherapy with children and adolescents revisited: A meta-analysis of treatment outcome studies. *Psychological Bulletin, 117,* 450–468.

Welch, B. L. (1947). The generalization of student's problem when several different population variances are involved. *Biometrika, 34,* 28–35.

Wertz, F. J. (2005). Phenomenological research methods for counseling psychology. *Journal of Counseling Psychology, 54,* 166–177.

Whiston, S. C., Brecheisen, B. K., & Stephens, J. (2003). Does treatment modality affect career counseling effectiveness. *Journal of Vocational Behavior, 62,* 390–410.

Whiston, S. C., Feldwisch, R., & James, B. (2015). Outcomes research on school counseling interventions and programs. In B. T. Erford (Ed.), *Transforming the school counseling profession* (4th ed.). Columbus, OH: Pearson Merrill.

Whiston, S. C., & Oliver, L. (2005). Career counseling process and outcome. In W. B. Walsh, & M. Savickas (Ed.), *Handbook of vocational psychology* (3rd ed., pp. 155–194). Hillsdale, NJ: Erlbaum.

Whiston, S. C., & Sexton, T. L. (1993). An overview of psychotherapy outcome research: Implications for practice. *Professional Psychology: Research and Practice, 24*(1), 43–51.

Whiston, S. C., & Sexton, T. L. (1998). A review of school counseling outcome research: Implications for practice. *Journal of Counseling and Development, 76,* 412–426.

Whiston, S. C., Sexton, T. L., & Lasoff, D. L. (1998). Career intervention outcome: A replication and extension of Oliver and Spokane (1988). *Journal of Counseling Psychology, 45,* 150–165.

Whiston, S. C., Tai, W. L., Rahardja, D., & Eder, K. (2011). School counseling outcome: A meta-analytic examination of interventions. *Journal of Counseling & Development, 89,* 37–55.

Wiggins, J. D., & Wiggins, A. H. (1992). Elementary students' self-esteem and behavioral ratings related to counselor time-task emphases. *The School Counselor, 39,* 377–381.

Wilcox, R. R. (1993). Robustness in ANOVA. In E. Edwards (Ed.), *Applied analysis of variance in the behavioral sciences* (pp. 345–374). New York, NY: Marcel Dekker.

Wilcox, R. R. (1997). Some practical reasons for reconsidering the Kolmogorov-Smirnov Test. *British Journal of Mathematical and Statistical Psychology, 50*(1), 9–20.

Wilcoxen, F. (1945). Individual comparisons by ranking methods. *Biometrics, 1,* 80–83.

Wilkinson, G., & Robertson, G. J. (2006). *Manual for the Wide-Range Achievement Test* (4th ed.). Lutz, FL: Psychological Assessment Resources.

Wilson, D. B., Gottfredson, D. C., & Najaka, S. S. (2001). School-based prevention of problem behaviors: A meta-analysis. *Journal of Quantitative Criminology, 17,* 247–272.

Wilson, K. B. (1999). Vocational rehabilitation acceptance: A tale of two races in a large midwestern state. *Journal of Applied Rehabilitation Counseling, 30,* 25–31.

Wilson, N. S. (1986). Effects of a classroom guidance unit on sixth graders' examination performance. *Journal of Humanistic Education and Development, 25*(2), 70–79.

Wilson, S. J., Lipsey, M. W., & Derzon, J. H. (2003). The effects of school-based intervention programs on aggressive behavior: A meta-analysis. *Journal of Consulting and Clinical Psychology, 71,* 136–149.

Winslow, B. W. (1998). Family caregiving and the use of formal community support services: A qualitative case study. *Issues in Mental Health Nursing, 19,* 11–27.

Woodcock, R., Mather, N., & McGrew, K. (2001). *The Woodcock-Johnson: Tests of Achievement (WJ-III)* (3rd ed.). Itasca, IL: Riverside Publications.

Yin, R. K. (2009). *Case study research, design, and methods* (4th ed.). Thousand Oaks, CA: Sage.

Zimmerman, D. W. (1995). Increasing the power of nonparametric tests by detecting and down-weighting outliers. *Journal of Experimental Education, 64,* 71–78.

Zimmerman, D. W. (1996). A note on homogeneity of variance of scores and ranks. *Journal of Experimental Education, 64,* 351–362.

Zimmerman, D. W. (1998). Invalidation of parametric and nonparametric statistical tests by concurrent violation of two assumptions. *Journal of Experimental Education, 67,* 55–68.

Zinck, K., & Littrell, J. M. (2000). Action research shows group counseling effective with at-risk adolescent girls. *Professional School Counseling, 4,* 50–59.

# NAME INDEX

# SUBJECT INDEX